Pregnancy and Infants: Medical, Psychological and Social Issues Series

INFECTIOUS PREGNANCY COMPLICATIONS

Pregnancy and Infants: Medical, Psychological and Social Issues Series

Focus on Milk and Infants
Viroj Wiwanitkit
2009. ISBN: 978-1-60741-106-2

Infectious Pregnancy Complications
Richard N. Canfield (Editor)
2009. ISBN: 978-1-60471-038-6

Pregnancy and Infants: Medical, Psychological and Social Issues Series

INFECTIOUS PREGNANCY COMPLICATIONS

RICHARD N. CANFIELD
EDITOR

Nova Biomedical Books
New York

For permission to use material from this book please contact us:
Telephone 631-231-7269; Fax 631-231-8175
Web Site: http://www.novapublishers.com

Library of Congress Cataloging-in-Publication Data

Infectious pregnancy complications / [edited by] Richard N. Canfield.
p. ; cm.
Includes bibliographical references and index.
ISBN 978-1-60741-038-6 (hardcover)
1. Communicable diseases in pregnancy. I. Canfield, Richard N.
[DNLM: 1. Pregnancy Complications, Infectious. 2. Communicable Diseases--complications. 3. Genital Diseases, Female--complications. WQ 256 I445 2009]
RG578.I545 2009
618.3'6--dc22

2009004979

Published by Nova Science Publishers, Inc. ✢ New York

Contents

Preface		**vii**
Chapter 1	Complications of Infections in Pregnancy *Dushyant Maharaj*	**1**
Chapter 2	Infection Related Recurrent Late Abortions and Preterm Birth: Early Total Cervix Occlusion (ETCO) Versus Cerclage *Erich Saling and Monika Dräger*	**83**
Chapter 3	Virulence of Influenza Virus on Human Fetal Membrane Tissues *Noboru Uchide and Hiroo Toyoda*	**111**
Chapter 4	Serological Response to Rubella, Herpes Simplex 2 and Cytomegalovirus in Pregnant Women with Unexplained Recurrent Abortions *Maysaa El Sayed Zaki and Ahmmed Badawy*	**139**
Chapter 5	Appendicitis during Pregnancy: A Serious Disease and a Diagnostic Problem *L. Penninga and E.I. Penninga*	**151**
Chapter 6	Mediastinal End Subcutaneous Emphysema as a Complication of Labor *Arkadiusz Praski, Włodzimierz Kupis, Marek Florczak and Małgorzata Szpetnar*	**159**
Chapter 7	Program for the Prevention of Infection-Related Premature Births: The Role of the *Lactobacilli* System and Vaginal pH *Erich Saling and Monika Dräger*	**167**
Chapter 8	Challenges for the Management of HIV-Infected Pregnant Women in Resource Constrained Settings *Stephen Mepham, Ruth Bland and Marie-Louise Newell*	**199**

Chapter 9	Impact of Materno-Placental Malaria, Anaemia and HIV Infection on Perinatal Outcome in Nigeria *C. J. Uneke, I. Sunday-Adeoye, F. E. Iyare, O. G. Asieghu and D. D. Duhlinska*	**235**
Chapter 10	*Toxoplasma gondii* and Pregnancy: Priorities for Diagnostics of Congenital Infection *Alessandra Sensini*	**289**
Chapter 11	Screening for *Toxoplasma gondii* Infection in Pregnancy in an Urban Area of Northern Italy: Management and Problems *Massimo De Paschale and Pierangelo Clerici*	**319**
Chapter 12	Rickettsioses in Pregnancy *Maria Bitsori and Emmanouil Galanakis*	**331**
Chapter 13	Infectious Diseases of the Urinary Tract during Pregnancy *Nándor Ács, Ferenc Bánhidy and Andrew E. Czeizel*	**345**
Chapter 14	Dengue Infection in Pregnancy: Pattern of Hematological Disturbance *Viroj Wiwanitkit*	**373**
Chapter 15	Infectious Diseases of the Respiratory System during Pregnancy *Andrew E. Czeizel, Nándor Ács and Ferenc Bánhidy*	**383**
Chapter 16	Maternal Outcomes in Pregnancy with Smallpox: Epidemiologic Investigations of Case Fatality, Miscarriage and Premature Birth Based on Previous Outbreaks *Hiroshi Nishiura*	**407**
Chapter 17	Chicken Pox Infection in Pregnancy *Viroj Wiwanitkit*	**421**
Index		**427**

Preface

Infectious Pregnancy Complications deal with the co-occurrence of pregnancy and an infection. The infection may precede or follow fertilization. This new book presents the latest research in the field.

Chapter 1- Epidemiological reports estimate that 7.7 million perinatal deaths occur annually worldwide, including 4.3 million that take place in late pregnancy, while the remaining neonates die in the first weeks of life. Reports attribute the majority of these consequences to infections of the fetus in utero. Infections during pregnancy affect the mother, and often some infections may be transmitted to the fetus in utero, during the intrapartum period or, postnatally, with potentially serious consequences. Many infections have been linked to increased risks of premature delivery and low birth weight, and associated morbidity and mortality of both mother and child. Acute or chronic specific infectious diseases may be contracted during the course of pregnancy, and conception may occur in women already subject to an infection. The coexistence of pregnancy may aggravate the risk to maternal life in cases of the more serious of these diseases. In pregnancy most infections are no more common, nor more serious than in a non-pregnant population of women of similar age. The effects on pregnancy depend on the degree of pyrexia, its duration, and the stage of fetal development when it occurs. Mild exposures during the preimplantation period, and more severe exposures during embryonic and fetal development often result in miscarriage, premature labor, growth restriction, or stillbirth. Hyperthermia may also cause a wide range of fetal structural and functional defects, with the central nervous system (CNS) being most at risk. While there is a greater incidence of neonatal morbidity and mortality with transmitted infections, not all maternal infections lead to transmission to the fetus, nor does transmission to the fetus lead to disease or sequelae. During the puerperium, parturient women are particularly susceptible to serious infections of the genital tract and childbed fever remains one of the most important causes of maternal death. Infections in pregnancy may be viral, bacterial or protozoal, affecting both mother and fetus. Some of the infections cause fevers, while others may not; this chapter will concentrate on infections resulting in maternal pyrexia, and some other infections which may not result in maternal pyrexia, but have important implications for the pregnancy and the fetus.

Chapter 2 - Recurrent late abortions and early prematurity continue to be two of the main problems of modern obstetrics and perinatal medicine which remain to be fully solved. The patients concerned often suffer increasingly.

Ascending genital infection is the main preventable cause for late abortions or early premature births. In recurrent cases, the Early Total Cervix Occlusion (ETCO) is an early preventive measure particularly for women with a history of ≥ 2 late abortions or early premature births (< 32+0 weeks gestation). The operative technique, our own results, and results from a multi-center-enquiry undertaken in Germany are subjects of our present discussion. In both evaluations, the women within this high risk group had a surviving infant in about 70% of cases after a Total Cervix Occlusion (TCO). Differentiated according to „early“ TCO (ETCO) and „late“ TCO, the success rate has been 80% and 40% respectively.

Cerclage is still a frequently employed measure in cases with recurrent preterm births, but it has increasingly become the subject of controversy. ETCO is quite different from cerclage. The cerclage only tightens the canal. Whereas ETCO really closes the cervical canal: After the epithelium of the lower cervical canal and of the lower portio has been removed these parts are sutured. This allows the lower cervix to heal up and close totally. This is a complete barrier which thus prevents ascension of organisms The much poorer results inevitably achieved by cerclage are compared with the results of ETCO. In our sample of women treated with ETCO we found that, in 51 previous pregnancies in which cerclage was performed, only 13 infants survived. This is a survival rate of only 26% (as compared to a survival rate of 80% with ETCO).

ETCO was developed by us in 1981 in Germany and is widespread in Germany and also used in other German-speaking countries, but it is still rarely performed on an international level. This might partly be due to the fact that randomized studies with ETCO have up to now never been performed. But—considering the excellent results of ETCO—performing such a study now in Germany would raise serious ethical issues.

Another possible indication for the future may be in the area of multiple pregnancies: With ETCO, generally performed in multiple pregnancies, Schulze [40] was able to achieve a prematurity rate of only 17% as against a rate of 29% in cases without ETCO. In the group of infants at very high risk (< 28 weeks gestation), the rate with ETCO was 1% as opposed to 4% without.

More information on: http://www.saling-institut.de/eng/04infoph/04tmv.html.

Chapter 3 - An increase of the risk of premature delivery, abortion and stillbirth has been observed during the past pandemics of influenza. The occurrence of intrauterine influenza virus infection during pregnancy is substantiated. Human fetal membranes are appendages of placenta and compose of amnion, chorion and decidua tissues. They play a critical role as defensive barriers in order to maintain normal pregnancy. Recent *in vitro* studies have demonstrated that influenza A/H1N1 virus infection induced apoptosis and the gene expression of a set of pro-inflammatory cytokines, such as interleukin (IL)-6, tumor necrosis factor (TNF)-α and interferon (IFN)-β in cultured chorion cells. IL-6, TNF-α and IFN-β molecules in culture supernatants of the virus-infected chorion cells induced the differentiation of monocytes to well-matured macrophages. It should be noted that these phenomena were not observed in cultured amnion cells after influenza virus infection, yet viral replication was observed in the cells. It has been known that apoptosis of the constituent cells and macrophage activation in the tissues are implicated in the pathogenesis of fetal membrane rupture. Therefore, accumulating evidence suggests that fetal membrane chorion and amnion cells play a pivotal role in the pathogenesis of influenza-associated complications during pregnancy. This article reviews the virulence of influenza virus against human fetal membrane tissues in order to understand the molecular pathogenesis of intrauterine influenza virus infection during pregnancy.

Chapter 4 - Bad obstetric history (BOH) implies previous unfavorable foetal outcome in terms of two or more consecutive spontaneous abortions, history of early neonatal death, intrauterine growth retardation, stillbirths, intrauterine fetal death and/or congenital anomalies. Recurrent pregnancy wastage due to maternal infections transmissible *in utero* at various stages of gestation can be caused by a wide array of organisms that include *Toxoplasma gondii*, rubella virus, cytomegalovirus, herpes simplex virus and other agents.

Herpes simplex virus (HSV) is classified in the alpha virinae subfamily within the family Herpesviridae. Two closely-related viruses are designated HSV types 1 and 2. Both can be transmitted in utero to fetus, with more complications associated with herpes simplex 2.

Another important viral cause of BOH is cytomegaloviruses (CMV). Cytomegaloviruses are ubiquitous and species-specific. Humans are believed to be the only reservoir of this virus, and transmission occurs by direct or indirect person-to-person contact. Vertical transmission can lead to serious congenital infections.

Rubella virus causes serious disease after vertical transmission. Most maternal infections remain subclinical or cause a trivial infection that may remain unrecognized. Its vaccination coverage is not sufficient throughout the world, so new cases are still reported. Clinical diagnosis of rubella is difficult and unreliable, as rubella virus infection can be asymptomatic in up to 50% of infected patients.

Several modalities are available for the diagnosis of those infections. The benchmark method is viral culture. Serology can establish current and past infection. Recently, molecular techniques have become available for rapid diagnosis.

Testing of pregnant women for HSV, CMV and rbella antibodies is usually done with a type-specific assay for their antibodies.

The objective of the present study was to explore the prevalence of herpes simplex virus 2, cytomegalovirus and rubella in pregnant with repeated spontaneous abortions (RSA) in first trimester. The diagnosis was performed by polymerase chain reaction, serological study for specific immunoglobulins G and M for herpes simplex 2 and cytomegalovirus and rubella. There was also an attempt to discover the accuracy of serological diagnosis for herpes simplex 2 and cytomegalovirus compared to polymerase chain reaction.

Patients recruited in the study were complaining of repeated first trimester abortions without obvious medical or gynecological etiology. Laboratory screenings for immunoglobulin M for toxoplasmosis were negative. The study also included pregnant women with normal obstetric history as a control group. Complete medical and obstetric evaluations were performed for patients and control subjects. Furthermore, specific virological diagnosis was performed to measure specific immunoglobulins M and G for CMV and herpes simplex 2 by enzyme linked immunosorbant assay with detection of their DNA in maternal serum by polymerase chain reaction. Diagnosis of rubella was performed by measurement of specific immunoglobulin M by enzyme linked immunosorbant assay.

There was a statistically significant difference between the RSA group and the pregnant women without RSA in frequency of rubella IgM (44.7%), herpes simplex IgM (39.1%) and CMV 10.9% ($P < .001$) . However, there was insignificant difference in IgG for herpes simplex 2, CMV and rubella between patients and control. Herpes simplex 2 viremia was positive in 26% RSA and cytomegalovirus was positive in 10.9% RSA patients. There was a significant association between viremia for cytomegalovirus and herpes simplex 2 ($P<0.009$).

The present study highlights the significant association of rubella, herpes simplex and cytomegalovirus with bad obstetric history. There may be persistence of rubella virus related to repeated early abortions. Moreover, combined viral infections in those patients were found that could even further aggravate intrauterine infections. The study allows the idea that serological tests for IgM are a rapid and accurate method for laboratory diagnosis.

Chapter 5 - The incidence of appendicitis during pregnancy is equal to that in the normal population. However, during pregnancy appendicitis may occur with a variety of clinical presentations, thereby causing severe diagnostic difficulties, especially during the second half of gestation. As a result, appendicitis during pregnancy is associated with an increase in perforation rate, morbidity and mortality compared to that in the normal population. In addition, it may cause pre-term birth and/or fetal loss.

In this chapter we review diagnostic and treatment strategies and complications of appendicitis occuring during pregnancy

Chapter 6 - Mediastinal emphysema and subcutaneous emphysema are rare complications of labor. We describe a case of mediastinal and subcutaneous emphysema observed in the II stage of labor, otherwise known as healthy primigravida. The diagnosis was confirmed clinically through X-ray, and endoscopic examination in District Hospital, as well as in the Clinical Department of Surgery. The etiology of this condition was not established. The mediastinal and subcutaneous emphysema disappeared spontaneously. It was confirmed within 3 months by a check-up.

Chapter 7 - Prevention of early preterm birth (<32 weeks of gestation) and of very-low-birth- weight infants (<1500 g) is one of the most urgent priorities of perinatal medicine. Ascending genital tract infection is an important preventable cause of early preterm birth. The protective effect of the *Lactobacillus* system and a low vaginal pH are important to maintain a normal microbial ecosystem in the lower genital tract and in the prevention of ascending intrauterine infections. Bacterial vaginosis, other changes in the microbial ecosystem and infections can lead to ascending intrauterine infection. They all often begin with a disturbance of this vaginal milieu—which we consider a precursor.

We recommend an assessment of the risk of preterm birth that includes obstetrical history, the early detection of warning signs (including screening for pre-infection states or overt infection by regular determinations of the vaginal pH) and, if indicated, the implementation of appropriate therapeutic measures.

Our prematurity prevention program includes measures taken by physicians and by midwives; "self-care" measures taken by the women themselves (preferably for all pregnant women); and additional special measures for women at risk.

The self-care measures for pregnant women are additional to regular prenatal care. They include information about risk factors and warning signs as well as regular measurement of the vaginal pH by the women themselves. With this self-care, the rate of premature births in the up-to-now published studies could be reduced. Most interesting are the results concerning preterm neonates at particularly high risk: In our experience the rate of very-low-birth-weight infants (<1500 g) was successfully reduced from 7.8% in the immediate previous pregnancy to 1.3%. In Thuringia, the rate of infants born <32+0 weeks was reduced from 1.36 % to 0.94%. Several health insurance companies in Germany are currently offering and evaluating the self-care measures for their clients.

Further information can be found on:

General information : http://www.saling-institut.de/eng/04infoph/01allg.html

Prematurity Prevention Program: http://www.saling-institut.de/eng/04infoph/02programm.html

Self-care measures: http://www.saling-institut.de/eng/04infoph/03selbst.html

Chapter 8 - Pregnant women are at significant risk of acquiring HIV, particularly in areas of high prevalence such as sub-Saharan Africa. HIV in pregnancy results in mother-to-child transmission (MTCT) rates of up to 35% in breast feeding populations as well as relative increases in antenatal death, spontaneous abortion, stillbirth, and low birth weight infants. The identification of HIV-infected women is crucial in the prevention of maternal and infant morbidity and mortality. Whilst most countries recommend 1st or 2nd trimester screening of pregnant women for HIV, the recognition that pregnant women are at risk of primary HIV infection has led to recommendations to repeat testing in the 3rd trimester or during delivery itself. In resource rich countries the use of combination highly active antiretroviral therapy (HAART), avoidance of breastfeeding, and caesarean section delivery has resulted in transmission rates of less than 2%. However, such preventive interventions have been associated with adverse consequences for women and their uninfected infants.

Effective interventions are difficult to implement in developing countries where breastfeeding is critical to infant survival and resources for costly drugs and surgical procedures are scarce. The health of HIV-infected pregnant women in these settings is further compounded by inter-current conditions, notably sexually transmitted infections, tuberculosis, anaemia, and malaria, which also require appropriate management.

A number of trials have shown the benefit of antiretrovirals alone in reducing mother-to-child transmission (MTCT) of HIV, with WHO recommendations for resource-poor settings potentially associated with significantly reduced perinatal and early post-partum transmission. However, women subsequently face a significant dilemma in the postpartum period where the benefits of breastfeeding but attached risks of HIV vertical transmission need to be balanced against the risk of gastroenteritis and malnutrition associated with replacement feeding and earlier cessation of breastfeeding. Recently evaluated strategies allowing safer breastfeeding include exclusive breastfeeding for six months and neonatal prophylaxis with either lamivudine or nevirapine. The use of prolonged maternal HAART during the breastfeeding period is currently under investigation.

Unfortunately many HIV-infected women remain undetected or fail to benefit from effective and affordable interventions as a result of inequitable access to health care. The greatest challenge of implementing Prevention of Mother-to-Child (PMTCT) interventions remains the provision of integrated, accountable healthcare systems with effective procedures of governance driven by strong leadership.

Chapter 9 - Malaria, HIV infection and anaemia constitute major public health problems during pregnancy and are important factors associated with increased risk for adverse pregnancy outcomes. The objective of this study was to evaluate the impact of maternal and placental malaria, HIV infection and anaemia on perinatal outcome. Pregnant women were enrolled at labour ward (LW) at full pregnancy term at Ebonyi State University Teaching Hospital (EBSUTH), Abakaliki Nigeria. The study was conducted from November 2006 to November 2007. At childbirth, fetal length and head circumference, birth weight and placental weight were determined using standard techniques. Maternal peripheral, placental, and cord blood samples were obtained. Peripheral and placental malaria was detected using microscopy. Haemoglobin concentration (HbC), ABO blood group and genotype were performed using standard techniques. HIV infection was screened using ELISA and confirmed by Immunoblot analysis. Prevalence of malaria was 16.0% and *P. falciparum* was the only species identified. Individuals of younger age, primigravidae and those who never attended antenatal clinic (ANC) were more likely to have malaria. Prevalence of malaria significantly decreased with increase in HbC (χ^2=23.8, P<0.05). Individuals with HbAA genotype and those with blood group O had higher prevalence of malaria infection. Prevalence of HIV infection at childbirth was 3.6% and malaria prevalence was significantly higher among HIV-positive women (χ^2=13.3, P<0.05). Malaria infected women had a significantly higher proportion of LBW babies (P<0.05). A higher proportion of LBW was recorded among anemic women, primigravidae, those with HIV infection, blood group O and HbAA genotype and those who never attended ANC. Prevalence of placental malaria was 12.2%. Women with peripheral malaria infection had significantly higher proportion (54.2%) of placental infection than those without peripheral malaria infection (3.5%) (χ^2=94.4, P<0.05). A significantly higher proportion (33.3%) of malaria infected placentas had the lowest placental weight (0.4kg) (χ^2=6.99, P<0.05) and a higher proportion of babies born by mothers with malaria infected placenta had low birth weight (<2.5kg), lower fetal length and head circumference. Prevalence of fetal anaemia (cord HbC<12.5g/dl) was 65.6%. Babies of malaria infected, HIV-positive, and anaemic mothers had a higher proportion of FA. There is need to strengthen ANC services to ensure delivery of malaria, HIV and anaemia interventions within existing health systems, to reduce adverse perinatal outcome.

Chapter 10 - Toxoplasmosis is a disease of considerable public health impact. As the transmission, occurrence and phenotype of this disease are influenced in a complex way by host genetics, immunity, behavior and by the agent characteristics, prevention is not simple. Primary toxoplasmosis is a relatively benign disease usually acquired by ingestion of food contaminated by a protozoan parasite with a complex life cycle. However, in the case of primary infection during pregnancy, the parasite can be transmitted to the fetus, causing visual or neurological impairment or even death. The main risk factors for toxoplasmosis in pregnant women are unsanitary feeding habits, poor immune system, contact with cats, contact with soil, pregnancy, number of births, older age, race, travelling outside the country, drinking beverages prepared with unboiled water, consumption of municipal or uncontrolled water and *T. gondii* strain virulence. The severity of congenital *T. gondii* infection underlines the need for a precise diagnosis of acute infection during pregnancy. The microbiological diagnosis is primarily based upon serological tests, since the recovery of the parasite from biological samples is often unpractical due to its particular life cycle. Infection in the mother or congenital infection in the child are usually asymptomatic and can only be detected by serological screening for *Toxoplasma* specific antibodies. The search for specific IgM has been widely used for this purpose, but their possible early disappearance or persistence over time limits their meaning. This has led to the search of additional serological biomarkers which include the detection of specific IgA, IgE and IgG avidity. Identifying acute infection through repeated antenatal tests facilitates fetal diagnosis through polymerase chain reaction amplification of DNA in amniotic fluid and ultrasonography to monitor fetal development. Eventually, the presence of IgM and IgA antibodies and/or persistence of IgG at one year of life in neonatal serum samples confirm congenital infection. As prenatal treatment of women and postnatal treatment of infants are hampered by the lack of proven efficacy, prenatal serological screening, although a matter of debate, should be considered in a constructive approach to better monitor and reduce the impact of toxoplasmosis on pregnant women and their newborn infants.

Chapter 11 - Italian law requires serological screening for toxoplasmosis by the 13th week of pregnancy, with further screenings for seronegative women every 30-40 days until delivery (a total of 5-7). In order to make this protocol effective, full cooperation is required between physician and patient, and its implementation is particularly problematic in the case of women coming from countries with different languages, cultures and health conditions. Italy has recently seen an increase in immigration from countries outside the European Union, which means that a growing number of extra-Community women are involved in the screening programme. An audit of how such screening is carried out is of paramount importance in order to assess its effectiveness, identify its weaknesses, and plan focused interventions.

We considered the data regarding 3395 pregnant women referred for serological screening for anti-*Toxoplasma* IgG antibodies in the three years 2005-2007: 2465 Italians (72.6%) and 930 (27.4%) of foreign origin. Among the latter, 337 (36.2%) came from Eastern Europe, 213 (22.9%) from the Middle East and the Maghreb, 158 (17.0%) from Latin America, 94 (10.1%) from China and the Far East, 66 (7.1%) from the Indian subcontinent, and 62 (6.7%) from Equatorial and Southern Africa.

By the end of the first trimester, 85.0% of the Italians and 81.2% of the foreign women ($p<0.01$) had undergone their first screening. With reference to origin, the differences from Italians were statistically significant only in the case of the African (96.8%), Latin American (77.2%) and Chinese women (71.3%). The prevalence of anti-*Toxoplasma* IgG ranged from 3.2% in the women of Chinese origin to 54.4% in those of Latin America: comparison with the Italian prevalence (19.4%) showed that all of the differences were statistically significant ($p<0.01$) except for that relating to the women of the Indian subcontinent (13.6%). Five or more screenings (as indicated by the Italian Ministry of Health) were undergone by 32.2% of the seronegative Italians and 30.4% of the seronegative foreign women, among whom the differences from the Italians were statistically significant only in the case of the Latin American (20.8%, $p<0.05$) and Chinese women (18.7%, $p<0.01$). In conclusion, our study shows that screening is active in recruiting both Italian and foreign women by the end of the first trimester of pregnancy, when it is easier to assess and manage a possible acute infection. However, it seems to be more difficult to implement the full screening programme as indicated by the Ministry of Health as only about one-third of the seronegative women underwent five or more screenings. Furthermore, the management of screening is particularly problematic in the case of Chinese and Latin American women, which should stimulate more health education campaigns.

Chapter 12 - The term "rickettsioses" traditionally has included the diseases caused by 23 species of the genus *Rickettsia* up-to-date recognized to be pathogenic to humans as well as diseases caused by *Coxiella, Ehrlichia, Anaplasma* and *Orientia* species, which belong to different genera, families or even orders. Infections caused by rickettsiae and related pathogens are of major morbidity worldwide; additionally, new pathogens are continuously recognized and consideration has recently been given to their potentiality as biological weapons.

Pregnant women, especially those living in endemic areas, are of considerable risk for rickettsioses, but very little is known about the natural course of infections caused by rickettsiae and related pathogens during pregnancy. Transplacental passage has not been documented for any of the pathogens of the genus *Rickettsia,* the youngest serologically confirmed case having been a *R. ricketsii* infection a 6-month-old infant. By contrast, transplacental transmission is likely, for *Orientia* and *Anaplasma* species, thus treatment of the newborn should be considered in such cases. *C burnettii*, a major cause of infertility and abortions in animals has been associated with obstetric complications, abortions and stillbirths in humans as well and perinatal infection with this pathogen is considered possible.

The treatment of infections caused by rickettsiae and related pathogens in pregnancy raises serious safety issues. Tetracyclines, which are the treatment of choice for non-pregnant adults can be toxic for both, the mother and the fetus and the alternative choice of chloramphenicol has been associated with the rare but life-threatening complication of "gray baby syndrome" if given near term. Macrolides have been safely used in pregnancy for the treatment of other infections and seem to be an attractive option but their efficacy against the most serious of these infections, i.e., *R rickettsii*, is questioned. Moreover, macrolides alone are not sufficient for the management of *C burnettii* infection, which has the potential of chronicity and can complicate future pregnancies.

Rickettsioses in pregnancy are associated with complications both for the mother and fetus/infant. Treatment of these infections remains challenging and controversial and should be carefully considered on case-by-case basis until further investigation elucidates the natural course of the infections in pregnancy and the efficacy and safety issues. Prevention, principally by avoiding ticks and contact to infected animals, is of paramount significance.

Chapter 13 - The objective of our studies was to estimate the association between maternal glomerulonephritis / urinary tract infections (UTI) during pregnancy and structural birth defects, i.e. congenital abnormalities or adverse pregnancy outcome. The prevalence of these maternal diseases during the first trimester of pregnancy in cases with different congenital abnormalities was compared to that of matched controls without congenital abnormalities in the population-based Hungarian Case-Control Surveillance System of Congenital Abnormalities. Of 22,843 cases with congenital abnormalities, 309 (1.35%) had mothers with glomerulonephritis during pregnancy, compared to 479 (1.26%) of 38,151 controls (adjusted POR with 95% CI = 1.0, 0.9-1.2). Specified groups of congenital abnormalities were also assessed versus controls. Cases with isolated intestinal atresia/stenosis (adjusted POR with 95% CI: 6.8, 1.3-37.4) based on five cases were more likely to have mothers with prospectively and medically recorded glomerulonephritis. A total of 1542 (6.75%) mothers in the case group had UTI during the entire pregnancy compared with 2188 (5.74%) mothers in the control group (adjusted prevalence odds ratios [POR] with 95% CI: 1.15, 1.06-1.24). We did not find a higher prevalence of UTI during the second and/or third months of pregnancy in total case group (adjusted POR with 95% CI: 1.1, 0.9-1.2) and in any group of CAs including atrial septal defect type II. In conclusion a higher rate of congenital isolated intestinal atresia/stenosis may be associated with maternal glomerulonephritis. However, this finding is considered only as signal and further studies are needed to confirm or reject this possible association. Maternal urinary tract infections during pregnancy increase pre-eclampsia and polyhydramnios, and in addition the rate of preterm birth; however, the latter is preventable by appropriate drug treatments. No evidence was found for the teratogenic effect of maternal UTI and related drug treatments during early pregnancy.

Chapter 14 - Dengue infection is a common arboviral infection that poses a significant threat to tropical countries. The serious forms of this infection are called dengue hemorrhagic fever and dengue shock syndrome. These serious forms of dengue infection can lead to a high rate of fatality. Pregnant women in the endemic area of dengue infection can be infected and can develop many signs and symptoms. In this chapter, the author will focus on dengue infection in pregnancy, especially on the pattern of hematological disturbance. The co-manifestation with other common hematological disorders in pregnancy will also be mentioned.

Chapter 15 - Infectious diseases of respiratory system frequently complicate pregnancy. This review evaluates the possible association between maternal infectious diseases of the respiratory system during pregnancy and preterm birth or structural birth defects, i.e., congenital abnormalities (CAs), in addition to their pregnancy complications based on the data set of the Hungarian Case-Control Surveillance of Congenital Abnormalities.

At the evaluation of a *common cold*, it is necessary to differentiate the usual common cold (with short duration and without fever) and the common cold with secondary complications (i.e., with longer duration and frequently high fever). Pregnant women with a common cold mainly with secondary complications did not have a higher incidence of pregnancy complications. The gestational age at delivery was 0.1 week shorter with a somewhat higher rate of preterm birth, but these differences had no real clinical importance. However, an association of common cold (mainly with secondary complications) in the second and/or third gestational month of pregnancy with a higher rate of newborns with congenital cataract, cleft lip ± palate and possibly some other specific congenital abnormalities was found, and this association was preventable with antifever drug treatments.

Acute infectious diseases of the respiratory system cover a wide spectrum of diseases, from sinusitis to pneumonia. These diseases during pregnancy have no obvious effect of pregnancy complications. Infectious respiratory diseases in the severe lower catetory were associated with a higher risk for preterm birth, but their mild upper category seems to reduce indirectly the rate of preterm birth. Acute infectious diseases of the respiratory system during the second and third gestational months of pregnancy were not associated with a higher risk for the total group or any specific group/entity of congenital abnormalities. However, frequently high-fever–related tonsillitis in pregnant women was associated with a higher risk for congenital cataract, neural-tube defects, cleft lip ± palate and unclassified multiple congenital abnormalities. We may suppose that the association between these fever-sensitive defect groups and tonsillitis may be caused by high fever, because the parallel antifever treatment was able to prevent this risk.

Finally, *influenza* during pregnancy was evaluated. The short duration of influenza in pregnant women did not increase the risk for pregnancy complications. Our study showed that the appropriately treated pregnant women affected with influenza in the first and second trimester of pregnancy have no higher risk for preterm birth. However, the high- fever–related influenza in the second and/or third gestational month of pregnancy may associate with a higher risk of some hyperthermia-sensitive CAs such as neural-tube defects, congenital cataract, cleft lip ± palate, cleft palate only, cardiovascular CAs, and unclassified multiple CAs. The main finding of our study is that this higher risk for these major CAs can be prevented by the parallel use of antifever drugs.

Chapter 16 - *Objective:* To assess the maternal outcomes and the characteristic features of pregnancy with smallpox.

Design: Retrospective collection and review of literature on previous smallpox outbreaks.

Setting: Case fatalities in 16 outbreaks and miscarriage and premature birth in 15 outbreaks in Europe, Australia and the United States during the 19th and 20th centuries.

Population: Pregnant smallpox cases at various gestational periods and with various vaccination histories.

Methods: Overall crude estimates of the outcomes were obtained based on the collected publications. Stratifications were then performed by gestational period, clinical classification of smallpox, and vaccination status.

Main outcome measures: Case fatality, and miscarriage and premature birth.

Results: Overall case fatality and the proportion of miscarriage and premature birth were estimated as 34.3% (95% confidence interval (CI); 31.4, 37.1) and 39.9% (36.5, 43.2), respectively. Although the estimate of case fatality was highest during the third trimester (40.5% (26.8, 54.2)), miscarriage and premature birth did not show a clear localised pattern according to gestational stage. Vaccination prior to pregnancy effectively reduced the risk of death in three outbreaks ($p < 0.01$, $p = 0.02$ and $p < 0.01$, respectively). Miscarriage and premature birth were frequently observed even among those with mild classifications of smallpox.

Conclusions: Despite the extremely high estimates of both outcomes, fatality can be lowered by vaccination prior to pregnancy. Nevertheless, it might be difficult to prevent cases from miscarriage and premature birth using vaccination only. The historical records appeared useful for clarifying the examined outcomes and in characterising the common patterns.

Chapter 17 - Chicken pox infection is a common viral infection. Fever with skin abnormality is the common presentation. Pregnant women in areas with poor hygienic conditions can become infected and can develop many signs and symptoms. In this chapter, the author will focus on chicken pox infection in pregnancy. Important reports are reviewed and presented.

In: Infectious Pregnancy Complications
Editor: Richard N. Canfield
ISBN 978-1-60741-038-6

Chapter 1

Complications of Infections in Pregnancy

Dushyant Maharaj *
MBBS, Dip Tert Teach, D.MAS, FCOG (S.A.), FRANZCOG
University of Otago, Wellington. New Zealand; and Consultant,
Wellington Women's Hospital, Wellington, New Zealand

Abstract

Epidemiological reports estimate that 7.7 million perinatal deaths occur annually worldwide, including 4.3 million that take place in late pregnancy, while the remaining neonates die in the first weeks of life. Reports attribute the majority of these consequences to infections of the fetus in utero. Infections during pregnancy affect the mother, and often some infections may be transmitted to the fetus in utero, during the intrapartum period or, postnatally, with potentially serious consequences. Many infections have been linked to increased risks of premature delivery and low birth weight, and associated morbidity and mortality of both mother and child. Acute or chronic specific infectious diseases may be contracted during the course of pregnancy, and conception may occur in women already subject to an infection. The coexistence of pregnancy may aggravate the risk to maternal life in cases of the more serious of these diseases. In pregnancy most infections are no more common, nor more serious than in a non-pregnant population of women of similar age. The effects on pregnancy depend on the degree of pyrexia, its duration, and the stage of fetal development when it occurs. Mild exposures during the preimplantation period, and more severe exposures during embryonic and fetal development often result in miscarriage, premature labor, growth restriction, or stillbirth. Hyperthermia may also cause a wide range of fetal structural and functional defects, with the central nervous system (CNS) being most at risk. While there is a greater incidence of neonatal morbidity and mortality with transmitted infections, not all maternal infections lead to transmission to the fetus, nor does transmission to the fetus lead to disease or sequelae. During the puerperium, parturient women are particularly

* Telephone: +64 4 385 5999; Fax: +64 4 389 5943; e-mail: dean.maharaj@otago.ac.nz

susceptible to serious infections of the genital tract and childbed fever remains one of the most important causes of maternal death. Infections in pregnancy may be viral, bacterial or protozoal, affecting both mother and fetus. Some of the infections cause fevers, while others may not; this chapter will concentrate on infections resulting in maternal pyrexia, and some other infections which may not result in maternal pyrexia, but have important implications for the pregnancy and the fetus.

Introduction

Infections during pregnancy affect the mother and often some infections may be transmitted to the fetus in utero, during the intrapartum period or, postnatally, with potentially serious consequences. Epidemiological reports estimate that 7.7 million perinatal deaths occur annually worldwide, including 4.3 million that take place in late pregnancy, while the remaining neonates die in the first weeks of life [1, 2, 3, 4, 5]. Reports attribute the majority of these consequences to infections of the fetus in utero [6, 7]. Acute or chronic specific infectious diseases may be contracted during the course of pregnancy, or conception may occur in women already infected. The coexistence of pregnancy may aggravate the risk to maternal life in cases of the more serious of these diseases. In pregnancy most infections are no more common, nor more serious than in a non-pregnant population of women of similar age. The effects on pregnancy depend on the degree of pyrexia, its duration, and the stage of fetal development when it occurs. Many infections have been linked with increased risks of premature delivery and low birth weight, and associated morbidity and mortality. Hyperthermia acts as a teratogen in some animals where it can induce resorption of the fetus and fetal death. Fever during pregnancy, especially in the period of embryogenesis, is also suspected as being a risk factor for fetal death. Drawing on the large Danish Birth Cohort study involving over 24 000 women identified about 4500 women (18·5% of those enrolled) who recalled having a fever during the first 16 weeks of pregnancy, which shows that in early pregnancy maternal fever is a common event [8]. In general, perinatal infections have more severe fetal consequences when they occur early in gestation, because first-trimester infections may disrupt organogenesis. Second- and third-trimester infections can cause neurologic impairment or growth disturbances. In utero infection may be associated with certain ultrasound findings, including intrauterine growth restriction, echogenic bowel, intracranial or intrahepatic calcifications, hydrocephalus, microcephaly, isolated ascites, pericardial or pleural effusions, or nonimmune hydrops, although congenital infections may be asymptomatic [9]. The effects on pregnancy depend on the extent of temperature elevation, its duration, and the stage of fetal development when it occurs. Mild exposures during the preimplantation period and more severe exposures during embryonic and fetal development often result in miscarriage, premature labour, growth restriction and stillbirth. Hyperthermia may also cause a wide range of fetal structural and functional defects, with the central nervous system (CNS) being most at risk. While there is a greater incidence of neonatal morbidity and mortality with transmitted infections, not all maternal infections lead to transmission to the fetus, nor does transmission to the fetus lead to disease or sequelae.

During the puerperium, parturient women are particularly susceptible to serious infections of the genital tract and childbed fever remains one of the most important causes of maternal death. Infections in pregnancy may be viral, bacterial or protozoal, affecting both mother and fetus. Some of the infections cause fevers, while others may not, but have important implications for the pregnancy and the fetus (Table 1).

Table 1. Causative agents, transmission, and effects on mother and fetus/neonate

Infecting agent	Transmission	Potential effects on mother	Potential effects on fetus/newborn
1) Viral			
Coxsackie A and B	Mostly intrauterine	Herpangina; hand, foot, mouth disease; myocardiopathy, aseptic meningitis, Bornholm disease	Abortion, stillbirth, neonatal sepsis, myocarditis-meningoencephalitis, ? gastrointestinal, cardiac and urogenital defects,
Cytomegalovirus	Mostly intrauterine. 50% in primary maternal infection (25% symptomatic)	Usually asymptomatic. Sometimes moderate to high fever in primary infection	Deafness, microcephaly, hepatosplenomegaly, hydrops fetalis
Echovirus		Rash may resemble rubella; mimics appendicits and abruption placenta	Neonatal sepsis, disseminated infection (hepatic necrosis), late stillbirth,
Enteroviruses		Non-specific febrile illness, abdominal pains	Neonatal sepsis
Hepatitis B	Intrauterine, postnatal, mostly perinatal. Risk of perinatal infection if mother HBAg +ve is 90%	Asymptomatic chronic carrier state, acute hepatitis	Chronic carrier, rarely acute fulminant neonatal hepatitis
Hepatitis C	Intrauterine, mostly perinatal. 0%-6.2% depending on HCV RNA-titres. Upto 19.4% in HCV/HIV +ve patients	Acute hepatitis, cirrhosis, hepatocellular carcinoma.	?effects
Herpes simplex	Intrauterine and perinatal. 40-50% risk of severe neonatal infection after primary maternal genital infection, and 8% risk after secondary infection	Oral or genital papular eruptions; more severe in pregnancy	Abortion after primary infection, fatal disseminated infection, prematurity, congenital malformations, stillbirth, intrauterine growth restriction ?Infantile disease, viremia

Table 1. (Continued)

Infecting agent	Transmission	Potential effects on mother	Potential effects on fetus/newborn
Human Immunodeficiency viruses (HIV-1 and HIV-2)	Intrauterine, postnatal, mostly perinatal. 2%-40% transmission depending on treatment, and breastfeeding	Asymptomatic, unless had AIDS	Uncertain. ?CNS malformations, neural tube defects, ?circulatory malformations, ?cleft lip, ?reductive deformities
Influenza	Intrauterine and postnatal	Upto 54% mortality in pandemics	Congenital disease Congenital measles, ?increased mortality
Lymphocytic choriomeningitis virus	Mostly intrauterine	Meningitis/meningoencephalitis	?increased mortality, ?endocardial fibroelastosis
Measles	Mostly intrauterine	May be complicated by pneumonia and CCF. More severe. May be fatal	Stillbirth, neonatal disease
Mumps	Intrauterine	Nonspecific effects	Congenital malformations, abortions, fetal death, chronic infection
Poliomyelitis		Increased severity, mortality	
Rubella (German measles)	Mostly intrauterine, postnatal. 40%-60% risk of severe defects in months 1and2, 30%-35% in month 3, 10% in month 4. rare fetal damage after 20 weeks	Mild nonspecific symptoms	Second trimester abortions, hydrops fetalis due to severe anemia, ?myocarditis, ?hepatitis, haematological effects in late pregnancy,
Parvovirus B19	Intrauterine	Asymptomatic, "slapped-cheek" rash, erythema infectiosum (Fifth disease)	Varicella embryopathy, congenital varicella syndrome, infantile zoster, microcephaly, focal brain calcification, optic atrophy, skin scarring, limb atrophy
Varicella zoster (Chickenpox)	Intrauterine and perinatal. No accurate figures; estimated 0.7%-2.2% transmission	More severe; maternal death	Abortion, stillbirth, premature birth, non-immune hydrops, intrauterine growth restriction, perinatal death, congenital disease

Table 1. (Continued)

Infecting agent	Transmission	Potential effects on mother	Potential effects on fetus/newborn
2) Bacterial Treponema pallidum	Intrauterine. 0.02%–4.5%, but varies in regions	Primary (asymptomatic, chancre, lymphadenopathy), secondary (rash, condylomata, alopecia, arthritis, periostitis, optic neuritis, intersitial keratitis, iritis, uveitis, meningitis) and tertiary (cardiovascular, neurological, joint disorders, gummas, dementia)	Abortion, premature birth, stillbirth Fetal death, chronic intrauterine, congenital or perinatal infection, prematurity, meningoencephalitis.
Mycobacterium tuberculosis	Mostly intrauterine, postnatal.	9% of all deaths of women of reproductive age. Malaise, night sweats, weight loss, usually respiratory symptoms	Miscarriage, stillbirth, neonatal deaths, congenital Lyme disease hydrocephalus, cardiovascular anomalies, neonatal respiratory distress, hyperbilirubinemia, intrauterine growth restriction, cortical blindness
Listeria moncytogenes	Mostly intrauterine, perinatal. Soil, food, animals.	Headache, myalgia, fever, loin pains, pharyngitis, gastrointestinal symptoms	
Borrelia burgdorferi (Lyme disease)	Intrauterine	3 stages: early localized, early disseminated, and late disease. Erythema migrans, rash, palsies of the cranial nerves, meningitis, conjunctivitis, carditis, arthritis, Meningoradiculoneuritis (Bannwarth syndrome). Systemic symptoms, such as arthralgia, myalgia, headache, fatigue	Hydrocephalus, intracranial calcification, chorioretinitis. Jaundice, anemia, hepatosplenomegaly, lymphadenopathy
3) Protozoal Toxoplasma gondii	Intrauterine. 15% - 40%. Acquired through eating raw or undercooked meat or ingesting soil contaminated with toxoplasma oocysts, which are excreted in the faeces of infected cats.	Usually asymptomatic or mild, non-specific symptoms. Posterior cervical lymphadenopathy	Abortion, stillbirth, premature delivery, intrauterine growth restriction, low birth weight.
Plasmodium species	Intrauterine. Placental malaria rates 4.7%-74% in endemic areas	Increased susceptibility. Maternal death, anemia	

Pre-Pregnancy Counselling and Antenatal Screening

Ideally, all women should consult their health-care provider before conception. Pre-pregnancy testing for infections should include an assessment of rubella immunity, syphilis status, human immunodeficiency virus (HIV) status, and immunity to hepatitis B. Some countries test for varicella IgG antibody to exclude previous infection with chickenpox. Women in close contact with children, such as childcare workers, may be at increased risk of cytomegalovirus (CMV) infection during pregnancy, and should be tested for CMV IgG before conception. A pre-pregnancy visit is also an opportunity to give dietary and other advice on how to reduce the risk of contracting listeriosis and toxoplasmosis, ie. avoid raw or undercooked meat and meat products; peel or wash raw fruit and vegetables thoroughly to remove contaminating soil, and to wash hands after disposing of cat litter or gardening. The pre-pregnancy session also provides an opportunity for counselling of both partners to avoid casual sexual contact, and intravenous drug use and consequent risk of infection. Women who lack immunity to rubella, hepatitis B, or varicella, should be advised vaccinations, and pregnancy should be postponed for at least two months after completion of the vaccination [10].

Table 2. CDC Recommendations for STI Screening in Pregnancy [13]

Condition	Screening recommended?	Preferred test
Bacterial vaginosis*	No	-
Chlamydia	Yes: all pregnant women	NAAT
Gonorrhea	Yes: women who are at risk† or living in a high-prevalence area	NAAT or culture on Thayer-Martin media
Hepatitis B	Yes: all pregnant women	HBsAg serology
Hepatitis C	Yes: women who are at high risk‡	Anti-HCV
Herpes	No (culture lesions if present)	Culture, PCR
HIV	Yes: all pregnant women	EIA, Western blot
HPV	No	-
Syphilis	Yes: all pregnant women	RPR or VDRL
Trichomoniasis	No	-

NOTE: "Yes" indicates screening is recommended at the first prenatal visit, with repeat screening in the third trimester for those at risk.

CDC = Centers for Disease Control and Prevention; STI = sexually transmitted infection; NAAT = nucleic acid amplification test; HBsAg = hepatitis B surface antigen; HCV = hepatitis C virus; PCR = polymerase chain reaction; HIV = human immunodeficiency virus; EIA = enzyme immunoassay; HPV = human papillomavirus; RPR = rapid plasma reagin; VDRL = Venereal Disease Research Laboratories.

*-Bacterial vaginosis is not an STI, but it is more common in sexually active women. †-Women who have a new or more than one sex partner.

‡-Women with a history of injection drug use, repeated exposure to blood products, or blood transfusion or organ transplant before 1992.

Screening should generally be applied to all pregnant women [11]. Selective screening based on risk factors is unreliable — eliciting risk factors for all relevant infections is time-consuming and unlikely to identify all those at risk — and women are generally more willing to accept routinely offered tests than to acknowledge, if they are aware of it, being at high risk [12]. Informed consent should be obtained for routine antenatal screening, which implies that women have the option of refusing. The Centers for Disease Control and Prevention (CDC) recommends screening for some sexually transmitted infections (STI's) at the first prenatal visit, then again in the third trimester for mothers at high risk (Table 2) [13].

Screening tests should be conducted as early as possible during pregnancy. Tests that are recommended include those for human immunodeficiency virus (HIV) infection, hepatitis B and C, syphilis, and *Chlamydia trachomatis.* Women at risk should be tested for *Neisseria gonorrhea*. Women younger than 25 years and those who are at risk of chlamydia (e.g., those who have multiple sex partners) should be rescreened in the third trimester. Women who continue to be at risk of gonorrhea should also be rescreened in the third trimester [13]. In cases of current infection, treatment should be instituted immediately, and physicians should counsel the patient to use condoms and avoid sexual contact until her partner has been treated.

Effects of Hyperthermia in Pregnancy

Persistent elevation of body temperature above normal levels in an individual is defined as fever. The normal body temperature usually lies between 37.0 and 37.5°C with diurnal variations. Disturbances of temperature regulation in disease can be explained by shifts in body water, inadequate hydration, and changes in metabolism. The pattern of febrile response may be intermittent (falling to normal each day), remittent (falling each day, but still remaining above the normal), sustained (without significant diurnal variation), or relapsing (alternating with periods of one to several days of normal temperatures). The underlying sequence of events seems to be the removal of endotoxins from the circulation by fixed phagocytes of the reticuloendothelial system, followed by margination of polymorphonuclear leukocytes along the margins of the vessels. These two types of cells undergo activation to release endogenous pyrogen in to the circulation. The pyrogen produced in response to toxic, immunological or infectious stimuli, is induced through the release of lymphocytic lymphokines arising in response to antigenic recognition, and acts on the hypothalamic thermoregulatory center, transmitting information to the vasomotor center, possibly through production of prostaglandin [14].

The release of endogenous pyrogen by phagocytic cells appears to be the common factor in the pathogenesis of fever, irrespective of its cause (Table 3).

Modes of transmission of infective agents include transplacental transfer via umbilical blood flow, or by direct spread to the amniotic fluid, ascending transmission from the cervix and uterus to the amniotic fuid, intrapartum exposure to maternal vaginal secretions and blood, or by postpartum exposure to maternal respiratory secretions or breast milk. There is a clear association between antenatal infection/inflammation and preterm labour, with intrauterine infection complicating up to one third of preterm deliveries [15]. In addition to this, there is now accumulating evidence that intrauterine infection and inflammation can lead to the development of a systemic inflammatory response in the fetus and subsequent tissue injury. The fetal inflammatory response is characterized by funisitis, high levels of pro-inflammatory cytokines in the amniotic fluid and cord blood, and systemic immune activation [16]. A hyperthermic episode during pregnancy can result in embryonic death, abortion, growth retardation, and defects of development [17]. During a sensitive stage of development, hyperthermia can cause apoptosis, interruption of the normal sequence of developmental gene activities and damage to the embryonic vascular system. The thermal dose delivered to an embryo is a product of the elevation of temperature above normal and the duration of that elevation.

Table 3. Infectious and non-infectious causes of fever in the mother

Systemic diseases	Non-infectious diseases	Bacterial infections
1. Tuberculosis 2. Gall bladder • cholecystitis • cholangitis • empyema 3. Abscesses • subphrenic • hepatic • pelvic • cerebral • dental • breast 4. Gastrointestinal • appendicitis • diverticulitis 5. Urinary tract infections 6. Retroperitoneal infection 7. Septicemia • meningococcal • streptococcal • staphylococcal • gonococcal • listeriosis • vibriosis • brucellosis 8. Endocarditis 9. Breast • mastitis 10. Other • Q-fever • amebiasis • leptospirosis	1. Neoplasms • Lymphoma • Leukemia • Melanoma • Metastasis • Retroperitoneal sarcoma • Tumors of the lung, kidney, pancreas, liver 2. Connective tissue disease • Rheumatic fever • Systemic lupus erythematosis • Rheumatoid arthritis 3. Other • Drug fever • Thromboembolism • Sarcoidosis • Hemolytic disease	1. Gonococcal • septicaemia • salpingitis • arthritis 2. Secondary syphilis 3. Gas gangarene 4. Tetanus 5. Opportunistic – associated with immune deficiency syndrome – • candidiosis • cryptococcosis • histoplasmosis • aspergillosis • coccidiomycosis

As the temperature is increased, the time required to cause a defect is reduced. There are several ways in which maternal infection might lead to inflammation within the fetal tissue and the loss of vulnerable cell populations. Bacterial products could cross to the fetal circulation, bind specific cell-membrane receptors such as CD14 and toll-like receptors [18], both on inflammatory cells within the systemic circulation and the brain, initiating a cascade of intracellular events and activating transcription factors such as nuclear factor κ-B and production of proinflammatory cytokines (e.g. TNF-α, IL-1β and IL-6).

These proinflammatory cytokines have a variety of cerebral effects including a direct toxic effect on neurones and vulnerable oligodendrocyte precursor populations, [19], gliosis with release of nitric oxide and mitochondrial dysfunction, [20], as well as microglial activation [21].

Animal studies describe clearly the direct correlation between increasing brain temperature and susceptibility to a variety of neurotoxic factors. Hypothermia can be neuroprotective after hypoxia–ischemia in neonatal animals, while hyperthermia increases brain injury after ischemia in adult rats [22, 23].

Maternal pyrexia, resulting from both microbial infection as well as noninfective causes such as epidural anaesthesia, could therefore augment the deleterious effects of hypoxia on the fetal brain, possibly by increasing the cerebral metabolic rate and demand for oxygen.

Systemic fetal hypotension, endothelial injury and leukocyte aggregation may all contribute to local tissue ischemia, especially in vulnerable areas such as deep white matter. Many of these mechanisms could lead directly to cell death. They may also have an indirect neurotoxic effect by sensitising the brain and lowering the threshold at which hypoxia triggers apoptosis [24].

Hyperthermia interferes with protein synthesis via heat-shock proteins, inducing cell death in the S-phase of the cell cycle by apoptosis and delay of mitotic activity in M-phase cells, and causing vascular disruption and placental infarction. All these mechanisms can lead directly to death of the embryo or to severe and lethal malformations. Furthermore, heat-induced increased uterine contractility can lead to expulsion of the fetus at a non-viable stage of gestation [25]. Studies have found that children of mothers who experienced infectious fevers in pregnancy were more likely to have neurological problems than children whose mothers had the infection without fever. [26].

The association between maternal influenza, or fever, in the second trimester of pregnancy, and the later onset of schizophrenia in the offspring raises the possibility of hyperthermia being one of the initiating factors in this condition, and perhaps, a number of other neurological conditions of uncertain etiology such as cerebral palsy and autism. Inflammation (leukocytic invasion) of the chorioamnion (chorioamnionitis) and/or umbilical cord (funisitis) marks the maternal and fetal immune responses, respectively. While these histologic markers may result from numerous insults (hypoxic injury, trauma, meconium or allergens), by far the most common is the immune response to subclinical or clinical infection [27, 28, 29, 30].

The immune status of an individual may be innate or acquired. Innate immunity is genetically or constitutionally determined, and is not a function of cells of the immune system or antibodies, but of physiological, biochemical or anatomical differences between species. The response of adults to antigen stimulation consists of production of IgM, followed by production of IgG.

The pattern of response in the neonate is different; IgM is produced as a first response, and persists for several weeks before IgG is released. The fetus elaborates IgM in response to antigen exposure in utero, and it is the detection of the specific antibody in the IgM fraction of cord blood that is used for detection of congenital infections. The poor response of newborns to certain infections are not clearly understood, however, there is evidence that in addition to physiological dysglobinemia, the cellular response to infection varies, and the phagocytes are less active.

Further, there is a lack of antigen-presenting macrophages. Immunity acquired either passively or actively, follows the transfer of immune antibody of the IgG class from mother to fetus by the transplacental route, and the ingestion of IgA antibody in colostrum.

Artificially acquired passive immunity follows injection of immune products such as antitoxins, antisera, or immune globulin [31].

Investigation of Infection in Pregnant Women

Possible or Confirmed Exposure

If a pregnant woman is exposed to an infection known to be transmissible to the fetus or infant, she should be investigated as soon as possible to determine her susceptibility.

In susceptible women, determining the basis for diagnosis in the contact may help in assessing the risk of infection. Serological testing should be repeated up to three weeks after contact to detect seroconversion. Pregnant women at risk for contracting a sexually transmitted infection should be re-tested, even if routine antenatal screening has already been done [10].

Presentation with Symptoms

Symptoms of infection in pregnant women should be investigated unless the cause is obvious. Diagnosis may be based on clinical grounds, and confirmed by laboratory tests (table 4).

The best serological evidence of recent systemic infection is IgG seroconversion, or a significant increase in IgG level, when measured quantitatively, and serially. The first serum specimen should be collected as soon as possible after contact or symptom onset. A negative specific IgG result early in the illness does not exclude recent infection. Testing should be repeated up to three weeks after contact. Specific IgM (or sometimes IgA) may be present without IgG early in the infection. If IgG seroconversion does not occur, the IgM result is likely to be a false positive. If both IgG and IgM are present, and their levels remain unchanged in sequential specimens, IgM testing should be repeated using a different method. In general, IgM tests should not be performed in the absence of a suggestive clinical illness or contact, as the positive predictive value can be relatively low. It is important to note that infection should not be diagnosed on the basis of a single positive IgM result [10].

Table 4. Investigation of symptomatic infective illness during pregnancy

Diagnosis	Diagnostic tests
Primary CMV infection, primary toxoplasmosis	IgG and IgM (paired sera)
Listeriosis	Culture of faeces, blood and/or urine
Other viral infections	Culture, serology
Rubella, Parvovirus infection	IgG and IgM (paired sera)
Enterovirus infection	Throat swab or faecal culture
Varicella	Lesion swab and serology
Urinary tract infection (cystitis, pyelonephritis)	Urine microscopy and culture
Genital herpes	First episode: lesion swab, HSV1 and HSV2 IgG and IgM (paired with stored serum if available)
Chlamydia, gonorrhoea	Cervical swab, Gram stain and culture; urine PCR (if positive, check syphilis, HBVand HIV serology)
Chorioamnionitis	Vaginal Gram stain and culture (for group B streptococci or abnormal vaginal flora associated with bacterial vaginosis)
Pneumonia	Chest x-ray, sputum for stain and culture
Malaria	Peripheral blood smear, antigen detection techniques (PfHPR-2), fluorescent staining, PCR based assay, antibody test
Typhoid	Antigen detection
Hepatitis	HBsAg, HBeAg, Hepatitis C-RNA (PCR)

If a vertically transmissible infection is confirmed, or cannot be excluded in a pregnant woman, the risk to the fetus depends on the stage of pregnancy and the type of infection. For some infections, it may be appropriate to determine whether the fetus has been infected (eg, CMV infection, toxoplasmosis and, in some circumstances, varicella), as the diagnosis has important implications for the pregnancy. These infections require specialised tests, such as culture or nucleic acid testing of amniotic fluid obtained at amniocentesis [10].

Sexually Transmitted Infections

Sexually transmitted infections (STI) have been associated with a number of adverse pregnancy outcomes including spontaneous abortion, stillbirth, prematurity, low birth weight (LBW), postpartum endometritis, and various sequelae in surviving neonates [32].

Though sexually transmitted infections (STI's) often do not cause fevers in pregnancy, they may predispose to co-infections, and have implications for the fetus and neonate. When infection is detected, the physician must inform the woman, ensure adequate and safe treatment, and advise partner notification and treatment. The principles of management of all STI's are:

- Treat the patient
- Treat the partner
- Contact tracing and treatment
- Investigate for other STI's
- Evaluate response to treatment
- Patient education

A summary of treatment of STI's in pregnancy is shown in table 5 [13].

Table 5. Treatment of STI's in Pregnancy [13]

Infection	Treatment options
Chlamydia	Azithromycin 1 g orally in a single dose Amoxicillin 500 mg orally three times per day for seven day
Gonorrhea	Ceftriaxone 125 mg intramuscularly in a single dose Cefixime 400 mg orally in a single dose
HSV First episode Recurrent Suppressive therapy	 Acyclovir 400 mg orally three times per day or 200 mg orally five times per day for seven to 10 days Valacyclovir 1 g orally two times per day for seven to 10 days Acyclovir 400 mg orally three times per day for five days Valacyclovir 1 g orally once per day for five days Acyclovir 400 mg orally two times per day Valacyclovir 500 mg orally once per day
HIV	Highly active antiretroviral therapy
Syphilis	Benzathine penicillin G 2.4 million units intramuscularly Primary: single dose Positive serology, no symptoms: three doses one week apart Desensitization recommended in patients who are allergic to penicillin
Trichomoniasis	Metronidazole 2 g orally in a single dose
Bacterial vaginosis*	Metronidazole 500 mg orally two times per day for seven days

STI = sexually transmitted infection; HIV = human immunodeficiency virus; HSV = herpes simplex virus.

**Bacterial vaginosis is not an STI, but it is more common in sexually active women.*

Chlamydia

Chlamydia trachomatis infection in pregnancy leads to cervicitis and cervical discharge but a high proportion of women are asymptomatic. *Chlamydia trachomatis* is the most common sexually transmitted bacterial pathogen in the United States, and as many as 5% to 15% of pregnant women are infected [33]. The infection has been associated with stillbirth, premature delivery, premature rupture of the membranes, and LBW [32]. Mother-to-child transmission of *C. trachomatis* can occur at the time of birth and may result in ophthalmia neonatorum or pneumonitis in the newborn, or postpartum endometritis in the mother. The nucleic acid amplification test (NAAT) is the preferred test for chlamydia because of its high sensitivity and specificity and its use on specimens obtained noninvasively [34]. It can be performed using cervical or urine specimens. Nonamplified nonculture tests, such as the DNA probe test, remain an option when the NAAT is not available or is too expensive. Repeat testing three weeks after completion of therapy is recommended for pregnant women [13]. Tetracyclines are contraindicated in pregnancy because of the risk of bone and tooth abnormalities; azithromycin (Zithromax) in a single 1-g dose azithromycin is U.S. Food and Drug Administration pregnancy category B drug, and is recommended as first-line treatment for chlamydia in pregnancy [13].

Gonorrhea

Gonococcal infection is associated with spontaneous abortion, premature labor, preterm premature rupture of membranes, and increased neonatal morbidity and mortality [35]. Further, gonococcal ophthalmia neonatorum occurs in 30–50% of infants born to infected mothers, and if untreated, may lead to corneal ulceration or perforation, and blindness [32]. The clinical pattern of gonorrhoea in pregnant women is similar to non-pregnant women, with up to 45% of cases being asymptomatic [36]. *Neisseria gonorrhea* can be transmitted to the newborn from the mother's genital tract at the time of birth and can cause ophthalmia neonatorum, systemic neonatal infection, maternal endometritis, or pelvic infection [37]. The risk of vertical transmission is between 30% and 47% [38].

Screening can be performed using a culture on Thayer-Martin media; nucleic acid hybridization tests of cervical specimens and NAAT's of cervical specimens or urine, with NAAT's being the most sensitive and specific [34, 39]. A repeat test is recommended in the third trimester for those at continued risk [13]. A Cochrane review of treatment for gonorrhea in pregnancy concluded that ceftriaxone 125 mg intramuscularly and spectinomycin 2 g intramuscularly have similar cure rates to oral amoxycillin plus probenecid [38]. One randomized trial found cefixime (Suprax) 400 mg orally to be as effective as ceftriaxone 125 mg intramuscularly for the treatment of gonorrhea in pregnancy [40]. The CDC recommends either of these as the treatment of choice for gonorrhea [13].

Hepatitis

Hepatitis A

Hepatitis A (HAV) is caused by a picorna (RNA) virus. It is particularly common in areas of the world where sanitation is poor, and causes disease in all age groups. In the developed world it is less common. Hepatitis A is mostly transmitted by the oral-fecal route, linked to oro-anal or digital-rectal contact. Outbreaks have also been reported amongst intravenous drug users, and following the use of contaminated blood products [41]. Patients are infectious for approximately two weeks before, and one week after the onset of jaundice. Incubation period ranges from 15 to 45 days. Up to half of adults are asymptomatic or have mild non-specific symptoms with little or no jaundice. In the more 'typical' case there are two phases of symptoms

- *The prodromal illness*: flu-like symptoms (malaise, myalgia, fatigue), often with right upper abdominal pain, lasting for 3-10 days. This is followed by -
- *The icteric illness:* jaundice (mixed hepatic and cholestatic) associated with anorexia, nausea and fatigue which usually lasts for 1-3 weeks. It can persist for 12 or more weeks in a minority of patients who have cholestatic symptoms (pruritis and deep jaundice). Fever is not found in this phase.

Signs are non-specific in the prodromal phase, however, in the icteric phase there is jaundice with pale stools and dark urine. Hepatomegaly with tenderness, and signs of dehydration are also common. Complications of HAV are fulminant hepatitis, with an overall case–fatality ratio among reported cases of less than 1% [42]. If a pregnant woman becomes infected with HAV, generally her baby is not affected. Intra-uterine transmission of hepatitis A virus is rare, but perinatal transmission could occur [43, 44]. HAV infection during pregnancy has been associated with preterm labor, and though rare, has been implicated in congenital infections [45, 46].

The diagnosis of hepatitis A cannot be made on clinical grounds alone and requires serologic testing. The presence of IgM antibody to HAV is diagnostic of acute HAV infection. A positive test for total anti-HAV indicates immunity to HAV infection but does not differentiate current from previous HAV infection. Although usually not sensitive enough to detect the low level of protective antibody after vaccination, anti-HAV tests might be positive after hepatitis A vaccination.

Other tests that aid in the diagnosis include:

- Serum/plasma amino-transferases (AST/ALT) 500-10,000iu/l.
- Bilirubin up to 500μmoles/l.
- Alkaline phosphatase levels < 2x the upper limit of normal, but higher if there is cholestasis.
- Prothrombin time (PT) prolongation by more than 5 seconds suggests developing hepatic decompensation.

Patients with acute hepatitis should be hospitalized if they have encephalopathy, coagulopathy, or severe debilitation. Nutritional needs should be addressed, as should fluid and electrolyte abnormalities. If a coagulopathy is present, administration of erythrocytes, platelets, and clotting factors such as fresh frozen plasma or cryoprecipitate may be necessary. Activity should be limited, and the patient should be protected from upper abdominal trauma [13]. According to the American Academy of Pediatrics Work Group on Breastfeeding, hepatitis A infection, even during the acute infectious period, is not a contraindication to breastfeeding [47].

Hepatitis B

Hepatitis B (HBV) is a partially double-stranded deoxyribonucleic acid (DNA) virus. Viral particles appear in large quantities in the serum in two forms: the complete virion, and the empty viral envelope, which contains only the hepatitis B surface antigen (HBsAg). The hepatitis 'e' antigen (HBeAg) is a peptide and normally detectable in the bloodstream when the hepatitis B virus is actively reproducing, and is a serum marker that is used to identify highly infectious mothers. HBV infection may run an acute course with complete recovery, or a fulminant course due to hepatic failure with a high mortality rate. Alternatively it may last for more than 6 months and become a chronic infection. HBV infection may lead to acute, fulminant or chronic hepatitis, liver cirrhosis and liver carcinoma [48]. In Asia, Africa, Southern Europe and Latin America the prevalence of HBsAg carriers in the general population ranges from 2–20%; whereas in North America, Northern Europe and the Oceanic areas the prevalence rate is around 0.1% in the general population [49].

HBV can be transmitted either perinatally or horizontally to the child. Acute hepatitis B or exacerbation of chronic HBV disease may occur during pregnancy. The frequency of vertical transmission also depends on the time during gestation that maternal infection occurs. When it occurs in the first trimester, up to 10% of neonates will be seropositive for HBsAg. In women acutely infected in the third trimester, 80–90% of offspring will be infected [50]. Pregnancy does not increase maternal mortality or morbidity from HBV. However, pre-term labor has been reported to be increased in mothers with acute hepatitis B during pregnancy. Although infection is rarely symptomatic, 70–90% of infected babies will remain chronically infected into adult life if immunoprophylaxis is not given [49]. Transplacental leakage of HBeAg-positive maternal blood, which is induced by uterine contractions during pregnancy and the disruption of placental barriers, is the most likely route for intrauterine tramsmission. The age at which HBV infection occurs is an important factor affecting the outcome; the earlier the infection occurs, the higher is the risk for chronicity [51]. The CDC recommends routine screening of all pregnant women for HBsAg to detect maternal disease and avoid perinatal transmission.

The presence of immunoglobulin M antibody to hepatitis B core antigen is diagnostic of acute or recently acquired infection. HBsAg is the first detectable virologic marker for HBV infection. Pregnant women seeking STI treatment who have not previously been vaccinated should be vaccinated against hepatitis B. Infants of HBsAg-positive mothers should receive hepatitis B immune globulin as well as hepatitis B vaccine at birth.

In addition to active immunisation with HBV vaccines, passive immunisation with hepatitis B immunoglobulin (HBIG) can neutralise HBV transmitted from the mother during perinatal period. Prophylaxis must be given within 24 h of birth.

In the USA, pregnant women are screened for HBsAg but not HBeAg. Every infant is recommended to receive 3 doses of HBV vaccines. In addition, all infants of HBsAg positive mothers, regardless of their HBeAg status, should receive HBIG within 24 h of birth [52].

Hepatitis C

Studies show that 90% of all adult patients with chronic non-A, non-B hepatitis are Hepatitis C (HCV) infected [53]. The risk of developing chronic HCV infection once the patient is infected is 60–80% [53]. The long-term risks are development of liver damage, cirrhosis and hepatocellular carcinoma. The detection of HCV-RNA, i.e. the viral genome, by polymerase chain reaction (PCR) in the serum, indicates an ongoing infection. The prevalence of chronic HCV infection in the adult general population varies from 0.5–2% in Western Europe, North America and Asia, to 5–15% in certain areas of Africa [54, 55]. The prevalence among pregnant women does not seem to differ from that of the general adult population [56]. Chronic HCV infection also has been associated with an increased risk of developing both B-cell lymphomas and cryoglobulinemia. Although at least 20% of chronic HCV infections lead to chronic active hepatitis or cirrhosis, whether a link to hepatocellular carcinoma exists is controversial and may vary by geographic region [57]. Hepatitis C and HIV share common transmission routes, and concomitant infection is reported to accelerate the progression and severity of hepatic injury [58].

Data indicates that approximately 5% of all infants born to HCV infected mothers become infected [59, 60]. In most studies, the HCV infection in infants born to infected mothers is defined by the detection of HCV-RNA by PCR in serum in at least two samples and/or the detection of anti-HCV in serum when the infant is at least 15 months old. Maternal antibodies are passively transferred to the fetus during pregnancy. The exact mechanism(s) for mother-to-child transmission (MTCT) of HCV is unknown and there are currently no relevant animal models available to establish this [61].

Routine screening for HCV in pregnancy is not recommended [13]. Women with known risk factors (e.g., history of injection drug use, blood transfusion or organ transplant before 1992) should be offered counseling and testing for hepatitis C antibodies. Approximately 5 % of infants whose mothers are infected with HCV become infected [13]. As in adults, pediatric HCV infection becomes chronic in a majority of cases. Chronic HCV infection, including infection very early in life, is most often asymptomatic in children [61]. The data concerning viral content in breast milk are contradictory [13, 61]. There is currently no vaccine or protective immunoglobulin available against hepatitis C.

Herpes Simplex Virus

Herpes simplex virus (HSV) infection, a sexually transmissible disease, is prevalent worldwide, particularly among women of childbearing age. In the United States, more than 600,000 new cases of herpes occur every year [62]. HSV is a double-stranded DNA enveloped virus, which is a member of the Herpesviridae family. HSV-1 and HSV-2 belong to the Alphaherpesvirinae subfamily and the genus *Simplexvirus*. Primary HSV-1 is largely a childhood disease affecting the mucosal surfaces of the mouth, pharynx, lips, and eyes. HSV-2 is primarily responsible for genital tract disease spread through sexual contact. Seroepidemiology studies suggest that a large number of individuals infected with HSV-2 also have HSV-1 [63]. Herpes simplex virus is an extremely common STI that has potentially devastating effects on perinatally infected neonates. The risk of transmission is 30% to 50% higher among women who acquire genital HSV near the time of delivery [64].

The primary-episode of genital HSV manifests as multiple painful vesicles in clusters on an inflamed surface. These vesicles rapidly become painful ulcers. They may be associated with pruritus, dysuria, vaginal discharge, and tender regional lymphadenopathy. Many women experience fever, malaise, and myalgia 1 to 2 days before the appearance of lesions. The lesions may last 4 to 5 days before crusting, but the skin may not re-epithelialize for almost 10 days. Viral shedding begins approximately 2 days after the onset of the lesions and ceases when re-epithelialization occurs. Symptomatic recurrent HSV episodes are characterized by a prodrome (eg, local pain or paresthesia) followed by vesicular lesions. They are generally fewer in number, may be painful, and often unilateral.

The presentation of primary HSV in pregnancy is similar to that in the nonpregnant state. As in the nonpregnant state, 92% of lesions in patients with recurrent disease in pregnancy are caused by HSV-2, which has potential neonatal implications [65]. There are several important features of maternal- fetal transmission of HSV. The most common mode of transmission is direct contact of the fetus with infected vaginal secretions during delivery. Studies have shown that the rate of maternal- fetal transmission is 10 times higher among infants of women with recently acquired first-episode infection than those with recurrent disease [66, 67]. First-episode HSV in early gestation may be associated with spontaneous abortion [68]. Several studies have found an increased risk of preterm birth and low birthweight in pregnancies complicated by HSV infection, particularly late acquisition of the disease [69, 70]. However, recurrent HSV has not been associated with spontaneous abortion or embryopathy [71]. HSV neonatal infection may be acquired through the birth canal during the intrapartum period and accounts for 90% of cases. Only 5% of neonatal cases are acquired through close contact during the postpartum period. Congenital or intrauterine HSV infection acquired transplacentally accounts for approximately 5% of cases of neonatal HSV disease. Congenital HSV is defined as the presence of skin vesicles or scarring, chorioretinitis, hydranencephaly, microphthalmia, microcephaly, or an abnormal computed tomography (CT) scan of the brain within the first week of life [72]. Many of these children will have symptoms within the first 24 to 48 hours of life. Most babies who become infected acquire the disease from mothers who are asymptomatic. Of infected neonates, as many as 60% to 70% are caused by HSV-2. The outcome of neonatal HSV is highly variable, and includes prematurity, pneumonitis, disseminated intravascular coagulation, and coma.

Morbidity in survivors was highest among those with encephalitis. Likewise, seizures, and disseminated disease leads to significant long-term morbidity such as psychomotor retardation, spasticity, blindness, and learning disabilities [65].

The gold standard for diagnosis of acute HSV is viral culture, which may become positive within 2 to 3 days after inoculation. This process may be shortened to 18 to 24 hours when viral culture and antigen detection methods are combined [73]. Screening is performed clinically by visualization of lesions or by patient history. Diagnosis is by culture or polymerase chain reaction assay of an active lesion. Although the highest yield is from vesicular fluid of skin lesions, cultures may be obtained from the eyes, mouth, cerebrospinal fluid (CSF), rectum, urine, and blood. Routine serologic testing is not recommended [13]. Administration of acyclovir, vidarabine or valacyclovir in addition to supportive care starting at 36 weeks of gestation has been shown to significantly reduce the recurrence of herpes simplex lesions and viral shedding at the time of delivery in patients at risk of active lesions, and to reduce the number of cesarean deliveries performed because of genital herpes [74, 75, 76]. Acyclovir therapy is the CDC's recommended treatment for active HSV infection during pregnancy, as well as in pregnant women who have recurrent genital herpes near term [13]. Cesarean delivery should be offered to women who have active lesions at the time of labor [77, 78]. Prophylactic cesarean delivery is not recommended for women with a history of recurrent HSV but no evidence of active lesions at the time of labor [79]. If cultures performed at birth in the neonate become positive following discharge, or there are abnormal CSF findings, intravenous acyclovir therapy should be instituted [65].

Human Immunodeficiency Virus

The global impact of the human immuno-deficiency virus (HIV) on children has been enormous, with an estimated 1800 children becoming infected with HIV every day, mostly acquiring infection vertically from their mothers [80]. Mother-to-child transmission is almost entirely preventable with a combination of prophylactic interventions. In resource-rich settings the number of new pediatric infections has reached an all-time low due to broad application of these interventions [80]. Mother-to-child transmission can take place in utero, during labour, at delivery, and postnatally through breastfeeding. Before the widespread use of prophylactic MTCT (PMTCT) interventions, transmission rates ranged from 15–20% in Europe to 16–30% in the USA, 25–40% in Africa and 13–48% in South and South East Asia [81].

In utero acquisition of infection may occur through HIV infection in the placenta or fetal exposure to cell-free and/or cell-associated HIV in amniotic fluid. Intrapartum transmission is understood to occur as a result of micro-transfusions between the maternal and fetal blood circulation during uterine contractions, or ascending HIV infection from the genital tract to the amniotic fluid and the fetus after rupture of membranes. In non-breastfeeding populations, in the absence of other interventions, most transmissions take place in late pregnancy or around the time of delivery. Prolonged breastfeeding (beyond 12 months of age) is associated with an approximate doubling of overall MTCT risk, with the risk remaining for as long as breastfeeding continues [82]. Maternal plasma HIV RNA level is the best individual predictor of MTCT risk; other risk factors reported include mode of delivery, duration of rupture of membranes, prematurity, cervico-vaginal viral load, low CD4 cell count, maternal symptomatic HIV disease/AIDS, viral sub-type and host genetic factors [81].

Antiretroviral drugs are prescribed to HIV-infected women in pregnancy for PMTCT and, in those requiring treatment for their own health to delay HIV disease progression. Antiretroviral prophylaxis reduces MTCT risk by reducing maternal viral load, and for drugs that cross the placenta (including zidovudine (ZDV), nevirapine (NVP) and lamivudine (3TC)) through per- and post-exposure prophylaxis of the neonate [81]. The ACTG 076 trial was the first clinical trial to investigate the efficacy of an antiretroviral (ZDV) in PMTCT [83]; the three component regimen was associated with a two-thirds reduction in MTCT risk and there was a subsequent rapid uptake in the developed world.

The U.S. Public Health Service and the U.S. Preventive Services Task Force recommend that all pregnant women in the United States be tested for HIV infection, ideally at the first prenatal visit [84, 85]. Women who are at high risk should be retested in the third trimester. Testing is done with an enzyme immunoassay for antibodies against HIV. Positive test results are confirmed with a Western blot or an immunofluorescence assay. Goals of therapy are to control maternal infection and reduce transmission to the fetus. Highly active antiretroviral therapy (HAART) is used during pregnancy to suppress viral load [84, 85, 86]. Elective cesarean delivery at 38 weeks reduces the risk of transmission in women not taking antiretrovirals or taking only zidovudine [87]. Further, studies reported that elective caesarean section (CS) before labor and before rupture of membranes appeared to be protective against MTCT and that long durations of ruptured membranes were associated with increased transmission risk in other deliveries [88, 89, 90]. Elective CS is associated with a higher rate of post-partum complications among HIV-infected women than is vaginal delivery [91]. However, infected women are generally at increased risk of post-partum complications compared to uninfected women, regardless of mode of delivery [92].

Around a fifth of vertically-infected children develop serious HIV disease or die in the first year of life, with the remaining children having a much slower disease progression [80]. Although the vast majority of infants born to HIV-infected mothers in developed country settings are now protected from vertical transmission, they are exposed to antiretroviral drugs for which there is only limited information on toxicity, particularly in the medium- to long-term.

Human Papillomavirus

Genital Warts

Human papillomavirus (HPV) is one of the most common causes of sexually transmitted infection (STI) in the world. Health experts estimate there are more cases of genital HPV infection than any other STI in the United States. According to the Centers for Disease Control and Prevention (CDC), approximately 6.2 million new cases of sexually transmitted HPV infections are reported every year, with about 20 million people in the USA already infected [13]. Genital warts (condylomata acuminata or venereal warts) are the most easily recognized sign of genital HPV infection. Many people, however, have a genital HPV infection without genital warts. HPV is spread by direct skin to skin contact during sexual activity with a person who has the virus. HPV types 6 and 11, causes around 90% of genital warts. Genital warts are soft, moist, or flesh-colored and appear in the genital area within weeks or months after infection. They sometimes appear in clusters that resemble cauliflower-like bumps, and are either raised or flat, small or large. Genital warts can show up in women on the vulva and cervix, and inside and surrounding the vagina and anus.

Diagnosis of genital warts is made by visual inspection. Biopsy may be needed if the diagnosis is uncertain, if the warts do not respond to standard treatment, or if there is suspicion of malignancy. Because genital warts can proliferate and become friable during pregnancy, it is recommended that they be removed [13]. Podofilox, imiquimod, and podophyllin are not recommended during pregnancy. Trichloroacetic acid 80-90% applied by a health care professional weekly has been used safely in pregnancy [64], as has cryotherapy and electrofulguration.

Syphilis

Syphilis is a sexually transmitted disease caused by a gram-negative spirochaete bacterium called Treponema *pallidum*. This motile spirochaete is generally acquired by close sexual contact, entering the host via breaches in squamous or columnar epithelium. The organism can also be transmitted to a fetus transplacentally during the later stages of pregnancy, giving rise to congenital syphilis. It has often been called "the great imitator" because many of the signs and symptoms are indistinguishable from those of other diseases. Treponema *pallidum* is highly infectious, even in the absence of any specific symptoms or clinical findings [93]. The World Health Organisation (WHO) estimates that 12 million people are infected with syphilis each year and more than 90% of infections occur in developing countries [94]. In high-income countries, until recently, very few babies were born with congenital syphilis but there has been resurgence over the past decade [95, 96].

Centers for Disease Control guidelines recommend that all women be screened serologically for syphilis during early pregnancy, and for populations where syphilis prevalence is high or patients are high risk, serological testing should also be performed twice during the third trimester, at 28–32 weeks' gestation, and at delivery [97]. All women delivering a stillborn after 20 weeks' gestation should be tested for syphilis [98]. About a million pregnancies globally are annually adversely affected by syphilis (about 270,000 babies are born with congenital syphilis, 460,000 pregnancies end in abortion or perinatal death and 270,000 babies are born prematurely or with low birthweight [99, 100]

The painless genital chancres of primary syphilis often go unnoticed. This is followed several weeks or months later by widespread cutaneous, mucosal and sometimes systemic manifestations of disseminated secondary syphilis. This contagious stage of syphilis can last for up to a year. Even without treatment both primary and secondary lesions resolve and the infection enters a 'latent' stage. During this latent phase there are no clinical manifestations but, as during the primary and secondary stages, the infection can still be passed to babies born to infected mothers. Left untreated, syphilis has a dramatic impact on pregnancy outcome. Spirochetes can cross the placenta and infect the fetus from about 14 weeks' gestation, with the risk of fetal infection increasing with gestational age [101]. The most common cause of fetal death is placental infection and vasculitis associated with decreasing blood flow to the fetus, although direct fetal infection also plays a role [102, 103]. Congenital syphilis is a multiorgan infection that may cause neurological or skeletal disabilities or death in the fetus or newborn. Historically, one third of pregnancies are believed to result in second trimester spontaneous abortion or perinatal death, one third in a congenitally infected infant, and one third in an uninfected infant [104]. Maternal syphilis has been associated with complications such as low birth weight, hydramnios, spontaneous abortion, and preterm delivery. Fetal complications such as infection in utero, hydrops, prematurity, fetal distress, and stillbirth also occur. Neonatal complications can include congenital syphilis, neonatal death, and late sequelae [105, 32].

The earliest sign that a baby is infected with syphilis is often a nasal discharge (snuffles) that occurs 1–2 weeks before the onset of a maculopapular rash. Other early stigmata include hepatosplenomegaly and jaundice. Screening is performed with a non-specific blood test - the rapid plasma reagin (RPR) or Venereal Disease Research Laboratories (VDRL) test and confirmed with specific tests such as the fluorescent treponemal antibody (FTA) serology and *T. pallidum* particle agglutination test (TPHA). A single serologic test is insufficient because false-positives may occur with other illnesses [64].

If syphilis is diagnosed after 20 weeks of gestation, ultrasonography should be performed to evaluate for evidence of fetal syphilis. Although fetal infection can be cured by treating the mother, treatment failure is much higher in the presence of fetal hepatomegaly, ascites, hydrops, polyhydramnios, and placental thickening, which are signs of fetal syphilis detected on ultrasonography [64]. The CDC recommends benzathine penicillin G, 2.4 million units intramuscularly, with desensitization in patients who are allergic to penicillin [13]. WHO, CDC and the UK recommend that infants with confirmed or highly probable congenital syphilis be treated with systemic benzylpenicillin 100,000 to 150,000 IU/kg/day for 10 days. WHO and CDC recommend asymptomatic babies born to seropositive mothers be treated with a single dose of benzathine benzylpenicillin 50,000 IU/kg [97, 106].

Vaginal Infections

Trichomonas *vaginalis*, an anaerobic, parasitic flagellated protozoan, is the causative agent of trichomoniasis. This sexually transmitted infection can occur in females if the normal acidity of the vagina shifts from a semi-acidic pH (3.8 - 4.2) to a more basic one (pH 5 - 6) that is conducive to its growth. It has been associated with preterm delivery and low birth weight [107]. *Trichomonas* infection may present with symptoms such as vaginal irritation, itching, copious discharge, and malodor. It also causes a chronic inflammation and may facilitate HIV transmission [108]. Women with symptoms of trichomoniasis should be evaluated with a saline wet mount or culture for the presence of trichomonads. Screening for *Trichomonas* in asymptomatic women is not recommended [13]. Metronidazole 2 g orally in a single dose or 500 mg twice per day for seven days is the treatment of choice in pregnancy, although many physicians wait until after the first trimester to initiate it [13]. Treatment of trichomoniasis has not been shown to reduce the incidence of preterm birth [107].

Bacterial vaginosis is sometimes called nonspecific vaginosis or Gardnerella vaginitis. It is caused by an imbalance of the normal vaginal flora, with an overgrowth of anaerobic bacteria and a lack of the normal lactobacillary flora. Though not an STI, it is prevalent in sexually active women. Bacterial vaginosis during pregnancy has been associated with poor perinatal outcome and, in particular, preterm birth. Other studies have shown an association between bacterial vaginosis and premature rupture of membranes, low birth weight early or late miscarriage, preterm pre-labour rupture of membranes, amniotic fluid colonization, chorioamnionitis, postpartum endometritis, increased efficiency of HIV seroconversion, and cerebral palsy [109, 110, 111, 112, 113, 114, 115, 116, 117, 118].

The precise pathophysiological mechanisms involved have yet to be fully elucidated. One hypothesis is that of the potential effect of bacterial vaginosis colonization results in endometrial inflammation. Such endometrial inflammation may disturb the immuno-endocrinological milieu during implantation and early embryological development, which may lead to miscarriage or preterm birth. Alternatively, lower genital tract organisms may ascend into the uterine cavity and reach the decidua causing endometrial inflammation. This event is associated with the activation of the cellular and molecular events involved in the pathway of preterm labor, including leukocyte recruitment, cytokine production, prostaglandin synthesis in the amnion, chorion and myometrium; this results in uterine contractions, cervical dilatation, membrane exposure, and further entry of microbes into the uterine cavity [119]. Bacteria may elaborate lytic enzymes such as sialidases and mucinases, which may weaken the protective cervical mucous and promote bacterial invasion of the upper genital tract [113]. Cytokines also stimulate chorionic and amnionic production of matrix metalloproteinases (MMP's) implicated in membrane degradation and cervical ripening. However, it is not known whether the bacterial overgrowth causes these complications, or if it is a marker for intrauterine colonization. Screening for and treating bacterial vaginosis in asymptomatic pregnant women does not appear to reduce the risk of pregnancy complications [64]. The majority of pregnant women with abnormal vaginal flora have a good pregnancy outcome, and in some populations the presence of bacterial vaginosis is not even associated with adverse outcome [120].

In a review to determine whether antibiotic treatment for bacterial vaginosis or *T. vaginalis* during pregnancy decreases the risk of preterm birth and associated adverse outcomes, the authors found no evidence to support the use of antibiotic treatment for bacterial vaginosis or *T. vaginalis* in pregnancy to reduce the risk of preterm birth or its associated morbidities in low- or high-risk women [121]. At present there is no consensus on the antibiotic of choice for the treatment of abnormal vaginal flora in pregnancy, or for its best route of administration, the optimal time for initiating therapy, or whether further treatment of persistent or recurrent cases improves outcome. Clindamycin exhibits a broad range of antimicrobial activity that makes it an attractive option for the treatment of abnormal vaginal flora in pregnancy. Oral or topical metronidazole is also effective in the treatment of bacterial vaginosis. Erythromycin and ampicillin are ineffective against anaerobes and are not recommended for bacterial vaginosis, in contrast to clindamycin and metronidazole [120].

Perinatal Viral and Parasitic Infections

Cytomegalovirus

Cytomegalovirus (CMV) belongs to the *Betaherpesvirinae* subfamily of *Herpesviridae*, a double-stranded DNA virus that is transmitted by sexual contact or by contact with infected blood, saliva, or urine. The incubation period of CMV is 28-60 days, with a mean of 40 days. Infection induces an immunoglobulin M (IgM) antibody response that disappears within 30-60 days. Viremia can be detected 2-3 weeks following primary infection. Primary CMV infection in adults generally is asymptomatic. Almost all CMV infections acquired in individuals with a normal immune response are clinically silent. Only 5% may experience a mononucleosis-like syndrome, and the pregnant woman is generally unaware of being infected with CMV [122].Occasionally, patients may be found to have a leukocytosis, lymphocytosis, abnormal liver function tests, fever, malaise, myalgia, and chills [123]. After the initial infection, CMV remains latent in host cells; recurrent infection can occur following reactivation of latent virus. In rare cases, recurrent CMV infection can occur by infection with a new strain of virus.

Prevalence of both primary and recurrent infection in pregnant women varies from 0.7% to 4% for primary infection and up to 13.5% for recurrent infection [124]. Vertical transmission of CMV may occur as a result of transplacental infection after primary or recurrent CMV infection, exposure to contaminated genital tract secretions at parturition, or from breastfeeding. During early pregnancy, CMV has a teratogenic potential in the fetus, as CMV infections may result in migrational disturbances in the brain. Later in pregnancy, when the gross morphology of the brain is completed and myelination is occurring, white matter lesions without cerebral cortical malformations can be seen. Visual impairment and strabismus are common in children with clinically apparent CMV infection and can be caused by chorioretinitis, pigmentary retinitis, macular scarring, optic atrophy and central cortical defects. Congenital CMV infection in a child may cause other disabilities, alone or in combination, such as mental retardation, autism, learning disabilities, cerebral palsy, and epilepsy [125]. About 10–15% of neonates with congenital CMV present symptoms recognisable as an infection. The classic clinical picture of cytomegalic inclusion disease (CID) is characterised by involvement of multiple organs, in particular the reticuloendothelial and central nervous system, with or without ocular and auditory damage. Other signs of CID could be jaundice, hepatosplenomegaly and petechiae in a growth impaired, often prematurely born baby [125]. The neurological involvement includes microcephaly, seizures, hypotonia and lethargy. The most severely affected infants have a mortality rate of about 30%. Death is usually due to hepatic dysfunction, bleeding, disseminated intravascular coagulation or secondary bacterial infections [126, 127]. Cytomegalovirus is the most common congenital infection, occurring in 0.2-2.2% of all neonates [128], and is the leading cause of congenital hearing loss. With primary maternal CMV infection, the risk of transmission to the fetus is 30-40% [129]. Of those infected in utero following a primary infection, 10% will have signs and symptoms of CMV infection at birth and develop sequelae [130]. Approximately 30% of severely infected infants die, and 80% of survivors have severe neurologic morbidity [131].

The incidence of severe fetal infection is much lower after recurrent maternal infection than after primary infection. Vertical transmission after a recurrent infection is 0.15-2% [132]. Infants infected after maternal CMV reactivation generally are asymptomatic at birth. Congenital hearing loss is typically the most severe sequela of secondary infection, and congenital infection following recurrent infection is unlikely to produce multiple sequelae [132]. Cytomegalovirus infection acquired as a result of exposure to infected cervical secretions or breast milk is typically asymptomatic and is not associated with severe neonatal effects. A vaccine is not available and therefore it is desirable to reduce the risk for CMV exposure in pregnant women. Prophylactic hygienic measures such as hand washing after contact with saliva or urine in children, are an important and simple way to diminish the risk for viral transmission [133, 134].

The policy for analysis of CMV-IgG in women during pregnancy is different in different western countries. Currently, there is no treatment for primary CMV infection during pregnancy and abortion may be an alternative. Administration of intravenous human immunoglobulin to the pregnant mother with a primary CMV infection has been claimed to protect the fetus [135].

Parvovirus B19

Parvovirus B19 infection, also known as fifth disease, is caused by a single-stranded DNA virus that results in childhood exanthem erythema infectiosum, described as a "slapped cheek" appearance. In immunocompetent adults, the most common symptoms of parvovirus B19 infection are a reticular rash on the trunk and peripheral arthropathy, although approximately 33% of infections are asymptomatic [136]. Adults may also present with an exanthem preceded by nonspecific symptoms to include fever, sore throat, and lymphadenopathy. In healthy adults and children the clinical course is self limited and requires no specific treatment. Although reticulocytopenia, lymphopenia, neutropenia, and thrombocytopenia can occur to some degree, it is usually clinically insignificant [137]. Another manifestation of parvovirus B19 infection is a transient aplastic crisis, which is more common in those with an underlying hemoglobinopathy. Most infections are mild; most individuals recover completely from parvovirus B19 infection and require only supportive care.

Parvovirus B19 has a unique affinity for erythroid progenitor cells due to a receptor commonly found on erythroid cells known as the P blood group antigen. Parvovirus B19 arrests erythropoiesis and has a cytopathic affect on erythroid precursors [138, 139]. Evidence suggests that the virus stimulates a cellular process initiating programmed cellular death (apoptosis), potentially accounting for the minimal inflammatory response noted in tissues infected with the virus [140].

Transmission of parvovirus B19 most commonly occurs through respiratory secretions and hand-to-mouth contact. The infected person generally is infectious 5-10 days after exposure prior to the onset of the rash or other symptoms and is no longer infectious with the onset of the rash [141]. Both IgM and IgG are produced in response to infection. The IgM response, which persists for 1 to several months, is indicative of a recent infection. IgG antibodies persist indefinitely and, in the absence of IgM, indicate prior infection and immunity. Prevalence of seropositivity to parvovirus B19 increases with age and is greater than 60% in adolescents and adults [141]. The risk of maternal infection of parvovirus B19 varies with level of exposure to the infected individual. Exposure to a household member infected with parvovirus B19 is associated with an approximate 50% risk of seroconversion [142, 143, 144]. As the fetus is capable of producing IgM by approximately 18 weeks gestation, either fetal blood or amniotic fluid can be tested for IgM. Polymerase chain reaction is a sensitive method for detecting small amounts of B19 DNA, so this is the preferred method for making the diagnosis in utero [145]. There is little data to support invasive testing such as amniocentesis if the mother has serologic evidence of recent infection [146, 147]. The risk of transmission in a child-care setting or classroom is lower, ranging from approximately 20% to 50% [148, 149].

Recent maternal infection with parvovirus B19 constitutes a low risk for fetal morbidity [150], although some cases have been associated with adverse fetal effects. Transplacental transmission has been reported to be as high as 33% [151], and fetal infection with parvovirus B19 has been associated with spontaneous abortion, and stillbirth. Several other pathological conditions also have been linked to this virus, including fetal anemia and nonimmune hydrops fetalis [152]. The rate of fetal loss among women with serologically proven parvovirus B19 infection ranges from 2% to 9%

[153, 154]. In utero, parvovirus B19 infection is responsible for up to 18% of cases of nonimmune hydrops fetalis in some series [155]. Hydrops fetalis results from aplastic anemia, myocarditis, or chronic fetal hepatitis. Severe effects are seen most frequently among fetuses when maternal parvovirus B19 infection occurs at less than 20 weeks of gestation. Stillbirth resulting from maternal infection has occurred from 1 to 11 weeks after maternal infection. However, hydrops is unlikely to develop if it has not occurred by 8 weeks after maternal infection [156]. It therefore appears that there may be an increase in fetal loss rate with maternal infection in the early second trimester, a time when the fetus has a rapidly expanding hematopoetic system and may be prone to viral-associated myocardial depression. When fetal death does occur after maternal infection, it usually takes place between 4 to 6 weeks after exposure, although it has been reported up to 12 weeks following exposure [147]. Reports confirm the association between maternal parvovirus B19 infection and fetal hydrops, and several possible mechanisms responsible for parvovirus B19-associated hydrops have been proposed [157, 158]. Because the fetus grows at a rapid rate, and the survival time for fetal red blood cells is decreased, it is dependent on adequate red blood cell production to ensure adequate oxygen transport to fetal cells. The resulting anemia due to fetal parvovirus B19 infection can result in hypoxia, high cardiac output failure and hydrops. Another proposed mechanism for fetal hydrops may be B19 myocarditis, because there have been reported cases of fetuses with parvovirus B19-associated hydrops who were found not to have severe anemia on fetal blood sampling and subsequently recovered without fetal transfusion [159,157]. Thus, it is possible that some of the infected fetuses may have acquired hydrops, which subsequently resolved without treatment. It would therefore seem reasonable to use a 1% risk of fetal hydrops for counseling purposes in women with acute infection in the second and third trimesters [152].

Long-term development appears to be normal in fetuses with congenital parvovirus B19 infection that do not succumb to the disease [160, 161]. However, there have been case reports of fetuses with hydrocephalus, craniofacial anomalies, encephaloclastic perinatal encephalopathy and eye anomalies born to women with serological evidence of parvovirus B19 infection during pregnancy [162, 163, 164, 165]. It has been postulated that parvovirus B19 may have a direct cytopathic effect on rapidly growing immature embryonic tissues [166]. Parvovirus B19 also is a known cause of vasculitis in infants, and it is possible that a fetal cerebral vessel vasculitis could have resulted in some of the above central nervous system disorders [162]. However, confirmative data establishing parvovirus B19 infection as a teratogenic agent are lacking, and there is no epidemiological information available that conclusively establishes parvovirus B19 intrauterine infection as a cause of birth defects [167, 168, 169].

Maternal parvovirus infection is usually a self-limiting illness that resolves without treatment. The arthropathy can last for several weeks and may require analgesics. Patients who are immunocompromised can have persistent infection that results in severe anemia [170]. Treatment with intravenous immunoglobulin (IVIg) has been reported to be successful in these patients [171]. Maternal infections in the first half of pregnancy should be expectantly managed with serial sonographic examinations to evaluate for fetal hydrops or intrauterine fetal demise. Ultrasound findings suggestive of fetal hydrops include hydramnios, placentomegaly, pericardial or pleural effusions, ascites, skin or scalp edema, and deranged middle cerebral artery doppler flows [147]. Since fetal anemia appears to be the major cause of the fetal pathophysiological process, intrauterine transfusion has been proposed and used in the treatment of nonimmune hydrops caused by parvovirus B19 infection in the latter half of pregnancy [172, 173]. As there are no other reliable markers of impending fetal death after the development of hydrops, it is reasonable that patients with parvovirus B19-associated hydrops fetalis be offered fetal blood sampling and intrauterine transfusion as indicated. Fetal hydrops usually resolves within 2 weeks after adequate intrauterine therapy. Repeat fetal blood sampling can be performed 3 to 4 weeks after transfusion to confirm adequate erythrocyte production. Weekly ultrasound scans should be performed for up to 12 weeks after exposure or diagnosis, to assess for the development of hydrops. Without evidence of fetal hydrops or compromise there is no need for invasive tests to evaluate for fetal infection [152]. If fetal hydrops develops after maternal infection, consideration should be given for delivery at term or near-term gestations. At gestational ages of 32 to 34 weeks, an amniocentesis test could be performed and delivery would be appropriate if pulmonary maturity is confirmed [152].

Varicella Zoster Virus

Varicella zoster virus (VZV) is a DNA herpes virus that is highly contagious and is transmitted by respiratory droplets or close contact. The incubation period after infection is 10-20 days, with a mean of 14 days [174]. The period of infectivity begins 48 hours before the appearance of the rash, and lasts until the vesicles crust over. The primary infection causes chickenpox, which is characterized by fever, malaise, and a maculopapular pruritic rash that becomes vesicular. Lesions may be at various stages in the same area of skin. The lesions initially appear on the face or trunk and spread centripetally to the extremities over 4 to 7 days. After the primary infection, VZV remains dormant in sensory ganglia and can be reactivated to cause a vesicular erythematous skin rash termed *herpes zoster*. The antibody to VZV develops within a few days after the onset of infection, and prior infection with VZV confers lifelong immunity.

Chickenpox (or primary VZV infection) is a common childhood disease that usually results in a mild infection, such that over 90% of the antenatal population are seropositive for VZV immunoglobulin G (IgG) antibody [175, 176]. For this reason, although contact with chickenpox is common in pregnancy, especially in women with young children, primary VZV infection is uncommon, i.e. it is estimated to complicate three in every 1 000 pregnancies [177]. Varicella-zoster virus is estimated in USA to affect up to 1% of pregnancies, or about 6,000 cases annually [178].Varicella infection is uncommon in pregnancy (occurring in 0.4-0.7 per 1 000 patients), because of the high prevalence of natural immunity [179]. Varicella national mortality data shows that although less than 5% of varicella cases occur among adults 20 years of age or older, that group contributes to 55% of varicella-related deaths [180].

All organ systems may be involved. Pneumonia is the primary serious complication and is more common in adolescents and adults. When varicella pneumonia does occur during pregnancy, however, the mortality rate may be as high as 40% in the absence of specific antiviral chemotherapy [181, 182, 183]. Varicella encephalitis is uncommon but can occur at any age. Other unusual complications of varicella include dysfunction of bowel and bladder sphincters, hepatitis, arthritis, orchitis, pericarditis, nephritis, and Reye's syndrome. The most common reason for hospitalization is a secondary bacterial infection causing a local cellulitis or focal pyogenic infection. Complications, such as encephalitis and pneumonia, are more common in adults than in children; VZV pneumonia in pregnancy is a risk factor for maternal mortality [184, 185].

Intrauterine infection can occur regardless of the severity of maternal varicella. In pregnancy, varicella may be transmitted transplacentally, resulting in congenital or neonatal chickenpox. The risk of congenital varicella syndrome is limited to exposure during the first 20 weeks of gestation, and occurs in up to 2% of cases. Specific anomalies associated with congenital varicella syndrome include cutaneous scars, limb hypoplasia, muscle atrophy, malformed digits, psychomotor retardation, microcephaly, cortical atrophy, and various eye abnormalities including cataracts, chorioretinitis and microophthalmia. [186, 187]. In addition, autopsy findings in these fetuses suggest other abnormalities such as intrauterine growth restriction, thoracic dysplasia, dextrocardia, limb atrophy, cerebellar dysplasia, and ocular anomalies might be detected by ultrasound scan [188].

Neonatal VZV infection is associated with a high neonatal death rate when maternal disease develops from 5 days before delivery up to 48 hours postpartum as a result of the relative immaturity of the neonatal immune system and the lack of protective maternal antibody [189]. The clinical course of varicella of the newborn can be quite variable in progression and severity. Clinical illness typically develops within 5 to 10 days of delivery. Some infants have only scattered skin lesions and no systemic signs of illness, whereas others have a biphasic course, initially presenting with a cluster of skin lesions, followed by later dissemination. Some have an acute illness accompanied by an extensive cutaneous eruption and visceral involvement. The most common life-threatening complication is pneumonia. Encephalitis and hepatitis also may occur. The mortality rate associated with varicella of the newborn may be 20% to 30% [190]. Occasionally, herpes zoster is present in the newborn. This condition is usually a benign manifestation of intrauterine varicella exposure; although in rare cases, it may be associated with encephalitis [191].

In situations of acute exposure, serologic testing must be completed within 24 to 48 hours because varicella-zoster immune globulin (VZIG) should be administered as soon as possible. If serologic testing cannot be performed quickly, VZIG should be administered empirically to exposed women who are not certain of their immune status [184]. Other supportive measures include adequate fluids and analgesics. Women should be observed for evidence of disseminated disease, including severe mucocutaneous infection, pneumonia, hepatitis, or encephalitis. If any of these events occur, the woman should be admitted to the hospital for treatment with intravenous acyclovir. In studies, acyclovir appeared to modify life-threatening maternal infection, reducing mortality rates to 14% compared with 41% in untreated historic controls [182]. However, acyclovir should be used with caution before 20 weeks of gestation, and women should be informed of the potential risk and benefits of treatment with acyclovir [185]. Oral acyclovir (800 mg five times a day for 7 days) reduces the duration of fever and symptomatology of varicella infection in immunocompetent adults if commenced within 24 hours of developing the rash when compared with placebo [192]. Data suggest that there is no increase in the risk of fetal malformation with acyclovir in pregnancy, although the theoretical risk of teratogenesis persists in the first trimester [193, 194].

Toxoplasmosis

Toxoplasma gondii occurs worldwide, but its incidence is higher in tropical areas and decreases with increasing latitude. Toxoplasmosis is caused by the intracellular parasite *T. gondii*, which exists in several forms: a trophozoite, which is the invasive form, and a cyst or an oocyst, which are latent forms. Human infection is acquired by consuming cysts in undercooked meat of infected animals, by insect contamination of food, by contact with oocysts from the feces of infected cats, which are the only definitive hosts, or by contact with infected soil. After an acute infection, IgM antibodies appear early and reach maximum levels in 1 month. IgG antibodies appear after IgM antibodies, are detectable within a few weeks after infection, and confer immunity. High titers of both IgG and IgM may persist for years. In the immunocompetent adult, the clinical course is benign and self-limited [195].

Infection with *T. gondii* usually is asymptomatic, although after an incubation of 5-18 days, some non-specific symptoms may occur, such as cervical lymphadenopathy, fever, malaise, night sweats, myalgias, and hepatosplenomegaly. Parasitemia can occur after infection, which, in pregnant women, can seed the placenta and cause subsequent fetal infection. Vertical transmission depends on the time of acquisition of maternal infection. The later in gestation that the infection occurs, the more likely transmission will occur. The rate of vertical transmission increases from 10% to 15% in the first trimester, to 25% in the second trimester, and to more than 60% in the third trimester [196, 197]. If a pregnant woman acquires primary infection in pregnancy, *T. gondii* may be transmitted to the fetus and cause inflammatory lesions that may lead to permanent neurological damage, with or without hydrocephalus. The pregnant woman and the infected newborn are often asymptomatic but the child is at risk of recurring chorioretinitis later in life [195]. The severity of infection depends on gestational age at the time of transmission. The earlier the fetus is infected, the more severe the disease. Most infected infants do not have clinical signs of infection at birth, but 55-85% will develop sequelae, including chorioretinitis, leading to severe impairment of vision, hearing loss, or mental retardation [198, 199]. Other clinical manifestations of congenital toxoplasmosis include rash, hepatosplenomegaly, ascites, fever, periventricular calcifications, ventriculomegaly, and seizures [200, 201].

It is a problem to diagnose whether women with specific IgM antibodies were infected before or after conception. This problem has been partly solved by obtaining repeat samples from pregnant women to see if there is any development of an immune response. It is generally agreed that there is development of *Toxoplasma*-specific IgG-antibody response within the first 8 weeks after infection, after which time the IgG levels are maintained at a high level [202, 203]. Samples are obtained during pregnancy and analysed for *Toxoplasma*-specific IgM- and IgG-antibodies. When seroconversion is detected, the mother is infected, and treatment is usually started. The biggest diagnostic challenge is the situation when *Toxoplasma*-specific IgG and IgM-antibodies are found in the first sample after conception, where the time of infection is the key to estimating whether the fetus is at risk or not [204]. Established congenital toxoplasmosis is treated with pyrimethamine, sulfadiazine and folic acid from second trimester until a year old [205].

Rubella (German Measles)

Rubella virus (RV) is a non-arthropod-borne member of the family *Togaviridiae* and the sole member of the genus, *Rubivirus.* The virus contains RNA, which is surrounded by a capsid and a lipoprotein envelope. The capsid is composed of the capsid protein (C), while the envelope contains two glycoproteins E1 and E2. These proteins induce the major immune responses. Rubella virus is only found in humans; there is no known animal reservoir. It is transmitted by aerosol via the respiratory tract. Rubella has recently been eliminated from the USA and Scandinavian countries, where there are effective vaccination programmes, and it is becoming a rare disease in many other industrialized countries [206]. In 2003, it was estimated that more than 100 000 infants with congenital rubella syndrome (CRS) were born worldwide [207].

Rubella is generally a mild disease in children, but may be more severe in adults. It has an incubation period of about 14 days (range 12–23 days), before the characteristic non-confluent maculopapular rash appears. Lymphadenopathy may be present before appearance of the rash, and persists for 10–14 days after the rash disappears. The suboccipital, postauricular and cervical lymph nodes are most frequently affected. Adults may experience a prodromal phase with malaise and low grade fever, headache, sore throat, cough and conjunctivitis. Depending on the population, 20–50% of infections are subclinical. A viremia occurs for about 7 days before the onset of rash, while virus excretion may be detected from 7 days before appearance of the rash until 7–12 days after onset of rash, thus the patient is potentially infectious for more than 2 weeks. Arthralgia and arthritis are the most common complications. Other serious complications are post-infectious encephalopathy (about 1 in 6000 cases) and bleeding disorders due to thrombocytopaenia (1 in 3000 cases) [206]. Infection prior to conception does not present a risk to the fetus [208], but when primary rubella infection occurs in the first 12 weeks of pregnancy rubella virus will cross the placenta and induce a generalized and persistent fetal infection in about 80% of cases [206], with multiple defects most likely to occur in those infected during the first 8 weeks. After 12 weeks the risk to the fetus declines rapidly, with only rare cases of deafness reported at 17–18 weeks' gestation. The risk of congenital defects may be less when maternal infection is subclinical. Spontaneous abortion may occur in up to 20% of cases when rubella occurs in the first 8 weeks of pregnancy [209]. Rubella reinfection is usually subclinical and most often detected by serology in pregnant women who are investigated following exposure to rubella or immunization [210]. Congenital infection occurs in about 8%, but the risk of defects is probably less than 5%, substantially less than the risk from primary rubella [211]. Maternal reinfection is usually suclinical and diagnosed by changes in antibody concentration (IgG and/or IgM) only. The risk to the fetus of subclinical maternal reinfection in the first 16 weeks gestation would suggest the risk of congenital damage is less than 10%, and probably less than 5% [212]. Thus, it is important to differentiate reinfection from primary rubella in pregnancy. No congenital defects have been reported when maternal reinfection has occurred after 12 weeks' gestation.

As a clinical diagnosis is unreliable, it is essential that pregnant women developing or exposed to a rubella-like illness in the first 16 weeks of pregnancy are investigated for rubella IgM and IgG in serum obtained as soon as possible, since a termination of pregnancy (TOP) should be offered when rubella is confirmed [212]. A positive rubella IgM and IgG result is strongly suggestive of rubella, but should be confirmed by testing a second serum taken 5–10 days later to detect rubella IgM and a rise in rubella IgG titers [206].

The outcome of rubella in pregnancy may be the birth of an infant with congenital abnormalities, birth of an apparently normal infant or spontaneous abortion. Early UK and Swedish studies suggested that 3–4% infants whose mothers had rubella in the first 12 weeks of pregnancy would die in the first 2 years of life [213]. In a US study, 35% of severely affected infants with thrombocytopenic purpura, low birth weight and heart disease died in the first 18 months of life [214].The abnormalities caused by congenital rubella infection are collectively known as congenital rubella syndrome (CRS). Congenital rubella infection (CRI) can provoke transient, permanent and late damage in organogenesis [215]. Permanent CRS includes sensorial hearing loss, heart abnormalities (ductus arteriosus), ocular defects (cataracts, micropthalmia, glaucoma), encephalopathy with mental retardation and motor impairment.

Delayed CRI includes organ pathology, endocrinopathies related to autoimmune phenomena triggered by persistent rubella infection (diabetes, thyroiditis, growth hormone deficiency), hearing loss, ocular damage, arteriosclerosis, hypertension and progressive rubella panencephalitis [216, 217, 218].

In spite of normal appearance of 50–70% infants with CRI at birth, one of the above listed abnormalities develops later in life. The overall mortality of infants in CRS is 5–35%; spontaneous abortions occur in 4–9% and stillbirths in 2–3% of pregnancies complicated by maternal rubella [6, 219]. In the first trimester the risk of damage in seropositive infants reaches 85%, in the second (13–16 weeks) it is lowered to 35%. The risk of maternal infection to the fetus are 90% before the 11th week of pregnancy, 33% for weeks 11–12, 11% for weeks 13–14 and 2–4% for weeks 15–16 [6, 220]. Early infected fetuses are of greater risk to *in utero* death or to congenital malformations and damages of organs and systems [221]. Fetal infection *in utero* is a consequence of maternal viremia which seeds the placenta, causes fetal viremia and damages fetal organs. Placentas may contain the virus even when the fetus does not [222].

It has been suggested that RV crosses to the fetus via the chorion during maternal viremia and virus-infected desquamated epithelial and endothelial cells are transported to the fetal circulation and fetal organs [223]. No inflammatory response is detected, which is characteristic of rubella embryopathy following maternal rubella in early pregnancy, as fetal immune responses have not developed. Suggested mechanisms for fetal damage include a RV-induced retardation in cell division, RV-induced apoptosis of essential cells, viral interference with the cell cycle, and tissue necrosis [224 225]. When maternal infection occurs after the first trimester, virus may cross the placenta, but a persistent infection is not established, because fetal immune responses have developed and these terminate infection [206]. If infection occurs in the first trimester of pregnancy, the risk of fetal infection and damage is high (about 90% in the first two months of pregnancy, and 50% in the third), and termination of pregnancy is usually recommended. Risk of fetal damage falls steeply after the first trimester and is negligible after 16 weeks; between 12 and 16 weeks, deafness has been reported [10]. If a pregnant woman has close contact with or develops rubella-like illness, her IgG and IgM titres should be measured, even if she was previously positive for rubella IgG; rarely, women with apparently adequate immunity can be reinfected, although the risk of fetal abnormality is probably less than 5% even in the first trimester [210]. If contact is in the second or third trimester and rubella IgG was detected in the first trimester, further investigation is not necessary. Women who remain susceptible to rubella should receive measles-mumps-rubella (MMR) vaccine postpartum [10].

Urinary Tract Infection

It is estimated that about 35% of healthy women suffer symptoms of urinary tract infection (UTI) at some time in their life [226]. UTI is the presence of bacteria in the urine (bacteriuria). For epidemiological purposes, 'significant' bacteriuria is defined as at least 10^5 bacteria/ml in a specimen of freshly-voided urine. Symptomatic infection is associated with inflammation and a urine WBC count higher than 8 cells/ml (pyuria, leukocyturia). The principal bacterial infections of the kidney and urinary tract occur in either the renal parenchyma (pyelonephritis), the bladder (cystitis) or the urethra (urethritis). The majority of UTI's are caused by gastrointestinal organisms. Bacteria most commonly enter via the urethra (ascending infection), but can enter via the bloodstream. Ascending infections account for most cases of uncomplicated cystitis and pyelonephritis, and usually involve organisms of the normal bowel flora – principally *Escherichia coli* (≥75% of cases). *Staphylococcus saprophyticus* is sometimes found in young women (5–10%), and *Proteus mirabilis* and *Klebsiella pneumoniae* are rare causes. The greater susceptibility of women to UTI is partly because of the short urethra and its proximity to the bowel [227]. The factors that predispose a woman to UTI in pregnancy appear to be related to the anatomical and physiological changes in the kidney and urinary tract that occur during pregnancy. The ureters become dilated above the pelvic brim and the bladder is displaced anteriorly and superiorly by the enlarging uterus. Renal blood flow and the glomerular filtration rate increase by about 30-40% during pregnancy and the kidneys become slightly enlarged and hyperaemic. Urine flow may be sluggish and the bladder may not empty completely [228].

Acute cystitis is associated with frequency, urgency and dysuria. The urine is discolored, appears hazy and may be offensive smelling. Microscopic hematuria is often present. Cystitis is not a systemic infection; therefore, patients are not febrile. Acute urethritis is associated with dysuria and urethral discharge. Infection is usually sexually transmitted and is caused by *Neisseria gonorrhoeae* (20%) or non-gonococcal organisms (80%) including *Chlamydia trachomatis*, *Mycoplasma genitalium* and *Ureaplasma urealyticum*. The latter infections (nonspecific urethritis) are often asymptomatic, and the organisms become permanent commensals [227]. Asymptomatic bacteriuria is often not associated with symptoms. Acute pyelonephritis is associated with fever, malaise, loin pain, bacteriuria and pyuria. There may be symptoms of cystitis. The condition can present as Gram-negative septicemia. Acute pyelonephritis is a systemic illness, so patients are commonly febrile and the C-reactive protein level is raised. Blood cultures are positive in 15–20% of patients admitted to hospital [227]. Patients with an abnormal urinary tract and recurrent episodes of pyelonephritis may simply feel unwell, suffering general malaise, headache, loss of appetite and backache. They may report that their urine is discolored and has an offensive odor [227].

Symptomatic UTI occurs in 1% to 2% of pregnancies, while asymptomatic bacteriuria has been reported in 2% to 13% of pregnant women, and is associated with premature delivery and low birth weight [229, 230]. Pyelonephritis develops in 30–40% of pregnant women with untreated bacteriuria, compared with 1–2% in non-bacteriuric pregnancies [227]. Most β-lactam antibiotics, including amoxicillin and cephalosporins, and nitrofurantoin are considered safe and effective in pregnancy. It is usual to treat the woman for 1 week and re-culture her urine on follow-up visits. If bacteriuria recurs, or if the women has vesico-ureteric reflux, prophylactic therapy may be necessary. Pyelonephritis is the most common severe bacterial infection that can lead to perinatal and maternal complications including premature delivery, infants with low birth weight, fetal mortality, preeclampsia, pregnancy-induced hypertension, anemia, thrombocytopenia, and transient renal insufficiency [228].

An MSU must be taken in patients with pyelonephritis or complicated UTI. Urine culture is not required in those with sporadic, uncomplicated UTI if the signs and symptoms are associated with hazy urine and microscopic hematuria. A leukocyte esterase dipstick can be used to detect pyuria, and sticks are available to detect nitrite (produced by bacterial metabolism of urinary nitrate). Most symptomatic UTI's in pregnant women present as acute cystitis, as occurs in non-pregnant women. Usually a 7-day treatment course is recommended, e.g. with nitrofurantoin, cefazolin, cephalexin, ceftriaxone, and gentamicin [231]. Existing data indicate that exposure to penicillins, cephalosporins, fluoroquinolones, nitrofurantoin, or phenazopyridine during pregnancy is not associated with increased risk of fetal malformations. Trimethoprim-sulfamethoxazole should be avoided, if possible, during the first trimester of pregnancy because of the anti-folate effect associated with neural tube defects [231].

Controversy exists as to the treatment period of asymptomatic bacteriuria. Some studies report that a single dose therapy is efficient [232], while others suggest three, five or seven days of treatment [233].The Infectious Diseases Society of America recommends that duration of antimicrobial therapy should be 3-7 days [234].Randomised trials indicate that drinking 200 ml to 750 ml of cranberry or lingonberry juice, or taking of cranberry concentrate tablets, reduces the risk of symptomatic, recurrent infection by 10% to 20% [235, 236, 237]. In cases of delayed defeverescence and upper tract dilatation, a ureteral stent may be indicated and antimicrobial prophylaxis until delivery, and including the puerperium should be considered. Follow-up urine cultures should be obtained after therapy to demonstrate eradication of the bacteriuria [230]. As in non-pregnant women, there is no advantage to be gained by using long-term prophylaxis except for recurrent infections. Low-dose cephalexin (125-250 mg) or nitrofurantoin (50 mg) at night is recommended for prophylaxis against re-infection if indicated, lasting up to and including the puerperium. Postcoital prophylaxis may be an alternative approach. The major causes of concern are the presence of underlying urological abnormalities and associated risks to the mother and fetus, such as toxemia, hypertension, prematurity and perinatal mortality. With the use of appropriate antimicrobial therapy almost all patients with uncomplicated pyelonephritis do well and become afebrile within a few days [234].

Complications of pyelonephritis during pregnancy can be devastating. Although complications such as pyonephrosis and perinephric abscesses most often occur in patients with obstruction, they are not prerequisites for severe complications. Complications may include the following: perinephric cellulitis and abscess, septicemic shock, renal dysfunction (usually transient, but as many as 25% of pregnant women with pyelonephritis have a decreased GFR), hematologic dysfunction (common but seldom of clinical importance) and pulmonary injury [238]. Approximately 1 in 50 women with severe pyelonephritis during pregnancy have evidence of pulmonary injury and respiratory insufficiency. Endotoxins that alter alveolar-capillary membrane permeability are produced; subsequently, pulmonary edema and acute respiratory distress syndrome develop [239].

Malaria in Pregnancy

Pregnant women are more likely than nonpregnant women to become infected with malaria and to have severe infection. The effects of malaria during pregnancy include spontaneous abortion, preterm delivery, low birth weight, stillbirth, congenital infection, and maternal death [240, 241, 242, 243]. Malaria is caused by the four species of the protozoa of the genus Plasmodium, which is transmitted by the bite of the female Anopheline mosquito, congenitally, or through exposure to infected blood products [244]. Malaria in humans is caused by the four species of the protozoa of the genus *Plasmodium* (*P. falciparum, P. vivax, P. ovale,* and *P. malariae*).

In high transmission areas, women have a level of immunity to malaria that wanes somewhat during pregnancy, and infection is more likely to result in severe maternal anemia and delivery of low birth-weight infants. On the other hand, in low transmission areas, women generally have developed no immunity to malaria, and infection is more likely to result in severe malaria disease, maternal anemia, premature delivery, or fetal loss [245]. The effects of malaria in pregnancy also are affected by the status of malaria in the community. Malaria endemic areas are defined as those with seasonal or perennial significant annual transmission. In areas of stable, endemic transmission, adult women usually have a protective semi-immunity against *P falciparum* acquired during the first 10 to 15 years of life [246]. Immunity is maintained through continued exposure to malarial illness. In these areas, most malaria infections are asymptomatic [247, 248]. In areas of unstable, non-endemic transmission, adult women have no significant level of immunity, are more likely to be symptomatic when parasitemic, and are at greater risk of developing severe disease and of death.

Malaria affects more than three million pregnant women per year in developing countries, where it commonly causes poor birth outcomes and maternal anemia.

[249, 250, 251]. Each year, approximately 50 million women living in malaria-endemic countries throughout the world become pregnant, of whom over half live in tropical areas of Africa with intense transmission of *P. falciparum*. An estimated 10 000 of these women and 200 000 of their infants die as a result of malaria infection during pregnancy [252, 247]. South and southeast Asia is another region that has the burden of malaria of varying endemicity [253]. Another estimate suggests that 11·4% of neonatal deaths and 5·7% of all infant deaths in malaria-endemic areas of Africa may be caused by malaria in pregnancy-associated low birthweight, which translates to around 100 000 infant deaths [254].

The transmission vector for the malarial parasite is the female Anopheles mosquito. The mosquito feeds on blood for the production of her eggs. The infected mosquito transfers the infective *Plasmodium* parasite, or sporozoite, from the salivary gland into the capillaries, causing parasitemia. The sporozoites penetrate liver cells within 30 minutes where they mature and amplify for 7 to 30 days into schizonts, which burst and release merozoites. The merozoites invade the erythrocytes and multiply and develop into their reproductive form, or gametocytes. This multiplication and periodic release from erythrocytes of new merozoites and malarial antigens forms the classical description of waves of fever. The duration of the asexual schizogonic cycle differs between human malarias. It is usually 48-50 hours in case of *P. vivax*, *P. ovale*, and *P. falciparum*, but 72 hours in *P. malariae*, which results in different species-based fever pattern. This fever pattern was used to distinguish between tertian (48 hours) and quartan (72 hours) malaria.The parasites can remain dormant in the liver for months to years. When in the liver and erythrocytes, the parasite is relatively protected from attack by the body's immune system. To prevent the circulating infected erythrocytes from being destroyed in the spleen, the parasite produces surface proteins which cause the erythrocytes to adhere to the walls of the blood vessels producing end-organ damage and other complications. A female mosquito bites an infected person and ingests blood containing the gametocytes. Fertilization occurs in the mosquito's gut, and within 10 to

18 days new sporozoites develop and travel to the mosquito's salivary gland, and the cycle repeats itself [255, 256].

Pregnancy-associated malaria is characterized by placental malaria and the sequestration of malaria parasites. Placental malaria is the accumulation of Plasmodium infected erythrocytes in the intervillious space of the placenta, causing changes and leukocyte-induced damage to the trophoblastic basement membrane. [257]. When a pregnant woman is infected with the malaria parasite, the infected erythrocytes bind to specific receptors in the placenta, especially chondroitin sulphate A, and interfere with oxygen and nutrient transport across the placenta. Anti-adhesion immunoglobulin G antibodies against chondroitin sulphate A–binding parasites are associated with protection from maternal malaria that develops only over successive pregnancies [246].

The symptoms of early malaria are non-specific, and include headache, myalgia, arthralgia, fever, anorexia, emesis, and malaise. The diagnosis of malaria depends on a high suspicion for the disease, and is typically confirmed by microscopic examination, the gold standard for routine laboratory diagnosis of malaria. The numbers of plasmodia are counted either on a stained thick film blood smear for low parasitemias or thin film blood smear for high parasitemias [258]. However, in the United States, where most medical laboratories are not familiar with the diagnosis of malaria, polymerase chain reaction (PCR)-based techniques are more accurate than microscopy and can detect 5 to 10 parasites per microliter of blood [259]. Where laboratory facilities and microscopy expertise are limited, rapid diagnostic tests (RDT) that detect the plasmodial antigens can be used [260]. The Centers for Disease Control and Prevention recommends that all RDT results in the United States be followed up with a confirmatory blood film.

If malaria treatment is delayed or if ineffective medications are given, uncomplicated malaria may progress rapidly to severe malaria such as cerebral malaria, severe anemia, hypoglycemia, and if untreated, death [258]. In addition, pregnant women, already prone to hypoglycemia because of enhanced pancreatic beta-cell function, have an increased risk of symptomatic hypoglycemia during *Plasmodium* infection because of maternal hyperinsulinemia, parasite glucose requirements, maternal glucose requirements during febrile illness, and decreased liver glycogen stores from decreased oral intake related to anorexia and emesis [261].

The burden of malaria in pregnancy is exacerbated by co-infection with HIV. Sub-Saharan Africa bears the brunt of this comorbidity, where approximately 25 million pregnant women are at risk of *P. falciparum* infection every year, and 77% (13·5 million) of the world's HIV-infected women reside [262, 263]. Studies from Africa highlight the deleterious effect of HIV on malaria, reporting higher risks of placental malaria, high-density parasitemia, and febrile illness in HIV-infected women [264]. HIV increases the degree to which malaria is associated with maternal severe anemia and low birthweight beyond the effect of HIV itself on anemia and birthweight [264].

The World Health Organization currently recommends a three-pronged approach to prevent these adverse effects in areas with high levels of transmission of *P. falciparum* malaria - intermittent preventive treatment (IPT) with antimalarial drugs, insecticide-treated bed nets (ITN), and febrile malaria case management [252].The selection of the specific drug for malaria treatment during pregnancy is based on the regional *Plasmodium* species, known drug sensitivities or resistance, consideration to the potential benefit versus potential risks, and any contraindications to the use in pregnancy. Chloroquine phosphate can be used safely in all trimesters and is recommended by the CDC as the treatment of choice for pregnant women in the United States with uncomplicated malaria caused by chloroquine- sensitive *P. falciparum* [265]. Hydroxychloroquine may be given as an alternative to chloroquine. The CDC recommends quinine plus clindamycin to treat uncomplicated chloroquine-resistant *P.*

Falciparum. Parenteral treatment with quinidine gluconate plus clindamycin, tetracycline, or doxycycline is required for severe infection [265]. According to the WHO, quinine plus clindamycin is the preferred regimen to treat uncomplicated *P falciparum* malaria in the first trimester of pregnancy [266]. If clindamycin is unavailable or unaffordable, quinine monotherapy should be given. Sulfadoxine-pyrimethamine in the second and third trimesters is safe and effective protection against peripheral and placental infection. It also reduces the incidence of anemia during pregnancy, and the incidence of LBW [262, 266].

The CDC recommends that pregnant travelers avoid malaria endemic areas [259, 265]. Pregnant women who do travel to endemic countries should begin prophylactic antimalarial medication—either mefloquine or chloroquine - before their travel and continue medication post-travel. The type of medication indicated depends on the country that the patient is visiting. All travelers, including pregnant women, are also encouraged to use personal protection measures to prevent mosquito bites. Inspite of recommendations, currently there is insufficient reliable research on malaria treatment options in pregnancy [267].

Tuberculosis in Pregnancy

Mycobacterium tuberculosis is an obligate aerobe bacilli (weakly Gram-positive mycobacterium, hence Ziehl-Neelsen staining [acid-fast staining] is used). The disease spreads from person to person through the air. Tuberculosis (TB) usually affects the lungs, but it can also affect other parts of the body, such as lymph nodes, brain, kidneys, bowel, or bones. Tuberculosis is frequently encountered among pregnant women and is responsible for 9% of all deaths of women of reproductive age. India accounts for 30% of the burden of all tuberculosis cases in the world [268]. More than 80% of the patients are in the economically productive age-group. An increased obstetric morbidity has been reported in pregnant women, with adverse pregnancy outcomes occurring in about 20% of untreated cases. Studies have also suggested no unusual increase in pre-term labor or other adverse pregnancy outcomes in treated cases [269, 270, 271]. The effects of TB on pregnancy depend upon various factors such as type, site and extent of the disease, stage of pregnancy, when management gets instituted, nutritional status of mother, presence of concomitant disease, immune status and co-existence of HIV infection, and availability of facilities for early diagnosis and treatment. The pulmonary and extra-pulmonary forms of TB effect pregnant women in the same way as the non-pregnant women [269].

If anti-tuberculosis treatment (ATT) is started early in pregnancy, the outcome is same as that in non-pregnant patients, whereas late diagnosis and care is associated with a four-fold increase in obstetric morbidity and nine-fold increase in pre-term labour [272]. Poor nutritional states, hypo-proteinemia, anemia and associated medical conditions add to maternal morbidity and mortality. Co-existing HIV infection is known to augment progression of TB and worsens the immunosuppression of the patient [269].The stage of pregnancy at which ATT is begun is the factor of paramount importance that chiefly determines the maternal outcomes in pregnancies associated with TB. This infection is believed to flare-up by the stress of pregnancy, especially in association with poor nutritional status, immunodeficient states, or co-existent diseases [269].

A fetus may contract TB infection either by hematogenous spread through the umbilical vein to the fetal liver or by ingestion or aspiration of infected amniotic fluid [273]. True congenital TB is believed to be rare. Cantwell et al. criteria for confirming neonatal TB include the demonstration of either primary hepatic complex or caseating hepatic granulomas at per cutaneous liver biopsy at birth, or presence of maternal genital tract or placenta TB, or the presence of lesions during first week of life by excluding postnatal transmission by a thorough investigation of all the contacts (including the attendants) [274]. The overall mortality for congenital TB is 38% in the untreated and 22% in the treated [274].There is a two-fold increase in the occurrence of pre-maturity, small-for-dates, and low-birth weight babies in women treated with ATT for 6-9 months during pregnancy [275].However, late prenatal diagnosis of disease, late institution of ATT, incomplete or irregular adherence to therapy, advanced lung lesions and poor maternal nutrition contribute to poor fetal health [269]. In those with a late diagnosis, obstetric morbidity is increased fourfold and preterm labour ninefold [272]. A higher frequency of abortion, toxemia, and intrapartum complications has also been reported [276]. In sub-Saharan Africa tuberculosis is an increasingly important cause of non-obstetric mortality. In some countries tuberculosis now accounts for 25% of all non-obstetric deaths, most in combination with HIV positivity, the dual epidemic being a major factor in an eightfold increase in maternal mortality [277].

Health-care workers must bear in mind similarities of symptoms between TB and pregnancy, such as tachycardia, anemia, raised ESR and low serum albumin level, as well as dissimilar parameters which may confuse the clinical presentation [269].The most common site of tuberculosis in pregnancy is pulmonary, associated with cough, weight loss, fever, malaise or fatigue, and hemoptysis; 20% may be asymptomatic but may have abnormal radiographs [278]. Five percent to10% of pregnant women may present with extrapulmonary disease, a proportion comparable with non-pregnant women of the same age and ethnicity [279]. The weight gain as well as the height of uterus as compared to the period of gestation in tuberculous pregnant women has been found to be significantly less in comparison with healthy pregnant women [280].

Sputum examination done for acid-fast bacilli is the preferred method for the diagnosis of pulmonary TB. A chest x-ray (performed after shielding the abdomen) is done if all 3 sputum smears are negative and symptoms persist despite treatment with antibiotics. In the USA tuberculin testing in high risk groups followed by chest radiography where appropriate is recommended [281]. The detection of latent infection by tuberculin skin testing is not affected by pregnancy [282]. A pregnant woman with extra-pulmonary TB has constitutional and organ-affection symptoms. Routine hematology and Mantoux test along with investigations specific for the site are carried out for the establishment of specific diagnosis. Co-existence of HIV infection should especially lead to a thorough search for any extrapulmonary tuberculous focus. Mediastinal or retro-peritoneal adenopathy, pleural effusion or parenchymal infiltrate may be detected on chest x-ray in late course of the disease, whereas cavitary lesions could exist in early HIV co-infection [269].

In almost all situations, tuberculosis discovered during pregnancy should be treated without delay. A pregnant woman with a positive skin test and abnormal chest x-ray findings compatible with tuberculosis should start treatment. Three samples of induced sputum should be submitted for smear, culture, and drug-susceptibility testing. The outcome of these tests will determine the regimen for continuation of treatment. As with any other medication, particularly in the first trimester, the main concern about tuberculosis treatment in pregnancy is the risk of teratogenicity. Short course chemotherapy trials have shown that 6 month regimens of rifampicin (RIF) and isoniazid (INH), supplemented by 2 months initial treatment with pyrazinamide (PZA) and either ethambutol (EMB) or streptomycin, is the treatment of choice for tuberculosis [283]. The trials, however, were not performed in pregnant subjects. There are four recommended regimens for treating patients with tuberculosis caused by drug-susceptible organisms [284]. Each regimen has an initial phase of 2 months followed by a choice of several options for the continuation phase of either 4 or 7 months. Because of the relatively high proportion of adult patients with tuberculosis caused by organisms that are resistant to isoniazid, four drugs are necessary in the initial phase for the 6-month regimen to be maximally effective. In most circumstances, the treatment regimen for all adults with previously untreated tuberculosis consists of a 2-month initial phase of INH, RIF, PZA, and EMB. When drug susceptibility test results are known and the organisms are fully susceptible, EMB need not be included. If PZA cannot be included in the initial phase of treatment, or if the isolate is resistant to PZA alone, the initial phase should consist of INH, RIF, and EMB given daily for 2 months (Regimen 4). The initial phase may be given daily throughout (Regimens 1 and 4), daily for 2 weeks and then twice weekly for 6 weeks (Regimen 2), or three times weekly throughout (Regimen 3). The continuation phase of treatment is given for either 4 or 7 months. The 4-month continuation phase should be used in the large majority of patients. The 7-month continuation phase is recommended only for three groups: (i) patients with cavitary pulmonary tuberculosis caused by drug-susceptible organisms and whose sputum culture obtained at the time of completion of 2 months of treatment is positive; (ii) patients whose initial phase of treatment did not include PZA; (iii) patients being treated with once weekly INH and RIF and whose sputum culture obtained at the time of completion of the initial phase is positive [281, 283].

For HIV-seronegative patients with noncavitary pulmonary tuberculosis (as determined by standard chest radiography), and negative sputum smears at completion of 2 months of treatment, the continuation phase may consist of rifampicin and INH given once weekly for 4 months by daily observed treatment (DOT). If the culture at completion of the initial phase of treatment is positive, the once weekly INH and RIF continuation phase should be extended to 7 months. The once-weekly continuation phase is contraindicated in patients with HIV infection because of a high rate of failure/relapse.

For the same reason twice weekly treatment, either as part of the initial phase or continuation phase, is not recommended for HIV-infected patients with $CD4^{+}$ cell counts <100 cells/μl. These patients should receive either daily (initial phase) or three times weekly (continuation phase) treatment

Although all of these drugs cross the placenta, they do not appear to have teratogenic effects. Streptomycin is the only anti-tuberculosis drug documented to have harmful effects on the human fetus (congenital deafness) and should not be used.

The low concentration of anti-TB medications in breast milk should not be considered effective treatment for disease or as treatment for latent TB infection in a nursing infant [285]. Because the small concentrations of anti-tuberculosis drugs in breast milk do not produce toxicity in the nursing newborn, breast feeding should not be discouraged for an HIV-seronegative woman who is planning to take or is taking INH or other anti-TB medications. Pyridoxine supplementation (25 mg/day) is recommended for all women taking INH who are either pregnant or breastfeeding.

Typhoid Fever (Enteric Fever, Salmonella Typhi)

Salmonella Typhi is a serovar of *Salmonella enterica*, a gram-negative rod found only in humans, and the cause of the disease typhoid fever. *Salmonella* Typhi possesses three main antigenic factors: the *O*, or somatic antigen; the *Vi*, or encapsulation antigen; and the *H*, or flagellar antigen. A similar, but less severe, disease is caused by *Salmonella paratyphi* A. In the US approximately 500 cases of typhoid fever are reported annually in the United States. More than two thirds of those cases are contracted during travel abroad, and involve children, adolescents, and young adults [286]. According to the best global estimates, there are at least 16 million new cases of typhoid fever each year, with 600 000 deaths, mostly in Asia, Africa, and Latin America. In the developing world on the other hand, though, accurate statistics may be lacking, the incidence of up to 13-22 per 100 000 persons per year has been documented [287]. Global incidence is about 0.5%, but incidence rates as high as 2% have been reported in hot spots [288].

Typhoid fever is most prevalent in developing countries where sanitary water and sewage systems are lacking. Transmission occurs most often by one of the following mechanisms: 1) ingestion of contaminated food or water, 2) contact with an acute case of typhoid fever, 3) contact with a chronic asymptomatic carrier. Following ingestion of an infectious dose of at least 10 000 bacteria, mucosal penetration occurs in the distal ileum resulting in a transient, asymptomatic bacteremia. The organisms survive and multiply within mononuclear phagocytes located in lymph nodes, spleen, liver, and bone marrow. The clinical phase of the disease begins within 1-3 weeks, resulting from persistent bacteremia. Hematogenous spread to ileal Peyer patches and the gall bladder reintroduces bacteria to the gut lumen and stool cultures again become positive, allowing continued fecal-oral spread of the disease. Mucosal ulceration overlying hyperplastic Peyer patches in the ileocecal region may result in pain, diarrhea, bleeding, and occasional perforation.

Constitutional symptoms include fever, chills, headache, sore throat, muscle pain, and weakness. Many patients complain of a skin rash and cervical adenopathy. Gastrointestinal symptoms include nausea, vomiting, anorexia, diarrhea, constipation, and abdominal pain. Neurologic symptoms include altered mental status and occasional seizures. Patients with ocular manifestations generally complain of pain and decreased vision. Relative bradycardia (less tachycardia than expected for the degree of fever) may occur in up to 50% of patients but is not a reliable diagnostic indicator. Faintly erythematous maculopapules or rose spots occur on the trunk and may become hemorrhagic. Cervical adenopathy and hepatosplenomegaly are often present. Intestinal bleeding may occur from ulceration of mucosa overlying hyperplastic ileal Peyer patches. Altered mental status and seizures may occur. Ocular manifestations are rare and occur in association with systemic illness [289, 290].

Rare fatal complications include intestinal perforation or severe hemorrhage. Localized infections such as cholangitis, urinary tract infection, pneumonia, osteomyelitis, arthritis, meningitis, and endophthalmitis occasionally are seen. Spontaneous splenic rupture and multiple brain abscesses also have been reported [286]. Recovery is characterized by diminishing fever and begins by the fourth week in patients without antibiotic treatment. In contrast, antibiotic use usually results in defervescence in less than 7 days. Relapse occurs in as many as 10% of patients, while 1-3% of patients become long-term carriers following recovery.

New diagnostic tests include those for immunoglobulin M (IgM) and immunoglobulin G (IgG) antibodies. The Typhidot-M® test has a specificity of 75% and a sensitivity of 95% [291, 292]. The Tubex® test is rapid and detects the O9 antigen [293, 294]. The classic Widal test is rarely used because of its low sensitivity and specificity [295]. Blood, urine, and stool cultures are still frequently used to isolate *S. typhi,* but the yield is only about 70%. Complete blood count may reveal anemia and thrombocytopenia. Liver function test results are commonly elevated. Renal dysfunction may occur, but chronic renal failure has not been reported. Abdominal radiographs demonstrate free air in cases of intestinal perforation. Bone marrow biopsy results are positive in as many as 90% of individuals who are affected; therefore, performing a bone marrow biopsy is useful in cases of diagnostic uncertainty [296, 298].

Amoxycillin, and trimethoprim–sulfamethoxazole remain appropriate for the treatment of typhoid fever in areas of the world where the bacterium is still fully susceptible to these drugs and where the fluoroquinolones are not available or affordable. The fluoroquinolones are widely regarded as optimal for the treatment of typhoid fever in adults [298]. They are relatively inexpensive, well tolerated and reliably effective than the former first-line drugs, viz. chloramphenicol, ampicillin, amoxycillin and trimethoprim-sulfamethoxazole. However, the emergence of multidrug resistant strains (MDR) strains has reduced the choice of antibiotics in many areas. In recent years, however, there have been many reports of reduced susceptibility and treatment failure with fluoroquinolones [299, 300]. In areas of the world where the bacterium is still fully sensitive to traditonal first-line drugs (chloramphenicol, amoxycillin or trimethoprim-sulfamethoxazole), these remain appropriate for the treatment of typhoid fever [295]. The third-generation cephalosporins (ceftriaxone, cefixime, cefotaxime, and cefoperazone) and azithromycin are also effective drugs for typhoid. The current drug of choice in pregnant women is parenteral ceftriaxone [301, 302]. There are few data on the treatment of pregnant women with typhoid. Typhoid fever diagnosed in the latter part of the second and third trimesters, and treated early, did not seem to alter the neonatal outcome [303].

Salmonellea typhi causes septicemia of digestive origin that can cross the placenta resulting in chorioamniotitis. Maternal-fetal infection with *S. typhi* can lead to miscarriage, fetal death, and neonatal infection [302, 304]. Patients in shock or with altered mental status may benefit from parenteral corticosteroid administration [305 306]. Supportive care often is required, including intravenous fluids and occasionally transfusion. Several vaccines are available and are effective in decreasing the risk of disease by 50-75% [307, 308] However, persons who have been vaccinated should still exercise dietary precautions.

Intraamniotic Infection

Intraamniotic infection (IAI) is a term used to describe a clinically diagnosed infection of the contents of the uterus, most often associated with rupture of membranes [309]. Most women with a clinically apparent IAI typically have histological evidence of chorioamnionitis but not all placentas with this finding come from women with IAI [310]. Although histological inflammation of the chorion and amnion is found in 20% of term and 60% of preterm pregnancies, the clinical diagnosis of IAI is made in only 0.5% to 10.5% of pregnancies [311, 312]. Another term, *microbial invasion of the amniotic fluid,* describes a preclinical phase of amniotic fluid infection. The distinction between histological chorioamnionitis and IAI is important because the histological diagnosis cannot be made while the patient is pregnant, and to diagnose microbial invasion of the amniotic fluid requires amniocentesis [309].

Risk factors for developing chorioamnionitis include preterm labor, prolonged active labor, prelabor rupture of membranes, rupture of membranes greater than 12 hours, and maternal chronic autoimmune disease [313]. The greatest risk for IAI occurs after rupture of the membranes. Although hematogenous spread is possible, pathogenic organisms more easily reach the amniotic cavity from the maternal vaginal tract once this barrier is breached. Bacterial access to the amniotic cavity by itself is not sufficient to produce an infectious process. The size of the inoculum, the pathogenicity of the organisms, and the susceptibility of the hosts (mother and fetus) affect the risk of IAI [314]. Factors that increase the exposure of the amniotic cavity to pathogenic bacteria from the vagina such as duration of ruptured membranes, transcervical instrumentation, vaginal examinations, and cerclage placement seem to further increase the risk of IAI [314, 315]. Intraamniotic infection has been described in some patients with intact membranes who undergo procedures such as amniocentesis and percutaneous umbilical blood sampling, however, these instances are rare [316 317]. Certain microorganisms, such as group B streptococcus, *Listeria monocytogenes,* fusobacterium, and group A streptococcus are implicated more frequently in IAI in spite of intact membranes. Other organisms that have been reported in association with IAI include *Ureaplasma urealyticum*, *Candida* sp, and *Haemophilus influenzae.* The most common high virulence isolates are *Bacteroides* species, group B streptococcus, and *Escherichia coli* [318, 319, 320, 321].

The diagnosis of IAI is typically made by clinical findings; which include maternal temperature, maternal and fetal tachycardia, uterine tenderness, or purulent amniotic fluid, in the absence of other signs of infection. In the majority of cases, an elevated maternal temperature may be the only symptom. Often, fetal heart rate changes (specifically tachycardia or variable decelerations) will accompany the diagnosis of chorioamnionitis

[313]. The accurate and timely diagnosis of IAI is important so that affected women may be treated without delay. Unfortunately, early diagnosis is difficult because clinical signs and symptoms of IAI occur late and are neither sensitive nor specific [322]. To avoid a delay in diagnosis, a high index of suspicion should be maintained. Patients with fever, and maternal or fetal tachycardia, especially in the presence of ruptured membranes, are likely to have IAI.

Many serological and amniotic fluid assays have been studied to diagnose IAI: leukocyte esteraseY, glucose levels, Limulus amebocyte assay, gas-liquid chromotography, and interleukins, however, there is no reliable gold standard against which to measure any of the diagnostic tests [323, 324, 325, 326, 327]. Gram's stain, culture, and cell count are the most commonly used tests on the amniotic fluid. Maternal leukocytosis, although found frequently, must be interpreted cautiously if the patient is in labor. In a non-laboring patient with intact membranes and fever, but otherwise no signs of IAI, it is reasonable to perform an amniocentesis to help exclude intrauterine infection. The amniotic fluid can be sent for white cell count, Gram staining, and culture tests [318].

Antibiotics, when given to patients with preterm premature rupture of membranes, may decrease the frequency of IAI and prolong the interval between rupture of membranes and delivery in addition to lowering neonatal morbidity [328]. Since most infections seem to be polymicrobial a combined regimen effective against Gram-positive and Gram-negative organisms based on the local flora and resistance patterns is recommended [329, 328]. The most established treatment regimen is intravenous ampicillin, and gentamicin; penicillin has also been used with gentamicin. Other antibiotics used include cephalosporins, erythromycin, amoxicillin, and amoxicillin-clavulinic acid [330, 331, 332, 333, 334, 335]. Induction of labor usually is indicated if this has not begun spontaneously. If cesarean section is necessary, intravenous clindamycin or metronidazole should be added after cord clamping to improve the coverage of anaerobic organisms [309]. Cesarean section should be reserved for the usual obstetric indications; although operative delivery occurs in up to 40% of affected women. Due to greater tissue injury from cesarean section, antibiotic coverage should be continued until the patient has been afebrile and asymptomatic for 24 to 48 hours [309].

Intraamniotic infection is a serious complication of pregnancy. It can lead to postpartum endometritis as well as systemic infection. Clinical and subclinical infections contribute to a sizeable proportion of preterm labor cases, neonatal sepsis and pneumonia [328, 312]. Antepartum antibiotics may decrease, but do not eliminate, the neonatal morbidity of IAI. The preterm fetus is most profoundly affected.

For example, the incidence of respiratory distress is doubled and the mortality rate increased fourfold among 28- to 32-week infants whose mothers had preterm premature rupture of membranes, and in whom IAI developed [336]. Other studies have found a higher rate of neonatal mortality, intraventricular hemorrhage, meningitis, necrotizing enerocolitis, and respiratory distress syndrome associated with the condition [337]. There has been a growing belief that intrauterine infections may predispose to pediatric neurodevelopmental impairment, and cerebral palsy [338, 312].

Appendicitis in Pregnancy

Appendicitis is one of the most common causes of an acute abdomen in pregnancy, occurring in approximately 1 in 1500 pregnancies [339, 340]. This represents an overall incidence of 0.05% to 0.07%, and does not appear to be any different in the non-gravid population [341 342]. While the incidence of appendicitis may arise in any of the trimesters, there is a higher incidence in the second trimester, ranging from 27% to 60% [343, 341]. Due to the lack of specificity of the preoperative evaluation the pathologic diagnosis of appendicitis is confirmed in only 30% to 50% of cases [344]. Delay in diagnosis is associated with a higher rate of complications such as perforation, infection, preterm labor, and fetal or maternal loss [345, 343]. Appendicitis occurs at the same rate in pregnant and nonpregnant women, but pregnant women have a higher rate of perforation [339, 341, 345]. Maternal mortality may be upto 2%. An unruptured appendix carries a fetal loss of 1.5% to 9%, while this rate increases to 36% with perforation [340, 343]. The risk of perforation increases with gestational age, and perforation in the third trimester often results in preterm labor [341]. Delay in surgical intervention carries increased fetal loss. The risk for premature delivery is the greatest during the first week after surgery [346].

Upon physical examination, findings may be less evident than in non-pregnant women with the same disorder [347, 348]. Peritoneal signs are often absent in pregnancy because of the lifting and stretching of the anterior abdominal wall. The underlying inflammation has no direct contact with the parietal peritoneum, which precludes any muscular response or guarding that would otherwise be expected. The uterus can also obstruct and inhibit the movement of the omentum to an area of inflammation, distorting the clinical picture [349]. When evaluating laboratory investigations in the gravid patient with acute abdominal pain, it is important to note that there may be altered reference ranges in pregnancy. Leukocytosis and a diminished tendency to develop hypotension and tachycardia, which are physiologic in pregnancy, add complexity to the diagnosis and can make the initial evaluation process more difficult [350, 351]. Ultrasound is also used with graded compression as a diagnostic aid in appendicitis. The size of the gravid abdomen may limit this approach in pregnancy, however, some researchers have reported success [352, 353].

Treatment of an acute abdomen in pregnancy depends on the specific diagnosis. Indications for emergency surgery during pregnancy are the same as they are for any other patients. If surgery is required but is considered elective, waiting until the postnatal period is prudent. If surgery is deemed necessary during pregnancy, it is best performed in the second trimester, as the risk of preterm labor and delivery is lower in the second trimester compared to the third, and the risk of spontaneous loss and risks due to medications such as anesthetic agents are lower in the second trimester compared to the first [354, 355, 356].Treatment of appendicitis is surgical; either laparotomy or laparoscopy can be performed depending on the surgeon's skill and expertise. Laparoscopic appendectomy has become increasingly utilized in the gravid patient since its introduction and is considered by many to be the standard of care [357, 358, 359, 360, 361]. Several studies have shown that pregnant patients may undergo laparoscopic surgery safely during any trimester without any appreciated increased risk to the mother or fetus [362, 363, 364]. Laparoscopic appendectomy have been successfully performed even late in the third trimester [362, 365, 366]. No statistical difference was found between open and laparoscopic appendectomy when compared for gestational duration, Apgar scores, and birth weights [367]. During surgery it is important to take precautions, ie., to tilt the operating table 30° to the patient's left to help bring the uterus away from the surgical site and to improve maternal venous return and cardiac output by avoiding mechanical compression of the great vessels.

Acute Cholecystitis in Pregnancy

Estimates of occurrence of acute cholecystitis vary widely. The case-to-delivery ratio varies between 1:1 130 and 1:12 890 [368, 369]. Asymptomatic gall bladder disease is more common, occurring in 3-4% of pregnant women. Chronic hemolytic conditions, such as sickle cell disease, increase the risk for gallstone formation. Initial treatment is supportive in nature. These include intravenous fluids, nasogastric suction, which may be necessary if vomiting has been significant, analgesia, and if symptoms persist or if systemic or local signs are prominent, broad-spectrum antibiotics [370, 371].

The timing of surgery for acute cholecystitis is controversial. Some advocate surgery during pregnancy to avoid recurrent episodes and hospitalization [372]; others delay surgery until the postpartum period [373]. When a choice is available regarding the timing of surgery, operating in the second trimester minimizes fetal risk. Complications can occur, including empyema, perforation, pancreatitis, and failure to respond to medical management. With conservative management, 62-84% of patients can continue through delivery without surgery [370, 371, 369]. As with appendectomy in pregnancy, laparoscopic cholecystectomy is not contraindicated in pregnancy [362, 363, 364].

Meningitis in Pregnancy

Bacterial meningitis has an annual incidence of 4–6 cases per 100 000 adults and results in approximately 135 000 deaths worldwide each year. Meningococcal disease is the most frequent cause of bacterial meningitis in infants, children, adolescents, and young adults in the United States. Of the approximately 2 800 cases of meningococcal disease in the United States each year, more than 60% are in individuals aged 11 years or older [374]. Since the development of the *Haemophilus influenzae* type B vaccine, the most common bacterial pathogen for community-acquired meningitis is *Streptococcus pneumoniae,* which has a fatality rate of 19% to 37% [375]. In patients who survive the initial insult, neurologic sequelae including seizures, hearing loss, impaired mental status and cognition may occur in as many as 30% of all cases [376].

Local extension from contiguous extracerebral infection (e.g., otitis media, mastoiditis, or sinusitis) is a common source. Patients with bacterial meningitis will usually present soon after the onset of symptoms with a classic triad of fever, neck stiffness, and altered mental status. Prompt recognition and treatment are key to reducing the morbidity and mortality associated with this infection. Bacterial meningitis is a medical emergency in which early diagnosis and institution of treatment is vital to prevent death and to reduce long-term complications. Lumbar puncture is used to confirm the diagnosis in patients presenting with clinically suspected meningitis; however, imaging should be completed initially in patients with new-onset seizures, an immunocompromised state, signs of possible mass lesion or altered level of consciousness. The choice of initial antimicrobial therapy is based on the most common bacteria causing the disease, the patient's age, the clinical setting, and on patterns of antimicrobial susceptibility. Combination therapy with vancomycin plus a third-generation cephalosporin, such as ceftriaxone or cefotaxime, has become the standard approach to empirical antimicrobial therapy [375]. Intravenous dexamethasone before or with the first dose of antibiotics has been shown to reduce the risk of death and neurologic disability in adults with pneumococcal meningitis [377].

An extended interval between the onset of maternal illness and delivery provides an important window of time for maternal and neonatal well-being. Of women diagnosed with bacterial meningitis during pregnancy, the mortality rate could be upto 27%, and the rate of neurologic sequelae in survivors upto 53%. The fetal loss rate from spontaneous abortion, stillbirth, and neonatal death may be upto 47% [378]. Although pregnancy does result in a diminished immune response, there is no data to conclude that there is increased risk specific to *S. pneumoniae* [375]. In general, meningococcal disease has a high mortality of 10% to 14%, with 11% to 19% of survivors left with long-term disabilities such as hearing loss, brain damage, cognitive impairment, renal failure, or limb amputations, most cases are potentially vaccine preventable [374].

Listeria

Listeria *monocytogenes* is a short, gram-positive rod that can occur singly or in short chains. The organism grows well at refrigerator temperatures (5°–10° C) and is a known food-borne pathogen. Listeria has also been recovered from a variety of foods including soft cheeses, raw milk, and processed meats. There are close to 2 000 cases of listeriosis which account for approximately 425 deaths each year [379, 380]. The infection usually occurs after ingestion of infected food products. The incubation period is between two and six weeks.

The consequences of foodborne illness can be particularly devastating during pregnancy because both the woman and her fetus are at risk. Escalated production of progesterone during pregnancy leads to down-regulation of cell-mediated immune functions. Many foodborne pathogens are intracellular pathogens, and infections caused by these are controlled by cell-mediated immunity. The pregnancy-induced decrease in cell-mediated immune functions leads to increased susceptibility of the pregnant woman to L. *monocytogenes* [379]. In the United States, L. *monocytogenes* is one of the most important foodborne pathogens in pregnancy, and can lead to preterm labor, chorioamnionitis, spontaneous abortion, and stillbirth. It can be passed from an infected mother to her fetus through hematogenous spread, crossing the placenta and causing early and late onset disease in the neonate, with the most severe manifestation being *granulomatosis infantiseptica*, however, it does not cause habitual abortion in humans. [380].

Signs and symptoms of Listeria include fever, chills, and back pain; a nonspecific flu-like illness is the most common symptom. Other clinical manifestations include sepsis, meningitis, rhomboencephalitis, brain abscess, endocarditis, acute gastrointestinal illness and a variety of focal infections [379]. Infection is diagnosed by culture from sterile body fluids such as blood, cerebrospinal fluid and amniotic fluid. The treatment of choice is ampicillin. The patient also should be treated with gentamicin if she has meningitis, endocarditis, or is severly immunocompromised [379]. Early treatment decreases mortality and residual morbidity so it is imperative that each clinician maintain a high index of suspicion for this unusual infection.

Puerperal Fever

Puerperal fever is defined in the International Classification of Diseases (ICD-10), as a "temperature rise above 38.0°C (100.4°F) maintained over 24 hours or recurring during the period from the end of the first to the end of the tenth day after childbirth or abortion" [381]. Alternatively, the United States Joint Commission on Maternal Welfare uses a standard definition for puerperal fever used for reporting puerperal morbidity as an "oral temperature of 38.0°C (100.4°F) or more on any 2 of the first 10 days postpartum" [382]. While puerperal infection is most commonly encountered within the first 2 weeks after delivery, the definition extends to 42 days postpartum [383]. Further, the World Health Organization (WHO) [384], defines puerperal sepsis as "infection of the genital tract occurring at any time between the onset of the rupture of membranes or labor and the 42nd day postpartum in which fever and one or more of the following are present:

1) pelvic pain
2) abnormal vaginal discharge
3) abnormal odor of discharge and
4) delay in the rate of reduction of size of the uterus.

Some authors further differentiate between "puerperal sepsis," which refers specifically to infection of the genital tract after delivery, and "puerperal pyrexia or fever" which encompasses all cases of significant pyrexia in the puerperium, and would include patients with puerperal sepsis, as well as those with other causes of pyrexia [385]. Overt infections can and do occur in the absence of these criteria, but fever of some degree remains the hallmark of puerperal infection, and the patient with fever can be assumed to have a genital infection until proven otherwise. Endometritis is the most frequent infective cause of puerperal fever. Other sources of postpartum infections include urinary tract infections, mastitis, post surgical wound infections, perineal cellulitis, respiratory infections, retained products of conception, and septic pelvic phlebitis [386]. Deaths related to puerperal infection are very rare in the developed world, however, the death ratio in developing countries may be 100 times higher [387]. Maternal mortality ratio due to puerperal infection is estimated to be around 3 maternal deaths for each 100 000 live births.

The predisposing factors or conditions leading to the development of sepsis are quite varied and include home birth in unhygienic conditions, low socioeconomic status, poor nutrition, primiparity, anemia, prolonged rupture of membranes, prolonged labor, multiple vaginal examinations in labor (more than 5), cesarean section, and obstetrical maneuvers. Maternal complications include septicemia, endotoxic shock, peritonitis, or abscess formation leading to surgery and compromised future fertility. Cesarean section is perhaps the greatest risk factor for postpartum endometritis, with a 20- to 30-fold relative risk compared with a vaginal delivery [388, 389, 390]. The modes of transmission of puerperal sepsis are typically categorized into nosocomial, exogenous, and endogenous factors. Nosocomial infections are acquired in hospitals or other health facilities and may come from the hospital environment or from the patient's own flora [391]. Exogenous infections come from external contamination, especially when deliveries take place under unhygienic conditions. Most cases of endometritis are due to usual bacteria of the bowel, vagina, perineum, and cervix [392].

Endometritis

The uterine cavity is usually sterile until the rupture of the amniotic sac. As a consequence of labor, delivery, and associated manipulations, anaerobic and aerobic bacteria can contaminate the uterus. In severe cases of puerperal fever the infection is almost always caused by group A streptococci. Often, however, infections tend to be polymicrobial; the most common pathogens include gram-positive cocci (group B streptococci, *Staphylococcus epidermidis,* and *Enterococcus* sp), anaerobes (peptostreptococci, *Bacteroides* sp, and *Prevotella* sp), and gram-negative organisms *(Gardnerella vaginalis, Escherichia coli, Klebsiella pneumoniae,* and *Proteus mirabilis)* [393, 394, 395, 396, 397, 398].

Endometritis usually develops on the second or third postpartum day. Fever and a soft, tender uterus are the most prominent signs. Also there is anorexia, malaise and headache. Abdominal tenderness is generally limited to the lower abdomen and does not lateralize. Bowel sounds may be decreased and the abdomen distended and tympanitic. Motion of the cervix and uterus may cause increased pain. Adnexal masses palpable on abdominal or pelvic examination are not seen in uncomplicated endometritis, but if these infections are not treated aggressively, the organisms may act synergistically to form complex abscesses or necrotizing infections. When the parametria are affected, pain and pyrexia are severe; the large, tender uterus is indurated at the base of the broad ligaments, extending to the pelvic walls or posterior cul-de-sac. Lochia may be decreased or profuse and malodorous. Leukocytosis, a shift to the left of the differential WBC, and markedly increased RBC sedimentation rate are typical of puerperal infections. In the absence of antibiotic treatment or in the more severe cases, puerperal infection may be complicated by chronic pelvic pain, pelvic inflammatory disease, and secondary infertility [399]. Also, the more severe cases are responsible for the high rates of mortality from sepsis especially in developing countries.

A common treatment for postpartum endometritis involves the use of combination antimicrobial coverage, including an aminoglycoside for coverage of Gram-negative organisms and clindamycin phosphate for coverage of Gram-positive and anaerobic organisms [400]. Although regimens effective against penicillin-resistant anaerobic bacteria (a combination of gentamicin and clindamycin) are recommended in systematic reviews, other regimens and protocols are used.

Second or third-generation cephalosporins in combination with metronidazole is another widespread and popular choice [383, 401]. Pelvic abscess should be suspected in patients with persistent spiking fever despite antibiotic coverage; the treatment of choice then is surgical drainage.

Puerperal Mastitis

Lactation predisposes patients to mastitis. The presence of milk in the duct, combined with nipple cracking, creates a favorable environment for infection. The initiating event is milk stasis, and if a heavy bacterial inoculum is introduced into the duct system infectious mastitis may develop. *Staphylococcus aureus* is the most common causative agent in patients with puerperal mastitis. Other organisms less frequently isolated include group A and group B-hemolytic streptococci, *Escherichia coli,* and *Bacteroides* species.

Puerperal mastitis tends to occur two to three weeks postpartum and is associated with fever and myalgia, presenting as a flu-like illness. The diagnosis is based on identification of a tender, erythematous, wedgeshaped area in the breast. Since milk stasis is often the initiating factor in mastitis, the most important management step is frequent and effective milk expression. This may be achieved either by breastfeeding more frequently, or expressing by hand or pump. Additional therapy for the treatment of mastitis includes local care such as ice-packs, analgesia and breast support, in addition to a penicillinase-resistant antibiotic. Breast-feeding should be continued unless an abscess develops. The treatment of a breast abscess requires incision and drainage. Mastitis should be distinguished from late engorgement caused by milk stasis, which can cause inflammation of the breast but is not associated with high fever or cracked nipples, and does not require antibiotic therapy [402].

Episiotomy Infection

In general, the more extensive the episiotomy, the greater the chances of infection and breakdown of the wound. *Staphylococcus* or *Streptococcus* species and gram-negative organisms, are the most common organisms associated with perineal cellulitis and episiotomy site infections. Patients with episiotomy infections have perineal pain, erythema, edema, tenderness, and a purulent discharge from the site. Inspection of the episiotomy site shows disruption of the wound and gaping of the incision. A necrotic membrane may cover the wound. Episiotomy infection is usually confined to the skin and surrounding subcutaneous tissue, and limited by Camper's fascia.

Extension of the infection should be suspected in patients with significant perineal pain, hip pain, or erythema and swelling beyond the episiotomy site. Pelvic examination may detect the presence of hematomas or abscesses. If no abscess or extension is suspected, Sitz baths are usually sufficient treatment. Deeper involvement to Colle's and Scarpa's fascia may result in necrotizing fasciitis [403]. If an abscess is suspected, CT scanning may be necessary to determine if the abscess is located in the retroperitoneal or gluteal muscle areas, as severe infections may spread to the levator ani, lumbosacral nerve plexus, hip capsule, and retropsoas space [404, 405].

Treatment consists of exploration of the episiotomy, drainage and debridement. The wound is then allowed to heal secondarily; however, early closure of a clean wound may be attemped in order to maintain perineal integrity [406]. An open infected episiotomy should not be sutured.

Cesarean Wound Infections

Post-cesarean wound infections are usually detected in the immediate post-operative period. Swelling, edema, erythema, tenderness and drainage of purulent material from the wound are present. Treatment consists of local care; the wound is opened, cleaned and debrided. In wound infections following cesarean section, it may be packed with saline-soaked gauze 2-3 times per day, which will help remove necrotic debris. The wound may be left open to heal, or it may be closed secondarily when granulation tissue has begun to form.

Necrotic Fasciitis

Necrotic fasciitis must be considered whenever infection of the fascia is suspected. This is a rare, life-threatening infection. The diagnosis of necrotic fasciitis can be made if the patient has a high fever resistant to antibiotics, with associated systemic toxicity and a hard, "woody" feel to the infected area. Necrotic fasciitis requires immediate aggressive treatment to reduce morbidity and mortality. Fundamental to the successful treatment of necrotic fasciitis is early diagnosis, early administration of broad-spectrum antibiotics, and urgent surgical debridement [407].

Urinary Tract Infections

Bacteriuria in the postpartum period is often asymptomatic, with only 21% of culture-positive women reporting symptoms [408)]. Of all risk factors, urethral catheterization contributes most to the incidence of nosocomial urinary tract infections. Failure to treat a urinary tract infection in the postpartum period results in persistence of the bacteriuria in about 30% of cases. A 3-day course of antibiotics is usually sufficient to eradicate the infection in uncomplicated cases [408]. Acute pyelonephritis during the puerperium is a serious systemic illness that can progress to maternal sepsis. Parenteral antibiotic treatment of pyelonephritis is the same as in the pregnant state, and should be continued until the patient becomes afebrile. Most patients respond to hydration and prompt antibiotic treatment within 24 to 48 hours.

Septic Pelvic Thrombophlebitis

Septic pelvic thrombophlebitis is an uncommon cause of postpartum pyrexia, occurring in 1 in 2 000 deliveries. The incidence increases to 1% to 2% among women with post-cesarean section endometritis [409]. Pelvic thrombophlebitis is more common after cesarean section than after vaginal delivery. The mechanism of action involves the presence of a hypercoagulable state and spread of infection from the myometrium to pelvic and ovarian veins.The patient often complains of flank and lower abdominal pain, typically described as non-colicky and constant, of variable intensity, and may radiate to the groin or upper abdomen. On physical examination, the patient usually does not appear toxic, there may be tenderness in the lower abdomen, and an occasional tender abdominal mass described as "rope-" or "sausage-shape" may rarely be identified. The diagnosis is suspected when a patient responds poorly to antibiotic treatment of endometritis and a mass is palpable on pelvic examination. In suspected cases, a trial of anticoagulation therapy with heparin may suggest the diagnosis, which is confirmed by CT of the pelvis or magnetic resonance imaging [410]. Frequently, the first sign is a pulmonary embolus. When thrombophlebitis is recognized early, the risk of pulmonary embolism can be greatly reduced with appropriate anticoagulant therapy [411].

Miscellaneous

An overview of the common infections and their complications have been outlined; the list is by no means complete. As with any patient with fever, in pregnancy, the possibility of other causes, such as viral infection, connective tissue disease, malignancy, or subacute bacterial endocarditis, should be considered if the course of illness is atypical or the patient is unresponsive to standard therapy. The principles of management in cases of puerperal infection include assessment of risk factors, a detailed history, a "head-to-toe" examination, appropriate laboratory and radiologic tests, and treatment of the cause [412].

Vaccines in Pregnancy

Routine vaccines that generally are safe to administer during pregnancy include diphtheria, tetanus, influenza, and hepatitis B. Other vaccines, such as meningococcal and rabies, may be considered. Vaccines that are contraindicated, because of the theoretic risk of fetal transmission, include measles, mumps, and rubella; varicella; and bacille Calmette-Guérin. A number of other vaccines have not yet been adequately studied; therefore, theoretic risks of vaccination must be weighed against the risks of the disease to mother and fetus [413].

The administration of vaccines during pregnancy poses a number of concerns to physicians and patients about the risk of transmitting a virus to a developing fetus. This risk is primarily theoretic. According to the CDC, if a live-virus vaccine is inadvertently given to a pregnant woman, or if a woman becomes pregnant within four weeks after vaccination, she should be counseled about potential effects on the fetus. Inadvertent administration of these vaccines, however, is not considered an indication for termination of the pregnancy [414].

There is no evidence that there is an increased risk from vaccinating pregnant women with inactivated virus or bacterial vaccines or toxoids. Therefore, if a patient is at high risk of being exposed to a particular disease, if infection would pose a risk to the mother or fetus, and if the vaccine is unlikely to cause harm, the benefits of vaccinating a pregnant woman usually outweigh the potential risks [413]. Physicians should consider vaccinating pregnant women on the basis of the risks of vaccination versus the benefits of protection in each particular situation, regardless of whether live or inactivated vaccines are used. Vaccines commonly administered by family physicians, and their indication for use during pregnancy, are summarized in table 6.

Women of childbearing age often are concerned about whether breastfeeding is safe during immunization. Physicians should reassure their patients that no vaccines are contraindicated during breastfeeding.

The following vaccines are considered safe to give to women who may be at risk of infection [414].

- *Hepatitis B* - Pregnant women who are at high risk for this disease and have tested negative for the virus can receive this vaccine. It is used to protect the mother and baby against infection both before and after delivery.
- *Influenza* -This vaccine can prevent serious illness in the mother during pregnancy, but should be received after the mother has been pregnant for more than 14 weeks. If you have a serious medical condition that can lead to flu-related complications, you can receive the vaccine at any stage of your pregnancy.
- *Tetanus/Diphtheria* -This combination of vaccines are routinely recommended for pregnant women, both those who have never been immunized and those who have not received a booster in 10 years.

Table 6. Immunizations during pregnancy Adapted from Guidelines for vaccinating pregnant women. Recommendations of the Advisory Committee on Immunization Practices (ACIP). Atlanta, Ga.: Centers for Disease Control and Prevention, 2002 [413]

Considered safe if otherwise indicated	Contraindicated during pregnancy or safety not established	Special recommendations pertain
Influenza BCG* Rubella* Hepatitis A Polio (IPV) Yellow fever*	Tetanus and diphtheria toxoids Meningococcal Measles* Varicella* Japanese encephalitis Typhoid (parenteral and Ty21a*)	Hepatitis B Rabies Mumps* Anthrax Pneumococcal Vaccinia*

*--Live, attenuated vaccine.
BCG = bacille Calmette-Guérin; IPV = inactivated polio virus.

Which Vaccines Should Pregnant Women Avoid

The following vaccines can potentially be transmitted to the unborn child and may result in miscarriage, premature birth or birth defects [414]

- *Hepatitis A* - The safety of this vaccine hasn't been determined and it should be avoided during pregnancy. Women at high risk for exposure to this virus should discuss the risks and benefits with their doctors.
- *Measles, Mumps, Rubella (MMR)* - Women should wait at least three months to become pregnant after receiving these live-virus vaccines. If the initial rubella test shows that you are rubella nonimmune, then you will be given the vaccine after delivery.
- *Varicella* - This vaccine, used to prevent chicken pox, should be given at least one month before pregnancy.
- *Pneumococcal* - Because the safety of this vaccine is unknown, it should be avoided in pregnancy except for women who are at high risk or have a chronic illness.
- *Oral Polio Vaccine (OPV) and Inactivated Polio Vaccine (IPV)* - Neither the live-OPV nor the IPV version of this vaccine is recommended for pregnant women. Also, the risk of getting polio in the United States is very low.

Side effects vary from none to those that can occur up to three weeks after vaccination. If you experience any severe side effects, be sure to tell your physician.

- *Hepatitis A* - Soreness and redness at injection site, headache, fatigue, severe allergic reaction in very rare cases
- *Hepatitis B* - Soreness at injection site, fever
- *Influenza* - Redness and swelling at injection site that can last up to two days, fever
- *Tetanus/Diphtheria* - Low-grade fever, soreness and swelling at injection site
- *Measles, Mumps, Rubella (MMR)* - Non-contagious rash, swelling of neck glands and cheeks, pain and stiffness of joints one to two weeks after vaccination
- *Varicella* - Fever, soreness or redness at injection site, rash or small bumps up to three weeks after vaccination
- *Pneumococcal* - Fever, soreness at injection site
- *Oral Polio Vaccine (OPV)* - None
- *Inactivated Polio Vaccine (IPV)* - Redness, discomfort at injection site

Diagnostic Imaging in Pregnancy

Various imaging modalities are available for diagnostic aid during pregnancy; these include X-ray, ultrasonography, magnetic resonance imaging (MRI), and nuclear medicine studies. Of these, diagnostic X-ray is the most frequent cause of anxiety for both the physician and the patient. Much of this anxiety is attributed to a belief that any radiation exposure is harmful and will result in fetal anomalies or death [415]. According to the

American College of Radiology, no single diagnostic X-ray procedure results in radiation exposure to a degree that would threaten the well-being of the developing embryo or fetus [416]. Exposure to a single X-ray during pregnancy is not an indication for therapeutic abortion [417, 418].

X-Ray Exposure

Maternal illness during pregnancy sometimes requires radiographic imaging for proper diagnosis and treatment, this may include imaging with ionizing radiation. Ionizing radiation (x-ray) is composed of high-energy photons that are capable of damaging DNA and generating caustic free radicals [418]. It can result in the following harmful effects: 1) cell death and teratogenic effects, 2) carcinogenesis, and 3) genetic effects or mutations in germ cells [417, 418]. Units traditionally used to measure the effects of X-ray include the rad and roentgen equivalents man (rem). Modern units include the gray (Gy) and sievert (Sv). Commonly during pregnancy, the uterus is shielded for non-pelvic procedures.

Data from animal studies suggest that exposure to high-dose ionizing radiation, much greater than that used in diagnostic procedures, before implantation will most likely be lethal to the embryo [417]. Fetal risks of anomalies, growth restriction, or abortions are not increased with radiation exposure of less than 5 rad, a level above the range of exposure for diagnostic procedures [417]. Radiation exposure from computed tomography (CT) varies depending on the number and spacing of adjacent image sections. Although CT pelvimetry can result in fetal exposures as high as 1.5 rad, exposure can be reduced to approximately 250 mrad by using a low-exposure technique [419]. Spiral (or helical) CT allows continuous scanning of the patient as the couch is moved through the scanner, providing superior speed and image quality. Under typical use with a pitch of 1 or greater, the radiation exposure to the fetus from spiral CT is comparable to conventional CT [420].

Numerous teratogenic effects have developed in animals exposed to large doses of radiation (ie, 100–200 rad). However, in humans, growth restriction, microcephaly, and mental retardation are the most common adverse effects from high-dose radiation [418, 421, 422]. A linear, dose-related association between severe mental retardation and radiation was found, with the important caveat that most cases followed exposure during weeks 10 to 17 of gestation [418, 423, 424]. Until more data becomes available delineating potential fetal risk, it is best to delay non-urgent radiographs during the sensitive period of 10 to 17 weeks of gestation (eight to 15 weeks after conception).

The risk of carcinogenesis as a result of in utero exposure to ionizing radiation is unclear. It is estimated that a 1–2 rad fetal exposure may increase the risk of leukemia by a factor of 1.5–2.0 over natural incidence, and that an estimated 1 in 2 000 children exposed to ionizing radiation in utero will develop childhood leukemia. This is increased from a background rate of approximately 1 in 3 000 [417, 425]. Although radiation is commonly believed to give rise to mutations, data show that usually it merely increases the frequency of mutations occurring naturally in the general population [418]. It is believed that if 10 000 persons were exposed to 1 rad, 10 to 40 new genetic mutations would be induced [426]. When a radiographic study is needed for appropriate management of a pregnant patient, the American College of

Radiology recommends that health care workers should tell patients that x-rays are safe and provide patients with a clear explanation of the benefits of x-ray examinations [427].

Ultrasonography

Ultrasonography involves the use of sound waves and is not a form of ionizing radiation. Ultrasound has a demonstrated record of safety for more than 50 years of clinical use. To date there have been no reports of documented adverse fetal effects for diagnostic ultrasound procedures, including duplex Doppler imaging. There are no known contraindications to ultrasound procedures during pregnancy, and this modality has largely replaced X-ray as the primary method of fetal imaging during pregnancy.

Although no independently replicated epidemiologic data exist to suggest harmful effects of ultrasonography in the fetus, ultrasonography is a form of energy with two main bioeffects in tissue: heat, a direct effect, and oscillatory movements, secondary to the alternating positive and negative pressure waves. These effects are inherent in the physical properties of ultrasonography and have not been shown to be harmful in humans [428]. The bioeffects of clinical ultrasound exams are approximated by the thermal index for heating and by the mechanical index for cavitation effects. Both are indices of exposure, but neither takes time into account.

Thermal index predicts potential for temperature increase, not actual rise, and it remains unknown whether there is a threshold for temperature-related bioeffects. Mechanical index expresses potential to induce inertial cavitation. Mechanical effects are less likely in the fetus, because foci susceptible to cavitation (ie, containing gas) are not present [428]. Evidence in animals shows that exposure to diagnostic ultrasonography can produce significant temperature increases in the fetal brain near bone.

The critical questions include whether the extent of ultrasound-induced temperature rise is sufficient to create a hazard and whether there is a threshold for hyperthermia-induced birth defects. In addition, the determination of possible neurophysiologic effects or responses to clinically relevant exposures is needed [429]. In a review of epidemiologic studies of human exposure to ultrasonography, there were no effects noted on childhood cancer, dyslexia, speech development, or congenital anomalies [430]. However, there is limited evidence that the frequent exposure of the human fetus to ultrasound waves may be associated with a nonsignificant decrease in newborn body weight, a reduction in the frequency of right-handedness, and delayed speech [431, 432. 433].

Magnetic Resonance Imaging

With MRI, magnets that alter the energy state of hydrogen protons are used instead of ionizing radiation [434]. Early studies using MRI in the evaluation of fetal morphology were hindered by fetal motion. Current software and hardware for MRI now allow performance of MR examinations with high-quality images obtained in less than 1 second. Fetal MRI using 1.5-T magnets may be performed in any trimester [435]. However, due to limited data, MRI in the first trimester is currently avoided whenever feasible. Even less is known about the safety of MRI with newer 3-T magnets, and even higher strength MRI systems [436]. When the fetus is imaged by MRI, it is exposed to a combination of three electromagnetic fields of varying strengths and frequencies: static magnetic fields, radiofrequency fields, and fast switching gradient fields.

Overall, there is no indication that the use of clinical MR procedures during pregnancy produces adverse effects, but the safety of such procedures during pregnancy has not been proven or fully evaluated. [429].

Nuclear Medicine

Nuclear studies such as pulmonary ventilation–perfusion, thyroid, bone, and renal scans are performed by "tagging" a chemical agent with a radioisotope. The fetal exposure depends on the physical and biochemical properties of the radioisotope [421]. Technetium Tc $_{99}$m is one of the most commonly used isotopes used for brain, bone, renal, and cardiovascular scans. In general, these procedures result in an embryonic or fetal exposure of less than 0.5 rad [421, 437]. One of the more common nuclear medicine studies performed during pregnancy is the ventilation –perfusion scan for suspected pulmonary embolism. The amount of radiation to which the fetus is exposed in this procedure is small - approximately 50 mrad [438]. Studies have found that the mean fetal doses associated with helical CT were even lower than that employed in a ventilation–perfusion scan [439]. Radioactive iodine readily crosses the placenta and can adversely affect the fetal thyroid, especially if used after 10–12 weeks of gestation. Radioactive isotopes of iodine used for treatment of hyperthyroidism are contraindicated during pregnancy, If a diagnostic scan of the thyroid is essential, $_{123}$I or Technetium Tc $_{99}$m should be used in place of $_{131}$I [438].

Guidelines

The following guidelines for X-ray examination or exposure during pregnancy are suggested by ACOG [415].

1. Women should be counseled that X-ray exposure from a single diagnostic procedure specifically, exposure to less than 5 rad, has not been associated with an increase in fetal anomalies or pregnancy loss.
2. Concern about possible effects of high-dose ionizing radiation exposure should not prevent medically indicated diagnostic X-ray procedures from being performed on a pregnant woman. However, other imaging procedures not associated with ionizing radiation (eg, ultrasonography, MRI) should be considered instead of X-rays when appropriate.
3. Ultrasonography and MRI are not associated with known adverse fetal effects.

4. Consultation with an expert in dosimetry calculation may be helpful in calculating estimated fetal dose when multiple diagnostic X-rays are performed on a pregnant patient.
5. The use of radioactive isotopes of iodine is contraindicated for therapeutic use during pregnancy.
6. Radiopaque and paramagnetic contrast agents are unlikely to cause harm and may be of diagnostic benefit, but these agents should be used during pregnancy only if the potential benefit outweighs the potential risk to the fetus.

Conclusion

Advances in screening, diagnostic evaluation, and treatment strategies of women with pregnancy-related infections have led to reductions in delay in diagnosis, and neonatal and maternal morbidity and mortality. Establishment of objective criteria for evaluating women who present with fever or other evidence of infection has been suggested as a means of improving care [440]. In all pregnant women, as in non-pregnant cases presenting with infections, there should be a complete history and physical examination. The examination should be "from head-to-toe"; with special note of the characteristics of the fever, maximum temperature, presence of diurnal variation, and recent travel. The challenge to the clinician is to select investigations with the highest sensitivity and specificity to increase the probability of a correct diagnosis. In cases of a fever in which the cause is unclear, a number of tests may be useful, depending on the history and physical examination findings. These tests include initial laboratory studies such as a complete blood count with a differential cell count, electrolytes, blood urea nitrogen and creatinine, glucose, calcium, urinalysis, urine cultures, liver function tests, and ESR. Other blood tests would include tests for human immunodeficiency virus (HIV), rapid plasma reagent (RPR), antistreptolysin-O (ASO) titer, rheumatoid arthritis (RA) factor, and antinuclear antibody (ANA), as well as acute and convalescent phase serology tests for various viruses. In addition bloods should be taken for culture, both aerobic and anaerobic, including thick smear of the blood to evaluate for parasites (e.g., malaria). Where appropriate, swabs such as nasal and throat, sputum, stool, or any body discharge should be taken for microscopy and culture.

Diagnostic imaging such as a chest film, abdominal ultrasound, abdominal computed tomography (CT) may aid in select cases. If required, certain specific tests may be required to clinch the diagnosis, such as a tuberculin skin test for the diagnosis of tuberculosis, a lumbar puncture for cerebrospinal fliud analysis in suspected meningitis, an echocardiogram if there is suspicion of infective endocarditis or aortitis, tagged white cell scans may be used to localize an abscess, and a bone marrow biopsy may be indicated if leukemia or a myelodysplastic syndrome is suspected. Other biopsies if indicated may include the liver, bone marrow, lymph node, skin, muscle, or temporal artery. If antibiotics are used to treat infections in pregnancy it is important to remember that some are contraindicated in pregnancy (table 7).

Table 7. Antibiotics that can cause problems during pregnancy

Antibiotic	Problem
Chloramphenicol	Gray baby syndrome In women or fetuses with glucose-6-phosphate dehydrogenase (G6PD) deficiency, the breakdown of red blood cells
Ciprofloxacin	Possibility of joint abnormalities (seen only in animals)
Kanamycin, Streptomycin Gentamycin	Damage to fetal ear, resulting in deafness
Nitrofurantoin	In women or fetuses with G6PD deficiency, the breakdown of red blood cells
Sulfonamides	Jaundice, and possibly brain damage in the newborn (much less with sulfasalazine). In women or fetuses with G6PD deficiency, the breakdown of red blood cells
Tetracycline	Deposit on bone causing reduced bone growth in fetus. Permanent yellowing of teeth, and increasing susceptibility to cavities in children. Occasionally, liver failure in pregnant women.

References

[1] World Health Organization. Maternal and child health. *Wkly. Epidemiol. Rec.* 1989; 24: 184–186.

[2] World Health Organization. New estimates of perinatal mortality. *Wkly. Epidemiol. Rec.* 1996; 71: 297–304.

[3] Stoll, BJ. The global impact of neonatal infection. *Clin. Peritanol.* 1997; 24: 1–21.

[4] Hurley, R. Serious infections in the newborn. *Clin. Obstet. Gynecol.* 1983; 10: 65–91.

[5] Grossman, M. Bacterial and viral infections. In: Rudolph AM, editor. *Rudolph's Pediatrics*. 20th ed. Stanford: Appleton and Lange, 1996; 629–696.

[6] Klein, J.O. and Remington, J.S. Current concepts of infections of the fetus and newborn infant. In: Remington JS, Klein JO, editors. *Infectious diseases of the fetus and newborn infant*. 4th ed. Philadelphia: Saunders, 1995; 1–19.

[7] Zeichner, S.L. and Plotkin, S.A. Mechanisms and pathways of congenital infections. *Clin. Perinatol.* 1988; 15: 163–188.

[8] Andersen, A.N; Vastrup, P; Wohlfahrt, J. *et al.,* Fever in pregnancy and risk of fetal death: a cohort study. *Lancet* 2002; 360:1552-1556.

[9] ACOG Practice Bulletin, No. 20, September 2000. Perinatal Viral and Parasitic Infections.

[10] Gilbert, G.L. Infections in pregnant women. *MJA* 2002; 176: 229–236.

[11] Gilbert, G.L. Routine antenatal screening and prenatal diagnosis of vertically transmissible infection. *Baillieres Clin. Obstet. Gynaecol.* 1993; 7: 1-23.

[12] Carusi, D; Learman, L.A. and Posner, S.F. Human immunodeficiency virus test refusal in pregnancy: a challenge to voluntary testing. *Obstet. Gynecol.* 1998; 91: 540-545.

[13] Workowski, K.A. and Berman, S.M. for the Centers for Disease Control and Prevention. Sexually transmitted diseases treatment guidelines, 2006 [Published correction appears in MMWR Recomm Rep 2006; 55: 997]. MMWR Recomm Rep 2006; 55(RR-11):1-94. Accessed June11, 2008, at: http://www.cdc.gov/mmwr/PDF/rr/rr5511.pdf.

[14] Dinarello, C.A. Thermoregulation and the pathogenesis of fever. *Infect Dis. Clin. North Am.* 1996; 10(2): 433 – 449.

[15] Berry, S.M; Romero, R; Gomez, R *et al.*, Premature parturition is characterized by in utero activation of the fetal immune system. *Am. J. Obstet. Gynecol.* 1995; 173 (4): 1315–1320.

[16] Murthy, V. Antenatal infection/inflammation and fetal tissue injury. *Best Practice and Research Clinical Obstetrics and Gynaecology* 2007; 21(3): 479- 489.

[17] Edwards, M.J. Review: Hyperthermia and fever during pregnancy. *Birth Defects Research* (Part A) 2006; 76: 507–516.

[18] Kopp, E.B. and Medzhitov, R. The Toll-receptor family and control of innate immunity. *Curr. Opin. Immunol.* 1999; 11: 13–18.

[19] Volpe, J.J. Neurobiology of periventricular leukomalacia in the premature infant. Pediatr Res 2001; 50:553–62.

[20] Bal-Price, A. and Brown, G.C. Inflammatory neurodegeneration mediated by nitric oxide from activated glia-inhibiting neuronal respiration, causing glutamate release and excitotoxicity. *J. Neurosci.* 2001; 21: 6480–6491.

[21] Raivich, G; Bohatschek, M; Kloss, C.U., *et al.* Neuroglial activation in the injured brain: graded response, molecular mechanisms and cues to physiological function. *Brain Res. Rev.* 1999; 30: 77–105.

[22] Dietrich, W.D; Busto, R; Valdes, I. *et al.* Effects of normothermic versus mild hyperthermic forebrain ischemia in rats. *Stroke* 1990; 21: 1318–1325.

[23] Bona, E; Hagberg, H; Loberg, E.M., *et al.* Protective effects of moderate hypothermia after neonatal hypoxia–ischemia: short- and long-term outcome. *Pediatr Res.* 1998; 43: 738–745.

[24] Peebles, D.M. Intrauterine Infection and Perinatal Brain Injury. Royal College of Obstetricians and Gynaecologists Scientific Advisory Committee Opinion Paper 3 2002. Accessed on 15 June 2008 from http://www.rcog.org.uk/index.asp?PageID=543.

[25] Graham, J.M. Jr. and Edwards, M.J. Teratogen update: gestational effects of maternal hyperthermia due to febrile illnesses and resultant patterns of defects in humans. *Teratology* 1998; 58: 209-221.

[26] Lynch, J.K; Hirtz, D.G; DeVeber, G. et al. Report of the National Institute of Neurological Disorders and Stroke Workshop on Perinatal and Childhood Stroke. *Pediatrics* 2002; 109:116-123.

[27] Brown AS, Schaefer CA, Wyatt RJ, *et al.* Maternal exposure to respiratory infections and adult schizophrenia spectrum disorders: a prospective birth cohort study. *Schizophr. Bull* 2000; 26: 287-295.

[28] Brown, A.S; Begg, M.D; Gravenstein, S. *et al.* Serologic evidence of prenatal influenza in the etiology of schizophrenia. *Arch. Gen. Psychiatry* 2004; 61: 774-780.

[29] Brown, A.S. Prenatal infection as a risk factor for schizophrenia. *Schizophr. Bull* 2006; 32: 200-202.

[30] Niswander, K.R. and Gordon, M. 1972. Collaborative Perinatal Study of the National Institute of the Neurological Diseases and Stroke. *The women and their pregnancies*. U.S. Dept of Education, Health and Welfare. Philadelphia: WB Saunders. pp. 252-256.

[31] Maldonado, Y.A. Impact of fetal and neonatal viral (and parasitic) infections on later development and disease outcome. In: Barker DJP, Bergmann RL, Ogra PL editors. *The Window of Opportunity: Pre-Pregnancy to 24 Months of Age.* Nestlé Nutr Workshop Ser Pediatr Program. Nestec Ltd., Vevey/S. Karger AG, Basel 2008, pp 225–242.

[32] Mullick, S; Watson-Jones, D; Beksinska, M., *et al.* Sexually transmitted infections in pregnancy: prevalence, impact on pregnancy outcomes, and approach to treatment in developing countries. *Sex Transm. Infect.* 2005; 81:294–302.

[33] Andrews, W.W; Klebanoff, M.A; Thom, E.A., *et al.,* for the National Institute of Child Health and Human Development Maternal-Fetal Medicine Units Network. Midpregnancy genitourinary tract infection with *Chlamydia trachomatis*: association with subsequent preterm delivery in women with bacterial vaginosis and *Trichomonas vaginalis. Am. J. Obstet. Gynecol.* 2006; 194:493-500.

[34] Olshen, E. and Shrier, L.A. Diagnostic tests for chlamydial and gonorrheal infections. *Semin. Pediatr. Infect. Dis.* 2005; 16:192-198.

[35] Handsfield, H.H. and Sparling, P.F. Neisseria gonorrhoeae. In: Mandell GL, Bennett JE, Dolin R editors. *Principles and Practice of Infectious Diseases* (Ed. 4). New York: Churchill Livingstone, 1995; pp 1909-1926.

[36] Farley, T.A. and Cohen, D.A. ElkinsW. Asymptomatic sexually transmitted diseases: the case for screening. *Prev. Med.* 2003; 36:502–509.

[37] Lacey, C.J. and Milne, J.D. Preterm labour in association with Neisseria gonorrhoeae: case reports. *Br. J. Vener Dis.* 1984; 60:123–124.

[38] Brocklehurst, P. Antibiotics for gonorrhoea in pregnancy. *Cochrane Database Syst. Rev.* 2002;(2): CD000098.

[39] Cook, R.L; Hutchison, S.L; Ostergaard, L., *et al.* Systematic review: noninvasive testing for *Chlamydia trachomatis* and *Neisseria gonorrhea*. *Ann. Intern. Med.* 2005; 142:914-925.

[40] Ramus, R.M; Sheffield, J.S; Mayfield, J.A., et al. A randomized trial that compared oral cefixime and intramuscular ceftriaxone for the treatment of gonorrhea in pregnancy. *Am. J. Obstet. Gynecol.* 2001; 185:629-632.

[41] Bell, B.P; Shapiro, C.N; Alter, M.J., *et al.* The diverse patterns of hepatitis A epidemiology in the United States—implications for vaccination strategies. *J. Infect. Dis.* 1998; 178:1579–1584.

[42] Viral hepatitis in pregnancy. ACOG Practice Bulletin No.86. *Obstet. Gynecol.* 2007; 110 (4): 941-955.

[43] Leikin, E; Lysikiewicz, A; Garry, D., *et al.* Intrauterine transmission of hepatitis A virus. *Obstet. Gynecol.* 1996; 88(4 Pt 2): 690-691.

[44] Duff, P. Hepatitis in pregnancy. *Semin. Perinatol.* 1998; 22(4): 277-283.

[45] Elinav, E; Ben-Dov, I.Z; Shapira, Y., *et al.* Acute hepatitis A infection in pregnancy is associated with high rates of gestational complications and preterm labor. *Gastroenterology* 2006; 130(4): 1129-1134.

[46] McDuffie, R.S. Jr. and Bader, T. Fetal meconium peritonitis after maternal hepatitis A. *Am. J. Obstet. Gynecol.* 1999; 180(4): 1031-1032.

[47] Breastfeeding and the use of human milk. American Academy of Pediatrics. Work Group on Breastfeeding. *Pediatrics* 1997; 100(6): 1035-1039.

[48] Ganem, D. and Prince, A.M. Hepatitis B virus infection natural history and clinical consequences. *N. Engl. J. Med.* 2004; 350:1118–1129.

[49] Chang, M.H. Hepatitis B virus infection. *Seminars in Fetal and Neonatal Medicine* 2007; 12(3): 160-167.

[50] Mast, E.E; Margolis, H.S; Fiore, A.E., *et al.* A comprehensive immunization strategy to eliminate transmission of hepatitis B virus infection in the United States: recommendations of the Advisory Committee on Immunization Practices (ACIP) part 1: immunization of infants, children, and adolescents. Advisory Committee on Immunization Practices (ACIP) [published erratum appears in MMWR Morb Mortal Wkly Rep 2006; 55:158–9]. MMWR *Recomm Rep.* 2005; 54(RR-16):1–31.

[51] Lin, H.H; Lee, T.Y; Chen, D.S., *et al.*, Transplacental leakage of HbeAg-positive maternal blood as the most likely route in causing intrauterine infection with hepatitis B virus. *J. Pediatr.* 1987; 111:877–881.

[52] Shepard, C.W; Simard, E.P; Finelli, L., *et al.* Hepatitis B virus infection: epidemiology and vaccination. *Epidemiol. Rev.* 2006; 28: 112–125.

[53] Alter, M.J. Epidemiology of hepatitis C in the West. *Semin. Liver. Dis.* 1995; 15 (1) 5–14.

[54] Mansell, C.J. and Locarnini, S.A. Epidemiology of hepatitis C in the East. *Semin Liver Dis* 1995; 15 (1): 15–32.

[55] Frank, C; Mohamed, M.K; Strickland, G.T., *et al.* The role of parenteral antischistosomal therapy in the spread of hepatitis C virus in Egypt. *Lancet* 2000; 355 (9207): 887–891.

[56] Roberts, E.A. and Yeung, L. Maternal-infant transmission of hepatitis C virus infection. *Hepatology* 2002; 36 (5 Suppl. 1): S106–S113.

[57] Jeffers, L.J; Hasan, F; De Medina, M., *et al.* Prevalence of antibodies to hepatitis C virus among patients with cryptogenic chronic hepatitis and cirrhosis. *Hepatology* 1992; 15:187–190.

[58] Recommendations for prevention and control of hepatitis C (virus HCV) infection and HCV-related chronic disease. Centers for Disease Control and Prevention. *MMWR Recomm Rep.* 1998; 47(RR-19): 1–39.

[59] Ohto, H; Terazawa, S; Sasaki N., *et al.*, Transmission of hepatitis C virus from mothers to infants. The Vertical Transmission of Hepatitis C Virus Collaborative Study Group. *N. Engl. J. Med.* 1994; 330 (11): 744–750.

[60] Thomas, S.L; Newell, M.L; Peckham, C.S., *et al.* A review of hepatitis C virus (HCV) vertical transmission: risks of transmission to infants born to mothers with and without

HCV viraemia or human immunodeficiency virus infection. *Int. J. Epidemiol.* 1998; 27 (1): 108–117.

[61] Fischler, B. Hepatitis C virus infection. *Seminars in Fetal and Neonatal Medicine* 2007; 12(3): 168-173.

[62] Whitley, R.J. and Gnann, J.W. The epidemiology and clinical manifestations of herpes simplex virus infections. In: Roizman B, Whifley RJ, Lopez C, editors. *The Human Herpesviruses*. New York: Raven; 1993; pp 69-105.

[63] Mertz, G. Epidemiology of genital herpes infections. *Infect. Dis. Clin. North Am.* 1993; 4:825-839.

[64] Majeroni, B.A. and Ukkadam, S. Screening and Treatment for Sexually Transmitted Infections in Pregnancy. *Am Fam Physician* 2007; 76(2). Available from: http://www.aafp.org/afp/20070715/265.html Accessed June11, 2008.

[65] Riley, L.E. Herpes Simplex Virus. *Semin. Perinatol.* 1998; 22 (4): 284-292.

[66] Brown, Z.A; Benedetti, J; Selke, S., *et al.* Asymptomatic maternal shedding of herpes simplex virus at the onset of labor: Relationship to preterm labor. *Obstet. Gynecol.* 1996; 87: 483-488.

[67] Forsgren, M. and Malm, G. Herpes simplex virus and pregnancy. *Scand J. Infect. Dis.* Suppl 1996;100:14-19.

[68] Brown, Z.A; Vontver, L.A; Benedetti, J., *et al.* Effects on infants of a first episode of genital herpes during pregnancy. *N. Engl. J. Med.* 1987; 312:1246-1251.

[69] Brown, Z.A. Is neonatal herpes a preventable disease? A review of the risks and mechanisms of neonatal transmission. *Am. J. Gynecol. Health* 1990; 4:17-25.

[70] Nahmias, A.J; Josey, W.E; Naib, Z.M., *et al.* Perinatal risk associated with maternal genital herpes simplex virus infection. *Am. J. Obstet. Gynecol.* 1971; 110:825-837.

[71] Harger, J.H; Amortegui, A.J; Meyer, M.P., *et al.* Characteristics of recurrent genital herpes simplex infections in pregnant women. *Obstet. Gynecol.* 1989; 73:367-372.

[72] Fagnant, R.J. and Monif, G.R. How rare is congenital herpes simplex? *J. Reprod. Med.* 1989; 34:417- 422.

[73] Kohl, S. Neonatal herpes simplex virus infection. *Clin. Perinatol.* 1997; 24:129-150.

[74] Sheffeld, J.S; Hollier, L.M; Hill J.B., *et al.* Acyclovir prophylaxis to prevent herpes simplex virus recurrence at delivery: a systematic review. *Obstet. Gynecol.* 2003; 102:1396-1403.

[75] Watts, D.H; Brown, Z.A; Money, D., *et al.* A double-blind, randomized, placebo-controlled trial of acyclovir in late pregnancy for the reduction of herpes simplex virus shedding and cesarean delivery. *Am. J. Obstet. Gynecol.* 2003; 188:836-843.

[76] Andrews, W.W; Kimberlin, D.F; Whitley, R., *et al.* Valacyclovir therapy to reduce recurrent genital herpes in pregnant women. *Am. J. Obstet. Gynecol.* 2006; 194:774-781.

[77] Prober, C.G; Corey, L; Brown, Z.A., *et al.* The management of pregnancies complicated by genital infections with herpes simplex virus. *Clin. Infect. Dis.* 1992; 15:1031-1038.

[78] Gibbs, R.S; Amstey, M.S; Sweet, R.L., *et al.* Management of genital herpes infection in pregnancy. *Obstet. Gynecol.* 1988; 71:779-780.

[79] Vontver, L.A; Hickok D.E; Brown, Z., *et al.* Recurrent genital herpes simplex virus infections in pregnancy: Infant outcome and frequency of asymptomatic recurrences. *Am. J. Obstet. Gynecol.* 1982; 143:75-84.

[80] Thorne, C. and Newell, M.L. HIV. *Seminars in Fetal and Neonatal Medicine* 2007; 12(3): 174-181.

[81] Thorne, C. and Newell, M.L., Mother-to-child transmission of HIV infection and its prevention. *Curr. HIV Res.* 2003; 1: 447–462.

[82] Nduati, R.W; John, G.C; Ngacha, D.A., *et al.* Effect of breastfeeding and formula feeding on transmission of HIV-1: a randomised clinical trial. *JAMA* 2000; 283: 1167–1174.

[83] Connor, E.M; Sperling, R.S; Gelber, R.D., *et al.* Reduction of maternal–infant transmission of human immunodeficiency virus type 1 with zidovudine treatment. *N. Engl. J. Med.* 1994; 331:1173–1180.

[84] Public Health Service Task Force. Recommendations for use of antiretroviral drugs in pregnant HIV-1-infected women for maternal health and interventions to reduce perinatal HIV-1 transmission in the United States. U.S. Department of Health and Human Services, October 12, 2006. Accessed June12, 2008, at: http://aidsinfo.nih.gov/ContentFiles/PerinatalGL.pdf.

[85] U.S. Preventive Services Task Force. Screening for HIV: recommendation statement. *Ann Intern Med* 2005; 143:32-37.

[86] Cooper, E.R; Charurat, M; Mofenson, L., *et al.* for the Women and Infants' Transmission Study Group. Combination antiretroviral strategies for the treatment of pregnant HIV-1-infected women and prevention of perinatal HIV-1 transmission. *J. Acquir. Immune. Defic. Syndr.* 2002; 29:484-494.

[87] Read, J.S. and Newell, M.K. Efficacy and safety of cesarean delivery for prevention of mother-to-child transmission of HIV-1. *Cochrane Database Syst. Rev.* 2005; (4): CD005479.

[88] European Collaborative Study, Caesarean section and risk of vertical transmission of HIV-1 infection. *Lancet* 1994; 343: 1464–1467.

[89] The European Mode of Delivery Collaboration, Elective caesarean section versus vaginal delivery in preventing vertical HIV-1 transmission: a randomised clinical trial. *Lancet* 1999; 353: 1035–1039.

[90] The International Perinatal HIV group. Mode of delivery and vertical transmission of HIV-1: a meta-analysis from fifteen prospective cohort studies. *N. Engl. J. Med.* 1999; 340: 977–987.

[91] Read, J.S. and Newell, M.L. Cesarean delivery for prevention of mother-to-child transmission of HIV. *Cochrane Database Syst. Rev.* 2005; 4.

[92] European HIV in Obstetrics Group. Higher rates of post-partum complications in HIV infected than in uninfected women irrespective of mode of delivery. *AIDS* 2004; 18: 933–938.

[93] Apea-Kubi, K.A; Yamaguchi, S; Sakyi, B., *et al.* *Neisseria gonorrhea, Chlamydia trachomatis,* and *Treponema pallidum* infection in antenatal and gynecological patients at Korle-Bu Teaching Hospital, Ghana. *Jpn J. Infect. Dis.* 2004;57:253-256.

[94] World Health Organization, Global prevalence and incidence of curable STIs, World Health Organization, Geneva (2001) WHO/CDS/CDR/EDC/2001.10.

[95] Fenton, K.A. A multilevel approach to understanding the resurgence and evolution of infectious syphilis in Western Europe. *Eurosurveillance* 2004; 9(10–11): 3–4.

[96] Simms, I. and Ward, H. Congenital syphilis in the United Kingdom. Are we prepared? *Sex Transm. Infect.* 2006; 82 (1):1.

[97] Centers for Disease Control and Prevention, Sexually transmitted diseases treatment guidelines, 2006; *MMWR* 55 (No. RR-11):1–100.

[98] Walker, G.J.A. and Walker, D.G. Congenital syphilis: A continuing but neglected problem. *Seminars in Fetal and Neonatal Medicine* 2007; 12(3): 198-206.

[99] Finelli, L; Berman, S.M; Koumans, E.H., *et al.* Congenital syphilis. *Bull World Health Organ.* 1998; 76 (Suppl. 2): 126–128.

[100] Schmid, G. Economic and programmatic aspects of congenital syphilis prevention. *Bull World Health Organ* 2004; 82: 402–409.

[101] Goldenberg, R.L. and Thompson, C. The infectious origins of stillbirth. *Am. J. Obstet. Gynecol.* 2003; 189 (3): 861–873.

[102] Sheffield, J.S; Sanchez, P.J; Morris, G., *et al.* Congenital syphilis after maternal treatment for syphilis during pregnancy. *Am. J. Obstet. Gynecol.* 2002; 186 (3): 569–573.

[103] Goldenberg, R.L; Culhane, J.F. and Johnson, D.C. Maternal infection and adverse fetal and neonatal outcomes. *Clin. Perinatol.* 2005; 32 (3): 523–559.

[104] Ingraham, N.R. The value of penicillin alone in the prevention and treatment of congenital syphilis. *Acta. Derm. Venereol.* Suppl 1950;31(Suppl 24):60–87.

[105] Wendel, G.D. Jr; Sheffield, J.S; Hollier, L.M., *et al.* Treatment of syphilis in pregnancy and prevention of congenital syphilis. *Clin. Infect. Dis.* 2002;35(suppl 2):S200-209.

[106] World Health Organization. *Guidelines for the management of sexually transmitted infections*. WHO, Geneva (2003).

[107] Riggs, M.A. and Klebanoff, M.A. Treatment of vaginal infections to prevent preterm birth: a meta-analysis. *Clin. Obstet. Gynecol.* 2004; 47:796-807.

[108] Klebanoff, M.A; Carey, J.C; Hauth, J.C., *et al.* for the National Institute of Child Health and Human Development Network Maternal-Fetal Medicine Units. Failure of metronidazole to prevent preterm delivery among pregnant women with asymptomatic *Trichomonas vaginalis* infection. *N. Engl. J. Med.* 2001; 345:487-493.

[109] Silver, H.M; Sperling, R.S; St Clair, P.J., *et al.* Evidence relating bacterial vaginosis to intraamniotic infection. *Am. J. Obstet. Gynecol.* 1989; 161: 808–812.

[110] Martius, J. and Eschenbach, D.A. The role of bacterial vaginosis as a cause of amniotic fluid infection, chorioamnionitis and prematurity–a review. *Arch. Gynecol. Obstet.* 1990; 247: 1–13.

[111] Watts, D.H; Krohn, M.A; Hillier, S.L., *et al.* Bacterial vaginosis as a risk factor for post-cesarean endometritis. *Obstet. Gynecol.* 1990; 75: 52–58.

[112] Kurki, T; Sivonen, A; Renkonen, O.V., *et al.*, Bacterial vaginosis in early pregnancy and pregnancy outcome. *Obstet. Gynecol.* 1992; 80: 173–177.

[113] McGregor, J.A; French, J.I; Jones, W., *et al.*, Bacterial vaginosis is associated with prematurity and vaginal fluid mucinase and sialidase: results of a controlled trial of topical clindamycin cream. *Am. J. Obstet. Gynecol.* 1994; 170:1048–1059.

[114] Hay PE, R.F; Lamont, R.F; Taylor-Robinson, D., *et al.*, Abnormal bacterial colonisation of the genital tract and subsequent preterm delivery and late miscarriage. *BMJ* 1994; 308: 295–298.

[115] Sewankambo, N; Gray, R.H; Wawer, M.J., *et al.* HIV-1 infection associated with abnormal vaginal flora morphology and bacterial vaginosis. *Lancet* 1997; 350: 546–550.

[116] Grether, J.K. and Nelson, K.B. Maternal infection and cerebral palsy in infants of normal birth weight. *JAMA* 1997; 278: 207–211.

[117] Ralph, S.G; Rutherford, A.J. and Wilson, J.D. Influence of bacterial vaginosis on conception and miscarriage in the first trimester: cohort study. *BMJ* 1999; 319: 220–223.

[118] McDonald, H.M; Brocklehurst. P. and Gordon, A. Antibiotics for treating bacterial vaginosis in pregnancy. *Cochrane Database of Syst Rev* 2007; Issue 1. Art. No.: CD000262.

[119] Keelan, J.A; Blumenstein, M; Helliwell, R.J., *et al.* Cytokines, prostaglandins and parturition–a review. *Placenta* 2003; 24 (supplement A): S33–S46.

[120] Ugwumadu, A. Role of antibiotic therapy for bacterial vaginosis and intermediate flora in pregnancy. *Best Practice and Research Clinical Obstetrics and Gynaecology* 2007; 21(3): 391- 402.

[121] Okun, N; Gronau, K.A. and Hannah, M.E. Antibiotics for bacterial vaginosis or Trichomonas vaginalis in pregnancy: a systematic review. *Obstet. Gynecol.* 2005; 105(4): 857-868.

[122] Zanghellini, S.B; Boppana, V.C; Emery, P.D., et al. Asymptomatic primary cytomegalovirus infection: virologic and immunologic features. *J. Infect. Dis.* 1999; 180: 702–707.

[123] Klemola, E. and Kaariainen, L. Cytomegalovirus as a possible cause of a disease resembling infectious mononucleosis. *BMJ* 1965; 5470:1099-1102.

[124] Fowler, K.B; Stagno, S and Pass, R.F. Maternal age and congenital cytomegalovirus infection: screening of two diverse newborn populations, 1980-1990. *J. Infect. Dis.* 1993; 168:552-556.

[125] Malm, G and Engman, M.L. Congenital cytomegalovirus infections. *Seminars in Fetal and Neonatal Medicine* 2007; 12(3): 154-159.

[126] Adler, S.P; Finney, J.W; Manganello, A.M., *et al.* Prevention of child-to-mother transmission of cytomegalovirus by changing behaviors: a randomized controlled trial. *Pediatr Infect. Dis.* J 1996; 15:240-246.

[127] Daniel, Y; Gull, I; Peyser, M.R., *et al.* Congenital cytomegalovirus infection. *Eur. J. Obstet. Gynecol. Reprod. Biol.* 1995; 63:7-16.

[128] Stagno, S; Pass, R.F; Dworsky, M.E., *et al.* Maternal cytomegalovirus infection and perinatal transmission. *Clin. Obstet. Gynecol.* 1982; 25:563-576.

[129] Stagno, S; Pass, R.F; Cloud, G., *et al.* Primary cytomegalovirus infection in pregnancy. Incidence, transmission to fetus, and clinical outcome. *JAMA* 1986; 256:1904-1908.

[130] Hagay, Z.J; Biran, G; Ornoy, A., *et al.* Congenital cytomegalovirus infection: a long-standing problem still seeking a solution. *Am. J. Obstet. Gynecol.* 1996; 174:241- 245.

[131] Stagno, S. and Whitley, R.J. Herpesvirus infections of pregnancy. Part 1: Cytomegalovirus and Epstein-Barr virus infections. *N. Engl. J. Med.* 1985; 313:1270-1274.

[132] Fowler, K.B; Stagno, S; Pass, R.F., *et al.* The outcome of congenital cytomegalovirus infection in relation to maternal antibody status. *N. Engl. J. Med.* 1992; 326:663-667.

[133] Stagno, S. and Britt, B. Cytomegalovirus. In: J.S. Remington, J.O. Klein, C.B. Wilson and C.J. Baker, editors. *Infectious diseases of the fetus and newborn infant* (6th ed.), Elsevier Saunders, Philadelphia (2006), pp. 740–781.

[134] Bale, J.F. Jr.; Zimmerman, B; Dawson, J.D., *et al.* Cytomegalovirus transmission in child care homes. *Arch. Pediatr Adolesc. Med.* 1999; 153: 75–79.

[135] Nigro, G; Adler, S.P; La Torre, T., *et al.* Congenital Cytomegalovirus Collaborating Group. Passive immunization during pregnancy for congenital cytomegalovirus infection. *N. Engl. J. Med.* 2005; 353: 1350–1362.

[136] Chorba, T; Coccia, P; Holman, R.C., *et al.* The role of parvovirus B19 in aplastic crisis and erythema infectiosum (fifth disease). *J. Infect. Dis.* 1986; 154:383-393.

[137] Rotbart, H. Human Parvovirus infection. *Ann. Rev. Med.* 1990; 41:25-34.

[138] Brown, K; Anderson, S. and Young, N. Erythrocyte P antigen: Cellular receptor for B19. *Science* 1993; 262:114-117.

[139] Young, N. and Mortimer, P. Viruses and bone marrow failure. *Blood* 1984; 63: 729-737.

[140] Morey, A; Ferguson, D. and Fleming, K. Ultrastructural features of fetal erythroid precursors infected with parvovirus B19 in vitro: Evidence of cell death by apoptosis. *J. Pathol.* 1993; 169: 213-220.

[141] Thurn, J. Human parvovirus B19: historical and clinical review. *Rev. Infect. Dis.* 1988; 10:1005-1011.

[142] Rice, P.S. and Cohen, B.J. A school outbreak of parvovirus B19 infection investigated using salivary antibody assays. *Epidemiol. Infect.* 1996; 116:331-338.

[143] Harger, J.H; Adler, S.P; Koch, W.C., *et al.* Prospective evaluation of 618 pregnant women exposed to parvovirus B19: risks and symptoms. *Obstet. Gynecol.* 1998; 91:413-420.

[144] Valeur-Jensen, A.K; Pedersen, C.B; Westergaard, T., et al., Risk factors for parvovirus B19 infection in pregnancy. *JAMA* 1999; 281:1099-1105.

[145] McCarter-Spaulding, D. Parvovirus B19 in Pregnancy. *JOGNN* 2002; 31: 107–112.

[146] Rodis, J. F; Borgida, A. F; Wilson, M.., *et al.* Management of parvovirus infection in pregnancy and outcomes of hydrops: A survey of members of the Society of Perinatal Obstetricians. *Am. J. Obstet. Gynecol.* 1998; 179: 985-988.

[147] Rodis, J.F; Quinn, D.L; Gary, G.W., *et al.* Management and outcomes of pregnancies complicated by human B19 parvovirus infection: A prospective study. *Am. J. Obstet. Gynecol.* 1990; 163:1168-1171.

[148] Gillespie, S.M; Cartter, M.L; Asch, S., *et al.* Occupational risk of human parvovirus B19 infection for school and day-care personnel during an outbreak of erythema infectiosum. *JAMA* 1990; 263: 2061-2065.

[149] Cartter, M.L; Farley, T.A; Rosengren, S., *et al.* Occupational risk factors for infection with parvovirus B19 among pregnant women. *J. Infect. Dis.* 1991; 163:282-285.

[150] Guidozzi, F; Ballot, D. and Rothberg, A.D. Human B19 parvovirus infection in an obstetric population. A prospective study determining fetal outcome. *J. Reprod. Med.* 1994; 39:36-38.

[151] Public Health Laboratory Service Working Party on Fifth Disease. Prospective study of human parvovirus (B19) infection in pregnancy. *BMJ* 1990; 300:1166-1170.

[152] Markenson, G.R. and Yancey, M.K. Parvovirus B 19 infections in pregnancy. *Semin. Perinatol.* 1998; 22(4): 309-317.

[153] Risks associated with human parvovirus B19 infection. *MMWR Morbid Mortal Wkly Rep.* 1989; 38:81-88, 93-97.

[154] Gratacos, E; Torres, P.J; Vidal, J., *et al.* The incidence of human parvovirus B19 infection during pregnancy and its impact on perinatal outcome. *J. Infect. Dis.* 1995; 171:1360-1363.

[155] Jordan, J.A. Identification of human parvovirus B19 infection in idiopathic nonimmune hydrops fetalis. *Am. J. Obstet. Gynecol.* 1996; 174:37-42.

[156] Yaegashi, N; Okamura, K; Yajima, A., *et al.* The frequency of human parvovirus B19 infection in nonimmune hydrops fetalis. *J. Perinat. Med.* 1994; 22: 159-163.

[157] Pryde, P.G; Nugent, C.E; Pridjian, G., *et al.* Spontaneous resolution of nonimmune hydrops fetalis secondary to human parvovirus B19 infection. *Obstet. Gynecol.* 1992; 79:859-861.

[158] Sheikh, A.U; Ernest, J.M. and O'Shea, M. Long-term outcomein fetal hydrops from parvovirus B19 infection. *Am. J. Obstet. Gynecol.* 1992; 167:337-341.

[159] Humphrey, W; Magoon, M. and O'Shaughnessy, R. Severe nonimmune hydrops secondary to parvovirus B-19 infection: Spontaneous reversal in utero and survival of a term infant. *Obstet. Gynecol.* 1991; 78:900-902.

[160] Miller, E; Fairley, C.K; Cohen, B.J., *et al.* Immediate and long term outcome of human parvovirus B19 infection in pregnancy. *Br. J. Obstet. Gynaecol.* 1998; 105:174-178.

[161] Rodis, J.F; Rodner, C; Hansen, A.A., *et al.* Long-term outcome of children following maternal human parvovirus B19 infection. *Obstet. Gynecol.* 1998; 91:125-128.

[162] Katz, V.L; McCoy, C; Kuller, J.A., *et al.* An association between fetal parvoviru.s B19 infection and fetal anomalies: A report of two cases. *Am. J. Perinatol.* 1996; 13:43- 45.

[163] Tiessen, R.G; Van Elsacker-Niele, A.M.W; Vermeij-Keers, C., *et al.* A fetus with a parvovirus B19 infection and congenital anomalies. *Prenat. Diag.* 1994; 14:173-176.

[164] Weiland, H.T; Vermeij-Keers, C; Salimans, M.M.M., *et al.* Parvovirus B19 associated with fetal abnormality. *Lancet* 1987; 1: 682-683.

[165] Conry, J; Torok, T. and Andrews, I. Perinatal encephalopathy secondary to in utero human parvovirus B19 (HPV) infection. *Neurol.* 1993; 43:A346.

[166] Hartwig, N.G; Vermeij-Keers, C; Van Elsacker-Niele, A.M.W., *et al.* Embryonic malformations in a case of intrauterine parvovirus B19 infection. *Teratol.* 1989; 39:295 302.

[167] Torok, T. Human parvovirus B19, in Remington J, Klein J, editors. *Infectious diseases of the fetus and newborn infant*. Philadelphia: PA, Saunders, 1995, pp 668-702.

[168] Schwartz, T.F; Roggendorf, M; Hottentrag, B., *et al.* Human parvovirus B19 infection in pregnancy. *Lancet* 1988; 2:566-567.

[169] Kinney, J; Anderson, L; Farrar, J., *et al.* Risk of adverse outcomes of pregnancy after human parvovirus B19 infection. *J. Infect. Dis.* 1988; 157:663-667.

[170] Cohen, B. Parvovirus B19: An expanding spectrum of disease. *BMJ* 1995; 311:1549-1552.

[171] Kurtzman, G.J; Cohen, B; Meyers, P., *et al.* Persistent B19 parvovirus infection as a cause of severe chronic anaemia in children with acute lymphocytic leukaemia. *Lancet* 1988; 2:1159-1162.

[172] Peters, M. and Nicolaides, K. Cordocentesis for the diagnosis and treatment of human fetal parvovirus infection. *Obstet. Gynecol.* 1990; 75:501-504.

[173] Sahakian, V; Weiner, C.P; Naides, S.J., *et al.* Intrauterine transfusion treatment of nonimmune hydrops fetalis secondary to human parvovirus B19 infection. *Am. J. Obstet. Gynecol.* 1991; 164:1090-1091.

[174] Centers for Disease Control and Prevention: Recommendations of the immunization practices advisory committee: Varicella-zoster immune globulin for the prevention of chickenpox. *MMWR* 1984; 33: 84-99.

[175] O'Riordan, M; O'Gorman, C; Morgan, C., *et al.* Sera prevalence of varicella zoster virus in pregnant women in Dublin. *Ir. J. Med. Sci.* 2000; 169:288.

[176] World Health Organization. Epidemiology of chicken-pox. *Weekly Epidemiology Record.* 1992; 67:118 –119.

[177] Miller, E; Marshall, R. and Vurdien, J.E. Epidemiology, outcome and control of varicella zoster virus infection. *Rev. Med. Microbiol.* 1993; 4:222–230.

[178] Shlyakhov, E; Segev, S. and Rubinstein, E. Main viral diseases with in utero transmission of pathogen during pregnancy: epidemiology, pathological features and outcome *Acta Obstet. Gynecol. Scand* 1998; 77: 875–882.

[179] Enders, G. Serodiagnosis of Varicella-Zoster virus infection in pregnancy and standardization of the ELISA IgG and IgM antibody tests. *Dev. Biol. Stand.* 1982; 52:221-236.

[180] Varicella-related deaths among adults-United States, 1997. *MMWR Morb Mortal Wkly Rep.* 1997; 46:409- 412.

[181] Harris, R.E. and Rhoades, E.R. Varicella pneumonia complicating pregnancy: Report of a case and review of the literature. *Obstet. Gynecol.* 1965; 25:734-740.

[182] Smego, R.A. Jr. and Asperilla, M.O. Use of acyclovir for varicella pneumonia during pregnancy. *Obstet. Gynecol.* 1991; 78:1112-1116.

[183] Paryani, S.G. and Arvin, A.M. Intrauterine infection with varicella-zoster virus after maternal varicella. *N. Engl. J. Med.* 1986; 314:1542-1546.

[184] Chapman, S.J.Varicella in Pregnancy. *Semin. Perinatol.* 1998; 22(4): 339-346.

[185] Chickenpox in pregnancy. RCOG 2007; Guidelines No.13. Available from: http://www.rcog.org.uk/resources/Public/pdf/greentop13_chickenpox0907.pdf. Accessed on 22 June, 2008.

[186] Jones, K.L; Johnson, K.A. and Chambers, C.D. Offspring of women infected with varicella during pregnancy: a prospective study. *Teratology* 1994; 49:29-32.

[187] Pastuszak, A.L; Levy, M; Schick, B., *et al.* Outcome after maternal varicella infection in the first 20 weeks of pregnancy. *N. Engl. J. Med.* 1994; 330:901-905.

[188] Pretorius, D.H; Hayward, I; Jones, K.L., *et al.* Sonographic evaluation of pregnancies with maternal varicella infection. *J. Ultrasound. Med.* 1992; 11:459- 463.

[189] Brunell, P.A. Placental transfer of varicella-zoster antibody. *Pediatrics* 1966; 38:1034-1038.

[190] Meyers, J.D. Congenital varicella in term infants: Risk reconsidered. *J. Infect. Dis.* 1974; 129:215-217.

[191] Gilbert, G.L. *Varicella in Infectious Disease in Pregnancy and the Newborn Infant.* Chur, Switzerland: Harwood Academic Publishers; 1991, pp 339-347.

[192] Wallace, M.R; Bowler, W.A; Murray, N.B., *et al.* Treatment of adult varicella with oral aciclovir. A randomized placebo controlled trial. *Ann Intern Med* 1992; 117: 358–363.

[193] Stone, K.M; Reiff-Eldridge, R; White, A.D., *et al.* Pregnancy outcomes following systemic prenatal acyclovir exposure: conclusions from the international acyclovir pregnancy registry, 1984–99. Birth Defects. *Res. A Clin. Mol. Teratol.* 2004; 70: 201–207.

[194] Ratanajamit, C; Vinther Skriver, M; Jepsen, P., *et al.* Adverse pregnancy outcome in women exposed to acyclovir during pregnancy; a population based observational study. *Scand J. Infect. Dis.* 2003; 35:225–229.

[195] Petersen. E. Toxoplasmosis. *Seminars in Fetal and Neonatal Medicine* 2007; 12(3): 214-223.

[196] Foulon, W; Villena, I; Stray-Pedersen, B., *et al.* Treatment of toxoplasmosis during pregnancy: a multicenter study of impact on fetal transmission and children's sequelae at age 1 year. *Am. J. Obstet. Gynecol.* 1999; 180:410-415.

[197] Hohlfeld, P; Daffos, F; Costa, J.M., *et al.* Prenatal diagnosis of congenital toxoplasmosis with a polymerase-chain-reaction test on amniotic fluid. *N. Engl. J. Med.* 1994; 331:695-699.

[198] Stray-Pedersen, B. Toxoplasmosis in pregnancy. *Baillieres Clin. Obstet. Gynaecol.* 1993; 7:107-137.

[199] Wilson, C.B; Remington, J.S; Stagno, S., *et al.* Development of adverse sequelae in children born with subclinical congenital Toxoplasma infection. *Pediatrics* 1980; 66:767-774.

[200] Desmonts, G. and Couvreur, J. Congenital toxoplasmosis. A prospective study of 378 pregnancies. *N. Engl. J. Med.* 1974; 290:1110-1116.

[201] Daffos, F; Forestier, F; Capella-Pavlovsky, M., *et al.* Prenatal management of 746 pregnancies at risk for congenital toxoplasmosis. *N. Engl. J. Med.* 1988; 318:271-275.

[202] Liesenfeld, O; Press, C; Montoya, J.G., *et al.* False-positive results in immunoglobulin M (IgM) toxoplasma antibody tests and importance of confirmatory testing: the Platelia Toxo IgM test. *J. Clin. Microbiol.* 1997; 35:174–178.

[203] Liesenfeld, O; Montoya, J.G; Kinney, S., *et al.* Effect of testing for IgG avidity in the diagnosis of *T. gondii* infection in pregnant women: experience in a U.S. reference laboratory. *J. Infect. Dis.* 2001; 183: 1248–1253.

[204] Robert-Gangneux, F; Commerce, V; Tourte-Schaefer, C., *et al.* Performance of a Western blot assay to compare mother and newborn anti-Toxoplasma antibodies for the

early neonatal diagnosis of congenital toxoplasmosis. *Eur. J. Clin. Microbiol. Infect. Dis.* 1999; 18:648–654.

[205] McLeod, R; Boyer, K; Karrison, T., *et al.* Outcome of treatment for congenital toxoplasmosis, 1981–2004: the National Collaborative Chicago-Based Congenital Toxoplasmosis Study. *Clin. Infect. Dis.* 2006; 42: 1383–1394.

[206] Best, J.M. Rubella. *Seminars in Fetal and Neonatal Medicine* 2007; 12(3):182-192.

[207] Robertson, S.E; Featherstone, D.A; Gacic-Dobo, M., *et al.* Rubella and congenital rubella syndrome: global update. *Pan. Am. J. Public. Health* 2003; 14 (5): 306–315.

[208] Adler, S. and Koch, W.C. Human parvovirus infections. In: J.S. Remington, J.O. Klein, C.B. Wilson and C.J. Baker, Editors. *Infectious diseases of the fetus and newborn infant* (6th ed.), Elsevier Saunders, Philadelphia (2006), pp. 868–892.

[209] Miller, E; Cradock-Watson, J.E. and Pollock, T.M. Consequences of confirming maternal rubella at successive stages of pregnancy. *Lancet* 1982; 2: 781–784.

[210] Best, J.M; Banatvala, J.E; Morgan-Capner, P., *et al.* Fetal infection after maternal reinfection with rubella: criteria for defining reinfection. *BMJ* 1989; 299: 773-775.

[211] Morgan-Capner, P; Miller, E; Vurdien, J.E., et al. Outcome of pregnancy after maternal reinfection with rubella. *Commun. Dis. Rep.* (Lond Engl Rev) 1991; 1 (6): R57–R59.

[212] Morgan-Capner, P. and Crowcroft, N.S., on behalf of the PHLS Joint Working Party of the Advisory Committees of Virology and Vaccines and Immunisation. Guidelines on the management of, and exposure to, rash illness in pregnancy (including consideration of relevant antibody screening programmes in pregnancy). *Commun. Dis. Public Health* 2002; 5(1): 59-71.

[213] Hanshaw, J.B; Dudgeon, J.A. and Marshall, W.C. *Viral diseases of the fetus and newborn* (2nd ed.), Saunders, Philadelphia, London, Toronto (1985).

[214] Cooper, L.Z. and Alford, C.A. Rubella. In: J.S. Remington, J.O. Klein, C.B. Wilson and C.J. Baker, editors. *Infectious diseases of the fetus and newborn infant* (6th ed.), Elsevier, Saunders, Philadelphia (2006), pp. 894–926.

[215] Saltzman, R.L. and Jordan, M.C. Viral infections. In Burrow GN, Ferris TF, editors. *Medical complications during pregnancy.* 3rd ed. Philadelphia: Saunders, 1988; 372–388.

[216] Slater, P.E; Roitman, M; Leventhal, H., *et al.* Control of rubella in Israel: progress and challenge. *Publ. Hlth. Rev.* 1996; 24: 183–192.

[217] Gumpel, S.M; Hayes, K. and Dudgeon, J.A. Congenital perceptive deafness: role of intrauterine rubella. *BMJ* 1971; 2: 300–304.

[218] Yadav, S; Gupta, S. and Kumari, S. Seroprevalence of rubella in women of reproductive age. *Indian J. Pathol. Microbiol.* 1995; 38: 139–142

[219] Robinson, J; Lemay, M. and Vaudry, W.L. Congenital rubella after anticipated maternal immunity: two cases and a review of the literature. *Pediatr. Infect. Dis.* 1994; 13: 812–815.

[220] Aboudy,Y; Fogel, A; Barnea, B., *et al.* Subclinical rubella reinfection during pregnancy followed by transmission of virus to the fetus. *J. Infect.* 1997; 34: 273–276.

[221] Control of communicable diseases manual. Benenson A, editor. 16th ed. Washington, DC: *Am. Publ. Hlth. Assn.*, 1995.

[222] Zeichner, S.L. and Plotkin, S.A. Mechanisms and pathways of congenital infections. *Clin. Perinatol.* 1988; 15: 163–188.

[223] Töndury, G. and Smith, D.W. Fetal rubella pathology. *J. Pediatr.* 1966; 68: 867–879.

[224] Lee, J.Y. and Bowden, D.S. Rubella virus replication and links to teratogenicity. *Clin. Microbiol. Rev.* 2000; 13:571–587.

[225] Banatvala, J.E. and Brown, D.W.G. Rubella. Lancet 2004; 363: 1127–1137.

[226] Stamm, W.E. and Hooton, T.M. Management of urinary tract infections in adults. *N. Engl. J. Med.* 1993; 329: 1328–1334.

[227] Lee, J.B.L. and Neild, G.H. Urinary tract infection. *Medicine* 2007; 35(8): 423-428.

[228] Le, J; Briggs, G.G; McKeown, A.., et al. Urinary tract infections during pregnancy. *Ann. Pharmacother.* 2004; 38 (10): 1692-1701.

[229] Smaill, F. and Vazquez, J.C. Antibiotics for asymptomatic bacteriuria in pregnancy. *Cochrane Database Syst. Rev.* 2007; Issue 2. Art. No.: CD000490.

[230] Dwyer, P.L. and O'Reilly, M. Recurrent urinary tract infection in the female. *Curr Opin Obstet. Gynecol.* 2002; 14(5): 537- 543.

[231] Lee, M; Bozzo, P; Einarson, A., et al. Urinary tract infections in pregnancy. *Can. Fam. Physician* 2008; 54: 853-854.

[232] Krcmery, S; Hromec, J. and Demesova, D. Treatment of lower urinary tract infection in pregnancy. *Int. J. Antimicrob. Agents* 2001; 17: 279-282.

[233] Mikhail, M.S. and Anyaegbunam, A. Lower urinary tract dysfunction in pregnancy: a review. *Obstet. Gynecol. Surv.* 1995; 50: 675-683.

[234] Nicolle, L.E; Bradley, S; Colgan, R., *et al.* Infectious diseases society of america guidelines for the diagnosis and treatment of asymptomatic bacteriuria in adults. *Clin. Infect. Dis.* 2005; 40: 643-654.

[235] Car, J. Urinary tract infections in women: diagnosis and management in primary care. *BMJ* 2006; 332: 94-97.

[236] Kontiokari, T; Sundqvist, K; Nuutinen, M., *et al.* Randomised trial of cranberry-lingonberry juice and Lactobacillus GG drink for the prevention of urinary tract infections in women. *BMJ* 2001 322: 1571.

[237] Jepson, R.G; Mihaljevic, L. and Craig, J. Cranberries for preventing urinary tract infections. *Cochrane Database Syst. Rev.* 2008;(1): CD001321.

[238] Miller, J.M. and Raimer, K.A. Urinary tract infection and pyelonephritis. In: Posterek JG, editor. *Obstetric and Gynecologic Infectious Diseases*. 2nd ed. New York: Raven Press, 1994: 274-293.

[239] Schieve, L.A; Handler, A; Hershow, R., *et al.* Urinary tract infection during pregnancy: its association with maternal morbidity and perinatal outcome. *Am. J. Public Health* 1994; 84(3): 405- 410.

[240] Steketee, R.W; Nahlen, B.L; Parise, M.E., *et al.* The burden of malaria in pregnancy in malaria-endemic areas. *Am. J. Trop. Med. Hyg.* 2001; 64 (suppl): 28.

[241] Luxemburger, C; McGready, R; Kham, A., *et al.* Effects of malaria during pregnancy on infant mortality in an area of low malaria transmission. *Am. J. Epidemiol.* 2001; 154: 459-465.

[242] Guyatt, H.L. and Snow, R.W. Malaria in pregnancy as an indirect cause of infant mortality in sub-Saharan Africa. *Trans R Soc. Trop. Med. Hyg.* 2001; 95: 569-576.

[243] Murphy, S.C. and Breman, J.G. Gaps in the childhood malaria burden in Africa: cerebral malaria, neurological sequelae, anemia, respiratory distress, hypoglycemia, and complications of pregnancy. *Am. J. Trop. Med. Hyg.* 2001; 64 (suppl): 57-67.
[244] Lesko, C.R; Arguin, P.M. and Newman, R.D. Congenital malaria in the United States: a review of cases from 1966 to 2005. *Arch. Pediatr. Adolesc. Med.* 2007; 161:1062-1067.
[245] Centers for Disease Control and Prevention. Malaria during pregnancy. Available from: http://www.cdc.gov/malaria/pregnancy.htm Accessed on June 29, 2008.
[246] Dorman, E.S.C. Malaria in pregnancy. *Curr. Obstet. Gynaecol.* 2000;10:183–189.
[247] Desai, M; ter Kuile, F.O; Nosten, F., *et al.* Epidemiology and burden of malaria in pregnancy. *Lancet Infect. Dis.* 2007; 7:93–104.
[248] Sirima, S.B; Sawadogo, R; Moran, A.C., *et al.* Failure of a chloroquine chemoprophylaxis program to adequately prevent malaria during pregnancy in Koupéla District, Burkina Faso. *Clin. Infect. Dis.* 2003; 36:1374–1382.
[249] Brabin, B.J. An analysis of malaria in pregnancy in Africa. *Bull World Health Organ.* 1983; 61:1005-1016.
[250] Menendez, C; Ordi, J; Ismail, M.R., *et al.* The impact of placental malaria on gestational age and birth weight. *J. Infect. Dis.* 2000; 181:1740-1745.
[251] Menendez, C; Fleming, A.F. and Alonso, P.L. Malaria-related anaemia. *Parasitol. Today* 2000; 16:469-476.
[252] World Health Organization. Global Malaria Programme. Impact of Malaria during pregnancy in sub-Saharan Africa. Available from: http://www.who.int/malaria/pregnantwomenandinfants.html. Accessed on June 29, 2008.
[253] Singh, N; Awadhia, S.B; Dash, A.P., *et al.* Malaria during pregnancy: a priority area for malaria research and control in South-East Asia. *WHO-SEARO Regional Health Forum* 2005; 9 (1).
[254] Guyatt, H.L. and Snow, R.W. Impact of malaria during pregnancy on low birth weight in sub-Saharan Africa. *Clin Microbiol Rev* 2004; 17: 760-769.
[255] Parmet, S; Lynm, C. and Glass, R. Malaria: JAMA patient page. *JAMA* 2007; 297:2310.
[256] Alvarez, J.R; Al-Khan, A. and Apuzzio, J.J. Malaria in pregnancy.*Infect Dis Obstet. Gynecol.* 2005; 13:229 –236.
[257] Uneke, C.J. Impact of placental Plasmodium falciparum malaria on pregnancy and perinatal outcome in sub-Saharan Africa: Introduction to placental malaria. *Yale J. Biol. Med.* 2007; 80: 39-50.
[258] Lagerberg, R.E. Malaria in Pregnancy: A Literature Review. *JMWH* 2008; 53(3): 209-214.
[259] Centers for Disease Control and Prevention. Malaria. 2007. Available at: http://www.cdc.gov/malaria/. Accessed on June 29, 2008.
[260] World Health Organization. The use of malaria rapid diagnostic tests. Available from: www.wpro.who.int/sites/rdt Accessed June 29, 2008.
[261] Bouyou-Akotet, M.K; Ionete-Collard, D.E; Mabika-Manfoumbi, M., *et al.* Prevalence of *Plasmodium falciparum* infection in pregnant women in Gabon. *Malar. J.* 2003; 2:18 (Published online).

[262] World Health Organization. A strategic framework for malaria prevention and control during pregnancy in the African region. Brazzaville: WHO Regional Office for Africa, 2004. Available from: www.cdc.gov/malaria/pdf/strategic framework mip_04.pdf Accessed June 29, 2008.

[263] UNAIDS. AIDS epidemic update: December 2005. UNAIDS. Available from: http://www.unaids.org/epi/2005 Accessed June 29, 2008.

[264] ter Kuile, F.O; Parise, M.E; Verhoeff, F.H., *et al.* The burden of co-infection with human immunodeficiency virus type 1 and malaria in pregnant women in sub-Saharan Africa. *Am. J. Trop. Med. Hyg.* 2004; 71 (suppl): 41-54.

[265] Griffith, K.S; Lewis, L.S; Mali, S., *et al.* Treatment of malaria in the United States: A systematic review. *JAMA* 2007; 297:2264 –2277.

[266] World Health Organization Website. Guidelines for the treatment of malaria. Available from: www.who.int/malaria/docs/ TreatmentGuidelines2006.pdf. Accessed June 29, 2008.

[267] Orton, L. and Garner, P. Drugs for treating uncomplicated malaria in pregnant women. *Cochrane Database Syst Rev* 2005, Issue 3. Art. No.: CD004912.

[268] World Health Organisation. Research for Action: understanding and controlling tuberculosis in India. 2000; 12.

[269] Arora, V.K. and Gupta, R. Tuberculosis and pregnancy. *Ind. J. Tub.* 2003; 50:13-16.

[270] Riley, L. Pneumonia and tuberculosis in pregnancy. *Infect. Dis. Clin. North Am.* 1997 11(1) 119-133.

[271] Robinson, C.A. and Rose, N.C. Tuberculosis: current implications and management in obstetrics. *Obstet. Gynecol. Surv* 1996; 51: 115-124.

[272] Figueroa-Damien, R. and Arredondo–Garcia, J.L. Pregnancy and tuberculosis: influence of treatment on perinatal outcome. *Am. J. Perinatol.* 1998; (15): 303-306.

[273] Hamadeh, M.A. and Glassroth, J. Tuberculosis and pregnancy. *Chest* 1992; 101(4): 1114-1120.

[274] Cantwell, M.F; Shehab, Z.M. and Costello, A.M. Brief report: Congenital tuberculosis. *N. Engl. J. Med.* 1994; 330 1051-1054.

[275] Jana, N; Vasishta, K; Jindal, S.K., *et al.* Perinatal outcome in pregnancies complicated by pulmonary tuberculosis. *Int. J. Gynecol. Obstet.* 1994; 44: 119-124.

[276] Bjerkedal, T; Bahna, S.L. and Lehmann, E.H. Course and outcome of pregnancy in women with pulmonary tuberculosis. *Scand J. Respir. Dis.* 1975;56:245–250.

[277] Ahmed, Y; Mwamba, P; Chintu, C., *et al.* A study of maternal mortality at the University Teaching Hospital, Lusaka, Zambia: the emergence of tuberculosis as a major non-obstetric cause of maternal death. *Int. J. Tuberc. Lung Dis.* 1999; 3:675–680.

[278] Good, J.T; Iseman, M.D; Davidson, P.T., *et al.* Tuberculosis inassociation with pregnancy. *Am. J. Obstet. Gynecol.* 1981; 140:492–498.

[279] Wilson, E.A; Thelin, T.J. and Dilts, P.V. Tuberculosis complicated by pregnancy. *Am. J. Obstet. Gynecol.* 1972; 115:526–529.

[280] Jain, N.K. (Safety of anti-tuberculosis drugs in pregnancy) and Kishan, J., Sailaja, Kaur, S. (Tuberculosis and pregnancy); *Abstracts; NAPCON;* Nov 2001, Mumbai, 33.

[281] Centres for Disease Control. Initial therapy for tuberculosis in the era of multiple drug resistance: recommendations of the Advisory Committee on the Elimination of Tuberculosis. *MMWR* 1993; 42:1–8.

[282] American Thoracic Society and Centers for Disease Control. Treatment of tuberculosis and tuberculosis infection in adults and children. *Am. J. Respir. Crit. Care Med.* 1994; 149:1359–1374.

[283] Ormerod, L.P. Chemotherapy of tuberculosis. *Eur Respir J* 1997; 12(Suppl 4): 273–297.

[284] American Thoracic Society, CDC, and Infectious Diseases Society of America. Treatment of Tuberculosis. MMWR 2003; 52(112): 1-77.Available from: http://www.cdc.gov/mmwr/preview/mmwrhtml/rr5211a1.htm. Accessed June 29, 2008.

[285] Committee on Drugs, American Academy of Pediatrics. The transfer of drugs and other chemicals into human milk. *Pediatrics* 1994; 93:137–150.

[286] New Jersey Department of Health and Senior Services. Typhoid Fever (Salmonella typhi) 2003. Available from: http://www.state.nj.us/health/cd/manual/typhoid.pdf. Accessed on June 30, 2008.

[287] Akinyemi, K.O; Smith, S.I; Oyefolu, A.O., *et al.* Multidrug-resistance in *Salmonella enterica serovar typhi* isolated from patients with typhoid fever complications in Lagos, Nigeria. *Public Health* 2005; 119(4): 321-327.

[288] Bhan, M.K; Bahl, R. and Bhatnagar, S. Typhoid and paratyphoid fever. *Lancet* 2005; 366(9487): 749-672.

[289] Riggall, F; Salkind, G. and Spizllacy, W. Typhoid Fever Complicating Pregnancy. *Obstet. Gynecol.* 1974; 44:117-121.

[290] Sulaiman, K. and Sarwari, A.R. Culture-confirmed typhoid fever and pregnancy. *Int J. Infect. Dis.* 2007; 11(4):337-341.

[291] Choo, K.E Davis, T.M.E; Ismail, A., *et al.* Rapid and reliable serological diagnosis of enteric fever: comparative sensitivity and specificity of Typhidot and Typhidot-M tests in febrile Malaysian children. *Acta. Tropica.* 1999; 72(2):175-183.

[292] Olsen SJ, Pruckler J, Bibb W, et al. Evaluation of Rapid Diagnostic Tests for Typhoid Fever. *J. Clin. Microbiol.* 2004; 42(5): 1885–1889.

[293] Tam, F.C.H; Ling, T.K.W; Wong, K.T., *et al.* The TUBEX test detects not only typhoid-specific antibodies but also soluble antigens and whole bacteria. *Med. Microbiol.* 2008; 57: 316-323.

[294] Oracz, G; Feleszko, W; Golicka, D., *et al.* Rapid Diagnosis of Acute Salmonella Gastrointestinal Infection. *Clin. Infect. Dis.* 2003; 36(1):112-115.

[295] Background document: The diagnosis, treatment and prevention of typhoid fever Communicable Disease Surveillance and Response. Vaccines and Biologicals. World Health Organization. Available from: http://www.who.int/vaccine_research/documents/en/typhoid_diagnosis.pdf. Accessed on June 30, 2008.

[296] Lien-Keng, K. and Odang, O. The bone marrow picture of typhoid fever in childhood. *J. Trop. Pediatr.* 1959 5(2): 35-44.

[297] Gower, N.D._Marrow biopsy in the diagnosis of pyrexia of undetermined origin *J. Clin. Pathol.* 1963; 16(3): 227–231.

[298] Chinh NT, Parry CM, Ly NT, et al. A randomised controlled comparison of azithromycin and ofloxacin for multidrug-resistant and nalidixic acid resistant enteric fever. *Antimicrob Agents Chemother.* 2000; 44: 1855-1859.

[299] Brown, J.C; Shanahan, P.M; Jesudason, M.V., *et al.* Mutations responsible for reduced susceptibility to 4-quinolones in clinical isolates of multi-resistant *Salmonella typhi* in India. *J. Antimicrob. Chemother.* 1996; 37: 891-900.

[300] Threlfall, E.J; Ward, L.R; Skinner, J.A., *et al.* Ciprofloxacin-resistant *Salmonella typhi* and treatment failure. *Lancet* 1999; 353: 1590-1591.

[301] Islam, A; Butler, T; Kabir, I., *et al.* Treatment of typhoid fever with ceftriaxone for 5 days or chloramphenicol for 14 days: a randomized clinical trial. *Antimicrob. Agents Chemother* 1993; 37(8): 1572–1575.

[302] Carles, G; Montoya, Y; Seve, B., *et al.* Typhoid fever and pregnancy. *J. Gynecol. Obstet. Biol. Reprod.* (Paris) 2002; 31(5): 495-499.

[303] Seoud, M; Saade, G; Uwaydah, M., *et al.* Typhoid Fever in Pregnancy. *Obstet. Gynecol.* 1988; 71:711-714.

[304] Amster, R; Lessing, J.B; Jaffa, A.J., *et al.* Typhoid fever complicating pregnancy. *Acta. Obstet. Gynecol. Scand.* 1985; 64(8):685-686.

[305] Long, W.M. and Sprung, C.L. Corticosteroids, nonsteroidal anti-inflammatory drugs, and naloxone in the sepsis syndrome. *World J. Surg.* 1987; 11(2): 218-225.

[306] Lamberts, S.W.J; Bruining, H.A. and de Jong, F.H. Corticosteroid Therapy in Severe Illness. *N. Engl. J. Med.* 1997; 337:1285-1292.

[307] Engels, E.A; Falagas, M.E; Lau, J., *et al.* Typhoid fever vaccines: a meta-analysis of studies on efficacy and toxicity. *BMJ* 1998; 316:110-116.

[308] Fraser, A; Goldberg, E; Acosta, C.J., *et al.* Vaccines for preventing typhoid fever. *Cochrane Database Syst. Rev.* 2007, Issue 2. Art. No.: CD001261.

[309] Riggs, J.W. and Blanco, J.D. Pathophysiology, diagnosis, and management of intraamniotic infection. *Sem. Perinatol.* 1998; 22(4): 251-259.

[310] Dong, Y; Clair, P.J.S; Ramzy, I., *et al.* A microbiologic and clinical study of placental inflammation at term. *Obstet. Gynecol.* 1987; 70:175-182.

[311] Hillier, S.L; Martius, J; Krohn, M., *et al.* A case-controlled study of chorioamnionitic infection and histologic chorioamnionitis in prematurity. *N. Engl. J. Med.* 1988; 319:972-978.

[312] Fahey, J.O. Clinical management of intra-amniotic infection and chorioamnionitis: a review of the literature. *J. Midwifery Womens Health* 2008; 53(3):227-235.

[313] Briggs, G.G. and Wan, S.R. Drug therapy during labor and delivery (Part 1). *Am J Health-Syst Pharm* 2006; 63(11): 1038-1047.

[314] Newton, E.R; Prihoda. T.J. and Gibbs, R.S. Logistic regression analysis of risk factors for intra amniotic infection. *Obstet. Gynecol.* 1989; 73:571-575.

[315] Aarnoudse, J.G. and Huisjes, H.J. Complications of Cerclage. *Acta Obstet. Gynecol. Scand* 1979; 58:255-257.

[316] Burnett, R.G. and Anderson, W.R. The hazards of Amniocentesis. *J. Iowa. Med. Soc.* 1968; 58:130-137.

[317] Wilkins, I; Mezrow, G; Lynch, L., *et al.* Amnionitis and life-threatening respiratory distress after percutaneous umbilical blood sampling. *Am. J. Obstet. Gynecol.* 1989; 160:427- 428.

[318] Gibbs, R.S; Blanco, J.D; Clair, P.J.S., *et al*. Quantitative bacteriology of amniotic fluid from women with clinical intraamniotic infection at term. *J. Infect. Dis.* 1982; 145:1-8.

[319] Silver, H.M; Sperling, R.S; St. Clair, P.J., *et al.* Evidence relating bacterial vaginosis to intraamniotic infection. *Am. J. Obstet. Gynecol.* 1989; 161:808-812.

[320] Blanco, J.D; Gibbs, R.S; Malherbe, H., *et al.* A controlled study of genital mycoplasmas in amniotic fluid from patients with intra-amniotic infection. *J. Infect. Dis.* 1983; 147:650- 653.

[321] Maher, C.F; Haran, M.V; Farrell, D.J., *et al.* Ureaplasma urealyticum chorioamnionitis. *Aust. N Z J. Obstet. Gynaecol.* 1994; 34:477-479.

[322] Sweet, R.L. and Gibbs, R.S. Infectious Diseases of the Female Genital Tract. Intraamniotic infection. *Intrauterine infection in late pregnancy.* Baltimore: Williams and Wilkins, 1990, pp 337-347.

[323] Egley, C.C; Katz, V.L. and Herbert, W.N.P. Leukocyte esterase: A simple bedside test for the detection of bacterial colonization of amniotic fluid. *Am. J. Obstet. Gynecol.* 1988; 159:120- 122.

[324] Romero, R; Jimenez, C; Lohda, A.K., *et al.* Amniotic fluid glucose concentration: A rapid and simple method for the detection of intraamniotic infection in preterm labor. *Am. J. Obstet. Gynecol.* 1990; 163:968-974.

[325] Romero, R; Kadar, N; Hobbins, J.C., *et al.* Infection and labor: The detection of endotoxin in amnotic fluid. *Am. J. Obstet. Gynecol.* 1987; 157:815-819.

[326] Gravett, M.G; Eschenbach, D.A. and Speigel-Brown, C.A. Rapid diagnosis of amniotic-fluid infection by gas-liquid chromatography. *N. Engl. J. Med.* 1982; 306:725-728.

[327] Cox, S.M; Roberts, S; Roussis, P., *et al.* Prematurity, subclinical intraamniotic infection, and fetal biophysical parameters: Is there a correlation? *Infectious Diseases in Obstetrics and Gynecology* 1993; 1:76-81.

[328] Yusuf, L. Antibiotic regimens for management of intra-amniotic infection: RHL commentary. 2004. *The WHO Reproductive Health Library*; Geneva: World Health Organization. Available from: http://www.who.int/rhl/pregnancy_childbirth/complications/infection/ylcom/en/index.html. Accessed on July 1, 2008.

[329] Hopkins, L. and Smaill, F. Antibiotic regimens for management of intraamniotic infection. *Cochrane Database of Syst Rev* 2002, Issue 3. Art. No.: CD003254.

[330] Gilstrap, L.C; Leveno, K.J; Cox, S.M., *et al.* Intrapartum treatment of acute chorioamnionitis: Impact on neonatal sepsis. *Am. J. Obstet. Gynecol.* 1988; 159:579-583.

[331] Gibbs, R.S; Castillo, M.S. and Rodgers, P.J. Management of acute chorioamnionitis. *Obstet. Gynecol.* 1980; 136:709-713.

[332] Casey, B.M. and Cox, S.M. Chorioamnionitis and endometritis. *Infect. Dis. Clin. North Am.* 1997; 11(1): 203-222.

[333] Charles, D. Dynamics of antibiotic transfer from mother to fetus. *Sem. Perinatol.* 1977; 1(1): 89-100.

[334] Kenyon, S; Taylor, D.J. and Tarnow-Mordi, W. On behalf of the ORACLE Collaborative Group. Broad-spectrum antibiotics for preterm, prelabour rupture of fetal membranes: the ORACLE I randomised trial. *Lancet* 2001; 357: 979–988.

[335] Kenyon, S; Taylor, D.J. and Tarnow-Mordi, W. On behalf of the ORACLE Collaborative Group. Broad-spectrum antibiotics for spontaneous preterm labour: the ORACLE II randomised trial. *Lancet* 2001; 357:989–994.

[336] Garite, T.J. and Freeman, R.K. Chorioamnionitis in the preterm gestation. *Obstet. Gynecol.* 1982; 59:539-545.

[337] Morales, W.J. The effect of chorioamnionitis on the developmental outcome of preterm infants at one year. *Obstet. Gynecol.* 1987; 70:183-186.

[338] Grether, J.K. and Nelson, K.B. Maternal infection and cerebral palsy in infants of normal birth weight *JAMA* 1997; 278:207-211.

[339] Mourad, J; Elliott, J.P; Erickson, L., *et al.* Appendicitis in pregnancy: new information that contradicts long-held clinical beliefs. *Am. J. Obstet. Gynecol.* 2000; 182:1027–1029.

[340] Hee, P. and Viktrup, L. The diagnosis of appendicitis during pregnancy and maternal and fetal outcome after appendectomy. *Int. J. Gynaecol. Obstet.* 1999; 65:129–135.

[341] Tracey, M. and Fletcher, H.S. Appendicitis in pregnancy. *Am Surg* 2000; 66: 555–560.

[342] Liu, C. and McFadden, D. Acute abdomen and appendix. In: *Surgery: Scientific Principles and Practice*, 2nd ed. Grennfield L, Mulholland M, Oldham K, editors. Philadelphia: Lippincott-Raven 1997; pp. 1246 – 1261.

[343] Al-Mulhim, A.A. Acute appendicitis in pregnancy. A review of 52 cases. *Int. Surg.* 1996; 81:295–297.

[344] Andersen, B. and Nielsen, T.F. Appendicitis in pregnancy: diagnosis, management and complications. *Acta Obstet. Gynecol. Scand* 1999; 78:758–762.

[345] Tamir, I.L; Bongard, F.S. and Klein, S.R. Acute appendicitis in the pregnant patient. *Am. J. Surg.* 1990; 160:571– 576.

[346] Pastore, P.A; Loomis, D.M. and Sauret, J. Appendicitis in Pregnancy. *J. Am. Board Fam. Med.* 2006; 19:621– 626.

[347] Cunningham, F.G. and McCubbin, J.H. Appendicitis complicating pregnancy. *Obstet. Gynecol.* 1975; 45(4): 415-420.

[348] McGee, T.M. Acute appendicitis in pregnancy. *Aust. N Z J. Obstet. Gynaecol.* 1989; 29 (4):378-385.

[349] Sivanesaratna, V. The acute abdomen and the obstetrician. *Baillieres Best Pract. Res. Clin. Obstet. Gynaecol.* 2000; 14(1): 89-102.

[350] Somani, R.A; Kaban, G; Cuddington, G., *et al.* Appendicitis in pregnancy: a rare presentation. *CMAJ* 2003; 168:1020.

[351] Bailey, L.E; Finley, R.K. Jr.; Miller, S.F., *et al.* Acute appendicitis during pregnancy. *Am. Surg.* 1986; 52(4): 218-221.

[352] Lim, H.K; Bae, S.H. and Seo, G.S. Diagnosis of acute appendicitis in pregnant women: value of sonography. *Am. J. Roentgenol.* 1992; 159(3): 539-542.

[353] Puylaert, J.B; Rutgers, P.H; Lalisang, R.I., *et al.* A prospective study of ultrasonography in the diagnosis of appendicitis. *N. Engl. J. Med.* 1987; 317(11): 666-669.

[354] Allen, J.R; Helling, T.S. and Langenfeld, M. Intraabdominal surgery during pregnancy. *Am. J. Surg.* 1989; 158 (6): 567-569.

[355] Saunders, P. and Milton, P.J. Laparotomy during pregnancy: an assessment of diagnostic accuracy and fetal wastage. *BMJ* 1973; 3(872): 165-167.

[356] Kammerer, W.S. Nonobstetric surgery during pregnancy. *Med. Clin. North Am.* 1979; 63(6): 1157-1164.

[357] Schwartzberg, B.S; Conyers, J.A. and Moore, J.A. First trimester of pregnancy laparoscopic procedures. *Surg. Endosc.* 1997; 11(12): 1216-1217.

[358] Thomas, S.J. and Brisson, P. Laparoscopic appendectomy and cholecystectomy during pregnancy: six case reports. *JSLS* 1998; 2(1): 41-46.

[359] Barnes, S.L; Shane, M.D; Schoemann, M.B., *et al.* Laparoscopic appendectomy after 30 weeks pregnancy: report of two cases and description of technique. *Am. Surg.* 2004; 70 (8):733-736.

[360] de Perrot, M; Jenny, A; Morales, M., *et al.* Laparoscopic appendectomy during pregnancy. *Surg. Laparosc Endosc. Percutan. Tech.* 2000; 10(6): 368-371.

[361] Schreiber, J.H. Laparoscopic appendectomy in pregnancy. *Surg. Endosc.* 1990; 4(2): 100-102.

[362] Affleck, D.G; Handrahan, D.L; Egger, M.J., *et al.* The laparoscopic management of appendicitis and cholelithiasis during pregnancy. *Am. J. Surg.* 1999; 178(6): 523-529.

[363] Barone, J.E; Bears, S; Chen, S., *et al.* Outcome study of cholecystectomy during pregnancy. *Am. J. Surg.* 1999; 177(3): 232-236.

[364] Rollins, M.D; Chan, K.J. and Price, R.R. Laparoscopy for appendicitis and cholelithiasis during pregnancy: a new standard of care. *Surg. Endosc.* 2004; 18(2): 237-241.

[365] Geisler, J.P. and Rose, S.L. Non-gynecologic laparoscopy in second and third trimester pregnancy: obstetric implications. *JSLS* 1998; 2(3): 235-238.

[366] Stepp, K. and Falcone, T. Laparoscopy in the second trimester of pregnancy. *Obstet. Gynecol. Clin. North Am.* 2004; 31(3): 485- 496.

[367] Conron, R.W. Jr.; Abbruzzi, K; Cochrane, S.O., *et al.* Laparoscopic procedures in pregnancy. *Am. Surg.* 1999; 65:259-263.

[368] Hill, L.M; Johnson, C.E. and Lee, R.A. Cholecystectomy in pregnancy. *Obstet. Gynecol.* 1975; 46(3): 291-293.

[369] Landers, D; Carmona, R; Crombleholme, W., *et al.* Acute cholecystitis in pregnancy. *Obstet. Gynecol.* 1987; 69(1): 131-133.

[370] Friley, M.D. and Douglas, G. Acute cholecystitis in pregnancy and the puerperium. *Am. Surg.* 1972; 38(6): 314-317.

[371] Hiatt, J.R; Hiatt, J.C; Williams, R.A. *et al.* Biliary disease in pregnancy: strategy for surgical management. *Am. J. Surg.* 1986; 151(2): 263-265.

[372] Dixon, N.P; Faddis, D.M. and Silberman, H. Aggressive management of cholecystitis during pregnancy. *Am. J. Surg.* 1987; 154(3): 292-294.

[373] Swisher, S.G; Schmit, P.J; Hunt, K.K., et al. Biliary disease during pregnancy. *Am. J. Surg.* 1994; 168(6): 576-579; 580-581.

[374] Barclay, L. CDC Issues New Guidelines for Meningococcal Vaccination. Available from http://www.medscape.com/viewarticle/559807. Accessed June 29, 2008.

[375] Landrum, L.M; Hawkins, A. and Goodman, J.R. Pneumococcal meningitis during pregnancy: a case report and review of literature. *Infect Dis Obstet. Gynecol.* 2007; 63624. Published online 2007 April 2. Available from: http://www.pubmedcentral.nih.gov/articlerender.fcgi?artid=1852901. Accessed on June 29, 2008.

[376] van de Beek, D; de Gans, J; Tunkel, A.R. *et al.* Community-acquired bacterial meningitis in adults. *N. Eng. J. Med.* 2006; 354(1): 44–53.

[377] de Gans, J. and van de Beek, D. Dexamethasone in adults with bacterial meningitis. *N. Eng. J. Med. 2002*; 347(20): 1549–1556.

[378] Lucas, A.O. Pneumococcal meningitis in pregnancy and the puerperium. *BMJ* 1964; 1(5375) 92–95.

[379] DiMaio, H. Listeria infection in women. *Primary Care Update for Ob/Gyns* 2000; 7(1): 40-45.

[380] Smith, J.L. Foodborne infections during pregnancy. *J. Food Prot.* 1999; 2(7): 818-829.

[381] The prevention and management of puerperal infections. Report of a technical working group. Geneva, 1992. WHO Problems, 10th Revision. Geneva, Switzerland: World Health Organization, 1992. (WHO/FHE/MSM//95.4). Available from: http://www.who.int/reproductivehealth/publications/MSM_ Accessed July 3, 2008.

[382] Wager, G.P; Martin, D.H; Koutsky, L. *et al.* Puerperal infectious morbidity: relationship to route of delivery and to antepartum *Chlamydia trachomatis* infection. *Am. J. Obstet. Gynecol.* 1980; 138(7 Pt 2): 1028–1033.

[383] Lindeque, B.G. Abnormalities of the puerperium. In: Cronje HS, Grobler CJF, editors. *Obstetrics in Southern Africa*. 2nd ed. Pretoria: Van Schaik Publishers; 2003:380–390

[384] World Health Organization. Maternal Health and Safe Motherhood Programme Division of Family Health. Mother–Baby Package: Implementing Safe Motherhood in Countries. WHO/ FHE/MSM/94.11. Geneva: WHO, 1994.

[385] van Gelderen, C.F. Puerperal sepsis. In: Chamberlain G, editor. *Turnbull's Obstetrics*. 2nd ed. London: Churchill Livingstone, 1995: pp.771–787.

[386] Maharaj, D. Puerperal pyrexia: A review. Part I. *Obstet. Gynecol. Surv* 2007; 62(6):393-399.

[387] Chaim, W.A; Bar-David, J; Shohan-Vardi, I. *et al.* Prevalence and clinical significance of postpartum endometritis and wound infection. *Infect. Dis. Obstet. Gynecol.* 2000; 8: 77-82.

[388] Dolea, C and Stein, C. Global burden of maternal sepsis in the year 2000. Evidence and Information for Policy (EIP). Geneva: World Health Organization; July 2003. Available from: http:// www.who.int/healthinfo/statistics/bod_maternalsepsis.pdf. Accessed July 3, 2008.

[389] Gibbs, R.S. Infection after cesarean section. *Clin. Obstet. Gynecol.* 1985; 28:697–707.

[390] Gilstrap, L.C. and Cunningham, F.G. The bacterial pathogenesis of infection following cesarean section. *Obstet. Gynecol.* 1979; 53:545–549.

[391] Charles, D. and Larsen, B. Puerperal sepsis. In: Turnbull A, Chamberlain G, editors. *Obstetrics*. London: Churchill Livingstone, 1989: pp.933–946.

[392] Hussein, J. and Fortney, J. A. Puerperal sepsis and maternal mortality: what role can new technologies play? *Int. J. Gynaecol. Obstet.* 2004; 85:S52–S61.

[393] Meis, J.F.G.M ; Muytjens, H.L ; Van den Berg, P.P., *et al.* Analysis of an outbreak of puerperal fever due to group A streptococci by random amplified polymorphic DNA fingerprinting. *Infect Dis Obstet. Gynecol.* 1997;5:232–236.

[394] Thewessen, E.A.P.M; Bontekoe-Hoornstra, J; Smelting- Nagtzaam, A.E., *et al.* A cluster of puerperal fever in Gouda; a renewed lesson of Seminmelweis. *Ned. Tijdschr. Geneeskd.* 1999; 143:1700–1705.

[395] Mead, P.B. Streptococcal screening in Obstetrics. *Obstet. Gynecol.* 2001; 98 (5 Pt 1):721–733.

[396] Stray-Pedersen, B. Is screening for genital infections in pregnancy necessary? *Acta Obstet. Gynecol. Scand* 1997; 76:116– 120.

[397] Mahon, B.E; Rosenman, M.B; Graham, M.F., *et al.* Postpartum Chlamydia trachomatis and Neisseria gonorrhoeae infections. *Am. J. Obstet. Gynecol.* 2002; 186:1320–1325.

[398] Duff, P. Pathophysiology and management of postcesarean endomyometritis. *Obstet. Gynecol.* 1986; 67:269–276.

[399] Abouzahr, C; Aaahman, E. and Guidotti, R. Puerperal sepsis and other puerperal infections. In: Murray CJL, Lopez AD, editors. *Health Dimensions of Sex and Reproduction: The Global Burden of Sexually Transmitted Diseases, Maternal Conditions, Perinatal Disorders, and Congenital Anomalies*. Geneva: WHO, 1998.

[400] American College of Obstetrics and Gynecology. Antimicrobial Therapy for Obstetric Patients. Washington, DC: The College, 1998. Education Bulletin No. 245.

[401] Kankuri, E; Kurki, T; Carlson, P. *et al.* Incidence, treatment and outcome of peripartum sepsis. *Acta. Obstet. Gynecol. Scand.* 2003; 82:730–735.

[402] Thomsen, A.C; Espersen, T. and Maigaard, S. Course and treatment of milk stasis, noninfectious inflammation of the breast, and infectious mastitis in nursing women. *Am. J. Obstet. Gynecol.* 1984; 149:492–495.

[403] Lowthian, J. and Gillar, D. Poatpartum necrotizing fasciitis. *Obstet. Gynecol.* 1980; 56:661–663.

[404] Shy, K. and Eschenbach, D. Fatal perineal cellulitis from an episiotomy site. *Obstet. Gynecol.* 1979; 54:292–298.

[405] Hibbard, L; Snyder, E. and McVann, R. Subgluteal and retropsoal infection in obstetric practice. *Obstet. Gynecol.* 1972; 39:137– 150.

[406] Ramin, S.M; Ramus R.M; Little B.B, et al. Early repair of episiotomy dehiscence associated with infection. *Am. J. Obstet. Gynecol.* 192; 167:1104-1107.

[407] Thompson, C.D; Brekken, A.L. and Kutteh, W.H. Necrotizing fasciitis: a review of management guidelines in a large obstetrics and gynecology teaching hospital. *Infect. Dis. Ob. Gyn.* 1993; 1: 16-22.

[408] Stray-Pedersen, B; Blakstad, M. and Bergan, T. Bacteriuria in the puerperium. Risk factors, screening procedures, and treatment programs. *Am. J. Obstet. Gynecol.* 1990; 162:792–797.

[409] Josey, W.E. and Staggers, S.R. Heparin therapy in septic pelvic vein thrombophlebitis: a study of 46 cases. *Am. J. Obstet. Gynecol.* 1974; 120:228–233.

[410] Lev-Toaff, A.S; Baka, J.J; Toaff, M.E., *et al.* Diagnostic imaging in puerperal febrile morbidity. *Obstet. Gynecol.* 1991; 78:50–55.

[411] Villasanta, U. Thromboembolic disease in pregnancy. *Am. J. Obstet. Gynecol.* 1965; 93:142–151.

[412] Maharaj, D. Puerperal Pyrexia: A Review. (Part 2). *Obstet. Gynecol. Surv* 2007; 62(6): 400-406.

[413] Centers for Disease Control and Prevention (CDC). General recommendations on immunization: recommendations of the Advisory Committee on Immunization Practices (ACIP). *MMWR* 2006; 55 (No. RR-15): 32-33.

[414] Centers for Disease Control and Prevention (CDC) and Department of Health and Human Services (DHHS). Guidelines for Vaccinating Pregnant Women.October 1998 (updated May 2007). Available from: http://www.cdc.gov/vaccines/pubs/preg-guide.htm. Accessed on July 1, 2008.

[415] ACOG Committee Opinion No. 299. Guidelines for diagnostic imaging during pregnancy. *Obstet. Gynecol.* 2004; 104:647–651.

[416] Gray, J.E. Safety (risk) of diagnostic radiology exposures. In: American College of Radiology. Radiation risk: a primer. Reston (VA): ACR; 1996. pp. 15–7.

[417] Brent, R.L. The effect of embryonic and fetal exposure to x-ray, microwaves, and ultrasound: counseling the pregnant and nonpregnant patient about these risks. *Semin. Oncol.* 1989; 16:347–368.

[418] Hall, E.J. Scientific view of low-level radiation risks. *Radiographics* 1991; 11:509–518.

[419] Moore, M.M. and Shearer, D.R. Fetal dose estimates for CT pelvimetry. *Radiology* 1989; 171:265–267.

[420] Parry, R.A; Glaze, S.A. and Archer, B.R. The AAPM/RSNA physics tutorial for residents. Typical patient radiation doses in diagnostic radiology. *Radiographics* 1999; 19:1289–1302.

[421] Cunningham, F.G; Gant, N.F; Leveno, K.J., et al. 3rd, Hauth JC, Wenstrom KD. *General considerations and maternal evaluation*. In: William's obstetrics. 21st ed. New York (NY): McGraw-Hill; 2001. pp. 1143–1158.

[422] Otake, M; Yoshimaru, H. and Schull, W.J. Severe mental retardation among prenatally exposed survivors of the atomic bombing of Hiroshima and Nagasaki: a comparison of the T65DR and DS86 dosimetry systems. Technical report; RERF TR 87-16. Hiroshima: Radiation Effects Research Foundation; 19.

[423] Yamazaki, J.N. and Schull, W.J. Perinatal loss and neurological abnormalities among children of the atomic bomb: Nagasaki and Hiroshima revisited, 1949 to 1989. *JAMA* 1990; 264:605-609.

[424] Otake, M. and Schull, W.J. In utero exposure to A-bomb radiation and mental retardation: a reassessment. *Br. J. Radiol.* 1984; 57:409-414.

[425] Miller, R.W. *Epidemiological conclusions from radiation toxicity studies*. In: Fry RJ, Grahn D, Griem ML, Rust JH, editors. Late effects of radiation: proceedings of the colloquium held at the Center for Continuing Education, the University of Chicago, Illinois, May 1969. New York (NY): Van Nostrand Reinhold; 1970. p. 245–256.

[426] Committee on Biological Effects of Ionizing Radiation, Board on Radiation Effects Research, Commission on Life Sciences, National Research Council. Health effects of

exposure to low levels of ionizing radiation: BEIR V. Washington, D.C.: National Academy Press, 1990.

[427] Gray, J.E. *Safety (risk) of diagnostic radiology exposures*. In: American College of Radiology. Radiation risk: a primer. Reston, Va.: American College of Radiology, 1996.

[428] Abramowicz, J.S. Technical advances in ultrasound equipment. *Clin. Obstet. Gynecol.* 2003; 46:839–849.

[429] Reddy, U.M; Filly R.A. and Copel J.A. Prenatal imaging ultrasonography and magnetic resonance imaging. *Obstet. Gynecol.* 2008; 112:145–157.

[430] Salvesen, K.A. and Eik-Nes, S.H. Is ultrasound unsound? A review of epidemiological studies of human exposure to ultrasound. *Ultrasound Obstet. Gynecol.* 1995; 6:293–298.

[431] Newnham, J.P; Evans, S.F; Michael, C.A., et al. Effects of frequent ultrasound during pregnancy: a randomised controlled trial. *Lancet* 1993; 342:887–891.

[432] Kieler, H; Cnattingius, S; Haglund, B., et al. Sinistrality—a side-effect of prenatal sonography: a comparative study of young men. *Epidemiology* 2001; 12:618–623.

[433] Campbell, J.D; Elford, R.W. and Brant, R.F. Casecontrol study of prenatal ultrasonography exposure in children with delayed speech. *CMAJ* 1993; 149:1435–1440

[434] Curry, T.S. 3rd; Dowdey, J.E. and Murry, R.C. Jr., editors. *Christensen's physics of diagnostic radiology*. 4th ed. Philadelphia (PA): Lea and Febiger; 1990.

[435] Shellock, F.G. and Crues, J.V. MR procedures: biologic effects, safety, and patient care. *Radiology* 2004; 232: 635–652.

[436] Levine, D. Obstetric MRI. *J. Magn. Reson. Imaging* 2006; 24:1–15.

[437] Mettler, F.A. Jr. and Guiberteau, M.J. Essentials of nuclear medicine imaging. 4th ed. Philadelphia (PA): WB Saunders; 1998.

[438] Ginsberg, J.S; Hirsh, J; Rainbow, A.J., et al. Risks to the fetus of radiologic procedures used in the diagnosis of maternal venous thromboembolic disease. *Thromb. Haemost.* 1989; 61:189–196.

[439] Winer-Muram, H.T; Boone, J.M; Brown, H.L., et al. Pulmonary embolism in pregnant patients: fetal radiation dose with helical CT. *Radiology* 2002; 224:487–492.

[440] Geller, S.E; Adams, M.G; Kominiarek, M.A., et al. Reliability of a preventability model in maternal death and morbidity. *Am. J. Obstet. Gynecol.* 2007; 196:57-58.

In: Infectious Pregnancy Complications
Editor: Richard N. Canfield
ISBN 978-1-60741-038-6

Chapter 2

Infection Related Recurrent Late Abortions and Preterm Birth: Early Total Cervix Occlusion (ETCO) Versus Cerclage

Erich Saling and Monika Dräger
Institute of Perinatal Medicine (charitable institute)
Located at Vivantes-Clinic Berlin-Neukoelln, Berlin, Germany

Abstract

Recurrent late abortions and early prematurity continue to be two of the main problems of modern obstetrics and perinatal medicine which remain to be fully solved. The patients concerned often suffer increasingly.

Ascending genital infection is the main preventable cause for late abortions or early premature births. In recurrent cases, the Early Total Cervix Occlusion (ETCO) is an early preventive measure particularly for women with a history of ≥ 2 late abortions or early premature births (< 32+0 weeks gestation). The operative technique, our own results, and results from a multi-center-enquiry undertaken in Germany are subjects of our present discussion. In both evaluations, the women within this high risk group had a surviving infant in about 70% of cases after a Total Cervix Occlusion (TCO). Differentiated according to „early“ TCO (ETCO) and „late“ TCO, the success rate has been 80% and 40% respectively.

Cerclage is still a frequently employed measure in cases with recurrent preterm births, but it has increasingly become the subject of controversy. ETCO is quite different from cerclage. The cerclage only tightens the canal. Whereas ETCO really closes the cervical canal: After the epithelium of the lower cervical canal and of the lower portio has been removed these parts are sutured. This allows the lower cervix to heal up and close totally. This is a complete barrier which thus prevents ascension of organisms The much poorer results inevitably achieved by cerclage are compared with the results of ETCO. In our sample of women treated with ETCO we found that, in 51 previous pregnancies in which cerclage was performed, only 13 infants survived. This is a survival rate of only 26% (as compared to a survival rate of 80% with ETCO).

ETCO was developed by us in 1981 in Germany and is widespread in Germany and also used in other German-speaking countries, but it is still rarely performed on an international level. This might partly be due to the fact that randomized studies with ETCO have up to now never been performed. But—considering the excellent results of ETCO—performing such a study now in Germany would raise serious ethical issues.

Another possible indication for the future may be in the area of multiple pregnancies: With ETCO, generally performed in multiple pregnancies, Schulze [40] was able to achieve a prematurity rate of only 17% as against a rate of 29% in cases without ETCO. In the group of infants at very high risk (< 28 weeks gestation), the rate with ETCO was 1% as opposed to 4% without.

More information on: http://www.saling-institut.de/eng/04infoph/04tmv.html.

Introduction

Recurrent late abortions and early prematurity continue to be two of the main problems of modern obstetrics and perinatal medicine which remain to be solved. The patients concerned often suffer considerably: On the one hand they deeply long for an infant but, on the other, they experience recurrent losses, which are often accompanied by increasing psychological problems. To help such patients successfully is a particularly important task, from both medical and psychological points of view.

Infection as Cause for Late Abortion and Prematurity

Ascending genital infection is the main preventable cause for late abortions and early premature births (≤ 32+0 weeks gestation). The first convincing and direct confirmation of the ascension infection genesis was found at the beginning of the 1980s when the operative Early Total Cervix Occlusion (ETCO) was introduced for patients with recurrent late abortions [1]. ETCO creates a complete barrier within the ascension area (see below), and leads to remarkably good results.

Back in 1991 [2, 3] we were able to find concrete signs of an infection in about three quarters of those infants with a birth weight of less than 2000g.

Fundamental biochemical studies later performed by Romero et al. [4] led to a great leap forward in understanding the mechanisms by which infections lead to premature birth. For a review of current developments in this area we recommend studying the publication by Romero et al. [5] and our contribution in chapter 6 in this volume.

According to microbiological studies, infection may account for 25–40% of preterm births, but this may be a conservative estimate, because—as Romero et al. [5] point out—infection is difficult to detect due to the limitations of standard microbiological techniques.

Another interesting finding supporting the ascension hypothesis is that, in twin gestations in which a microbial invasion of the amniotic cavity (MIAC) is detected, the presenting sac is frequently involved, whilst the other amniotic cavity may not have MIAC [6].

Other infections, particularly of the urinary tract, may also lead to premature births. A lot of research has been done in the last decades in order to try to prevent infection-related premature births, and some success has been achieved, e.g. in many countries, screening for urinary tract infection is now a standard component of prenatal care, and many physicians also screen for vaginal infections.

Our prematurity-prevention program, also discussed in this volume (see chapter 6), focuses on the early detection of disorders within the vaginal environment or already manifest vaginal infections. For some women, however, these screening measures seem not to be sufficient. Possible causes and operative solutions are discussed below.

Recurrence Risk of Premature Births

Reviewing the literature, it is rather difficult to estimate the recurrence risk of preterm birth, as the studies vary considerably particularly with regard to:

- sample population,
- inclusion/exclusion of special cases, such as multiple pregnancies, stillbirths or late abortions,
- whether the study distinguished between indicated or spontaneous premature birth,
- whether or not the gestational age was considered as well.

Therefore we only want to make some general remarks: once a patient has had one preterm birth the risk of a recurrent preterm birth is increased [7, 8, 9]. Both late miscarriages and premature births in the patient history increase the risk of preterm birth in the next pregnancy. For example, Künzel [10] analyzed the data of single pregnancies in the Hessian perinatal inquiry (n=150,591) and found that:

- one prior miscarriage increases the risk of a premature birth twofold,
- two prior miscarriages increases the risk of a premature birth 6.2 fold,
- one prior *premature birth* increases the risk of another premature birth 15.6 fold.

The risk increases even more with the next preterm birth (see table 1). But it also depends on whether or not the preterm birth has been induced or whether it occurred spontaneously [11], or whether and when there had been a term birth in the patient history and also on the gestational week of the previous preterm birth (some studies suggest that the risk of recurrence is higher the earlier the preterm birth has been). Also, in some studies additional comparisons between the historical findings and the current pregnancy, such as sonographically measured cervix length and markers of inflammation have been made, such as IL-8 and fetal fibronectine [8, 12, 13]. Just to give a general impression, we will show in table 1 some results from McManemy et al. [14].

Table 1. Recurrence risk of preterm birth (after McManemy et al. [14]). Sample population: 19,763 women from the Missouri maternally linked cohort who delivered 3 consecutive singleton live births. Multiple pregnancies, births before 20 gw and stillbirths had been excluded. Average rate of premature births in the US was 12.1 % (1993)

	Prior two deliveries			
	Preterm/Preterm	Term/Preterm	Preterm/Term	Term/Term
Prematurity Risk	**42%**	21%	13%	5%
	↓			
Prior **two preterm** deliveries (Very = 21-31 weeks; Moderate = 32-36 weeks)				
	Very/Very	Moderate/Very	Very/Moderat	Moderate/Mode rate
Prematurity Risk	57%	50%	40%	38%

The Terms "Cervical Incompetence" and "Cervical Insufficiency"

Gream used the term "cervical incompetence" for the first time in 1865 [15]. Romero and others suggested the term "cervical insufficiency" in order "to avoid the negative connotation that the term 'incompetence' implies to patients." [16]. Similarly, in Germany the term "*Zervixverschlussinsuffizienz*" (insufficiency of the cervical closure) is mostly used.

Despite the long history of the term, there is still no common definition, nor are there objective diagnostic criteria, for a review see: [16, 17]. Examples of definitions are: "the inability of the uterine cervix to retain a pregnancy in the absence of contractions or labor" [18] or, in the case of "*Zervixverschlussinsuffizienz*", " … the incompetence of the cervix to retain a intrauterine pregnancy until the period of due date. According to the textbook, it is characterized by a painless opening and shortening of the cervix uteri between 16 and 28 weeks of gestation." ([17], p. 727, translated by us).

Some authors suggest considering cervical sufficiency and insufficiency as a continuum (for a review see Romero et al. [16]). They also suggest considering "cervical insufficiency" as a syndrome. They list as reasons for cervical ripening in the mid-trimester:

1. the loss of connective tissue after a cervical operation such as conization
2. a congenital disorder such as cervical hypoplasia after diethylstilbestrol (DES) exposure
3. intrauterine infection
4. a suspension of progesterone action.

Of these reasons intrauterine infection is particularly relevant. According to Romero et al. [19], among women corresponding to the clinical picture of cervical insufficiency, the frequency of microbial invasion of the amniotic cavity is as high as 51% (please also compare chapter 6 in this volume).

Reasons for Operation: According to Vetter and Kilavuz [17] the reasons for performing operations at the cervix may roughly be divided into:

1. *A mechanical incompetence* of the cervix tissue which leads to a premature opening of the cervix. This is cervical incompetence or cervical insufficiency in the classical sense and is rather rare. Examples for diseases with these tissue changes are Marfan syndrome or Ehlers-Danlos Syndrome.
2. *A functional disturbance* of the closing system of the cervix, brought about for example by a smaller functional length, the lack of, or dysfunctional, cervical mucus, or after a lesion of the cervix. These may allow infections to ascend which then may be the basis for late abortions or premature births.

According to Vetter and Kilavuz, a *cerclage* is regarded as a solution for mechanical incompetence, whereas, for functional disturbance, *(Early) Total Cervix Occlusion* is recommended (the latter applies to date only to German speaking countries). But neither of the operations can prevent cervical changes due to labor.

Cerclage

History

Cervical cerclage was introduced in 1955 by Shirodkar and was first performed on women who had had at least 4 abortions or was confined to women in whom he could prove the existence of weakness of the internal os by ‘‘repeated internal examinations’’ [20]. McDonald [21] suggested a simplification, and there now exist a variety of modifications. During the last 50 years cerclage has been used in circumstances different from those originally intended, (eg, prevention of preterm birth after only one late abortion or preterm birth in the history or in women with a sonographically short cervix) and there is a lot of discussion about the efficacy of the more recently used indications. The last decade in particular has seen a decrease in the usage of cerclage [17].

Indications and Results

In contrast to “the early days” of cerclage, a cerclage is performed today either

- *prophylactically and electively,* according to the history of the patient or due to findings within the present pregnancy, or
- *therapeutically,* in cases with significant opening or shortening of the cervix.

Although cerclage has been performed quite frequently, it has increasingly become a subject of controversy. Harger [22] and the ACOG practice bulletin [18] give good overviews with regard to current recommendations. In the last decades, several randomized and controlled trials as well as meta-analyses have been performed (some examples are listed in table 2).

Randomized studies with cerclage have not proven to be of benefit for women with low risk of preterm delivery (by history) [24]. The effectiveness in women with high risk pregnancies is uncertain. For example, Rush [26] could not find any significant difference. The MRC/RCOG final report on cerclage [27] did find a significant difference only in one of 6 subgroups, namely with regard to births under 33 weeks gestation in the subgroup of women with 3 or more second trimester miscarriages or preterm births in the history.

Table 2. Meta-analyses with regard to cervical cerclage

Meta-analyses	No. of included randomized trials and objectives	Conclusion
Odibo et al. 2003 [23]	6 trials. Objective: To review the evidence on the use of cerclage to prevent preterm birth compared with expectant management.	Trend that cerclage prevents delivery before 34 weeks gestation, but not significantly. No improvement of neonatal mortality, but an increased risk of postpartum fever.
Drakely et al. 2003 [24]	6 trials. Objective: To estimate the effectiveness of prophylactic and therapeutic cerclage	The effectiveness of prophylactic cerclage in women at low and medium risk for second trimester pregnancy loss has not been proven. The role of cerclage in women whose ultrasound reveals short cervix remains uncertain.
Belej-Rak et al. 2003 [25]	6 trials. Objective: Effectiveness of cerclage for a shortened cervix on transvaginal ultrasound scanning.	The available evidence does not support cerclage for sonographically detected short cervix.

More current research tried to identify women who might benefit from cerclage by monitoring the cervical length and performing a cerclage only when the cervix is shortened or shortening. Although initial studies had been promising [28, 29] more recent studies do not support this [30, 25]. Hassan et al. [31] could even show in a retrospective cohort study, that, in patients with a shortened cervix ($\leq$ 15 mm), cervical cerclage did not only not reduce the rate of preterm delivery but it did increase the risk of preterm rupture of membranes. Obido et al. [32] compared Shirodkar versus McDonald cerclage in women with a short cervix and found no significant difference in the prevention of preterm delivery.

In conclusion: For women with low risk, cerclage does not appear to be indicated, but with regard to women at high risk (by history), the situation is not quite clear. Romero et al. conclude in their review: "The role of prophylactic cerclage in high-risk patients without a sonographic short cervix for the prevention of preterm delivery/mid-trimester abortion (by history) is unclear. While the largest trial conducted before the introduction of ultrasound evaluation of the cervix suggested a modest beneficial effect, other trials and systematic reviews before the use of ultrasound have indicated that the evidence of effectiveness is either weak or nonexistent." and further: "... patients with the clinical presentation of 'acute cervical insufficiency' and those with a previous history consistent with 'cervical insufficiency' and progressive shortening of the cervix demonstrated with ultrasound may benefit from cerclage placement. However, these conclusions are based on the results of one randomized clinical trial each." (Romero et al. [16], page 3).

When considering the possible benefits of cerclage, one has also to consider the possible complications, which are various: for example (besides the general risk of anesthesia), premature labor, rupture of membranes or placental abruption, local infections, infections of the amnion, lesions of the cervix, fistulas and even ruptures of the uterus [17].

Romero et al. [16] discuss a combination of cervical ultrasound and markers of endocervical inflammation (for example IL-8) to identify patients who may benefit from a cerclage. Referring to the results of Sakai et al. [33, 34], they suggest that

- patients with an elevated concentration of IL-8 and a short cervix (< 25 mm) may not benefit from cerclage, because they may have already an inflammation. In contrast,
- patients with a history of a preterm birth, a sonographically short cervix and an IL-8-levels of less than 360 ng/mL may benefit from cerclage [16].

Much more research seems to be necessary to identify women who may actually benefit from cerclage. Although we share the opinion (a) as stated by Romero et al, we would, however, rather recommend an ETCO for the cases described in (b), as it provides both some mechanical support for the cervix as well as preventing the ascension of microbes (see below).

ETCO

History

We introduced the Early Total Cervix Occlusion (ETCO) in 1981 [1]. Before that time there were very few publications in the literature about occlusions of the cervix[1]. Apart from this, the occlusion had been performed almost entirely in cases of threatened abortions, and always when an advanced stage in the abortion process had been reached. At that time the cervix occlusion was an emergency measure, particularly in cases with protruding membranes. In Germany, Szendi [36, 35] published in 1961 two articles on the subject prevention of advanced miscarriages and abortion through total cervix occlusion. In the USA, Baden and Baden [38] performed tracheloplasty in some cases with recurrent late abortions and dilatation of the cervix despite non-surgical therapy. Although they removed some of the cervix surface and then made the sutures, their occlusion was not complete, as they

[1] Also, some of theses reports are not complete occlusions in the strict sense. For example Hall [37] published the case report of an occlusive trachelorrhaphy in the case of women with amputed cervix and recurrent abortions. He used mattress sutures to occlude the cervix, but he did not remove the epithelium (which is important to allow the os uteri to grow completely together). Therefore we would rather classify this measure as a "tight" form of cerclage.

intentionally left open one small canal or, on occasion, two canals in the case of a "bridge" tracheloplasty.

ETCO as Preventive Measure

Our goal was completely different. We introduced the cervix occlusion as a preventive measure to prevent premature labor. The total cervix occlusion creates a complete barrier against ascending infections within the cervical canal und is as such, from our point of view, the most effective measure for preventing repeated late abortions and premature births. ETCO should be performed when:

- women have a poor past history (see below)
- the pregnancy is not advanced (at about 12 weeks gestation)
- the cervix is still in an anatomically undisturbed condition.

ETCO is quite different from cerclage (and in principle also from the occasionally used pessary). The cerclage only tightens the canal and leads to much poorer results (see below). ETCO on the other hand really closes the cervical canal: After the epithelium of the lower cervical canal and of the lower portio had been removed these parts are sutured. This allows the lower cervix to heal up and close totally. This is a total barrier which thus prevents ascension of organisms (Figure 1).

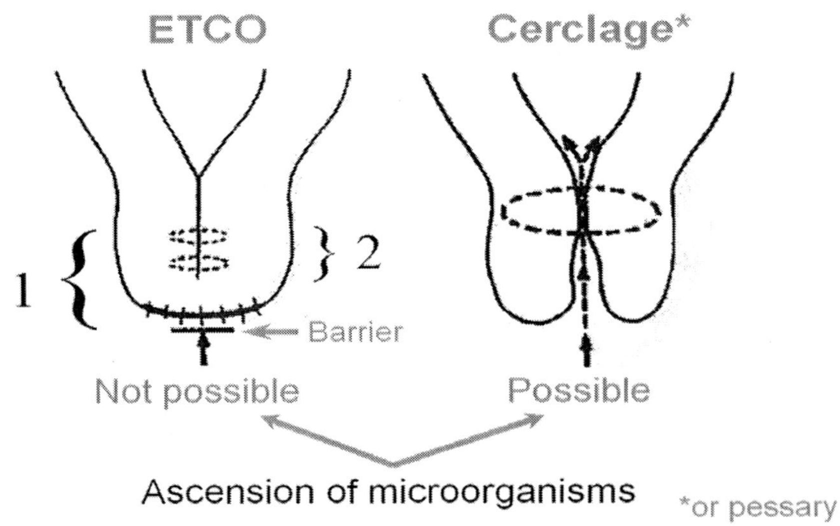

Figure 1. Early Total Cervix Occlusion (ETCO) versus Cerclage or pessary. ETCO = Early Total Cervix Occlusion ("early" means: operation performed at < 16+0 weeks gestation and before anatomic changes at the cervix are detectable); 1) "Extensive" ETCO; 2) "Small" ETCO.

All three measures provide some mechanical support for the cervix. In the case of ETCO this support is due to scars that develop as a result of the circular intracervical stitches and also of the two transverse rows of sutures in the region of the external os uteri. ETCO therefore has a double benefit, whereas cerclage and pessary mainly give mechanical support.

Definitions

With regard to the Total Cervix Occlusion (TCO) we differentiate between "early" and "late" and between "small" and "extensive" (table 3). Because the results in the prevention of prematurity are much better (see below) we recommend performing the TCO "early" (ETCO) rather than "late" (LTCO).

Table 3. Definitions with regard to Total Cervix Occlusion (TCO)

Description	Definition, resp. performance
Early Total Cervix Occlusion (ETCO)	performed at < 16+0 weeks *and* with an almost normal anatomical state of the portio: • no critical sonographic cervix finding* or • modified** Bishop score of $\leq$ 4)
Late Total Cervix Occlusion (LTCO)	performed at $\geq$16+0 weeks *or* critical state of the portio diagnosed sonographically*: • cervix length <30 mm • funneling of the isthmical part • prolapse of amniotic sac or, if sonography is not available: diagnosed by palpation modified** Bishop score of > 4 (s. table 4).
Extensive TCO	After removing both the glandular epithelium in the lower cervical canal and the epithelium of the lower portio, the cervix is closed by 2-3 circular internal sutures followed by 2 transverse rows of knotted stitches to close and adapt the surface of the portio (see figurc 1, brackct 1) For most cases we recommend an *extensive* occlusion. Best is the Early Total Cervix Occlusion (ETCO), or, if this is not possible anymore, the late TCO.
Small TCO	Only the cervical canal is closed after removing the glandular epithelium by 2-3 circular sutures (see figure 1, bracket 2).
*The sonographic measurement of the cervical length is more reliable than the assessment using the Bishop score and is therefore the method of choice. **Saling and Schumacher [39], see table 4	

Table 4. Modified Bishop Score according to Saling [39] (nowadays recommendable only at places, where ultrasonography is not available)

Length of the portio	*Points*
3 cm (Portio intact)	0
2 cm (partially effaced)	1
1 cm (considerably effaced)	2
0 cm (completely effaced)	3
Consistency of the portio	
Hard	0
Medium	1
Soft	3
External os uteri	
Closed	0
Open for finger tip	1
Accessible for the finger	2
Opened for ≥ 2 cm	3

Indications and Contraindication

1. Indications for an ETCO are :

- two or more late abortions (≥ 12+0 weeks gestation)
- or two or more early premature births (<32+0 weeks gestation)
- or one late abortion and one early premature birth

in the patient's history with

- either infection as cause for these events
- or when no other cause has been found, but when for instance PROM occurred. Please note that the main reason for premature rupture of the membranes is ascending vaginal infection.

2. Up to now no study is available to indicate whether, in cases with only one previous late abortion or early premature birth, consistent screening for vaginal infection (see chapter 6) will lead to similar good results as ETCO. Therefore, in some cases, one might consider an ETCO even after only *one* late abortion or premature birth,

particularly when additional risks exist, for instance, when the patient is older or when there had been problems with fertility. In these cases a *"small" occlusion of the cervix* (see table 3 and figure 1) may be sufficient.

3. *In multiple pregnancies* Schulze [40] was able to achieve a clear reduction in the number of premature births (see below) by performing an ETCO as a general preventive measure, even when there were no historical risks. When considering the existing data, it is perhaps too early to recommend that ETCO be performed generally in all multiple pregnancies before equally good results have been confirmed by other studies. Nevertheless, in multiple pregnancies and when additional risks factors are present (e.g. after In-vitro fertilisation, or in a pregnant woman nearing the end of her possible reproductive time), we are of the opinion that the possibility of performing an ETCO should certainly be taken into consideration.

A *contraindication* is dilatation of the cervix with apparent signs of infection and labor activity which cannot be inhibited.

Preoperative Diagnostics and Measures

Choice of Clinical Department and Informing the Patient

Although ETCO is now quite widespread in Germany and also performed in Switzerland and Austria, it is still not a standard operation. The operation is not especially difficult to perform (see below) but we nonetheless recommend choosing a clinical department with experience in this procedure. Also, the patient should be informed accordingly, and she should also be informed that, for patients with otherwise poor chances of bearing a live child ETCO offers very good chances (80-88 %)—but is no guarantee for success.

Screening for Infections and Pap-Test

If the last Pap-test dates back a longer period, it is recommended to perform one before admission to the hospital, as the portio surface will partially be removed and then, after the occlusion, the concerning area is covered for a longer period.

Examinations for infections are compulsory: for example vaginal, cervical and urethral smears with microscopic and/or bacteriologic examinations. Furthermore, should pathological findings be present—such as bacterial vaginosis, candida, Trichomonas or Chlamydia infection, the patient should be given an appropriate local or a systemic therapy. Furthermore it is recommended to perform an egg-pole lavage (see below) directly before the operation (right on the operating table).

Pre-Operative Disinfection

2 to 3 days before the operation a pre-operative disinfection or germ-reducing vaginal therapy should be performed by means of:

- one Hexetidine vaginal tablet e.g. VagiHex® taken twice daily or
- a twice daily intravaginal application of Octenidine-2HCL solution for local antiseptic treatment.

It is advisable to continue the disinfection measures for 2-3 days after the operation. After this has finished a Lactobacillus acidophilus preparation should be administered for several days to help rebuild the normal vaginal flora.

Egg-Pole Lavage (EPL, Isthmical Lavage) as Immediate Preoperative Diagnostic

After an ETCO has been performed there is no further chance to examine whether any organisms may already have ascended to the intrauterine space. Therefore we recommend performing a so-called egg-pole lavage (isthmical lavage, this means a lavage of the lower uterine extra-amniotic space) directly before the operative occlusion of the cervix. We introduced the EPL in 1992 [42] and reported on the first experiences [41].

With this method, by which fluid is obtained from the lower egg-pole and bacteriologically examined, important information can be obtained without the necessity of having to do a more invasive amniocentesis. If necessary the appropriate antibiotics can be administered. The egg-pole lavage is explained in detail on *www.saling-institute.org* at the site for professionals/Early Total Cervix Occlusion. In departments where the egg-pole lavage is not performed, they often applicate broad-band antibiotics around the time of the operation as a preventive measure. We are not in favor of this, because this might lead unnecessarily to antibiotic resistance and because of other side effects of antibiotics. Whereas taking samples for culture via an egg-pole lavage allows specific antibiotic therapy and only when necessary.

Operation Technique

Before starting the operative occlusion, we highly recommend that the portio should be tied off as high as possible to prevent bleeding, in such a way that there is a nearly complete stoppage of the circulation. This measure has two distinctive advantages:

- The blood loss, which in pregnant patients can be considerable, due to the intense vascularisation, can be reduced to a minimum and

- the visibility during the operation and later when the wound is being stitched is much better than if continuous, diffuse bleeding had occurred.

We have developed a special loop instrument for this purpose [43], see figures 2 and 3

Ligature with the loop instrument

There is a ratchet on the loop instrument [43] on the traction stick with a blocking spring (Figure 3). This allows the stainless steel braided wire loop (Figure 2), to be attached in a circle around the portio and to be fixed up in a tightened state. We always try to clamp the loop so tightly that only minimal bleeding remains.

This is a sign that the tissue circulation is not completely interrupted. When the hemostasis has to be suspended at the end of the operation, the traction stick is turned about 90°. The blocking spring slides out of the traction and the loop is set free. The loop instrument can be obtained from Willi Falk KG, Berlin (info@faromed.de).

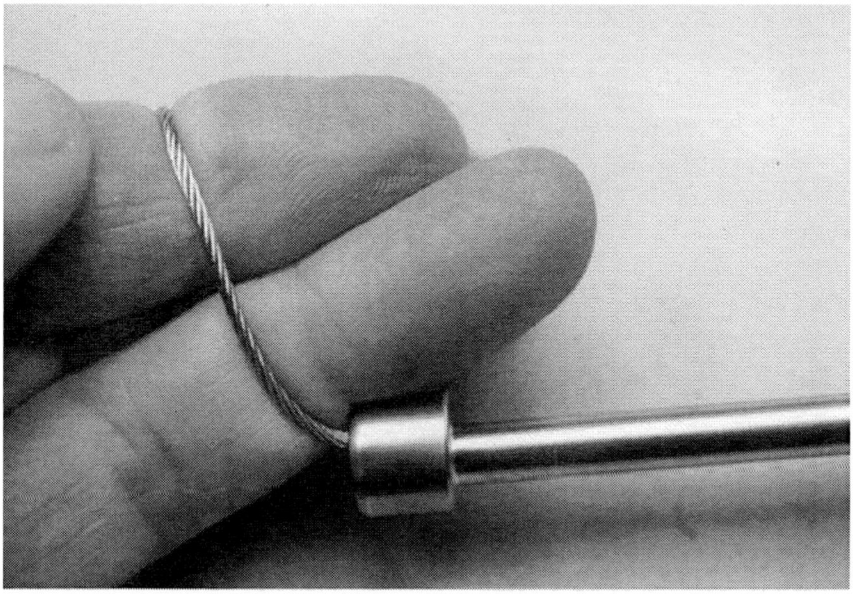

Figure 2. Loop instrument to reduce bleeding: Loop demonstrated on two fingers.

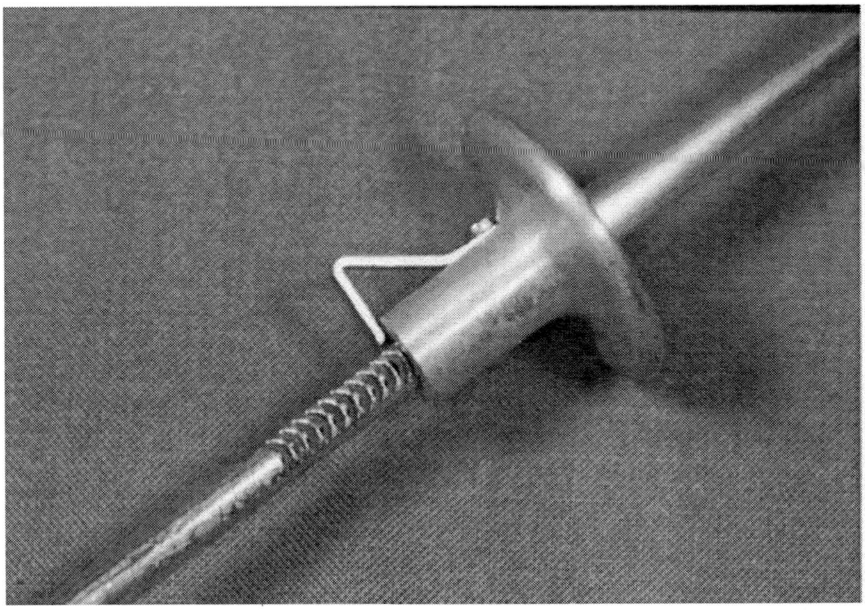

Figure 3. Loop instrument to reduce bleeding: blocking device.

Removal of the epithelium

In order to allow the lower part of the cervix to grow completely together, the upper surface of the portio (about 1.5 cm around the external os) has to be dissected, that is to say, the epithelium has to be removed completely. It is essential to remove this epithelium, because otherwise the portio tissue will not grow together. And the better the portio tissue grows together in such critical cases - namely when the portio remains completely occluded right until near term - the better are the chances that a good result can be achieved.

It used to be the case that the epithelium was removed from the portio surface by sharp dissection with a scalpel.

In the meantime a better method has been introduced: by smoothing down the surface of the portio with a high-speed rotating simple sterile wire brush (see Figure 4), as is used in dermatology to smooth out scars.

Possible is also a special metal rasp (see Figure 5). With this method only the superficial layer of the epithelium is gently removed and therefore the tissue is given a considerably better and more certain chance of regeneration.

So as to clearly mark the surface to be removed, but also to find the exact positioning of the wounded area later for the row of stitches adapting the upper surface of the portio, we make a circular incision with a scalpel one millimeter deep with a radius of 10 - 15 mm round the external os uteri (Figure 6).

Then we remove the portio epithelium with the fast rotating wire brush or the special metal rasp. This wire brush is powered by a small battery-operated electric engine over a flexible wavelength. A high-speed rotating instrument powered by compressed air (for example from Aesculap Co.) can also be used.

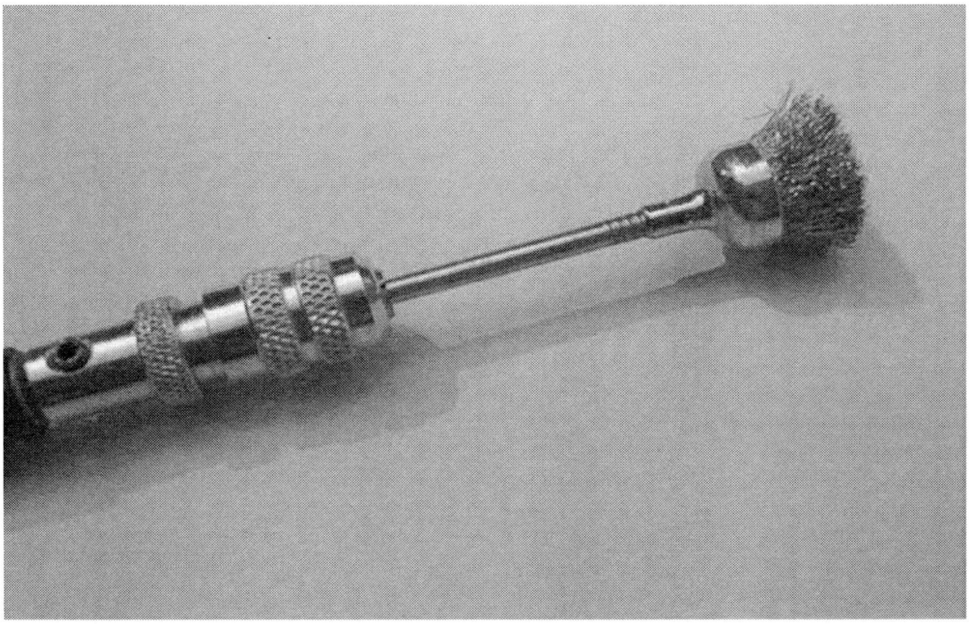

Figure 4. Rotating brush.

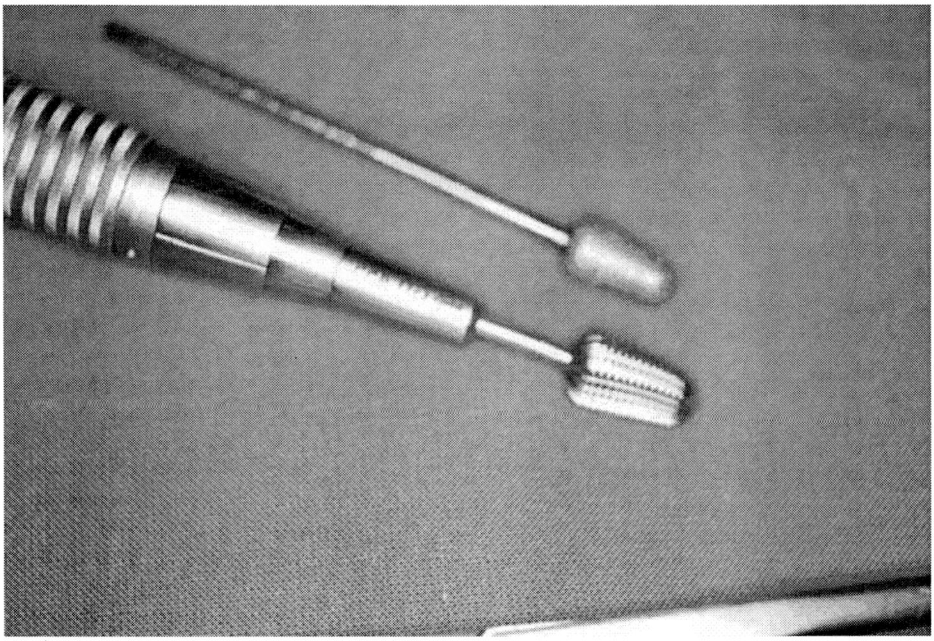

Figure 5. Rotating metal rasp.

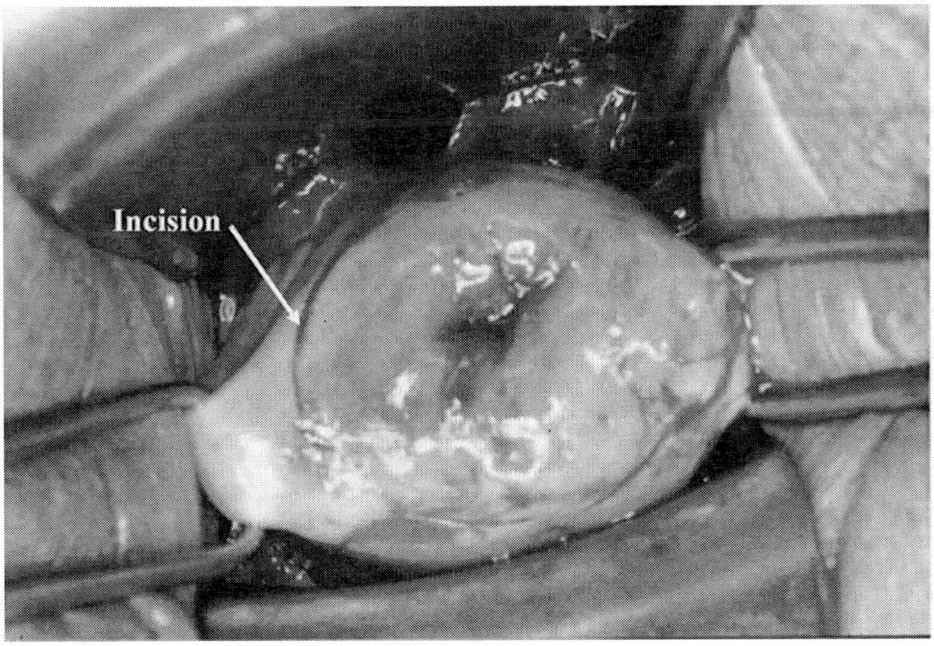

Figure 6. Marking by a circular incision.

This has the advantage that the patient is never connected to any electric source. However, this equipment is more expensive to obtain. Afterwards, the glandular epithelium of the cervical canal is also removed, as far as possible about 1 to 2 cm above the external os using the same rotating device, whilst the os uteri is spread using mosquito clamps (Figure 7).

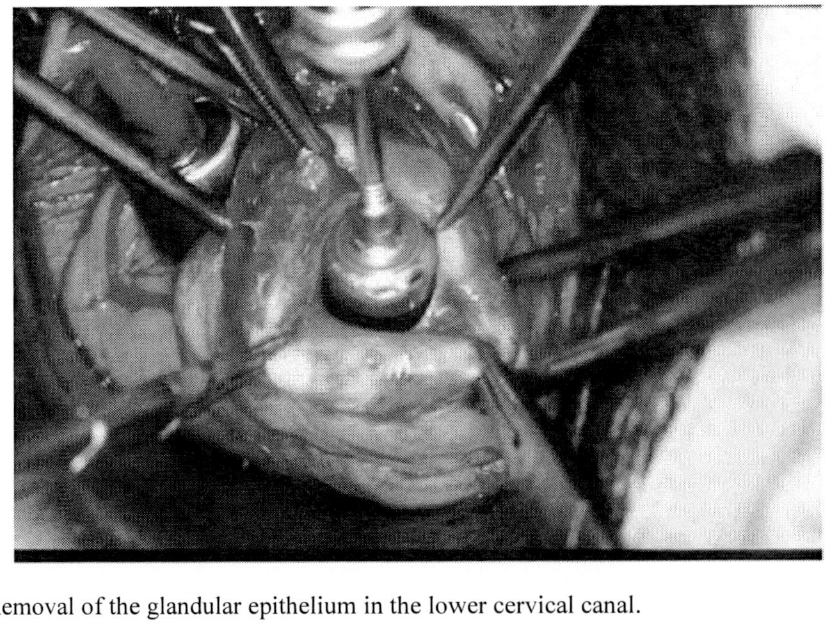

Figure 7. Removal of the glandular epithelium in the lower cervical canal.

Stitching Techniques

The stitching technique is shown in Figure 8. After the removal of the epithelium (Figure 8, No. 1) first 2-3 inner circular stitches are made to close the cervical canal (Figure 8, No. 2). Subsequently two rows of knotted stitches are made, which close the outer os uteri completely (Figure 8, No. 3-5).

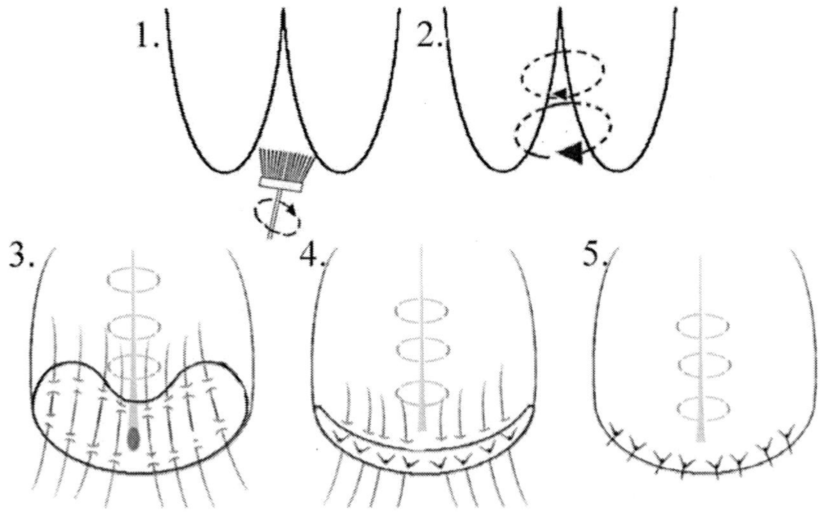

Figure 8. Stitching technique: schematic diagram. (1) removal of the epithelium, (2) 2-3 circular internal cervical sutures, (3) transverse stitching of the whole dissected area for deep adaptation, (4) after the first row has been knotted second row of stitches adapting the surface tissue, (5) situation after operation.

We use synthetic monofile thread like PDS or braided thread, such as Vicryl. These threads, when compared to catgut, are much better for the healing process and are reabsorbed much more slowly.

Measures at the End of Pregnancy

When the pregnancy has reached a sufficient number of weeks (for example 36-37 gestational weeks), when spontaneous labor starts or induction is indicated, an attempt must be made to recanalize the cervix.

This is particularly difficult when the portio is not significantly effaced (still 2-3 cm). The scar should be opened at latest when:

- labor starts spontaneously,
- an induction of labor is planned, or
- 37 weeks of gestation are completed.

A prior ultrasonic examination of the cervix is recommended to clarify the anatomical proportions. We generally cut the portio scar with scissors (Figure 9) under local or peridural anesthesia (if this was placed for labor). Then we penetrate with the finger to a depth of about 1-2 cm into the loose cervical tissue in the assumed direction of the cervical canal (Figure 10).

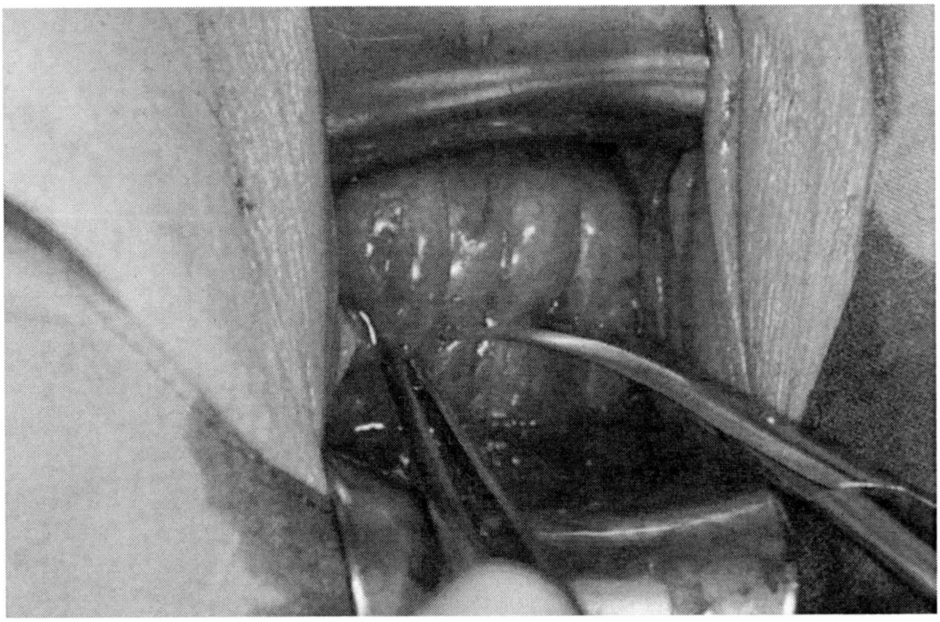

Figure 9. Opening of the portio scar.

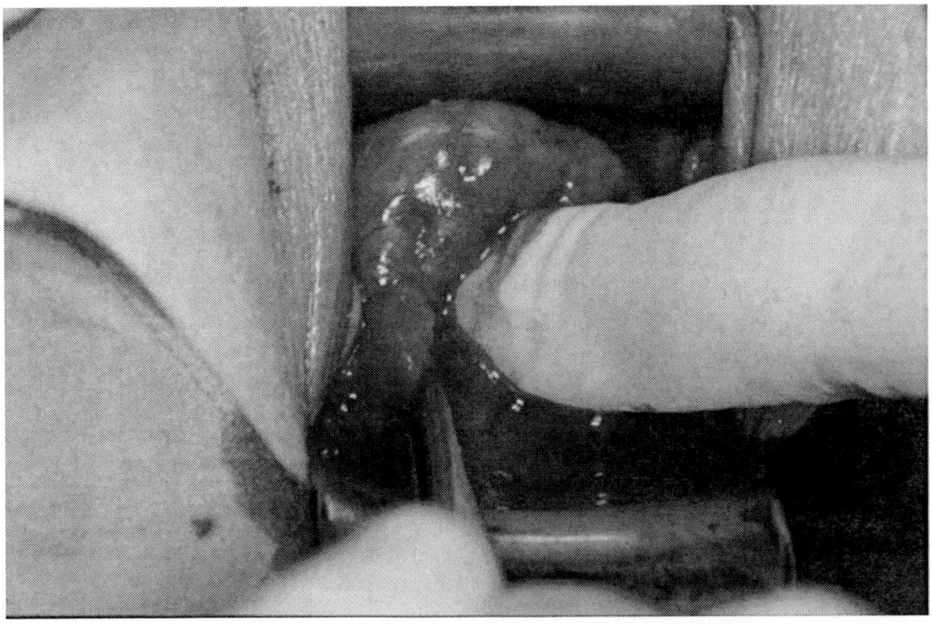

Figure 10. Introduction of the finger in the assumed direction of the internal os uteri.

If the patient wants to leave the hospital after the scar has been opened to wait until labor starts spontaneously, we see no reason why she should not do so, provided there are no signs of any increased risk.

We do not think that a primary cesarean section is necessary at all. Quite the contrary: When a recanalization of the cervix takes place during a vaginal delivery, this is in fact a good prerequisite for the reestablishment of normal anatomic conditions. We know from our own experience that after a primary cesarean section it can be extremely difficult to achieve recanalization of the cervix which has not been opened or dilated before, due to complex anatomical conditions.

In all those patients who had a vaginal delivery after ETCO, the epithelium tissue around the wounded area of the portio recovered during the puerperium within a short space of time (a few weeks) and it is surprising—particularly since the introduction of the gentle epithelium removal technique—how little of the operational scar is to be seen later on after regeneration during the puerperium (please see the pictures at www.saling-institute.org).

Results

To assess the results of ETCO, particularly in comparison to those of cerclage, one should only look at high-risk-groups such as those matching the above mentioned indications for an ETCO ($\geq$ 2 late abortions or early premature births). We have no knowledge of any randomized study concerning ETCO. On the basis of the results published so far we do not think that the operation can be withheld from any woman with such a critical history (for ethical discussion see below). Therefore, an acceptable solution is to compare the outcome of pregnancies after performing an ETCO with the outcome of these patients' former pregnancies [45, 44, 39, 46]. While doing this, we should also consider that the chances of giving birth to a surviving infant are reduced the more late abortions or premature births the woman has previously had (see above).

In 1990 we evaluated retrospectively the data of a group of 113 patients with previous recurrent abortions. From a total of 389 wanted pregnancies only 101 infants were born alive (26%). However, 35 of these infants died in the neonatal period. In total 66 survived, which means that only 17 % of all these pregnancies resulted in a surviving infant. Through the introduction of the total cervical occlusion (either early or late TCO) the same patients achieved 132 pregnancies with 94 live and surviving infants (71% !). We could also show, that the results in cases with an "early" TCO are twice as good as with a "late" TCO (80% vs. 40%) [47, 48].

If one considers the 38 cases where the pregnancy was unsuccessful, there were 10 premature deliveries with an extremely low birth weight, and who all died shortly after birth. In the remaining cases there were miscarriages, 13 of which occurred after a late occlusion, and 15 after an early occlusion. So the rate of abortions after the "late" occlusion amounted to 43% against only 15% after the "early" occlusion [49].

Similarly good results have been obtained by other clinicians performing the TCO: In 1996 we reported the results of a multi-center evaluation, in which 11 German hospitals took part [39], and the outcome of a total of 819 pregnancies with TCO was assessed. We showed that the rate of surviving infants in the pregnancies before TCO had been performed was 21% compared to 74% in the pregnancies with TCO. Hormel and Künzel [46] reported similarly good results.

Some years later Vetter and Kilavuz [17] achieved even better results; their success rate for Early Total Cervix Occlusion (indicated by the patients history) was 88 %, the success rate of late Cervix Occlusion due to critical cervix finding was 84 % and an occlusion of an opened cervix after the pushing back of the amniotic sac plus cerclage according to Shirodkar was still 74 %.

As far as the mode of delivery is concerned, 71% of the patients in our study with a total cervical occlusion had a spontaneous delivery and 15 % had an operative vaginal delivery. The rate of cesarean sections was 14% in comparison to 9% for the whole department at that time [48].

This relatively low cesarean rate shows that, in most cases after ETCO, vaginal delivery can be achieved without any problems (once the scar has been opened). This is actually recommendable, since the cervix is stretched, which can be regarded as advantageous for the regeneration process after the operative occlusion, particularly to facilitate future conception.

In 1997 we reported the results of a follow-up examination carried out on 52 women who had previously had a total cervical occlusion [50]. On the basis of these results generally we can conclude that up to now no notable negative effects have been proven in connection with the operative total cervical occlusion.

So far there have been no studies with a control group without ETCO. But Vetter and Kilavuz [17] reported some cases in which women had a successful pregnancy with ETCO; in the next pregnancy without ETCO they had a late abortion and after that with ETCO again successful pregnancies.

Multiple Pregnancy and ETCO

All the results published up to now concern women who had already had at least one or several early premature birth, or late abortion in the past. In the meantime more recent results have become available in cases where ETCO was performed as a general preventive measure in multiple pregnancies (which are known to have a higher risk of prematurity), even if the women concerned had not had a poor history: Since 1990 Schulze [40] has, in the cases of those patients who consented, been performing ETCO as a prophylactic measure in the Women's Hospital in Cottbus (Germany) on multiple pregnancies—and has achieved remarkable success: from a total of 219 multiple pregnancies he performed an ETCO on 96 of the women, and 123 did not have the operation. The rate of very early prematures (< 32 weeks gestation) was 24% in the cases without ETCO and 13.5% in those with ETCO. In the group of infants at very high risk—those who were born at less than 28 completed weeks of gestation - the rate with ETCO was 1% and without ETCO it was 4%. Consequently, it can be seen that the perinatal mortality in cases after ETCO was almost half as much. After ETCO it was 2.5% and without ETCO 4.1%.

When considering the existing data, before the good results seen above have been confirmed at other places it is perhaps too early to recommend that an ETCO should be performed in all multiple pregnancies. Furthermore there has not yet been a study on whether ETCO or the Self-Care-Program for pregnant women is more successful in multiple pregnancies in cases without poor history. Nevertheless, the ETCO should be seriously considered—particularly in multiple pregnancies with additional risk factors (e.g. after In-vitro fertilisation, or in the case of a pregnant woman near the end of her potential reproductive time).

ETCO versus Cerclage

To assess the results of ETCO, particularly in comparison to cerclage, one should only look at high-risk-groups such as those corresponding to the above mentioned indications for an ETCO (2 or more late abortions or early premature births). Cerclage is still a widespread measure despite controversial discussion. Some authors reported good results—but one should look at these reports very closely and verify whether or not the cerclage had been performed on women at similar high risk (see above).

Up to now there is no trial comparing ETCO and cerclage within the same study group (apart from our small group of ETCO patients with Cerclage in the history, see below) Therefore, the only option is to compare the data from different studies. But even this is difficult, particularly because the study groups are often disparate. For example Rush et al. [26] compared the pregnancy outcome in 194 women with or without cerclage within a high risk group. In their publication they gave the details of the obstetrical history of the women (e.g. how many women had none, one, two, three or more preterm deliveries), but they did not analyze the outcome of pregnancies according to these subgroups. They only evaluated all pregnancies together and found no significant difference between the cerclage and non-cerclage group (< 37weeks gestation: 34.4% vs. 31.6%).

The MRC/RCOG final report on cerclage [27] had six sub groups, three of them where either one, two or three and more second trimester miscarriage or preterm deliveries. Only in the subgroup with ≥ 3 second trimester miscarriage or preterm deliveries and birth with < 33 weeks gestation was there a significant difference (with cerclage 15%, without 32%; $p \geq 0.05$). The ACOG practice bulletin [18] therefore only recommends to consider elective cerclage for this subgroup. As the recurrence risk seems to be higher the earlier in pregnancy the preterm birth had been (see above), from our point of view, it would have been better, to differentiate the subgroups even further, according to the weeks gestation.

However, neither in our own study with regard to ETCO nor in the publications of Hormel and Künzel [46] or Vetter and Kilavuz [17] such a differentiated analysis with regard to subgroups has been made. This is something that future research should take into account.

Up to now, there are no studies comparing ETCO with cerclage. But in our sample of women treated with ETCO several women did previously have a cerclage with very limited benefit: In 51 previous pregnancies in which cerclage had been performed, only 13 infants survived. This is a survival rate of only 26% (as compared to a survival rate of 80% with ETCO). These results underline how advisable it is to give ETCO preference over cerclage in cases with such a critical history. In any case, cerclage is hardly capable of preventing ascending infections because this method only tightens the cervical canal and does not close it (see above, Figure 1)—although, theoretically, in a few cases of cerclage there could be an improvement of the immunological function of the cervical mucus achieved by tightening the cervical canal [51]. Noori et al [52] performed in addition to a cerclage an "external os occlusion suture". But as they didn't remove the epithelium, from our point of view, they still performed a very tight cerclage. Nonetheless, they report good results and discussed the concept, that their suture might allow "the build up of mucus plug, thus preventing the ingress of vaginal bacterial flora" (p. 534). It would be interesting to compare the results of their measure with the results after ETCO in a controlled study.

Some obstetricians combine the *Early Total Cervix Occlusion* with an additional cerclage. We, however, have not found any reason why this should be done—at least not when performed as a preventive measure. As has been explained already, the creation of a total barrier by the total occlusion is much more effective than a cerclage in the prevention of an ascending infection—the main cause of early prematurity. The combination might, however, be useful in cases with prolapse of the membranes. Vetter and Kilavuz [17] reported a success rate of 74% in such cases of a combination of Total Cervix Occlusion and additional cerclage according to Shirodkar.

Randomized Trials – Ethical Questions

We are aware that, in times of evidence-based medicine, prospective randomized trials are—or at least seem to be—"gold standard" when it comes to proving the effectiveness of a given measure. But we should not rely too much on the current, prevalent opinion that "randomized controlled studies" and the so-called "evidence based medicine" are the only reliable ways to differentiate between efficient and inefficient medical measures.

Also, one should bear in mind that, for example, randomized controlled trials:

- need considerable amounts of funds,
- need to be academically attractive,
- need a considerable amount of patients, which often can be only achieved by multi-center studies and
- there should be no benefit previously known to exist for either study or control group, as the patients would otherwise not be willing to take part (this is particularly the case for serious diseases)
- within the groups, there should not be a too extensive heterogenity, which is unfortunately often the case.

ETCO was developed in 1981 in Germany and is now widespread in Germany (currently, in more than 50 obstetrical departments and clinics the ETCO is performed regularly). It is also used in other German speaking countries, but it is still rarely performed on an international level. This might partly be due to the fact that randomized studies with ETCO have never yet been performed. But—considering the excellent results of ETCO—performing such a study now would raise serious ethical issues. Therefore, although it would be possibly more convincing for the international community if we had randomized trials for ETCO, we do not think that this is absolutely necessary to prove its efficiency.

On the basis of the results published so far we do not think that the operation can be withheld from any woman with such a critical history. A randomized study would hardly receive the approval of any council of ethics—at least not in Germany—and no woman with such a history is likely to agree to being integrated into a control group anyway. Also, our own ethical conscience would not permit such a study to be devised. Vetter and Kilavuz [17] express a similar opinion.

Therefore, an acceptable solution is to compare the outcome of pregnancies after performing an ETCO with the outcome of these patients' former pregnancies [44, 45, 39, 46]. While comparing these results, one should also consider that the chances of giving birth to a surviving infant are reduced the more late abortions or premature births the woman has previously had (see above).

The situation may be different in countries where ETCO is not performed at all. If a randomized study were to be performed there, at least some of the women would have the option of an ETCO (as opposed to now having only the option of cerclage or conservative measures). Therefore, if individual scientists or study groups consider a randomized trial with ETCO, we would welcome it and would support them with any advice or assistance, if necessary.

Conclusion

Recurrent premature births and late miscarriages are still a major problem in obstetrical and perinatal care. Infections, particularly ascending genital infections, may be responsible for a large proportion of these events.

Cerclage is still a widespread measure for cases with recurrent preterm births, but is increasingly becoming a subject of controversy. Due to the fact that it only tightens the cervical canal, but does not completely close it, cerclage may not sufficiently prevent infection-related premature births. Some results suggest, however, that it might be useful for other indications. A combination of poor history, shortening of the cervix and absence of elevated inflammation markers may possibly identify women who might actually benefit from it. More research in this area is necessary.

From our point of view, however, Total Cervix Occlusion (TCO), and, particularly, Early Total Cervix Occlusion (ETCO) are the better choice. It provides some mechanical support (as does the cerclage), but, more importantly, it completely closes the cervical canal and thus prevents the ascension of microorganisms.

On the basis of previous experiences and available results the Total Cervix Occlusion—in particular the early occlusion—is a convincingly efficient operative measure for the prevention of late abortions and early prematurity, particularly in cases where such events had previously recurrently happened.

Further Information

Our Website *www.saling-institute.org* contains information about ETCO both for medical professions as well as for patients. The following can be found:

- *detailed explanation of the operation* (including egg-pole-lavage) with more pictures than in this volume at: http://www.saling-institut.de/eng/04infoph/04tmv.html
- *Video about TMV:* the complete course of the Total Cervix Occlusion operation is available for a small fee in the form of a self-made video with commentaries in German or English. The amount that exceeds the production costs benefits the non-profit making Erich-Saling-Institute of Perinatal Medicine: http://www.saling-institut.de/eng/04infoph/04tmv.html#Video
- *address list* of clinics performing ETCO: Here we currently have a list of more than 60 obstetrical departments and clinics, mainly in German-speaking countries, where Early Total Cervix Occlusions are performed regularly. We are making efforts to get hold of more addresses. If a clinic performing this operation is not included in the list, please let us know. http://www.saling-institut.de/eng/06contact/04clin.html

References

[1] Saling E (1981): Der frühe totale Muttermundverschluß zur Vermeidung habitueller Aborte und Frühgeburten. *Z. Geburtshilfe Perinat.* 185: 259-261

[2] Saling E, Brandt-Niebelschütz S, Schmitz C (1991): Vermeidung von Spätaborten und risikoreichen Frühgeburten - für die Routine geeignete Maßnahmen. *Z. Geburtshilfe Perinat.* 195: 209-221

[3] Saling E (1991): Program for the Prevention of Prematurity. In: Hirsch HA: Infection and Preterm Labor (International Symposium Tübingen, 1990) Thieme, Stuttgart - New York.

[4] Romero R, Gomez R, Baumann P, Mazor M, Cotton D (1993): The role of the infection and cytokines in preterm parturition. In: Chwalisz K and Garfield RE: Basic Mechanismus controlling term and preterm birth; Ernst Schering Research Foundation, workshop 7; Springer, Berlin Heidelberg, New York: 197-240.

[5] Romero R, Espinoza J, Kusanovic JP, Gotsch F, Hassan S, Erez O, Chaiworapongsa T, Mazor M (2006b): The preterm parturition syndrome. *Br. J. Obstet. Gyneacol.* 113 (Suppl. 3): 17-42.

[6] Mazor M, Hershkovitz R, Ghezzi F, Maymon E, Horowitz S, Leiberman, JR (1996): Intraamniotic infection in patients with preterm labor and twin pregnancies. *Acta Obstet. Gynecol. Scand.* 75: 624–627.

[7] Bakketeig LS, Bergsjø P (1998): The epidemiology of preterm birth. In: Kurjak A (ed.): Textbook of Perinatal Medicine. London, New York: 1331-1336.

[8] Iams JD, Goldenberg RL, Mercer BM, Moawad A, Thom E, Meis PJ, McNellis D, Caritis SN, Miodovnik M, Menard MK, Thurnau GR, Bottoms SE, Roberts JM. (1998):

The preterm prediction study: recurrence risk of spontaneous preterm birth. *Am. J. Obstet. Gynecol.* 178: 1035-1040.

[9] Mercer, Brian M. MD; Goldenberg, Robert L. MD et al. (1999): The Preterm Prediction Study: Effect of gestational age and cause of preterm birth on subsequent obstetric outcome. *Am. J. Obstet. Gynecol.* 181 (5, Part 1): 1216-1221.

[10] Künzel W (1995): Epidemiologie der Frühgeburt, *Gynäkologe* 28: 130-135.

[11] Mazaki-Tovi S, Romero R, Kusanovic JP, Erez O, Pineles BL, Gotsch F, Mittal P, Than NG, Espinoza J, Hassan S (2007): Recurrent Preterm Birth. *Semin. Perinatol.* 31: 142-158.

[12] Durnwald CP, Walker H, Lundy JC, Iams JD (2005): Rates of recurrent preterm birth by obstetrical history and cervical length. *Am. J. Obstet. Gynecol.* 193, 1170-1174.

[13] Spong, CY (2007): Prediction and prevention of recurrent spontaneous preterm birth. *Obstet. Gynecol.* 110 (2): 405-415.

[14] McManemy, J, Cooke, E, Amon E, Leet T (2007): Recurrence risk for preterm delivery. *Am. J. Obstet. Gynecol.* 196: 567.e1-567.e7.

[15] Gream GT (1865): Dilatation or division of the cervix uteri. Lancet 1: 381 (quoted from: Vetter K, Kilavuz Ö (2001): Zervixinsuffizienz: operative Möglichkeiten. *Gynäkologe* 34: 726-731).

[16] Romero R, Espinoza J, Erez O, Hassan S (2006a): The role of cervical cerclage in obstetric practice: Can the patient who could benefit from this procedure be identified? *Am. J. Obstet. Gynecol.* 194: 1-9.

[17] Vetter K, Kilavuz Ö (2001): Zervixinsuffizienz: operative Möglichkeiten. *Gynäkologe* 34: 726-731.

[18] American College of Obstetricians and Gynecologists (2004): ACOG Practice Bulletin. Cervical insufficiency. *Int. J. Gynaecol. Obstet.* 85: 81-89.

[19] Romero R, Gonzalez R, Sepulveda W, Brandt F, Ramirez M, Sorokin Y, et al (1992): Infection and labor. VIII. Microbial invasion of the amniotic cavity in patients with suspected cervical incompetence: prevalence and clinical significance. *Am. J. Obstet. Gynecol.* 167: 1086–1091.

[20] Shirodkar VN (1955): A new method of operative treatment for habitual abortions in the second trimester of pregnancy. *Antiseptic* 1955; 52: 299-300.

[21] McDonald IA (1957): Suture of the cervix for inevitable miscarriage. *J. Obstet. Gynaecol. Br. Emp.* 64: 346-50.

[22] Harger JH (2002): Cerclage and ''cervical insufficiency'': an evidence based analysis. *Obstet. Gynecol.* 100: 1313-1327.

[23] Odibo AO, Elkousy M, Ural SH, Macones GA (2003): Prevention of preterm birth by cervical cerclage compared with expectant management: a systematic review. *Obstet. Gynecol. Surv.* 58 (2): 130-136.

[24] Drakeley AJ, Roberts D, Alfirevic Z (2004): Cervical cerclage for prevention of preterm delivery: meta-analysis of randomized trials. *Obstet. Gynecol.* 102 (3): 621-627.

[25] Belej-Rak T, Okun N, Windrim R, Ross S, Hannah ME (2003): Effectiveness of cervical cerclage for a sonographically shortened cervix: a systematic review and meta-analysis. *Am. J. Obstet. Gynecol.* 189 (6): 1679-1687.

[26] Rush RW, Isaacs S, McPherson K, Jones L, Chalmers I, Grant A (1984): A randomized controlled trial of cervical cerclage in women at high risk of spontaneous preterm delivery. *Br. J. Obstet. Gynaecol.* 91 (8):724-30.

[27] MRC/RCOG Working Party on Cervical Cerclage (1993): Final report of the medical research council/royal college of obstetricans and gynaecologists multicentre randomised trial of cervical cerclage. *Br. J. Obstet. Gynaecol.* 100: 516-523.

[28] Berghella V, Haas S, Chervoneva I, Hyslop T (2002): Patients with prior second-trimester loss: prophylactic cerclage or serial transvaginal sonograms? *Am. J. Obstet. Gynecol.* 187 (3): 747-751.

[29] To MS, Palaniappan V, Skentou C, Gibb D, Nicolaides KH (2002): Elective cerclage vs. ultrasound-indicated cerclage in high-risk pregnancies. *Ultrasound Obstet. Gynecol.* 19 (5): 475-477.

[30] To MS, Alfirevic Z, Heath VC, Cicero S, Cacho AM, Williamson PR, Nicolaides KH; Fetal Medicine Foundation Second Trimester Screening Group (2004): Cervical cerclage for prevention of preterm delivery in women with short cervix: randomised controlled trial. *Lancet* 363: 1849-1853.

[31] Hassan SS, Romero R, Maymon E, Berry SM, Blackwell SC, Treadwell MC, Tomlinson M (2001): Does cervical cerclage prevent preterm delivery in patients with a short cervix? *Am. J. Obstet. Gynecol.* 184: 1325-1329.

[32] Odibo AO, Berghella V, To MS, Rust OA, Althuisius SM, Nicolaides KH (2007): Shirodkar versus McDonald cerclage for the prevention of preterm birth in women with short cervical length. *Am. J. Perinatol.* 24 (1): 55-60.

[33] Sakai M, Sasaki Y, Yoneda S, Kasahara T, Arai T, Okada M, Hosokawa H, Kato K, Soeda Y, Saito S. (2004): Elevated interleukin-8 in cervical mucus as an indicator for treatment to prevent premature birth and preterm, pre-labor rupture of membranes: a prospective study. *Am. J. Reprod. Immunol.* 51: 220-225.

[34] Sakai M, Shiozaki A, Tabata M, Sasaki Y, Yoneda S, Arai T, Kato K, Yamakawa Y, Saito S. (2006): Evaluation of effectiveness of prophylactic cerclage of a short cervix according to interleukin-8 in cervical mucus. *Am. J. Obstet. Gynecol.* 194: 14-19.

[35] Szendi B (1961): Vollständiges Zusammennähen des äußeren Muttermundes auf blutigem Wege zur Verhinderung von vorgeschrittenen Abortus und Frühgeburten. *Zentralbl. Gynakol.* 83: 1083-1087.

[36] Szendi B (1961): Verhinderung von fortgeschrittenen Fehl- und Frühgeburten durch vollkommenen Muttermundverschluss auf blutigem Weg. Acta Chirurgica II: 413-418.

[37] Hall, HH (1956): Occlusive trachelorrhaphy for repeated abortion due to cervical incompetence. *Am. J. Obstet. Gynecol.* 71: 225-226.

[38] Baden WF and Baden EE (1960): Cervical invompetence: current therapy. *Am. J. Obstet. Gynecol.* 79: 545-551.

[39] Saling E, Schumacher E (1996): Der operative Totale Muttermund-Verschluß (TMV). Erhebung von Daten einiger Kliniken, die den TMV einsetzen. *Z. Geburtshilfe Neonatol.* 200: 82-87.

[40] Schulze G (2008): Ergebnisse des Frühen Totalen Muttermundverschlusses nach Saling (FTMV) bei Mehrlingsschawangerschaften – eine retrospektive Studie der Jahre 1995-2005 [Results of Early Total Cervix Occlusion (ETCO) According to Saling in

Multiple Pregnancies – a retrospective study of the period 1995-2005.] *Z. Geburtshilfe Neonatol.* 2008 212: 13-17.

[41] Brandt-Niebelschütz S, Saling E, Küchler R (1992): Weitere Erfahrungen mit der Eipol-Lavage (EPL) im Zusammenhang mit der Vermeidung von Frühgeburten. *Z. Geburtshilfe Perinat.* 196: 229-237.

[42] Saling E (1992): Current Measures to Prevent Late Abortion or Prematurity. In: Saling, E.: Nestlé Nutrition Workshop Series, Vol. 26. Raven Press, New York.

[43] Saling E, Lescinski R (1989): Schlingeninstrument zur Blutstillung bei operativen Eingriffen an der Portio. *Z. Geburtshilfe Perinat.* 193(5): 241-242.

[44] Saling, E (1984): Der frühe totale operative Muttermundverschluß bei anamnestischem Abort- und Frühgeburtrisiko. *Gynäkologe* 17: 225-227.

[45] Saling E (1984): Prevention of habitual abortion and prematurity by early total occlusion of the external os uteri. *Eur. J. Obstet. Gynecol. Reprod. Biol.* 17: 165-170.

[46] Hormel K, Künzel W (1995): Der totale Muttermundverschluss. Prävention von Spätaborten und Frühgeburten. *Gynäkologe* 28, 181-186.

[47] Giffei JM (1990): Der totale operative Muttermundverschluß. Ein neues Verfahren zur Vermeidung der wiederholten Spätaborte und Frühgeburten. Inauguraldissertation, Medizinische Fachbereiche der Freien Universität Berlin.

[48] Saling E (1993): Infektiologische Spätabortursachen und operativer Muttermundverschluss. *Arch. Gynecol. Obstet.* 254: 1265-1271.

[49] Saling E (1990): Der totale operative Muttermundverschluß zur Vermeidung habitueller Spätaborte und sich wiederholender Frühgeburten - Fortentwicklung der Technik, weitere Erfahrungen und Ergebnisse. In: Dudenhausen JW, Saling E (Hrsg): Perinatale Medizin, Bd. XIII. (14. Deutscher Kongreß für Perinatale Medizin, Berlin, 1989). Thieme: Stuttgart, New York, S. 65-67.

[50] Saling E, Schumacher E (1997): Ergebnisse einer Nachuntersuchung von Müttern nach vorausgegangenen operativen "Totalen Muttermund-Verschlüssen" (TMV) unter Berücksichtigung auch der Daten ihrer Kinder. Z. Geburtshilfe Neonatol. 201: 122-127.

[51] Hein M (2002): The immunology of the cervical mucus plug. Ph. D. thesis. Faculty of Helath Sciences.

[52] Noori M, Helmig RB, Hein M, Steer PJ (2007): Could a cervical occlusion suture be effective at improving perinatal outcome? BJOG 114: 532-536.

Reviewed by:
Amos Grunebaum, MD, FACOG,
Director of Clinical Maternal Fetal Medicine,
CORNELL UNIVERSITY, New York.

In: Infectious Pregnancy Complications
Editor: Richard N. Canfield

ISBN 978-1-60741-038-6

Chapter 3

Virulence of Influenza Virus on Human Fetal Membrane Tissues

Noboru Uchide * ***and Hiroo Toyoda***
Department of Clinical Molecular Genetics, School of Pharmacy,
Tokyo University of Pharmacy and Life Sciences, 1432-1 Horinouchi,
Hachioji, Tokyo 192-0392, Japan

Abstract

An increase of the risk of premature delivery, abortion and stillbirth has been observed during the past pandemics of influenza. The occurrence of intrauterine influenza virus infection during pregnancy is substantiated. Human fetal membranes are appendages of placenta and compose of amnion, chorion and decidua tissues. They play a critical role as defensive barriers in order to maintain normal pregnancy. Recent *in vitro* studies have demonstrated that influenza A/H1N1 virus infection induced apoptosis and the gene expression of a set of pro-inflammatory cytokines, such as interleukin (IL)-6, tumor necrosis factor (TNF)-α and interferon (IFN)-β in cultured chorion cells. IL-6, TNF-α and IFN-β molecules in culture supernatants of the virus-infected chorion cells induced the differentiation of monocytes to well-matured macrophages. It should be noted that these phenomena were not observed in cultured amnion cells after influenza virus infection, yet viral replication was observed in the cells. It has been known that apoptosis of the constituent cells and macrophage activation in the tissues are implicated in the pathogenesis of fetal membrane rupture. Therefore, accumulating evidence suggests that fetal membrane chorion and amnion cells play a pivotal role in the pathogenesis of influenza-associated complications during pregnancy. This article reviews the virulence of influenza virus against human fetal membrane tissues in order to understand the molecular pathogenesis of intrauterine influenza virus infection during pregnancy.

---

* Tel.: +81-42-676-5760, Fax: +81-42-676-5738, E-mail: uchide@toyaku.ac.jp

1. Introduction

Historical perspectives have described that influenza during pregnancy is implicated as one of the causes of fetal loss and maternal death. The risk of premature delivery, abortion and stillbirth has increased during the past pandemics of A/H1N1 Spanish virus in 1918, A/H2N2 Asian virus in 1957 and A/H3N2 Hong Kong virus in 1968. A new pandemic outbreak of A/H5N1 virus infection in humans poses potentially pregnant woman and fetus serious complications. The studies using human influenza virus type A may help to predict the potential effect of avian influenza on human pregnancy.

Human fetal membranes are appendages of placenta, which are composed of fetus-derived amnion and chorion tissues, and maternal decidua tissue (Lavery, 1987; Malak and Bell, 1994). They form boundaries between the fetus and the external world and play a critical role as defensive barriers in order to maintain normal pregnancy (Grossman and Dennis, 1987). The etiology of premature rupture of membranes is not completely established, but appears to be related to the biochemical processes, including apoptotic cell death and macrophage activation, during intrauterine infection.

Recently, we have demonstrated that influenza virus infection induced apoptosis in cultured chorion cells, which secrete heat-stable peptidyl macromolecules with monocyte differentiation-inducing (MDI) activity during apoptosis-mediated cellular degradation (Uchide et al., 2002a, 2002c, 2006b; see section 4 in detail). Interleukin (IL)-6, tumor necrosis factor (TNF)-α and interferon (IFN)-β were identified as a member of the MDI factors (Uchide et al., 2002b, 2006a; our unpublished data). A series of our studies, therefore, suggests that the induction of apoptosis and gene expression of a set of pro-inflammatory cytokines in chorion cells by influenza virus infection represents part of the mechanism for pregnancy-associated complications during intrauterine infection with the virus (Uchide et al., 2005a). This article highlights the virulence of influenza virus on human fetal membranes in order to understand the molecular pathogenesis of influenza-associated complications during pregnancy.

2. Overview of Influenza Infection

2.1. Epidemics and Pandemics of Influenza

Every year, the global burden of influenza epidemics is believed to be 3-5 million cases of severe illness and 300,000-500,000 deaths (Kamps and Reyes-Teran, 2006). New epidemic influenza A strains arise every 1 to 2 years by the introduction of selected point mutations within two surface glycoproteins: hemagglutinin (HA) and neuraminidase (NA). In contrast to epidemics, pandemics are rare events that occur every 10 to 50 years. During the 20th century, three pandemics have been occurred. The 1918 pandemic was caused by a A/H1N1 Spanish virus of apparently avian origin (Reid et al., 1999), whereas the subsequent pandemic strains – A/H2N2 Asian virus in 1957 and A/H3N2 Hong Kong virus in 1968 – were reassortant viruses containing genes from avian viruses (Kawaoka et al., 1989).

Avian influenza viruses do not typically replicate efficiently in humans, indicating direct transmission of avian influenza virus to humans is unlikely. However, since 1997, several cases of human infections with different subtypes (H5N1, H7N7 and H9N2) of avian influenza viruses have been identified and raised the pandemic potential of avian influenza virus in humans. Infection with a highly pathogenic avian influenza A/H5N1 virus in humans spreads out of Asia and into Europe and Africa. At the present day (May 28, 2008), there have been 383 cases infected with avian influenza A/H5N1 virus in Vietnam, Indonesia, Thailand, China, Cambodia, Bangladesh, Lao People's Democratic Republic, Myanmar, Azerbaijan, Iraq, Turkey, Pakistan, Egypt, Nigeria and Djibouti, the death rate of which was extremely high as 62.9% (World Health Organization, 2008). Person-to-person transmission of this virus is still very limited (Ungchusak et al., 2005). However, Smith and co-workers have provided insight into the ongoing evolution of H5N1 influenza viruses that are transmitting in diverse avian species and at the interface between avian and human hosts (Smith et al., 2006). Therefore, it has been expressed a warning that H5N1 virus evolves to become easily transmittable among humans (Patterson, 2005; Wong and Yuen, 2006). The human beings face the threat of a highly pathogenic avian influenza virus.

2.2. Virology

Influenza viruses belong to the Orthomyxoviridae family, which are classified as type A, B and C by serological properties of viral nucleoproteins (NP) and matrix proteins (M1). Among three types, influenza A viruses are clinically the most important pathogen since they are responsible for the most serious threat to public health. The influenza A virus particle is composed of a lipid envelope derived from the host cell, 9 structural viral proteins and 8 single-stranded virion RNA (vRNA) segments with negative-polarity. The components of the RNA-dependent RNA polymerase complex, PB2, PB1 and PA are associated with the ribonucleoprotein complex (RNP) and are encoded by the vRNA segments 1-3. The external glycoproteins HA and NA are expressed from vRNA segments 4 and 6, respectively. Influenza A viruses are categorized serologically according to the structural differences of the HA and NA proteins. Currently, 16 HA (H1-H16) and 9 NA (N1-N9) subtypes have been identified (Horimoto and Kawaoka, 2005). The NP associated with vRNA segments is encoded by segment 5, which is responsible for viral gene transcription and replication, and intracellular trafficking of the viral RNPs. The two smallest vRNA segments, each of which codes for two proteins. The M1 is derived from a colinear reading frame of segment 7 and forms an inner layer within the virion. A differential splicing of the same mRNA results in a third viral transmembrane component, the M2 protein, which functions as a pH-dependent ion channel. A similar mechanism of coding strategy for segment 8 harbors the sequence information for the nonstructural (NS1) protein and the nuclear export protein NS2. NS2 is a minor component of the virion and is found in association with the M1 protein. Recently, it has been reported that PB1-F2 protein, which is derived from a second open reading frame of *PB1*, associates with the mitochondria and induces apoptosis (Table 1) (Chen et al., 2001).

The viral replication cycle is initiated by the binding of the HA to sialic acid containing cellular receptors. The influenza virus binds to the cell surface by fixing the outer top of the

HA to the sialic acid of a cell's glycoproteins and glycolipids. The sialic acid linkage to the penultimate galactose, either α-2, 3 (in birds) or α-2, 6 (in humans), determines host specificity.

Table 1. Influenza A virus genome (Strain A/PR/8/34)

Segment	vRNA	Protein	Amino acid	Function(s)
1	2341	PB2	759	Subunit of viral RNA polymerase, cap-binding
2	2341	PB1	757	Catalytic subunit of viral RNA polymerase
		PB1-F2	87	Accumulation in mitochondria, apoptosis induction
3	2233	PA	716	Subunit of viral RNA polymerase
4	1778	HA	566	Hemagglutinin, surface glycoprotein, receptor binding, membrane fusion
5	1565	NP	498	Nucleprotein, encapsidation of viral genomic and anti-genomic RNA
6	1413	NA	454	Neuraminidase, particle release
7	1027	M1	252	Matrix protein
		M2	97	Ion channel activity, protecting HA conformation
8	890	NS1	230	Post-transcriptional regulator; inhibition of pre-mRNA splicing, polyadenylation, PKR activity
		NS2	121	Nuclear export factor

Since sialic acid-presenting carbohydrates are present on several cells of the organism, multiple cell types, such as airway epithelial cells, alveolar cells, vascular endothelial cells and macrophages, in an organism are infected with influenza virus. After attachment, the virus is taken up by the cell via a clathrin-coated receptor-mediated endocytosis process. When internalized, the clathrin molecules are liberated and the vesicle harbouring the whole virus fuses with endosomes. The contents of the vesicle are usually digested through a stepwise lowering of the pH within the phagosome. The lowering of the pH is stopped by the action of the M2 protein which induces the partial liberation of the fusion peptide of the HA. This allows the fusion of the HA with the membrane of the vesicle and liberation of the RNPs into the cytoplasm, as described above. The ion influx from the endosome to the virus particle leads to disconnection of the different viral proteins. M1-protein aggregation is disrupted and RNPs no longer adhere to the M1-protein complex. Uncoating is completed within 20-30 min of virus attachment.

The RNPs are transported to the nucleus, where the RNA polymerase complex binds to viral RNA, cleaves viral RNA by its endonuclease activity, and simultaneously leads to elongation. The production of viral RNA is limited by the NP in favour of mRNA. Both are transported to the cytoplasm, where viral proteins are generated at the ribosome. Part of the viral mRNA is spliced by cellular enzymes so that finally viral proteins, such as M1 and NS2, can be synthesised without any further cleavage. Some of the newly synthesised viral proteins are transported to the nucleus where they bind to viral RNA to form RNPs. Other newly synthesised viral proteins are processed in the endoplasmic reticulum and the Golgi apparatus where glycosylation occurs. These modified proteins are transported to the cell membrane where they stick in the lipid bilayer. When they reach a high enough concentration at the plasma membrane, RNPs and M1 proteins aggregate and condense to produce the viral particle. The precursor HA (HA0) protein is cleaved into two disulfide-liked chains, HA1 and HA2 by host trypsin-like proteases, which is essential for virus infectivity. Finally, the particle is extruded from the membrane and will be liberated by the neuraminidase activity. The time from entry to production of new virus is on average 6 h.

2.3. Viremia and Systemic Infection

Human influenza A viruses have been isolated directly from blood (Lehmann and Gust, 1971; Naficy, 1963; Ritova et al., 1979; Stanley and Jackson, 1966) and from various extrapulmonary tissues and fluids, such as brain, meninges, spinal cord, cerebrospinal fluid, heart, liver, kidney, adrenal, urine, spleen, tonsil, lymph node and muscle (Hakoda and Nakatani, 2000; Kaji et al., 1959; Lehmann and Gust, 1971; Nakai et al., 2003; Roberts and Roberts, 1976; Salonen et al., 1997; Yawn et al., 1971; Zhdanov and Ritova, 1959). Immunochemical analysis has demonstrated that viral proteins were detected in Purkinje cells, neurons, ependymocytes of plexus choriodeus in the brain, β cells in the pancreas, $CD8^+$ T lymphocytes in the spleen, hepatocytes and stellate endothelial cells in the liver, epithelial cells of convoluted tubules of the kidney and cerebrospinal fluid obtained from patients with influenza virus infection (Salonen et al., 1997; Takahashi et al., 2000; Zinserling et al., 1983). Viral RNAs were also detected in various tissues and fluids, such as brain, cerebrospinal fluid, heart, diaphragm, liver, lymph node and peripheral blood mononuclear cells obtained from patients with influenza virus infection (Nakai et al., 2003; Takahashi et al., 2000; Tsuruoka et al., 1997). Furthermore, in mouse model viral proteins and mRNAs have been detected in blood (both red blood cells and plasma), brain, liver, spleen, pancreas, salivary gland, kidney, heart and skeletal muscle after intranasal inoculation with influenza virus (Frankova and Rychterova, 1975; Mori et al., 1995a). These results substantiate the occurrence of viremia and systemic infection with human influenza A virus.

The virological course of avian influenza virus (A/H5N1) in human body is incompletely characterized. In a patient with fatal A/H5N1 influenza infection, viral RNA was detected by reverse transcription-polymerase chain reaction in the lung, intestine and spleen tissues, but positive-stranded viral RNA indicating virus replication was confined to the lung and intestine (Uiprasertkul et al., 2005). A recent case report has showed that A/H5N1 virus was isolated from the serum, cerebrospinal fluid and fecal samples in addition to the respiratory secretions (de Jong et al., 2005). Viral antigen was detected in pneumocytes by immunohistochemical tests (Uiprasertkul et al., 2005). These studies suggest that the virus replicates in the respiratory and gastrointestinal tracts, and that the major site of A/H5N1 viral replication is the pneumocyte.

2.4. Clinical and Pathological Manifestations

The symptoms observed during influenza virus infection are highly variable, ranging from mild respiratory disease with rhinitis or pharyngitis to primary viral pneumonia with fatal outcome (Cox and Kawaoka, 1989). In uncomplicated cases it is self-limited, while it is often accompanied by inflammation of the upper and lower respiratory tracts, myalgia, gastrointestinal disorders and neurological disorders (Gross-Schulmann et al., 1998). Much remains to be learned about the pathogenesis of influenza virus replication and its relationship to the clinical manifestation. Many studies on the pathogenesis of influenza infections were conducted during the 1957/1958 pandemic of Asian influenza type A (H2N2) (Hers and Mulder, 1961; Walsh e tal., 1961). These studies demonstrated that columnar epithelial cells are primary sites of replication. Histological studies indicate that viral replication occurs throughout the respiratory tracts. Infected ciliated columnar cells become vacuolated and lose their cilia, and infected mucosal and ciliated epithelial cells become necrotic and desquamate. In studies in which bronchoscopy was conducted on, or nasal and bronchial biopsy specimens were taken from, individuals with uncomplicated acute influenza infections, inflammation of the larynx, trachea and bronchi and desquamation of ciliated columnar epithelium into the lumen of the bronchus were observed.

In cases of severe influenza virus infection, pathological manifestations are as a result of complex biological consequences, such as apoptosis induction, macrophage activation and oxidative damage (Kash et al., 2004). An increased number of activated macrophages were found in the brain containing neurons and glial cells undergoing apoptosis in the patients with influenza-mediated encephalopathy (Nakai et al., 2003). The co-existence of macrophages and degraded cells, containing viral proteins, and pycnotic and fragmented nuclei, was also observed in other extrapulmonary tissues, such as liver, kidney and intestine, obtained from patients with influenza virus infection (Zinserling et al., 1983). The same phenomena were observed in mice infected with influenza virus intranasally (Zinserling et al., 1983). Intranasal influenza virus infection induced apoptosis in neurons in mouse brain, in which the virus protein-positive apoptotic bodies were phagocytosed by activated macrophages (Mori et al., 2002). The phagocytosis of influenza virus-infected cells undergoing apoptosis by macrophages plays a critical role in the presentation of viral antigen to T lymphocytes (Albert et al., 1998), the abortion of virus growth (Fujimoto et al., 2000) and the prevention of virus dissemination in the infected organs (Mori et al., 2002). Influenza virus-infected cells were phagocytosed by macrophages anchored with phosphatidylserine (PS) that appears on the surface of infected cells during the process of apoptosis (Shiratsuchi et al., 2000; Watanabe et al., 2002). The PS-mediated phagocytotic reaction is stimulated through the desialylation of macrophage surface by NA of influenza virus-infected cells (Watanabe et al., 2004). Two types of phogocytes (i.e. macrophages and granulocytes) equally contributed to the phagocytotic elimination of apoptotic cells in the lung of mice infected with influenza virus (Watanabe et al., 2005). The administration of Anexin V, PS-binding protein, reduced the level of phagocytosis, resulting in the augmentation of the lethality in mice and the extent of inflammation in the lung (Watanabe et al., 2005). Moreover, Fc receptor-mediated phagocytosis by macrophages contributes to the elimination of influenza virus particles *in vivo* (Huber et al., 2001). Subsequent to phagocytosis by macrophages, an abrupt increase in superoxide production by macrophages, known as the oxidative burst, occurs, which is catalyzed by reduced nicotinamide adenine dinucleotide phosphate (NADPH) oxidase enzyme complex (Park, 2003). The production of superoxide by phagocytes is necessary for remodeling tissues damaged by infectious agents (Cohen et al., 1981). However, an excessive production of superoxide is known to implicate in the lethal or toxic effect of influenza virus infection (Oda et al., 1989; Suliman et al., 2001). Therefore, a controlled superoxide production by phagocytes is critical for the pathogenesis of influenza virus infection as evidenced by a study using mouse model lacking functional phagocyte NADPH oxidase (Snelgrove et al., 2006).

Most patients with influenza virus (A/H5N1) infection have initial symptoms of high fever and an influenza-like illness with lower respiratory tract symptoms, and diarrhea, vomiting, abdominal pain, pleuritic pain, and bleeding from the nose and gums have also been reported early in the course of illness in some patients (Beigel et al., 2005; Tran et al., 2004). H5N1 influenza is still a relatively novel disease with poorly understood pathology and pathogenesis. The pathological findings including apoptotic cell death and macrophage activation are observed in the lung and some extrapulmonary tissues obtained from patients infected with H5N1 virus (Peiris et al., 2004; Ungchusak et al., 2005; To et al., 2001; Gu et al., 2007; Uiprasertkul et al., 2005, 2007; Chotpitayasunondh et al., 2004; Korteweg and Gu, 2008). Apoptosis was observed in alveolar epithelial cells, and numerous apoptotic leukocytes were observed in the lung of a patient (Uiprasertkul et al., 2007). Macrophages appeared to be the predominant cells within the alveoli, whereas in the interstitium T lymphocytes, with or without neutrophils, are present. Scattered histiocytes with hemophagocytic activity have been observed in the lungs of some cases. Reactive histiocytes with hemophagocytic activity have been noted in the spleen, lymph node, bone marrow, lungs, and liver. In liver tissue specimens, necrosis, activated Kupffer cells, cholestasis, and fatty changes have been observed. In most instances the brain is edematous without any significant histopathological change, whereas in two cases demyelinated areas and reactive histiocytes and foci of necrosis have been reported. In other organs no remarkable histological changes have been observed. Mice infected with highly pathogenic H1N1 and

H5N1 viruses exhibit significantly high numbers of macrophages and neutrophils in the lungs compared to mice infected with low pathogenic viruses (Perrone et al., 2008).

3. Influenza Virus Infection during Pregnancy

3.1. Influence of Influenza Virus on Pregnant Woman and Fetus

Infection during pregnancy occurs much more often than is recognized and disastrous for mother and/or fetus if proper care was not provided. Preterm premature rupture of the membranes complicates 3% of pregnancies and is responsible for approximately one third of all preterm births (Mercer, 2005).

The risk of premature delivery, abortion and stillbirth has increased during the past pandemics of A/H1N1 Spanish virus in 1918 (Harris, 1919), A/H2N2 Asian virus in 1957 and A/H3N2 Hong Kong virus in 1968 (Hardy et al., 1961; Freeman and Barno, 1959; Greengerg et al., 1958; Pleydell, 1960; McDonald, 1961). No increase of cases has been seen in the 1968-1969 pandemic of Hong Kong influenza (H3N2) (Sterner et al., 1990). Also even more recently in the presence of antibiotics, it has been demonstrated that a cluster of spontaneous abortions and stillbirths occurred within two or three weeks from the onset of influenza in 1985-1986 (Stanwell-Smith et al., 1994), yet some case reports were found. Within a week of hospitalization, the patient with pneumonia caused by influenza virus type A during 29 weeks' gestation developed regular uterine contractions. The cervix was 3 cm dilated, and an infant was delivered by cesarean section, but mother became severely hypotensive and bradycardic and died (Kort et al., 1986). Within two weeks of hospitalization, the patient with encephalopathy caused by influenza virus type A during 12 weeks' gestation underwent an abortion (Hakoda and Nakatani, 2000).

In the 1977-1978 pandemic of A/H1N1 Russian virus in Portland metropolitan area, the significant excess of acute respiratory disease among pregnant women was observed by reappearance of this type virus, that had circulated in the 1950s, and was confined to those under age of 25 who would not have been previously exposed to this type virus (Mullooly et al., 1986). An epidemiological study in the Tennessee from 1974 to 1993 estimated that 0.25% of pregnant women were hospitalized for the influenza infection (Neuzil et al., 1998). Another epidemiological study in the Tennessee from 1985 to 1993 demonstrated that 6.0% of pregnant women with asthma were hospitalized during influenza season, which was significantly higher than 0.51% of pregnant women without asthma (Hartert et al., 2003). Thus, influenza virus type A infection during pregnancy is still an etiological awareness at the present day even a multiple infection with bacteria is controllable by the treatment using antibiotics. It may be said that many pregnant women are exposed to the risk of influenza-associated complications of pregnancy. Therefore, it is important to study the mechanisms of virulence of influenza virus to pregnant woman and fetus.

3.2. Placental and Fetal Infection

Influenza virus type A has been isolated from placenta and amniotic fluid during the third trimester in fatal (Jewett, 1974; Yawn et al., 1971) and non-fatal cases (McGregor et al.,

1984). Placentitis caused by influenza virus type A and B has been observed in 32 of 186 placentas, which was characterized by hyperplasia and subsequent degeneration of amniotic cells, placental trophoblast cells, decidua cells and vascular endothelial cells and by the presence of viral proteins and fucsinophilic inclusions in the affected cells, and lymphoid cell infiltrations (Mel'nikova et al., 1987). Immunohistochemical analyses further demonstrated that influenza virus proteins were detected in astrocytes and neurons in the brain of infant who was delivered by cesarean section (Conover and Roessmann, 1990). Influenza virus has been isolated from the lung of a stillborn infant (Greenberg et al., 1958) and from fetal heart (Yawn et al., 1971). Immunoglobulin M type antibody against epidemic strain of influenza virus type A has been found in umbilical cord blood sera obtained from infants delivered after a community-wide epidemic, and lymphocytes isolated from umbilical cord blood were proliferated by the stimulation with epidemic strain of influenza virus type A (Ruben et al., 1975; Ruben and Thompson, 1981). These results substantiate that influenza viruses spread from the maternal respiratory tract to the fetus, placenta and amniotic fluid via viremia.

Both the placenta and the 4-month-old fetus have been studied on a fatal 24-year-old case with H5N1 virus infection (Shu et al., 2006; Gu et al., 2007). The placenta showed scattered foci of both syncytiotrophoblast necrosis and necrotizing deciduitis, and diffuse villitis. Both negative- and positive-strand viral RNAs for HA and NP were detected in Hofbauer and cytotrophoblastic cells but not syncytiotrophoblasts in the placenta by *in situ* hybridization. Immunohistochemical analysis consistently demonstrated that viral HA and NP proteins were detected in Hofbauer and cytotrophoblast cells but not syncytiotrophoblasts. Both negative- and positive-strand viral RNAs for HA were amplified from the placental tissue using reverse transcriptase-polymerase chain reaction techniques. Both negative- and positive-strand viral RNAs were detected in fetal bronchi, alveolar pneumocytes, Kupffer cells, and circulating mononuclear cells by *in situ* hybridization. The fetal tissues mostly showed no specific histopathological features, except for some edema and a few scattered interstitial neutrophils in the lungs. These results suggest that H5N1 viruses proliferate in Hofbauer and cytotrophoblastic cells but not syncytiotrophoblasts, and transplacental transmission of H5N1 virus results in infection of fetal organs.

Avian and human influenza viruses preferentially bind to α-2, 3-linked and α-2, 6-linked sialic acids, respectively. The expression of avian influenza (AIV-Rs) and human influenza virus receptors (HuIV-Rs) was analyzed by immunohistochemical stains using biotinylated *Maackia amurensis* lectin II and *Sambucus nigra* agglutinin, respectively (Yao L et al., 2008). In the placenta obtained from patients with H5N1 virus infection, endothelial cells expressed both HuIV-R and AIV-R, whereas Hofbauer cells stained positive only for HuIV-R. Both cytotrophoblasts and syncytiotrophoblasts were negative for both receptor types. The absence of AIV-Rs in several cell types, including cytotrophoblasts and Hofbauer cells, appears to be inconsistent with the detected H5N1-infection of these cells. Accordingly, Yao and co-workers have implied that other receptors or coreceptors might be involved in virus – target-cell interaction in H5N1 avian influenza (Yao et al., 2008).

In swine, some reports suggest that abortion and stillbirth can be associated with epidemics of swine influenza (Vannier, 1999; Wesley, 2004). Transplacental transmission of swine influenza virus has been also observed in pregnant gilts (Wallace and Elm, 1979). Influenza virus has been isolated from amnion and chorion tissues in pregnant guinea-pig models (Sweet et al., 1977) and amniotic fluid in pregnant ferret models (Rushton et al., 1983) after intracardial inoculation with the virus. These results demonstrate the occurrence of fetal membrane infection with this virus. In addition, influenza virus infection may preferably spread to chorion tissues adhered to decidua tissue via viremia, since human endometrial and decidua tissues provide a preferable environment for influenza virus replication than placental tissues (Rosztoczy et al., 1975).

4. Virulence of Influenza Virus on Human Fetal Membrane Tissues

4.1. Implication of Apoptosis in Pathology of Membrane Rupture

In our knowledge, Parmley has reported for the first time that apoptotic cells were detected in the chorionic trophoblast cell layer of human fetal membrane tissues (Parmley, 1990). The study using 121 specimens obtained from clinically heterogenouos patients has suggested that the trophoblastic cell layer of the chorion laeve showed widespread apoptotic cells and loss of the trophoblastic cell layer as term approached, and that the chorionic trophoblastic cells population of the chorion was prematurely destroyed by infiltrating maternal leukocytes in cases of chorioamnionitis (Parmley, 1990). The number of apoptotic cells was greater in the week of 37-42 group of uncomplicated cases at term than in the week of 23-30 group of complicated cases with preeclampsia and diabetes at preterm in chorionic trophoblast and decidual cell layers (Runic et al., 1998). The apoptotic bodies were quite abundant in the chorionic trophoblastic layer of fetal membranes located over the cervix (McLaren et al., 1999). Recent studies have revealed that the number of apoptotic cells was much higher in the chorion of fetal membranes with histological chorioamnionitis at term than those without chorioamnionitis (Murtha et al., 2002), and that the chorion of fetal membranes from patients with premature rupture of membranes had significantly more apoptotic cells than those without chorioamnionitis (George et al., 2008). It is likely that apoptotic cell death in broad area of fetal membrane tissue is responsible for rupture of membranes both at term under physiological conditions and at preterm with chorioamnionitis.

Elevated levels of IL-1β, IL-6 and TNF-α proteins can be found in the amniotic fluid of patients with preterm labor and intra-amniotic infection (Romero et al., 1989, 1990, 1992). Both IL-1α and IL-1β induced preterm delivery in mice, as demonstrated by the prevention of preterm delivery with the pretreatment with IL-1 receptor antagonist (Romero et al., 1992). Stress-triggered abortion was prevented by neutralizing TNF-α and IL-1 with soluble receptors in mice (Arck et al., 1997). Thus, pro-inflammatory cytokines, such as IL-1β, IL-6 and TNF-α, have been postulated to play a fundamental role in the pathogenesis of preterm delivery during intrauterine infection. Caspases (cysteinyl aspartate-specific proteinases) mediate highly specific proteolytic cleavage events in dying cells (Nicholson and Thornberry, 1997). It has been demonstrated that activities of pro-apoptotic caspase-3 and caspase-8, but not caspase-9, in later stages of gestation (40-41 weeks) were much higher than those in earlier stages (16-27 weeks) in fetal membranes (Kumagai et al., 2001). Pro-inflammatory cytokines, such as IL-1β, IL-6 and TNF-α, induced the expression of pro-apoptotic caspases mRNAs in isolated amniochorion tissues (Fortunato et al., 2001; Fortunato and Menon, 2003; Menon et al., 2002). Furthermore, these cytokines induced the cleavage of polyADP-ribose polymerase, a substrate for caspases, in isolated amniochorion tissues (Kumar et al., 2006). Consequently, it is likely that caspases, particularly caspase-3 and caspase-8, and pro-inflammatory cytokines (e.g. IL-1β, IL-6 and TNF-α) play a critical role in the molecular pathogenesis of premature rupture of fetal membranes associated with intrauterine infection through apoptosis induction (Fortunato et al., 2000, 2001, 2002; Fortunato and Menon, 2003; Kataoka et al., 2002; Kumar et al., 2006; McLaren et al., 1999; Menon et al., 2002; Murtha et al., 2002).

Apoptosis of chorionic trophoblast cells in the amniochorion tissues obtained at the end of pregnancy was progressed by the *in vitro* incubation, which was suppressed by the addition of glucocorticoids, antioxidative reagents [pyrrolidine dithiocarbamate (PDTC), *N*-acetyl-L-cysteine (NAC), nordihydroguaiaretic acid (NDGA), 6-hydroxyl-2, 5, 7, 8-tetramethylchroman-2-carboxylic acid (Trolox), a water-soluble analogue of vitamin E], general and selective cyclooxygenase (Cox)-2 inhibitors (indomethacin and nimesride, respectively) and inducible nitric oxide synthase (iNOS) inhibitor (2-amino-5, 6-dihydro-6-methyl-4H-1, 3-thiazine) to the medium (Ohyama et al., 1998, 2001; Yuan et al., 2006). The expression levels of Cox-2 and iNOS mRNAs as well as proteins were increased in the isolated chorion tissues during *in vitro* incubation (Yuan et al., 2006), resulting in the production of reactive oxygen species (ROS), such as superoxide and nitric oxide. Furthermore, apoptosis was induced in cultured chorion, but not amnion, cells by the treatment with a nitric oxide donor reagent, sodium nitroprusside (Yuan et al., 2006). It has been known that peroxynitrite, a strong oxidant, is formed when superoxide and nitric oxide are produced at near equimolar ratios (Virag et al., 2003). Moreover, Trolox inhibits peroxynitrite-mediated apoptosis in rat thymocytes (Salgo and Pryor, 1996). These results suggest that the induction of apoptosis in the chorionic trophoblast cells is mediated through peroxynitrite resulting from the induction of Cox-2 and iNOS gene expression. It has been known that bacterial toxin lipopolysaccharide (LPS) induces Cox-2 and iNOS gene expression simultaneously in macrophages (Swierkosz et al., 1995). On the basis of these results, it is possible that infiltrated maternal macrophages are a major source for Cox-2 and iNOS enzymes in isolated amniochorion tissues.

As described above, our previous study has identified the contribution of ROS production system (e.g., oxidant enzymes, such as iNOS and Cox-2) to the apoptosis induction in the chorion cells, suggesting an important role of the two inducible enzymes in the induction process (Yuan et al., 2006). Furthermore, we examined the role of ROS elimination system (e.g. antioxidant enzymes, such as glutathione peroxidase (GPx) and catalase) in the apoptosis induction of the cultured chorion cells (Yuan et al., 2008), since the apoptosis induction by oxidative stress is a result of imbalance between production and elimination of ROS. The treatment of cultured chorion and amnion cells with mercaptosuccinic acid (MS, GPx inhibitor) and 3-amino-1, 2, 4-triazole (ATZ, catalase inhibitor) resulted in an inhibition of GPx and catalase activity, respectively. The incubation with MS alone induced apoptosis in the chorion cells, the levels of which were enhanced by the addition of ATZ, while ATZ alone hardly induced apoptosis in the cultured chorion cells. However, none of these reagents induced apoptosis in the amnion cells. Therefore, we have concluded that GPx played a more critical role than catalase in the control of the apoptosis induction of the chorion cells, suggesting that the threshold levels of stress tolerance in the chorion cells are much lower than those in the amnion cells (Yuan et al., 2008).

4.2. Induction of Apoptosis in Fetal Membrane Chorion Cells by Influenza Virus Infection

We have investigated the virulence of influenza virus to human fetal membrane tissues in order to understand the pathogenesis of influenza-associated complications during pregnancy. *In vitro* study using primary cultured chorion and amnion cells has been conducted. Influenza A/PR/8/34 (H1N1) virus replicated both in the cultured chorion cells and in the cultured amnion cells (Uchide et al., 2002a). Significant cytopathic effects (CPEs), such as cell rounding and detachment, were observed in the cultured chorion cells after the virus infection (Uchide et al., 2002a). The detached chorion cells, which were stainable with trypan blue dye, were increased with time after the virus infection (our unpublished data). Simultaneously, lactate dehydrogenase (LDH) activity in the culture supernatants of chorion cells was enhanced by the virus infection (Uchide et al., 2002a). These results indicated that the intracellular LDH was leaked into the extracellular medium as a result of increasing permeability of cellular membrane. Chromosomal DNA in the cultured chorion cells was fragmented into oligonucleosomes by the virus infection (Uchide et al., 2002a). *In situ* the terminal deoxynucleotidyl transferase-mediated dUTP nick-end labeling (TUNEL) method demonstrated that numerous numbers of TUNEL-positive cells were detected in the cultured chorion cells after the inoculation with active influenza viruses, but not heat-inactivated viruses (Uchide et al., 2006b). In contrast, these phenomena were not observed in cultured amnion cells after influenza virus infection, yet the virus replicated in the cells (Uchide et al., 2002a, 2006b). The treatment with an antiviral reagent, ribavirin (1-β-D-ribofuranosyl-1, 2, 4-triazole-3-carboxamide), inhibited the induction of oligonucleosomal DNA fragmentation in the cultured chorion cells by the virus infection (Uchide et al., 2002a). Since oligonucleosomal DNA fragmentation and TUNEL-positive reaction are key features of apoptotic cell death (Gavrieli et al., 1992; Wyllie et al., 1980), these results suggest that influenza virus infection induces apoptosis in the cultured chorion cells but not in the cultured amnion cells, and moreover that influenza virus proliferation is prerequisite to the induction of apoptosis in cultured chorion cells by the virus infection. Consequently, the infection of chorion cells with influenza virus A/PR/8/34 is cytocidal accompanied with virus proliferation and cell lysis, but the infection of amnion cells with the cytopathogenic strain of influenza virus results in persistent accompanied with virus proliferation but without cell lysis.

Our unpublished study demonstrated that influenza virus infection induced the cleavage of pro-caspase-3 protein into an active form in primary cultured chorion, but not amnion, cells. A general caspase inhibitor, *N*-*t*-Boc-Asp(OMe)-fluoromethyl ketone (Boc-D-fmk), inhibited all of the cleavage of pro-caspase-3 protein to an active form and induction of DNA fragmentation in the influenza virus-infected chorion cells, and LDH leakage from the cells. The treatment with Boc-D-fmk did not interfere virus infection (e.g. NP expression) and virus particle release in the chorion cells. These results suggested that Boc-D-fmk inhibited the induction of apoptosis in the chorion cells by influenza virus infection through the inhibition of caspase-3 activation irrespective of virus proliferation. The induction of apoptosis in cultured amnion cells was not observed by the infection with cytopathogenic strain of influenza virus A/PR/8/34, although the virus proliferation occurred (Uchide et al., 2002a, 2002c, 2002d, 2006a). A precise mechanism for the persistent infection of cultured amnion cells with the cytopathogenic strain of influenza virus A/PR/8/34 is poorly understood. Apoptosis is a tightly regulated process involving several checkpoints before irreversible cellular degradation begins. The process consists of initiation, commitment and degradation phase (Kroemer et al., 1995; Oltvai and Korsmeyer, 1994). It is possible that amnion cells have neither initiation nor commitment of apoptotic cell death associated with influenza virus proliferation. In the amnion cells, pro-caspase-3 was not activated intrinsically by influenza virus infection, which might relate to the persistent infection. A previous study has proposed that the release of virus particles is responsible for the LDH leakage from influenza virus-infected cells, because several antiviral reagents inhibited the LDH leakage (Watanabe et al., 1995). Our results using antiviral reagents, such as ribavirin and PDTC, support the previous observation (our unpublished data). However, the treatment with Boc-D-fmk inhibited LDH leakage and apoptosis but not virus particle release (our unpublished data). These results indicated that LDH leakage occurs irrespective of the virus particle release. It has been well known that cellular membrane is degraded as a result of secondary necrosis after apoptosis (Wyllie et al., 1980). Accordingly, our study using Boc-D-fmk clearly demonstrated that LDH leakage from influenza virus-infected cells occurred as a result of the secondary necrosis after apoptosis rather than the virus particle release. Higher levels of LDH activity in amniotic fluid are associated with chorioamnionitis (Kidokoro et al., 2006) or preterm deliveries (Madazli et al., 2003), suggesting that LDH level in amniotic fluid is a useful marker in predicting fetal membrane damage. Therefore, our study provides a possibility that LDH is a useful marker of predicting fetal membrane damage through apoptosis induced by influenza virus infection.

Our *ex vivo* study has demonstrated that the infection with influenza virus A/PR/8/34 (H1N1) promoted apoptotic cellular degradation in organ cultured human amniochorion tissues (Uchide et al., 2006a). *In vivo* experiments have demonstrated that intranasal influenza virus infection induces apoptosis in bronchial/bronchiolar epithelial cells, alveolar cells, lymphoid cells in the lung, neurons in the brain and bone marrow B cells of mice (Mori et al., 1995b, 2000, 2002, 2003; Sedger et al., 2002) and vascular endothelial cells in the liver, pancreas, kidney and brain of chickens (Ito et al., 2002). Some postmortem studies have demonstrated that apoptotic cells were detected in various tissues, such as the brain, liver, kidney and intestine, obtained from patients with influenza virus infection (Nakai et al., 2003; Zinserling et al., 1983). These results suggest that influenza virus infection induces apoptosis in various types of cells when systemic infection occurred. Therefore, it has been postulated that a direct apoptosis-mediated CPE of influenza virus infection on human fetal membrane tissues is implicated in the pathogenesis of pregnancy-associated complications during intrauterine infection with the virus (Uchide et al., 2005a).

4.3. Implication of Macrophage Activation in Pathology of Membrane Rupture

Monocytes/macrophages are normally present in the maternal decidua tissue in large numbers but limited numbers in the fetal chorion and amnion tissues (Vince and Johnson, 2000). A recent study has demonstrated that maternal leukocytes invade the amnion and chorion during premature rupture as a result of chorioamnionitis (Steel et al., 2005). In particular, an increased numbers of infiltrated monocytes/macrophages was observed in choriodecidua tissues obtained from patients with chorioamnionitis as compared to normal samples (Hung et al., 2006). Furthermore, the expression levels of mRNAs for CD14, a cell surface marker for monocytes/macrophages; monocyte chemoattractive cytokines, such as macrophage inflammatory protein (MIP)-1α, MIP-1β, monocyte chemoattractant protein (MCP)-1, macrophage migration inhibitory factor (MIF) and regulated on activation, normal T cell expressed and secreted (RANTES), were increased in fetal membranes ruptured prematurely in patients with chorioamnionitis (Marvin et al., 2002). These results suggest that monocytes/macrophages are recruited from maternal decidua tissue to amniochorion tissue by monocyte chemoattractive cytokines described above, which play a critical role in the pathogenesis of premature rupture of membranes during intrauterine infection.

MIF immunoreactivity was found in fetal membranes, and concentration of MIF protein in amniotic fluid was increased at term labor (Ietta et al., 2002), suggesting that MIF contributes to the inflammatory events leading to labor. In addition, intra-amniotic infection and preterm parturition, but not term parturition, are associated with a significant increase in amniotic fluid MIF concentrations. Among patients with preterm labor with intact membranes, elevated amniotic fluid concentrations of MIF are associated with intra-amniotic inflammation and histologic chorioamnionitis. These changes in amniotic fluid were not reflected in maternal plasma. An increased expression of MIF protein and mRNA in chorioamniotic membranes was observed in patients with histologic chorioamnionitis. These observations suggest that MIF plays a role in histologic chorioamnionitis and preterm parturition associated with microbial invasion of the amniotic cavity (Chaiworapongsa et al., 2005). Recently, the importance of macrophage activation in rupture of membranes has been increasingly recognized (Marvin et al., 2002; Ietta et al., 2002).

4.4. Secretion of Monocyte Differentiation-Inducing (MDI) Factor from Fetal Membrane Chorion Cells after Influenza Virus Infection

Recent studies suggest that the phagocytosis of influenza-virus infected cells undergoing apoptosis by macrophages plays a critical role in the initiation of specific immune responses and in the elimination of viral pathogens in infected organs (Albert et al., 1998; Fujimoto et al., 2000; Mori and Kimura, 2000; Shiratsuchi et al., 2000; Watanabe et al., 2002, 2004, 2005). It has been postulated that immature monocytes in the bloodstream are able to differentiate to macrophages in order to phagocytose apoptotic cells as a result of virus infection. However, it is still not clear how monocytes are attracted to virus-infected cells and then differentiate to macrophages.

Apoptosis induction has been defined as the elimination of dying cells without inducing an inflammatory response (Wyllie et al., 1980). However, this conventional definition may not be fit in a certain situation. When pathogens invade, that induces an inflammatory response, resulting in the activation of an immune response (Restifo, 2000). Physiological program of monocyte differentiation to macrophage normally proceeds under the control of several cytokines in a coordinate manner. For example, IL-6 induces the differentiation of human monocytic leukemia cell lines including THP-1 cells to macrophages with the ability of superoxide production, the activity of which is synergistically enhanced in combination with either TNF-α or IFN-γ (Noda et al., 1991; Takeda et al., 1988). Therefore, we have been investigating the role of pro-inflammatory cytokines derived from influenza virus-infected chorion cells undergoing apoptosis in monocyte differentiation and macrophage activation (Uchide et al., 2002c, 2006b).

Our studies have demonstrated that influenza virus infection induced both apoptosis and mRNA expression of a set of pro-inflammatory cytokines, such as IL-1β, IL-6, TNF-α, IFN-β, IFN-γ and granulocyte macrophage colony-stimulating factor (GM-CSF), in cultured chorion cells (Uchide et al., 2002a, 2002b, 2002c, 2002d, 2005b, 2006a, 2006b, 2007). Immature form of IL-1β (proIL-1β) protein was accumulated within cultured chorion cells in response to influenza virus infection, although IL-1β protein was not secreted from the infected cells (Uchide et al., 2006a). Considerable amounts of IL-6, TNF-α and IFN-β proteins and a trace amount of IFN-γ protein were secreted from the virus-infected chorion cells undergoing apoptosis (Uchide et al., 2002b, 2006a, 2006b, 2007). Furthermore, influenza virus infection also promoted apoptotic cellular degradation in isolated amniochorion tissues and the secretion of IL-6 and TNF-α from the tissues (Uchide et al., 2006a, 2006b). It has been suggested that p38 mitogen-activated protein kinase pathway is involved in the process of TNF-α gene expression at a post-transcriptional level in influenza virus-infected chorion cells (Uchide et al., 2007). It should be noted that these phenomena were not observed in influenza virus-infected amnion cells, in which no apoptosis induction was occurred (Uchide et al., 2002a, 2002b, 2002c, 2006a, 2006b).

It has been shown that human monocytic leukemia THP-1 cells differentiate to macrophages in the presence of 12-*O*-tetradecanoylphorbol 13-acetate (TPA), and TPA-treated THP-1 cells adhere to a substrate and phagocytose yeasts and immunoglobulin G-coated sheep red blood cells (Tsuchiya et al., 1982). Therefore, we have developed a new simple adhesion assay using THP-1 cells in order to determine MDI activity quantitatively (Uchide and Toyoda, 2007). The effect of culture supernatants of influenza virus-infected chorion and amnion cells on monocyte differentiation to macrophages has been investigated (Uchide et al., 2002c, 2006b). The adhesion assay revealed that THP-1 cells became adherent to a substrate by incubation with heated culture supernatant of influenza virus-infected chorion cells (IV-C-sup), in which the extent of cell adhesion was much higher than that with culture supernatants of mock-infected chorion cells (Mock-C-sup). No adhesion induction was observed after treatment with culture supernatants of mock and influenza virus-infected amnion cells (Mock-A-sup and IV-A-sup, respectively). Microscopic analyses revealed that non-treated THP-1 cells were round, the nucleocytoplasmic ratio was >1, and the cytoplasm was highly basophilic with a few vacuoles. The THP-1 cells adhered to coverslips after incubation with IV-C-sup were irregularly shaped, the nucleocytoplasmic ratio decreased to

<1, and the cytoplasm was weakly basophilic with many vacuoles. The phagocytotic function of adhered THP-1 cells was examined. Fluorescence microscopy revealed that adhered THP-1 cells phagocytosed many fluorescent latex particles. These results demonstrated that monocytic THP-1 cells were morphologically and functionally differentiated to macrophages by incubation with heat-stable soluble factors in IV-C-sup. On the basis of our previous study, we suggested for the first time that influenza virus-infected chorion cells undergoing apoptosis secreted heat-stable soluble factors with MDI activity, MDI factors (Uchide et al., 2002c). This conclusion was further supported by another test for monocyte differentiation, such as the nitroblue tetrazolium (NBT) reduction test for measuring the ability of superoxide production (Baehner and Nathan, 1968). Treatment with IV-C-sup induced the ability of NBT reduction in human peripheral blood monocytes, the extent of which was much higher than that with Mock-C-sup (Uchide et al., 2006b). The NBT reduction was inhibited by the addition of excessive amounts of SOD and diphenyleneiodonium chloride, an inhibitor for NADPH oxidase (Uchide et al., 2006b), indicating that NBT is reduced by superoxide resulting from the activation of NADPH oxidase (Kobayashi et al., 1990; Shi et al., 2001). Therefore, these results suggested that the MDI factors induced the differentiation of monocytes to well-matured macrophages with the ability of superoxide production. The MDI factors also differentiated human monoblastic leukemia THP-1 and histiocytic leukemia U937 cells to superoxide producing cells but not promyelocytic leukemia HL-60 cells (Uchide et al., 2006b). No NBT reduction induction was observed after treatment with Mock-A-sup and IV-A-sup (Uchide et al., 2006b).

Characteristic features of macrophages induced by MDI factors have been further investigated. MDI factors derived from influenza virus-infected chorion cells induced both adherence and superoxide production abilities in THP-1 cells (Uchide et al., 2002c, 2006b). After the incubation with IV-C-sup, a large proportion (76%) of THP-1 cells acquired both adherence and superoxide production abilities, but a small proportion (24%) acquired only superoxide production ability (our unpublished data). Class A scavenger receptor (SR-A) on the cell surface of macrophages is one of the molecules recognizing apoptotic cell and adhesion molecules (Peiser and Gordon, 2001). The effect of MDI factors on mRNA expression for SR-A and NADPH oxidase subunits (i.e. gp91^{phox} and p22^{phox}) was examined (Uchide et al., 2002c; our unpublished data). Reverse transcriptase-polymerase chain reaction analysis revealed that the expression of SR-A mRNA was induced in only adhered, not suspended, THP-1 cells after incubation with IV-C-sup. In contrast, the mRNA expression of gp91^{phox}, a catalytic subunit of NADPH oxidase, was increased in both adhered and suspended THP-1 cells after incubation with IV-C-sup. The expression of p22^{phox} mRNA was not changed. These results indicated that the induction of SR-A and gp91^{phox} mRNA expression is critical for the acquisition of macrophage functions, such as adhesion and superoxide production, respectively. Accordingly, our results suggest that MDI factors derived from influenza virus-infected chorion cells induced the differentiation of monocytes to macrophages accompanied with the gene expression of SR-A and gp91^{phox}.

Phagocytosis of apoptotic chorion cell debris by MDI factors-induced macrophages has been investigated. Chorion cells were detached due to apoptosis resulting from influenza virus infection. The apoptotic chorion cell debris was collected by a centrifugation and suspended in 50% of IV-C-sup or 50% of fresh medium. IV-C-sup-induced adherent THP-1 cells were incubated for 24 hr with the apoptotic chorion cell debris in IV-C-sup or fresh medium. Viral NP-positive particles were detected within adhered THP-1 cells when THP-1 cells were incubated with IV-C-sup, but not with fresh medium. These results indicated that MDI factors-induced adherent THP-1 cells phagocytosed IV-infected apoptotic chorion cell debris. The incubation with fresh medium significantly decreased the total cell number of adhered THP-1 cells, and no phagocytosing THP-1 cells were observed. The incubation with heated Mock-C-sup did not change both numbers of total and phagocytosing THP-1 cells. Contrary, the incubation with non-heated IV-C-sup increased the total cell number of adhered THP-1 cells, accompanying by the increase in number of phagocytosing THP-1 cells. These results indicated that chorion cells secreted heat-stable soluble factors with the activity of maintaining macrophage adhesion irrespective of influenza virus infection, and that the activity was somewhat reduced by heating. It has bee shown that MIF maintains macrophage adhesion and is heat-stable (Weiss and Glaves, 1975). The activity in culture supernatants of chorion cells is similar to the activity of MIF. It has been demonstrated that MIF mRNA and protein were detected in amniochorion tissues (Marvin et al., 2002; Ietta et al., 2002), and moreover that treatment of macrophage-like RAW 264.7 cells with MIF increased the extent of phagocytosis (Onodera et al., 1997). Therefore, it is possible that the MIF-like activity secreted from chorion cells is critical for the phagocytosis by macrophages. As presented in this article, MDI factor-induced macrophages phagocytosed influenza virus-infected chorion cells undergoing apoptosis.

Both adhesion induction and NBT reduction activities were well correlated with the increase of IL-6 concentrations in IV-C-sup (Uchide et al., 2006b). It has been known that the IL-6 receptor α-chain (gp80) binds to IL-6 (Kishimoto et al., 1992), whereas IL-6 receptor β-chain (gp130) itself does not bind to IL-6, but associates with the α-chain/IL-6 complex and is responsible for signal transduction (Taga et al., 1989). The addition of respective antibodies against IL-6 and its receptor subunits, gp80 and gp130, inhibited the induction of adhesion and NBT reduction activities by MDI factors (Uchide et al., 2006b). The combination of these antibodies suppressed >60% of NBT reduction induced by IV-C-sup (our unpublished data). Moreover, the addition of respective antibodies against TNF-α and IFN-β also inhibited the induction of NBT reduction activity by IV-C-sup (our unpublished data). Although the addition of antibody against IFN-γ inhibited the induction of superoxide production by recombinant human (rh) IFN-γ, it did not inhibit the effect of IV-C-sup (our unpublished data). In addition, both superoxide production and adhesion activities were reconstituted with recombinant cytokines (e.g. rhIL-6, rhTNF-α and rhIFN-β) (our unpublished data). It has been known that IL-6, TNF-α and IFN-β are heat-stable at 56 °C for 30 min, but IFN-γ is labile (Roberts and Vasil, 1982; Uchide et al., 2006a; Wiedbrauk and Burleson, 1986). On the basis of these results, our studies suggest that IL-6 molecule predominantly contributed to the MDI activity derived from influenza virus-infected chorion cells, and TNF-α and IFN-β molecules also partly contributed, but IFN-γ did not. MDI activity was also detected in the supernatants of amniochorion tissue homogenate. Influenza virus infection induced the secretion of MDI factors containing IL-6 and TNF-α from organ cultured amniochorion tissues (Uchide et al., 2006a, 2006b). It is possible that chorionic trophoblast cells contribute to the production of MDI factors containing IL-6 and TNF-α by amniochorion tissues in response to influenza virus infection. Therefore, these results raise a possibility that chorion cell-derived MDI factors containing IL-6 and TNF-α induce the differentiation of maternal monocytes in decidua tissue to well-matured macrophages with superoxide production ability during intrauterine influenza virus infection.

Conclusion

Apoptosis induction is observed only in human fetal membrane chorionic trophoblast cells by influenza virus infection. The cells simultaneously secrete a set of pro-inflammatory cytokines, such as IL-6, TNF-α and INF-β, in the process of apoptosis. These cytokines induce the differentiation of monocytes to well-matured macrophages capable of generating toxic molecule (i.e. superoxide) accompanied by the induction of mRNA expression for $gp91^{phox}$, a catalytic subunit of NADPH oxidase. The macrophages phagocytose the virus-infected chorion cells undergoing apoptosis. It has been known that the production of superoxide by macrophages is stimulated as a result of the phagocytotic reaction. Superoxide produced by macrophages phagocytosing the virus-infected chorion cells may spread the damage in the fetal membranes as defensive barriers because ROS is responsible for the induction of apoptosis in the cells. These pathways represent part of the mechanism for pathological outcomes of intrauterine influenza virus infection during pregnancy. Therefore, the virulence of influenza virus on the fetal membranes may be responsible for the pregnancy complications during intrauterine infection with the virus. On the basis of this hypothesis described here, anti-inflammatory drugs and superoxide scavengers, which possess anti-influenza virus activity, can be potential candidates for a drug of choice for pregnancy complications associated with intrauterine influenza virus infection (Uchide and Toyoda, 2008a, 2008b).

Acknowledgements

This work was supported in part by grants from the Ministry of Education, Culture, Sports, Science and Technology and by the Promotion and Mutual Aid Corporation for Private School of Japan.

References

Albert, M. L., Sauter, B. and Bhardwaj, N. (1998). Dendritic cells acquire antigen from apoptotic cells and induce class I-restricted CTLs. *Nature,* 392, 86-89.

Arck, P. C., Troutt, A. B. and Clark, D. A. (1997). Soluble receptors neutralizing TNF-α and IL-1 block stress-triggered murine abortion. *Am. J. Reprod. Immunol.,* 37, 262-266.

Baehner, R. L. and Nathan, D. G. (1968). Quantitative nitroblue tetrazolium test in chronic granulomatous disease. *N. Engl. J. Med.,* 278, 971-976.

Beigel, J. H., Farrar, J., Han, A. M., Hayden, F. G., Hyer, R., de Jong, M. D., Lochindarat, S., Nguyen, T. K., Nguyen, T. H., Tran, T. H., Nicoll, A., Touch, S., Yuen, K. Y; Writing

Committee of the World Health Organization (WHO) Consultation on Human Influenza A/H5. (2005). Avian influenza A (H5N1) infection in humans. *N. Engl. J. Med.,* 353, 1374-1385.

Chaiworapongsa, T., Romero, R., Espinoza, J., Kim, Y. M., Edwin, S., Bujold, E., Gomez, R. and Kuivaniemi, H. (2005). Macrophage migration inhibitory factor in patients with preterm parturition and microbial invasion of the amniotic cavity. *J. Matern. Fetal Neonatal Med.,* 18, 405-416.

Chen, W., Calvo, P. A., Malide, D., Gibbs, J., Schubert, U., Bacik, I., Basta, S., O'Neill, R., Schickli, J., Palese, P., Henklein, P., Bennink, J. R. and Yewdell, J. W. (2001). A novel influenza A virus mitochondrial protein that induces cell death. *Nature Med.,* 7, 1306-1312.

Chotpitayasunondh, T., Ungchusak, K., Hanshaoworakul, W., Chunsuthiwat, S., Sawanpanyalert, P., Kijphati, R., Lochindarat, S., Srisan. P., Suwan, P., Osotthanakorn, Y., Anantasetagoon, T., Kanjanawasri, S., Tanupattarachai, S., Weerakul, J., Chaiwirattana, R., Maneerattanaporn, M., Poolsavathitikool, R., Chokephaibulkit, K., Apisarnthanarak, A. and Dowell, S. F. (2005). Human disease from influenza A (H5N1), Thailand, 2004. *Emerg. Infect. Dis.,* 11, 201-209.

Cohen, M. S., Isturiz, R. E., Malech, H. L., Root, R. K., Wilfert, C. M., Gutman, L. and Buckley, R. H. (1981). Fungal infection in chronic granulomatous disease. The importance of the phagocyte in defense against fungi. *Am. J. Med.,* 71, 59-66.

Conover, P. T. and Roessmann, U. (1990). Malformational complex in an infant with intrauterine influenza viral infection. *Arch. Pathol. Lab. Med.,* 114, 535-538.

Cox, N. J. and Kawaoka, Y. (1998). Orthomyxoviruses: influenza, In L. Collier, A. Balows and M. Sussman (Eds.), *Topley and Wilson's Microbiology and Microbial Infections, 9th edn.* (pp. 385-433). London: Arnold.

de Jong, M. D., Bach, V. C., Phan, T. Q., Vo, M. H., Tran, T. T., Nguyen, B. H., Beld, M., Le, T. P., Truong, H. K., Nguyen, V. V., Tran, T. H., Do, Q. H. and Farrar, J. (2005). Fatal avian influenza A (H5N1) in a child presenting with diarrhea followed by coma. *N. Engl. J. Med.,* 352, 686-691.

Fortunato, S. J., Menon, R., Bryant, C. and Lombardi, S. J. (2000). Programmed cell death (apoptosis) as a possible pathway to metalloproteinase activation and fetal membrane degradation in premature rupture of membranes. *Am. J. Obstet. Gynecol.,* 182, 1468-1476.

Fortunato, S. J., Menon, R. and Lombardi, S. J. (2001). Support for an infection-induced apoptotic pathway in human fetal membranes. Am. J. Obstet. Gynecol., 184, 1392-1398.

Fortunato, S. J., Menon, R. and Lombardi, S. J. (2002). Role of tumor necrosis factor-α in the premature rupture of membranes and preterm labor pathways. *Am. J. Obstet. Gynecol.,* 187, 1159-1162.

Fortunato, S. J. and Menon, R. (2003). IL-1β is a better inducer of apoptosis in human fetal membranes than IL-6. *Placenta,* 24, 922-928.

Frankova, V. and Rycheterova, V. (1975). Inhalatory infection of mice with influenza A0/PR8 virus. II. Detection of the virus in the blood and extrapulmonary organs. *Acta Virol.,* 19, 35-40.

Freeman, D. W. and Barno, A. (1959). Death from Asian influenza associated with pregnancy. *Am. J. Obstet. Gynec.,* 78, 1172-1175.

Fujimoto, I., Pan, J., Takizawa, T. and Nakanishi, Y. (2000). Virus clearance through apoptosis-dependent phagocytosis of influenza A virus-infected cells by macrophages. *J. Virol.,* 74, 3399-3403.

Gavrieli, Y., Sherman, Y. and Ben-Sasson, S. A. (1992). Identification of programmed cell death *in situ* via specific labeling of nuclear DNA fragmentation. *J. Cell Biol.,* 119, 493-501.

George, R. B., Kalich, J., Yonish, B., Murtha, A. P. (2008). Apoptosis in the chorion of fetal membranes in preterm premature rupture of membranes. *Am. J. Perinatol.,* 25, 29-32.

Greenberg, M., Lacobziner, H., Pakter, J. and Weist, B. A. G. (1958). Maternal mortality in the epidemic of Asian influenza, New York city, 1957. *Am. J. Obstet. Gynec.,* 76, 897-902.

Grossman, J. H. and Dennis, L. G. (1987). Infections affecting the placenta: In J. P. Lavery (Ed.), *The human placenta* (pp. 131-154). Maryland: Aspen Publishers Inc.

Gross-Schulman, S., Dassey, D. E. and Mascola, L. (1998). Influenza. *West J. Med.,* 169, 377-378.

Gu, J., Xie, Z., Gao, Z., Liu, J., Korteweg, C., Ye, J., Lau, L. T., Lu, J., Gao, Z., Zhang, B., McNutt, M. A., Lu, M., Anderson, V. M., Gong, E., Yu, A. C. and Lipkin, W. I. (2007). H5N1 infection of the respiratory tract and beyond: a molecular pathology study. *Lancet,* 370, 1137-1145.

Hakoda, S. and Nakatani, T. (2000). A pregnant woman with influenza A encephalopathy in whom influenza A/Hong Kong virus (H3) was isolated from cerebrospinal fluid. *Arch. Intern. Med.,* 160, 1041-1045.

Hardy, J. M., Azarowicz, E. N., Mannini, A., Medearis, D. N. and Cooke, R. E. (1961). The effect of Asian influenza on the outcome of pregnancy, Baltimore, 1957-1958. *Am. J. Public Health,* 51, 1182-1188.

Harris, J. W. (1919). Influenza occurring in pregnant women: A statistical study of thirteen hundred and fifty cases. *J. Am. Med. Assoc.,* 72, 978-980.

Hartert, T. V., Neuzil, K. M., Shintani, A. K., Mitchel, E. F., Snowden, M. S., Wood, L. B., Dittus, R. S. and Griffin, M. R. (2003). Maternal morbidity and perinatal outcomes among pregnant women with respiratory hospitalizations during influenza season. *Am. J. Obstet. Gynecol.,* 189, 1705-1712.

Hers, J. F. and Mulder, J. (1961). Broad aspects of the pathology and pathogenesis of human influenza. *Am. Rev. Respir. Dis.,* 83, 84-97.

Horimoto, T. and Kawaoka, Y. (2005). Influenza: lessons from past pandemics, warnings from current incidents. *Nat. Rev. Microbiol.,* 3, 591-600.

Huber, V. C., Lynch, J. M., Bucher, D. J., Le, J. and Metzger, D. W. (2001). Fc receptor-mediated phagocytosis makes a significant contribution to clearance of influenza virus infections. *J. Immunol.,* 166, 7381-7388.

Hung, T. H., Chen, S. F., Hsu, J. J., Hsieh, C. C., Hsueh, S. and Hsieh, T. T. (2006). Tumour necrosis factor-alpha converting enzyme in human gestational tissues from pregnancies complicated by chorioamnionitis. *Placenta,* 27, 996-1006.

Ietta, F., Todros, T., Ticconi, C., Piccoli, E., Zicari, A., Piccione, E. and Paulesu, L. (2002). Macrophage migration inhibitory factor in human pregnancy and labor. *Am. J. Reprod. Immunol., 48*, 404-409.

Ito, T., Kobayashi, Y., Morita, T., Horimoto, T. and Kawaoka, Y. (2002). Virulent influenza A viruses induce apoptosis in chickens. *Virus Res.,* 84, 27-35.

Jewett, J. F. (1974). Influenzal pneumonia at term. *N. Engl. J. Med.,* 291, 256-257.

Kaji, M., Oseasohn, R., Jordan, W. S. Jr. and Dingle, J. H. (1959). Isolation of Asian virus from extrapulmonary tissues in fatal human influenza. *Proc. Soc. Exp. Biol. Med.,* 100, 272-275.

Kamps, B. S. and Reyes-Terán, G. (2006). Influenza 2006, In B. S. Kamps, C. Hoffmann and W. Preiser (Eds), *Influenza Report 2006*; http://www.influenzareport.com/ (pp. 17-47). Flying Publisher.

Kash, J. C., Basler, C. F., Garcia-Sastre, A., Carter, V., Billharz, R., Swayne, D. E., Przygodzki, R. M., Taubenberger, J. K., Katze, M. G. and Tumpey, T. M. (2004). Global host immune response: pathogenesis and transcriptional profiling of type A influenza viruses expressing the hemagglutinin and neuraminidase genes from the 1918 pandemic virus. *J. Virol.,* 78, 9499-9511.

Kawaoka, Y., Krauss, S. and Webster, R. G. (1989). Avian-to-human transmission of the PB1 gene of influenza A viruses in the 1957 and 1968 pandemics. *J. Virol.,* 63, 4603-4608.

Kidokoro, K., Furuhashi, M., Kuno, N. and Ishikawa, K. (2006). Amniotic fluid neutrophil elastase and lactate dehydrogenase: association with histologic chorioamnionitis. *Acta Obstet. Gynecol. Scand.,* 85, 669-674.

Kishimoto, T., Akira, S. and Taga, T. (1992). Interleukin-6 and its receptor: a paradigm for cytokines. *Science,* 258, 593-597.

Kobayashi, S., Imajoh-Ohmi, S., Nakamura, M. and Kanegasaki, S. (1990). Occurrence of cytochrome b_{558} in B-cell lineage of human lymphocytes. *Blood,* 75, 458-461.

Kort, B. A., Cefalo, R. C., Baker, V. V. (1986). Fatal influenza A pneumonia in pregnancy. *Am. J. Perinatol.,* 3, 179-182.

Korteweg, C. and Gu, J. (2008). Pathology, molecular biology, and pathogenesis of avian influenza A (H5N1) infection in humans. *Am. J. Pathol.,* 172, 1155-1170.

Kroemer, G., Petit, P., Zamzami, N., Vayssière, J.-L. and Mignotte, B. (1995). *FASEB J.,* 9, 1277-1287.

Kumagai, K., Otsuki, Y., Ito, Y., Shibata, M-A., Abe, H. and Ueki, M. (2001). Apoptosis in the normal human amnion at term, independent of Bcl-2 regulation and onset of labour. *Mol. Hum. Reprod.,* 7, 681-689.

Kumar, D., Fung, W., Moore, R. M., Pandey, V., Fox, J., Stetzer, B., Mansour, J. M., Mercer, B. M., Redline, R. W. and Moore, J. J. (2006). Proinflammatory cytokines found in amniotic fluid induce collagen remodeling, apoptosis, and biophysical weakening of cultured human fetal membranes. *Biol. Reprod.,* 74, 29-34.

Lavery, J. P. (1987). Appendages of the placenta: In J. P. Lavery (Ed.), *The human placenta* (pp. 257-279). Maryland: Aspen Publishers Inc.

Lehmann, N. I. and Gust, I. D. (1971). Viremia in influenza. A report of two cases. *Med. J. Aust.,* 4, 1166-1169.

Madazli, R., Atiş, A., Uzun, H. and Aksu, F. (2003). Mid-trimester amniotic fluid angiogenin, lactate dehydrogenase and fibronectin in the prediction of preterm delivery. *Eur. J. Obstet. Gynecol. Reprod. Biol.,* 106, 160-164.

Malak, T. M. and Bell, S. C. (1994). Structural characteristics of term human fetal membranes: a novel zone of extreme morphological alteration within the rupture site. *Br. J. Obstet. Gynaecol.,* 101, 375-386.

Marvin, K. W., Keelan, J. A., Eykholt, R. L., Sato, T. A. and Mitchell, M. D. (2002). Use of cDNA arrays to generate differential expression profiles for inflammatory genes in human gestational membranes delivered at term and preterm. *Mol. Hum. Reprod.,* 8, 399-408.

McDonald, A. D. (1961). Maternal health in early pregnancy and congenital defect. Final report on a prospective inquiry. *Brit. J. Prev. Soc. Med.,* 15, 154-166.

McGregor, J. A., Burns, J. C., Levin, M. J., Burlington, B. and Meiklejohn, G. (1984). Transplacental passage of influenza A/Bangkok (H3N2) mimicking amniotic fluid infection syndrome. *Am. J. Obstet. Gynecol.,* 149, 856-859.

McLaren, J., Taylor, D. J. and Bell. S. C. (1999). Increased incidence of apoptosis in non-labour-affected cytotrophoblast cells in term fetal membranes overlying the cervix. *Hum. Reprod.,* 14, 2895-2900.

Mel'nikova, V. F., Tsinzerling, A. V., Aksenov, O. A., Vydumkina, S. P. and Kalinina, N. A. (1987). Involvement of the afterbirth in influenza. *Arkh. Patol.,* 49, 19-25.

Menon, R., Lombardi, S. J. and Fortunato, S. J. (2002). TNF-α promotes caspase activation and apoptosis in human fetal membranes. *J. Assist. Reprod. Genet.,* 19, 201-204.

Mercer, B. M. (2005). Preterm premature rupture of the membranes: current approaches to evaluation and management. *Obstet. Gynecol. Clin. North Am.,* 32, 411-428.

Mori, I., Komatsu, T., Takeuchi, K., Nakakuki, K., Sudo, M. and Kimura, Y. (1995a). Viremia induced by influenza virus. *Microb. Pathog.,* 19, 237-344.

Mori, I., Komatsu, T., Takeuchi, K., Nakakuki, K., Sudo, M. and Kimura, Y. (1995b). *In vivo* induction of apoptosis by influenza virus. *J. Gen. Virol.,* 76, 2869-2873.

Mori, I. and Kimura, Y. (2000). Apoptotic neurodegeneration induced by influenza A virus infection in the mouse brain. *Microbes Infect.,* 2, 1329-1334.

Mori, I., Goshima, F., Imai, Y., Kohsaka, S., Sugiyama, T., Yoshida, T., Yokochi, T., Nishiyama, Y., and Kimura, Y. (2002). Olfactory receptor neurons prevent dissemination of neurovirulent influenza A virus into the brain by undergoing virus-induced apoptosis. *J. Gen. Virol.,* 83, 2109-2116.

Mullooly, J. P., Barker, W. H. and Nolan, T. F. (1986). Risk of acute respiratory disease among pregnant women during influenza A epidemics. *Public Health Rep.,* 101, 205-211.

Murtha, A. P., Auten, R. and Herbert, W. N. (2002). Apoptosis in the chorion laeve of term patients with histologic chorioamnionitis. *Infect. Dis. Obstet. Gynecol.,* 10, 93-96.

Naficy, K. (1963). Human influenza infection with proved viremia. *N. Engl. J. Med.,* 269, 964-966.

Nakai, Y., Itoh, M., Mizuguchi, M., Ozawa, H., Okazaki, E., Kobayashi, Y., Takahashi, M., Ohtani, K., Ogawa, A., Narita, M., Togashi, T. and Takashima, S. (2003). Apoptosis and microglial activation in influenza encephalopathy. *Acta Neuropathol.,* 105, 233-239.

Neuzil, K. M., Reed, G. W., Mitchel, E. F., Simonsen, L. and Griffin, M. R. (1998). Impact of influenza on acute cardiopulmonary hospitalizations in pregnant women. *Am. J. Epidemiol.,* 148, 1094-1102.

Nicholson, D. W. and Thornberry, N. A. (1997). Caspases: killer proteases. Trends Biochem. Sci., 22, 299-306.

Noda, M., Takeda, K., Sugimoto, H., Hosoi, T., Takechi, K., Ishikawa, H., Arimura, H. and Konno, K. (1991). Purification and characterization of human fibroblast derived differentiation inducing factor for human monoblastic leukemia cells identical to interleukin-6. *Anticancer Res.,* 11, 961-968.

Oda, T., Akaike, T., Hamamoto, T., Suzuki, F., Hirano, T. and Maeda, H. (1989). Oxygen radicals in influenza-induced pathogenesis and treatment with pyran polymer-conjugated SOD. *Science,* 244, 974-976.

Ohyama, K., Oka, K., Emura, A., Tamura, H., Suga, T., Bessho, T., Hirakawa, S. and Yamakawa, T. (1998). Suppression of apoptotic cell death progressed *in vitro* with incubation of the chorion laeve tissues of human fetal membrane by glucocorticoid. *Biol. Pharm. Bull.,* 21, 1024-1029.

Ohyama, K., Yuan, B., Bessho, T. and Yamakawa, T. (2001). Progressive apoptosis in chorion laeve trophoblast cells of human fetal membrane tissues during *in vitro* incubation is suppressed by antioxidative reagents. *Eur. J. Biochem.,* 268, 6182-6189.

Oltvai, Z. N. and Korsmeyer, S. J. (1994). Checkpoints of dueling dimers foil death wishes. *Cell,* 79, 189-192.

Onodera, S., Suzuki, K., Matsuno, T., Kaneda, K., Takagi, M. and Nishihira, J. (1997). Macrophage migration inhibitory factor induces phagocytosis of foreign particles by macrophages in autocrine and paracrine fashion. *Immunology,* 92, 131-7.

Park, J. B. (2003). Phagocytosis induces superoxide formation and apoptosis in macrophages. *Exp. Mol. Med.,* 35, 325-335.

Parmley, T. H. (1990). Spontaneous cell death in the chorion laeve. *Am. J. Obstet. Gynecol.,* 162, 1576-1583.

Patterson, M. M. (2005). The coming influenza pandemic: lessons from the past for the future. *J. Am. Osteopath. Assoc.,* 105, 498-500.

Peiris, J. S., Yu, W. C., Leung, C. W., Cheung, C. Y., Ng, W. F., Nicholls, J. M., Ng, T. K., Chan, K. H., Lai, S. T., Lim, W. L., Yuen, K. Y. and Guan, Y. (2004). Re-emergence of fatal human influenza A subtype H5N1 disease. *Lancet,* 363, 617-619.

Peiser, L. and Gordon, S. (2001). The function of scavenger receptors expressed by macrophages and their role in the regulation of inflammation. *Microbes Infect.,* 3, 149-159.

Perrone, L. A., Plowden, J. K., García-Sastre, A., Katz, J. M. and Tumpey, T. M. (2008). H5N1 and 1918 pandemic influenza virus infection results in early and excessive infiltration of macrophages and neutrophils in the lungs of mice. *PLoS Pathog.,* 4, e1000115.

Pleydell, M. J. (1960). Anencephaly and other congenital abnormalities: An epidemiological study in Northamptonshire. *Br. Med. J.,* 1, 309-315.

Reid, A. H., Fanning, T. G., Hultin, J. V. and Taubenberger, J. K. (1999). Origin and evolution of the 1918 "Spanish" influenza virus hemagglutinin gene. *Proc. Natl. Acad. Sci. U S A.*, 96, 1651-1656.

Restifo, N. P. (2000). Building better vaccines: how apoptotic cell death can induce inflammation and activate innate and adaptive immunity. *Curr. Opin. Immunol.*, 12, 597-603.

Ritova, V. V., Schastnyi, E. I., Ratushkina, L. S. and Shuster, I. Y. (1979). Investigation of the incidence of influenza A viremia caused by virus strains circulating among children in 1968-1977. J. Hyg. Epidemiol. Microbiol. *Immunol.*, 23, 35-41.

Roberts, G. T. and Roberts, J. T. (1976). Postsplenectomy sepsis due to influenzal viremia and pneumococcemia. *Can. Med. Assoc. J.*, 115, 435-437.

Roberts, W. K. and Vasil, A. (1982). Evidence for the identity of murine gamma interferon and macrophage activating factor. *J. Interferon Res.*, 2, 519-532.

Romero, R., Brody, D. T., Oyarzun, E., Mazor, M., Wu, Y. K., Hobbins, J. C. and Durum, S. K. (1989). Infection and labor. III. Interleukin-1: a signal for the onset of parturition. *Am. J. Obstet. Gynecol.*, 160, 1117-1123.

Romero, R., Avila, C., Santhanam, U. and Sehgal, P. B. (1990). Amniotic fluid interleukin 6 in preterm labor. Association with infection. *J. Clin. Invest.*, 85, 1392-1400.

Romero, R., Mazor, M., Sepulveda, W., Avila, C., Copeland, D. and Williams, J. (1992). Tumor necrosis factor in preterm and term labor. *Am. J. Obstet. Gynecol.*, 166, 1576-1587.

Rosztoczy, I., Sweet, C., Toms, G. L. and Smith, H. (1975). Replication of influenza virus in organ cultures of human and simian urogenital tissues and human foetal tissues. *Br. J. Exp. Pathol.*, 56, 322-328.

Ruben, F. L., Winkelstein, A. and Sabbacha, R. E. (1975). In utero sensitization with influenza virus in man. *Proc. Soc. Exp. Biol. Med.*, 149, 881-883.

Ruben, F. L. and Thompson, D. (1981). Cord blood lymphocyte *in vitro* responses to influenza A antigens after an epidemic of influenza A/Port Chalmers/73 (H3N2). *Am. J. Obstet. Gynecol.*, 141, 443-447.

Runic, R., Lockwood, C. J., LaChapelle, L., Dipasquale, B., Demopoulos, R. I., Kumar, A. and Guller, S. (1998). Apoptosis and Fas expression in human fetal membranes. *J. Clin. Endocrinol. Metab.*, 83, 660-666.

Rushton, D. I., Collie, M. H., Sweet, C., Husseini, R. H. and Smith, H. (1983). The effects of maternal influenzal viremia in late gestation on the conceptus of the pregnant ferret. *J. Pathol.*, 140, 181-191.

Salgo, M. G. and Pryor, W. A. (1996). Trolox inhibits peroxynitrite-mediated oxidative stress and apoptosis in rat thymocytes. *Arch. Biochem. Biophys.*, 333, 482-488.

Salonen, O., Koskiniemi, M., Saari, A., Myllylä, V., Pyhälä R., Airksinen, L. and Vaheri, A. (1997). Myelitis associated with influenza A virus infection. *J. NeuroVirol.*, 3, 83-85.

Sedger, L. M., Hou, S., Osvath, S. R., Glaccum, M. B., Peschon, J. J., van Rooijen, N. and Hyland, L. (2002). Bone marrow B cell apoptosis during *in vivo* influenza virus infection requires TNF-α and lymphotoxin-α. *J. Immunol.*, 169, 6193-6201.

Shi, Y., Niculescu, R., Wang, D., Patel, S., Davenpeck, K. L. and Zalewski, A. (2001). Increased NAD(P)H oxidase and reactive oxygen species in coronary arteries after balloon injury. Arterioscler. Thromb. *Vas. Biol.,* 21, 739-745.

Shiratsuchi, A., Kaido, M., Takizawa, T. and Nakanishi, Y. (2000). Phosphatidylserine-mediated phagocytosis of influenza A virus-infected cells by mouse peritoneal macrophages. *J. Virol.,* 74, 9240-9244.

Shu, Y., Yu, H. and Li, D. (2006). Lethal avian influenza A (H5N1) infection in a pregnant woman in Anhui Province, China. *N. Engl. J. Med.,* 354, 1421-1422.

Smith, G. J., Naipospos, T. S., Nguyen, T. D., de Jong, M. D., Vijaykrishna, D., Usman, T. B., Hassan, S. S., Nguyen, T. V., Dao, T. V., Bui, N. A., Leung, Y. H., Cheung, C. L., Rayner, J. M., Zhang, J. X., Zhang, L. J., Poon, L. L., Li, K. S., Nguyen, V. C., Hien, T. T., Farrar, J., Webster, R. G., Chen, H., Peiris, J. S. and Guan, Y. (2006). Evolution and adaptation of H5N1 influenza virus in avian and human hosts in Indonesia and Vietnam. *Virology, 350,* 258-268.

Snelgrove, R. J., Edwards, L., Rae, A. J. and Hussell, T. (2006). An absence of reactive oxygen species improves the resolution of lung influenza infection. *Eur. J. Immunol.,* 36, 1364-1373.

Stanley, E. D. and Jackson, G. G. (1966). Viremia in Asian influenza. Trans Assoc Am Physicians 79, 376-387.

Stanwell-Smith, R., Parker, A. M., Chakraverty, P., Soltanpoor, N. and Simpson, C. N. (1994). Possible association of influenza A with fetal loss: investigation of a cluster of spontaneous abortions and stillbirths. *Commun. Dis. Rep. CDR Rev.,* 4, R28-32.

Steel, J. H., O'Donoghue, K., Kennea, N. L., Sullivan, M. H. F. and Edwards, A. D. (2005). Maternal origin of inflammatory leukocytes in preterm fetal membranes, shown by fluorescence *in situ* hybridization. *Placenta,* 26, 672-677.

Sterner, G., Grandien, M. and Enocksson, E. (1990). Pregnant women with acute respiratory illness at term. *Scand. J. infect. Dis.,* 71, 19-26.

Suliman, H. B., Ryan, L. K., Bishop, L. and Folz, R. J. (2001). Prevention of influenza-induced lung injury in mice overexpressing extracellular superoxide dismutase. *Am. J. Physiol., Lung Cell. Mol. Physiol.,* 280, L69-78.

Sweet, C., Collie, M. H., Toms, G. L. and Smith, H. (1977). The pregnant guinea-pig as a model for studying influenza virus infection in utero: infection of foetal tissues in organ culture and *in vivo*. *Br. J. Exp. Pathol.,* 58, 133-139.

Swierkosz, T. A., Mitchell, J. A., Warner, T. D., Botting, R. M. and Vane, J. R. (1995). Co-induction of nitric oxide synthase and cyclo-oxygenase: interactions between nitric oxide and prostanoids. *Br. J. Pharmacol.,* 114, 1335-1342.

Taga, T., Hibi, M., Hirata, Y., Yamasaki, K., Yasukawa, K., Matsuda, T., Hirano, T. and Kishimoto, T. (1989). Interleukin-6 triggers the association of its receptor with a possible signal transducer, gp130. *Cell,* 58, 573-581.

Takahashi, M., Yamada, T., Nakashita, Y., Saikusa, H., Deguchi, M., Kida, H., Tashiro, M. and Toyoda, T. (2000). Influenza virus-induced encepharopathy: Clinicopathologic study of an autopsied case. *Pediatr. Int.,* 42, 204-214.

Takeda, K., Hosoi, T., Noda, M., Arimura, H. and Konno, K. (1988). Effect of fibroblast-derived differentiation inducing factor on the differentiation of human monocytoid and myeloid leukemia cell lines. *Biochem. Biophys. Res. Commun.,* 155, 24-31.

To, K. F., Chan, P. K., Chan, K. F., Lee, W. K., Lam, W. Y., Wong, K. F., Tang, N. L., Tsang, D. N., Sung, R. Y., Buckley, T. A., Tam, J. S. and Cheng, A. F. (2001). Pathology of fatal human infection associated with avian influenza A H5N1 virus. *J. Med. Virol.,* 63, 242-246.

Tran, T. H., Nguyen, T. L., Nguyen, T. D., Luong, T. S., Pham, P. M., Nguyen, V. C., Pham, T. S., Vo, C. D., Le, T. Q., Ngo, T. T., Dao, B. K., Le, P. P., Nguyen, T. T., Hoang, T. L., Cao, V. T., Le, T. G., Nguyen, D. T., Le, H. N., Nguyen, K. T., Le, H. S., Le, V. T., Christiane, D., Tran, T. T., Menno, de J., Schultsz, C., Cheng, P., Lim, W., Horby, P. and Farrar, J.; World Health Organization International Avian Influenza Investigative Team. (2004). Avian influenza A (H5N1) in 10 patients in Vietnam. *N. Engl. J. Med.,* 350, 1179-1188.

Tsuchiya, S., Kobayashi, Y., Goto, Y., Okumura, H., Nakae, S., Konno, T. and Tada, K. (1982). Induction of maturation in cultured human monocytic leukemia cells by a phorbol diester. *Cancer Res.,* 42, 1530-1536.

Tsuruoka, H., Xu, H., Kuroda, K., Hayashi, K., Yasui, O., Yamada, A., Ishizaki, T., Yamada. Y., Watanabe, T. and Hosaka, Y. (1997). Detection of influenza virus RNA in peripheral blood mononuclear cells of influenza patients. *Jpn. J. Med. Sci. Biol.,* 50, 27-34.

Uchide, N., Ohyama, K., Bessho, T., Yuan, B. and Yamakawa, T. (2002a). Apoptosis in cultured human fetal membrane cells infected with influenza virus. *Biol. Pharm. Bull.,* 25, 109-114.

Uchide, N., Ohyama, K., Yuan, B., Sano, T., Bessho, T. and Yamakawa, T. (2002b). Differential mRNA expression of inflammatory cytokines in cultured human fetal membrane cells responding to influenza virus infection. *Biol. Pharm. Bull.,* 25, 239-243.

Uchide, N., Ohyama, K., Yuan, B., Bessho, T. and Yamakawa, T. (2002c). Differentiation of monocytes to macrophages induced by influenza virus-infected apoptotic cells. *J. Gen. Virol.,* 83, 747-751.

Uchide, N., Ohyama, K., Bessho, T., Yuan, B. and Yamakawa, T. (2002d). Effect of antioxidants on apoptosis induced by influenza virus infection: inhibition of viral gene replication and transcription with pyrrolidine dithiocarbamate. *Antiviral Res.,* 56, 207-217.

Uchide, N., Ohyama, K., Bessho, T. and Yamakawa, T. (2002e). Semi-quantitative RT-PCR-based assay, improved by Southern hybridization technique, for polarity-specific influenza virus RNAs in cultured cells. *J. Virol. Methods,* 106, 125-134.

Uchide, N., Ohyama, K., Bessho, T. and Toyoda, H. (2005a). Induction of pro-inflammatory cytokine gene expression and apoptosis in human chorion cells of fetal membranes by influenza virus infection: possible implications for maintenance and interruption of pregnancy during infection. *Med. Sci. Monit.,* 11, RA7-16.

Uchide, N., Ohyama, K., Bessho, T. and Toyoda, H. (2005b). Inhibition of influenza virus-induced apoptosis in chorion cells of human fetal membranes by nordihydroguaiaretic acid. *Intervirology,* 48, 336-340.

Uchide, N., Suzuki, A., Ohyama, K., Bessho, T. and Toyoda, H. (2006a). Secretion of bioactive interleukin-6 and tumor necrosis factor-α proteins from primary cultured human fetal membrane chorion cells infected with influenza virus. *Placenta,* 27, 678-690.

Uchide, N., Tadera, C., Sarai, H., Ohyama, K., Bessho, T. and Toyoda, H. (2006b). Characterization of monocyte differentiation-inducing (MDI) factors derived from human fetal membrane chorion cells undergoing apoptosis after influenza virus infection. *Int. J. Biochem. Cell Biol.,* 38, 1926-1938.

Uchide, N., Ohyama, K., Bessho, T. and Toyoda, H. (2007). Effects of mitogen-activated protein kinase inhibitors on tumor necrosis factor-α gene expression and apoptosis induction in cultured human fetal membrane chorion cells infected with influenza virus. *Intervirology,* 50, 99-107.

Uchide, N. and Toyoda, H. (2007). A new simple multi-well plate-based assay for monocyte differentiation using human monocytic leukemia THP-1 cells. *J. Immunol. Methods,* 328, 215-219.

Uchide, N. and Toyoda, H. (2008a). Future target molecules for influenza treatment. *Mini Rev. Med. Chem.*, 8, 491-495.

Uchide, N. and Toyoda, H. (2008b). Potential of selected antioxidants for influenza chemotherapy. *Anti-infect. Agents Med. Chem.*, 7, 73-83.

Uiprasertkul, M., Puthavathana, P., Sangsiriwut, K., Pooruk, P., Srisook, K., Peiris, M., Nicholls, J. M., Chokephaibulkit, K., Vanprapar, N. and Auewarakul, P. (2005). Influenza A H5N1 replication sites in humans. *Emerg. Infect Dis.,* 11, 1036-41.

Uiprasertkul, M., Kitphati, R., Puthavathana, P., Kriwong, R., Kongchanagul, A., Ungchusak, K., Angkasekwinai, S., Chokephaibulkit, K., Srisook, K., Vanprapar, N. and Auewarakul, P. (2007). Apoptosis and pathogenesis of avian influenza A (H5N1) virus in humans. *Emerg. Infect. Dis.,* 13, 708-712.

Ungchusak, K., Auewarakul, P., Dowell, S. F., Kitphati, R., Auwanit, W., Puthavathana, P., Uiprasertkul, M., Boonnak, K., Pittayawonganon, C., Cox, N. J., Zaki, S. R., Thawatsupha, P., Chittaganpitch, M., Khontong, R., Simmerman, J. M. and Chunsutthiwat, S. (2005). Probable person-to-person transmission of avian influenza A (H5N1). *N. Engl. J. Med.,* 352, 333-340.

Vannier, P. (1999). Infection causes of abortion in swine. Reprod. Dom. Anim., 34, 367-376.

Vince, G. S. and Johnson, P. M. (2000). Leucocyte populations and cytokine regulation in human uteroplacental tissues. *Biochem. Soc. Transact.,* 28, 191-195.

Virag, L., Szabo, E., Gergely, P. and Szabo, C. (2003). Peroxynitrite-induced cytotoxicity: mechanism and opportunities for intervention. *Toxicol. Lett.,* 140-141, 113-124.

Wallace, G.D. and Elm, J. L. Jr. (1979). Transplacental transmission and neonatal infection with swine influenza virus (Hsw1N1) in swine. *Am. J. Vet. Res.,* 40, 1169-1172.

Walsh, J. J., Dietlein, L. F., Low, F. N., Burch, G. E. and Mogabgab, W. J. (1961). Bronchotracheal response in human influenza. Type A, Asian strain, as studied by light and electron microscopic examination of bronchoscopic biopsies. *Arch. Intern. Med.,* 108, 376-388.

Watanabe, W., Sudo, K., Asawa, S., Konno, K., Yokota, T. and Shigeta, S. (1995). Use of lactate dehydrogenase to evaluate the anti-viral activity against influenza A virus. *J. Virol. Methods,* 51, 185-191.

Watanabe, Y., Shiratsuchi, A., Shimizu, K., Takizawa, T. and Nakanishi, Y. (2002). Role of phosphatidylserine exposure and sugar chain desialylation at the surface of influenza virus-infected cells in efficient phagocytosis by macrophages. *J. Biol. Chem.,* 277, 18222-18228.

Watanabe, Y., Shiratsuchi, A., Shimizu, K., Takizawa, T. and Nakanishi, Y. (2004). Stimulation of phagocytosis of influenza virus-infected cells through surface desialylation of macrophages by viral neuraminidase. *Microbiol. Immunol.,* 48, 875-881.

Watanabe, Y., Hashimoto, Y., Shiratsuchi, A., Takizawa, T. and Nakanishi, Y. (2005). Augmentation of fatality of influenza in mice by inhibition of phagocytosis. *Biochem. Biophys. Res. Commun.,* 337, 881-886.

Weiss, L. and Glaves, D. (1975). Effects of migration inhibiting factor(s) on the *in vitro* detachment of macrophages. *J. Immunol.* 115, 1362-1365.

Wesley, R. D. (2004). Exposure of sero-positive gilts to swine influenza may cause a few stillbirth per litter. *Can. J. Vet. Res.,* 68, 215-217.

Wiedbrauk, D. L. and Burleson, G. R. (1986). Production and characterization of poly(I):poly(C)-induced rat interferons *in vitro*. *J. Interferon Res.,* 6, 281-295.

Wong, S. S. and Yuen, K. Y. (2006). Avian influenza virus infections in humans. *Chest,* 129, 156-168.

World Health Organization. (2008). Cumulative Number of Confirmed Human Cases of Avian Influenza A/(H5N1) Reported to WHO. http://www.who.int/csr/disease/avian_influenza/ country/cases_table_2008_05_28/en/index.html

Wyllie, A. H., Kerr, J. F. and Currie, A. R. (1980). Cell death: the significance of apoptosis. *Int. Rev. Cytol.,* 68, 251-306.

Yawn, D. H., Pyeatte, J. C., Joseph, M. J., Eichler, S. L. and Garcia-Bunuel, R. (1971). Transplacental transfer of influenza virus. *J. Am. Med. Assoc.,* 216, 1022-1023.

Yao, L,, Korteweg, C., Hsueh, W. and Gu, J. (2007). Avian influenza receptor expression in H5N1-infected and noninfected human tissues. *FASEB J.,* 22, 733-740.

Yuan, B., Ohyama, K., Bessho, T. and Toyoda, H. (2006). Contribution of inducible nitric oxide synthase and cyclooxygenase-2 to apoptosis induction in smooth chorion trophoblast cells of human fetal membrane tissues. *Biochem. Biophys. Res. Commun.,* 341, 822-827.

Yuan, B., Ohyama, K., Bessho, T., Uchide, N. and Toyoda, H. (2008). Imbalance between ROS production and elimination results in apoptosis induction in primary smooth chorion trophoblast cells prepared from human fetal membrane tissues. *Life Sci.*, 82, 623-630.

Zhdanov, V. M. and Ritova, V. V. (1959). On the pathogenesis of influenza. *Klin. Med.* (Mosk.), 37, 45-48.

Zinserling, A. V., Aksenov, O. A., Melnikova, V. F. and Zinserling, V. A. (1983). Extrapulmonary lesions in influenza. *Tohoku J. Exp. Med.,* 140, 259-272.

In: Infectious Pregnancy Complications
Editor: Richard N. Canfield

ISBN: 978-1-60471-038-6

Chapter 4

Serological Response to Rubella, Herpes Simplex 2 and Cytomegalovirus in Pregnant Women with Unexplained Recurrent Abortions

***Maysaa El Sayed Zaki*[2a] *and Ahmmed Badawy*[b]**
[a]Clinical Pathology, [b]Gynaecology and Obstetrics,
Faculty of Medicine, Mansoura University, Mansoura, Egypt

Abstract

Bad obstetric history (BOH) implies previous unfavorable foetal outcome in terms of two or more consecutive spontaneous abortions, history of early neonatal death, intrauterine growth retardation, stillbirths, intrauterine fetal death and/or congenital anomalies. Recurrent pregnancy wastage due to maternal infections transmissible *in utero* at various stages of gestation can be caused by a wide array of organisms that include *Toxoplasma gondii*, rubella virus, cytomegalovirus, herpes simplex virus and other agents.

Herpes simplex virus (HSV) is classified in the alpha virinae subfamily within the family Herpesviridae. Two closely-related viruses are designated HSV types 1 and 2. Both can be transmitted in utero to fetus, with more complications associated with herpes simplex 2.

Another important viral cause of BOH is cytomegaloviruses (CMV). Cytomegaloviruses are ubiquitous and species-specific. Humans are believed to be the only reservoir of this virus, and transmission occurs by direct or indirect person-to-person contact. Vertical transmission can lead to serious congenital infections.

Rubella virus causes serious disease after vertical transmission. Most maternal infections remain subclinical or cause a trivial infection that may remain unrecognized. Its vaccination coverage is not sufficient throughout the world, so new cases are still

[2] Professor of Clinical Microbiology and Immunology, Faculty of Medicine–Mansoura University, Egypt. E-mail: may_s65@hotmail.com; Telephone: 0020502258877

reported. Clinical diagnosis of rubella is difficult and unreliable, as rubella virus infection can be asymptomatic in up to 50% of infected patients.

Several modalities are available for the diagnosis of those infections. The benchmark method is viral culture. Serology can establish current and past infection. Recently, molecular techniques have become available for rapid diagnosis.

Testing of pregnant women for HSV, CMV and rbella antibodies is usually done with a type-specific assay for their antibodies.

The objective of the present study was to explore the prevalence of herpes simplex virus 2, cytomegalovirus and rubella in pregnant with repeated spontaneous abortions (RSA) in first trimester. The diagnosis was performed by polymerase chain reaction, serological study for specific immunoglobulins G and M for herpes simplex 2 and cytomegalovirus and rubella. There was also an attempt to discover the accuracy of serological diagnosis for herpes simplex 2 and cytomegalovirus compared to polymerase chain reaction.

Patients recruited in the study were complaining of repeated first trimester abortions without obvious medical or gynecological etiology. Laboratory screenings for immunoglobulin M for toxoplasmosis were negative. The study also included pregnant women with normal obstetric history as a control group. Complete medical and obstetric evaluations were performed for patients and control subjects. Furthermore, specific virological diagnosis was performed to measure specific immunoglobulins M and G for CMV and herpes simplex 2 by enzyme linked immunosorbant assay with detection of their DNA in maternal serum by polymerase chain reaction. Diagnosis of rubella was performed by measurement of specific immunoglobulin M by enzyme linked immunosorbant assay.

There was a statistically significant difference between the RSA group and the pregnant women without RSA in frequency of rubella IgM (44.7%), herpes simplex IgM (39.1%) and CMV 10.9% ($P < .001$) . However, there was insignificant difference in IgG for herpes simplex 2, CMV and rubella between patients and control. Herpes simplex 2 viremia was positive in 26% RSA and cytomegalovirus was positive in 10.9% RSA patients. There was a significant association between viremia for cytomegalovirus and herpes simplex 2 ($P<0.009$).

The present study highlights the significant association of rubella, herpes simplex and cytomegalovirus with bad obstetric history. There may be persistence of rubella virus related to repeated early abortions. Moreover, combined viral infections in those patients were found that could even further aggravate intrauterine infections. The study allows the idea that serological tests for IgM are a rapid and accurate method for laboratory diagnosis.

Keywords: bad obstetric history, repeated spontaneous abortion, rubella, herpes simplex 2, cytomegalovirus

Introduction

Recurrent spontaneous abortion (RSA) is defined as three or more consecutive pregnancy losses prior to the 20th week of gestation. The etiology of recurrent spontaneous abortion is often unclear and may be multifactorial, with much controversy regarding diagnosis and treatment. Reasonably accepted etiologic causes include genetics; anatomical, endocrine, and placental anomalies; hormonal problems; infection; smoking and alcohol consumption;

exposure to environmental factors; psychological trauma and stressful life event; and certain coagulation and immunoregulatory protein defects. Detection of an abnormality in any of these areas may result in specific therapeutic measures, with varying degrees of success [1].

Several viruses are implicated as etiological infectious factors for RSA. Among those viruses is herpes simplex virus (HSV). Herpes simplex virus is classified in the alpha virinae subfamily within the family Herpesviridae. Two closely-related viruses are designated HSV types 1 and 2. HSV-1 is the usual cause of orolabial infection (gingivostomatitis or herpes labialis), whereas HSV-2 is the major cause of genital infection. However, either virus can infect either location [2-5].

Several modalities are available for the diagnosis of HSV infections [6-8]. The benchmark method is viral culture, but it is available in reference laboratory. Serology can establish current and past infection with HSV. It has also been used in research studies of the epidemiology of HSV and is very useful in unusual clinical situations [9, 10]. The antibody response to HSV glycoprotein G (gG) is highly specific, and gG-based assays can accurately determine whether individuals have past infection with HSV-1 and/or HSV-2 [11-13].

Because genital HSV-2 infection is much more likely to recur than genital HSV-1 infection, the presence of antibody to HSV-2 and a compatible clinical history would be strong presumptive evidence that the disease was recurrent genital herpes [13, 14].

Testing of pregnant women for HSV antibodies is usually done with a type-specific assay for HSV antibodies [15]. Studies of neonatal HSV infections have generally shown that most infected infants are born to women who have no clinical history of recurrent genital herpes but who are HSV-2 antibody positive at term [16]. Early identification of these women by serologic testing might be used as part of a strategy to prevent some perinatal transmission of HSV.

It is generally agreed that identification of both unrecognized HSV-2-positive pregnant women and pregnant women who are HSV antibody negative but in danger of becoming infected is essential [17].

When a primary HSV-2 infection is contracted during pregnancy, the fetus is at high risk of acquiring HSV-2 infection at delivery. In the study population of almost 200 infants, an estimated 5% of neonatal HSV infections were intrauterine [18].

Detection of HSV IgM antibody in cord blood obtained by cordocentesis and in the blood of the neonate during the first week of life is also diagnostic of in-utero HSV infection [19].

Another virus implicated in bad obstetric history is rubella virus. Rubella is usually presented as mild disease with few complications. However, when acquired in the first 12 weeks of pregnancy, it usually results in congenital infection associated with one or more severe defects in 80% to 90% of cases. When maternal infection occurs between 13 and 20 weeks, the risk of congenital anomalies declines to about 17%; in some cases, there is serological evidence of infection, but no virus is excreted and no anomalies occur [20].

As a result of effective immunization programs, postnatal acquired rubella and congenitally acquired rubella (CAR) have become rare in countries such as the United States and the United Kingdom, although outbreaks of rubella, including cases among pregnant women, have recently occurred in these countries [20, 21]. However, in many European countries, which have yet to achieve good vaccination coverage, rubella continues to occur in pregnant women [22]. Studies suggest that congenitally acquired rubella is responsible for such congenital defects as blindness and deafness in developing countries, and this imposes a considerable burden on scarce health care resources [23]. Moreover, vaccination programs are not adequately inserted with a booster immunization dose for young girls found to be negative for rubella antibodies.

Cytomegalovirus (CMV) is another virus that can cross the placenta and cause both fetal and placental infections. Most congenital infections are asymptomatic; only 10% of fetuses infected in utero will develop clinical signs of CMV infection. Studies have shown that infants congenitally infected with CMV as a result of primary infection of their mothers are more likely to have overt squeal than those infected from reactivated infections of the mothers [24, 25].

Transmission of CMV infection to the fetus has been identified in all trimesters of pregnancy. Abortion can result from ascending CMV endometritis and the virus has been isolated from post-abortion uterine discharge [26]. The usual manifestations of overt CMV infection at birth are hepatosplenomegaly, jaundice, thrombocytopenia and various congenital malformations, especially those involving the central nervous system [27]. Universal screening of pregnant women for CMV infection during an early prenatal visit is not yet recommended worldwide.

The objective of the present study was to explore the prevalence of herpes simplex virus 2, cytomegalovirus and rubella in pregnant with repeated spontaneous abortions (RSA) in first trimester. The diagnosis was performed by polymerase chain reaction, serological study for specific immunoglobulins G and M for herpes simplex 2 and cytomegalovirus and rubella. There was also attempt to discover the accuracy of serological diagnosis for herpes simplex 2 and cytomegalovirus compared to polymerase chain reaction.

The patients were recruited from an obstetric outpatient clinic at the Mansoura University Hospital, Egypt. Two different groups were evaluated. The first group (n =92) consisted of patients with medically unexplained recurrent spontaneous abortions (RSA) (women with a history of 3 or more consecutive spontaneous abortions including abortions up to 22 gestational weeks). The second group (n = 12) consisted of pregnant women without a history of RSA and with pregnancy duration of more than 32 weeks' gestation. The demographic, medical, and clinical data were collected in each case based on personal interviews and medical examination. The women signed an informed consent before they were included in this study. The study was approved by the ethics committee of Mansoura University, Egypt.

Blood samples were obtained from each patient and centrifuged, and the sera were kept frozen in aliquots at -20°C until analysis. Serologic study was performed for rubella, HSV-1/HSV-2, and CMV for specific qualitative IgG and IgM by enzyme linked immunosorbant assay (ELISA-Equipar Via G, Ferrari, Saronno, Italy).

Polymerase chain reaction (PCR) was performed for each patient and control to detect specific DNA of CMV and HSV-1/HSV-2 (Experteam Di De Bortoli Angelo and CSAS, Spain).

QiAamp DNA mini kit was used for DNA extraction of CMV (GmbH, Hilden, Germany). For each sample, we prepared the following mixture: buffer (2.5 μL), deoxynucleoside triphosphates (2.5 μL), primer P1 (1.0 μL), primer P2 (1.0 μL), *Taq* polymerase (0.3 μL), distilled water (7.7 μL), extracted DNA solution (10 μL), and overlaid mineral oil (30 μL).

PCR for detection of major immediate-early gene MIE region was performed as described. The nested primers of mtr II, wereCMTR (5′CTG TCG GTG ATG GTC TCT TC-′3) and CMTR (5′ CCC GACACG CGG AAA AGA AA ′3) for the first round and CMTR 3(5′TCT CTG GTC CTG ATC GTC TT ′3) and CMTR 4 (5′ GTG ACCTAC CAA CGT AGG TT ′3) for the second round [28].

Amplification program was 94°C for 1 minute, 30 cycles (55°C for 1 minute, 72°C for 1 minute). Following PCR, the amplicon (221 bp) for CMV was resolved on a 1.5% agarose gel, visualized using ethidium bromide (0.5 μg/ mL) under ultraviolet illumination.

For detection of HSV-1/HSV-2 DNA, multiplex nested PCR was used. DNA was extracted with the commercially available Qiagen kit (GmbH, Hilden). Primers were designed to bracket a well-conserved region in the DNA polymerase gene. Primer pair HSVP1 (5′-GTGGTGGACTTTGCCAGCCTGTACCC-′3) and HSV-P2 (5′-TAAACATGGAGTCCGTGTCGCCGTAGATGA-′3) were used to amplify HSV-1 and HSV-2 [29]. *Taq* (0.25 μL) and extracted DNA (10 μL) were added to each premixed supplied tube. Negative control was analyzed by adding sterile distilled water instead of DNA and positive control was performed by 5.0 μL of HSV-1 positive control and 5.0 μL of positive control HSV-2 DNA.

The following program was used for the thermal cycle for the first amplification: 1 cycle at 94°C for 2 minutes, 35 cycles (94°C for 30 seconds, 56°C for 30 seconds, 72°C for 30 seconds), and 1 cycle at 72°C for 5 minutes.

For the second amplification we added 1 μL from the amplified DNA and 0.25 μL of *Taq* polymerase in premixed tubes supplied with the kit. The program used in the thermal cycles was 1 cycle at 94°C for 2 minutes, 30 cycles (of 94°C for 30 seconds, 58°C for 30 seconds, 72°C for 30 seconds), and 1 cycle at 72°C for 5 minutes.

Following PCR, the amplicon (137 bp for HSV-1 and 100 bp for HSV-2) was resolved on a 1.5% agarose gel and visualized using ethidium bromide (0.5 μg/mL) under ultraviolet illumination.

Values were represented as means ±SD, median (range), or the number of subjects and proportions. One-way analysis of variance test and independent samples Student *t* test were used for group comparisons of normally distributed variables, and the Kruskal-Wallis test and Mann-Whitney *U* test were used for comparisons of variables with skewed distribution. The chi-square test was used to compare proportions.

Ninety-two patients with a history of recurrent abortions and 12 pregnant women without a history of recurrent abortions were studied. All studied cases were in the first trimester. The mean age ± SD of the patients was 28.8± 5.61 years and the mean± SD age of the control group was 29.2± 6.25 years with a statistically insignificant difference between both groups (P =0.80). The range of gravidity between both groups was 2 to 7 times.

In the study of serologic responses for the viruses in RSA, IgM for rubella had the highest rate (44.7%), followed by HSV-1/HSV-2 IgM (39.1%), and CMV IgM (10.9%) while for IgG the highest rate was for HSV1/2 IgG (54.3%), CMV 38% followed by rubella IgG 32.6%. In control subjects the highest rate was for rubella IgG and CMV 75% followed by HSV1/2 58%.

There was a statistically significant difference between the patients group and the control group in prevalence of rubella IgM and IgG (*P* = .001, *P* <0.05, respectively) HSV-1/HSV-2 IgM (*P*=0.001) and CMV IgM and IgG (*P* = .001, *P* <0.05, respectively) and insignificant difference for HSV IgG , P>0.05 (Table 1).

Polymerase chain reaction study for viral DNA, HSV-2 was positive in 24 RSA (25%), and CMV DNA was detected in 10 RSA (10.9%) patients. There was a statistically significant difference between RSA patients and pregnant women without RSA for CMV PCR and HSV-2 PCR (*P* = .002 and *P* = .02, respectively) (Table 2). Moreover, there was statistically significant association between positive IgM for herpes simples and CMV (*P*=0.009) and between viremia of HSV2 and CMV (*P*=0.013) (Table 3).

Table 1. Serological study for rubella, herpes simplex 1/2 and cytomegalovirus

	Patients Control P
	No. % No. %
Rubella IgM	42 44.7% 0 0% P=0.001
Rubella IgG	30 32.6% 9 75% P<0.05
Herpes simplex 1/2IgM	36 39.1% 0 0% P=0.001
Herpes simplex 1/2 IgG	50 54.3% 7 58% P>0.05
CMV IgM	10 10.9% 0 0% P=0.001
CMV IgG	35 38% 9 75% P<0.05

Table 2. Polymerase chain reaction (PCR) results of DNA detection for cytomegalovirus (CMV) and herpes simplex virus 1/ herpes simplex virus 2 (herpes 1/2)

Virus detection by PCR	Patients Control
	No. % No. %
Herpes simplex 2	26% 0 0% x^2=9.39 P=0.002
CMV	10 10.9% 0 0% x^2=1.59 P=0.2

Table 3. Association between virological markers for CMV and HSV

CMV and HSV IgM	P=0.009
CMV and HSV2 DNA	P=.013

The sensitivity of HSV-2 IgM was 100%, specificity was 91.3%, positive predictive value was 80%, and negative predictive value was 100%. The sensitivity, specificity, positive predictive value and negative predictive value of CMV IgM was 100% for each compared with PCR (Table 4).

Table 4. Values of serological markers for herpes simplex 2 and cytomegalovirus compared with polymerase chain reaction

	Sensitivity, %	Specificity,%	Accuracy, %	Positive Predictive Value, %	Negative Predictive Value, %
Herpes 2 IgM	100	91.3	93.5	80	100
CMV IgM	100	100	100	100	100

Rubella was the first virus demonstrated as a teratogen. There is a high risk for developing congenital rubella syndrome (CRS) if the infection occurs in the first part of pregnancy, particularly in women without specific immunological protection [30].

Infection with rubella virus was endemic worldwide until the advent of rubella immunization in the early 1980s. Most vaccines used currently contain the RA 27/3 strain, which induces long-lasting immunity, as an antibody response is detectable for >20 years in 95% of patients [31]. Because rubella vaccination coverage is not sufficient throughout the world, rubella cases are still reported, especially in less developed countries.

In our study, the highest frequency of viral markers in RSA was for rubella virus, followed by HSV 1/2 and CMV IgM in RSA patients. In India, various rates for rubella and CMV IgM were reported with ranges from 11% and 3.6% to 28.6% and 26.7%, respectively [32, 33, 34].

In Russia, a high prevalence rate of antibodies for rubella (59.8%) and for CMV (81.1%) was reported by Odland et al., 2001 [35]. In the United States, the number of cases of rubella has decreased 99%, from 57,686 cases in 1969 to 271 cases in 1999 [36]. The discrepancy between results of serologic tests in various studies for the studied viruses might be the result of the differences of the studied populations, in addition to the difference in practice of rubella immunization among developed and less developed countries. As rubella virus continues to circulate, surveillance and control strategies need further optimization [37].

Diagnosis of primary rubella infection rests on detection of specific IgM antibodies. The presence of rubella-specific IgM antibodies must be interpreted with caution: Specific IgM antibodies may occur following reinfection, and there have also been reports of rubella-specific reactivity in sera collected after infections with other viruses. In some cases, the presence of rubella-specific IgM antibodies cannot be ascribed to any of the reasons above and remains completely unexplained [38].

The lower rate of positive CMV IgM in the present study could be attributed to the fact that primary CMV infection is usually acquired during childhood, so the serosusceptibility and the risk of primary infection is lower during pregnancy than with other viruses [39].

On the other hand, high seroprevalence to herpes simplex virus 1/2 was found in this study. High prevalence rates were reported in various studies, from 32% to 80% in women with recurrent abortions [40,41]. It seems that the state of pregnancy predisposes to HSV reactivation, so pregnant females either with recurrent abortions or with normal pregnancy display serologic markers of HSV reactivation [42]. However, in our study there was a significant increase of HSV in patients with recurrent abortions compared with pregnant patients without recurrent abortions, which denotes that HSV may predispose to this condition.

Fragmentary evidence suggests that trophoblast viral infections may play a role in placental dysfunction, leading to complications including spontaneous miscarriage, preeclampsia, fetal growth restriction and preterm birth [43]. It is concluded that in utero infection and the associated cytokine up-regulation are responsible for many cases of unexplained fetal and neonatal loss [44].

We found a statistically significant increase of IgG for rubella and herpes simplex in control subjects compared with patients. Nevertheless, the rate of immunoglobulin G for rubella was less than other studies carried out in Turkey [45] and in the United States [46]. This might denote the need for strict implementation of immunization of young girls and their examination for the presence of effective neutralizing antibodies to the rubella virus. It may be even beneficial to recommend postpartum immunization for pregnant women with no immune response to rubella [47].

There was a significant association between herpes simplex and cytomegalovirus infections. A previous study reported that PCR analysis of biopsy specimens of the maternal-fetal interface revealed that DNA sequences from cytomegalovirus were commonly found with those of herpes simplex viruses and pathogenic bacteria [48].

Cytomegalovirus DNA and infected cell proteins were found more often in the decidua than in the placenta, suggesting that the uterus functions as a reservoir for infection. In women with low neutralizing titers, cytomegalovirus replicated in diverse decidual cells and placental trophoblasts and capillaries.

In women with intermediate to high neutralizing titers, decidual infection was suppressed and the placenta was spared. Overall, cytomegalovirus virions and maternal immunoglobulin G were detected in syncytiotrophoblasts, villus core macrophages, and dendritic cells. These results suggest that the outcome of cytomegalovirus infection depends on the presence of other pathogens and coordinated immune responses to viral replication at the maternal-fetal interface. In healthy adults, CMV reactivation is controlled predominantly by T cells which are underrepresented in the decidual leukocyte population in pregnant women. The cytokine milieu also diminishes adaptive responses to pathogens, presenting an opportunity for viral infection and/or bacterial colonization [48].

The serological study of HSV 2 and CMV IgM in diagnosis of active infections were sensitive, specific and accurate. Similar results were reported by Xu et al. (1993) [49] for CMV IgM and by El Sayed Zaki and Goda (2007) [50] for both CMV and HSV IgM..

Conclusion

The present study highlights the significant association of rubella, herpes simplex and cytomegalovirus with bad obstetric history. There may be persistence of rubella virus related to repeated early abortions. Moreover, combined viral infections in those patients were found that could even further aggravate intrauterine infections. The study gives an idea that serological tests for IgM are a rapid and accurate method for laboratory diagnosis of HSV2 and CMV compared with polymerase chain reaction.

References

[1] Pandey M K , Rani R and Agrawal S An update in recurrent spontaneous abortion. *Archives of Gynecology and Obstetrics* 2005. 272 (2): 95-108

[2] Whitley RJ, Roizman B: Herpes simplex viruses, In Richman DD, Whitley RJ, Hayden FG, editors: *Clinical virology,* New York, 1997, Churchill Livingstone.

[3] Reeves WC, Corey L, Adams HG, et al: Risk of recurrence after first episodes of genital herpes: relation to HSV type and antibody response, *N Engl J Med* 1981, 305-315.

[4] Wald A, Corey L, Cone R, et al: Frequent genital herpes simplex virus 2 shedding in immunocompetent women: effect of acyclovir treatment, *J Clin Invest.* 1997, 99:1092-1099.

[5] Alvin AM, Prober CG: Herpes simplex viruses. In Murray PM, Baron EJ, Pfaller MA, et al, editors: *Manual of clinical microbiologt,* ed 7, Washington, DC, 1999, ASM Press.

[6] Blank H, Burgoon CF; Baidridge GD, et al: Cytological smears in the diagnosis of herpes simplex, herpes zoster, and varicella. *JAMA* 1999 146:1410-1414.

[7] Nahass GT, Goldstein BA, Zhu WY, et al: Comparison of Tzanck smear, viral culture, and DNA diagnostic methods in detection of herpes simplex and varicella-zoster infection, *JAMA*. 1992 268:2541-2547.

[8] Kimberlin DW, Lakeman FD, Alvin AM, et al: Application of the polymerase chain reaction to the diagnosis and management of neonatal herpes simplex virus disease: National Institute of Allergy and Infectious Diseases Collaborative Antiviral Study Group. *J Infect Dis*, 1996, l74:1162-1166.

[9] Ashley RL, Militonij, Lee F; et al: Comparison of Western blot (immunoblot) and glycoprotein G specific immunodot enzyme assay for detecting antibodies to herpes simplex virus types 1 and 2 in human sera, *J Clin Microbiol*, 1988. *2:662-666.*

[10] Ashley R, Benedettij, Corey L: Humoral immune response to HSV-1 and HSV-2 viral proteins in patients with primary genital herpes, *J Med Virol,* 1985, 17:153-158.

[11] Ashley RE, Militonij, Lee F; et al: Comparison of Western blot (immunoblot) and glycoprotein G-specific immunodot enzyme assay for detecting antibodies to herpes simplex virus types 1 and 2 in human sera, *Clin Microbiol* , 1988. 26:662-667.

[12] Ashley RE, Wu L, Pickering JW, et al: Premarket evaluation of a commercial glycoprotein G-based enzyme immunoassay for herpes simplex virus type-specific antibodies. *J Clin Microbiol*, 1998, 36:294-297.

[13] Corey L, Adams HG, Brown ZA, Homes KK: Genital herpes simplex virus infections: clinical manifestations, course, and complications, *Ann Intern Med,* 1983. 98:958-965.

[14] Kulhanjianj A, Soroush V, Au DS, et al: Identification of women at unsuspected risk of primary infection with herpes simplex virus type 2 during pregnancy, *N Engl J Med*, 1992. 326:916-920.

[15] Brown ZA, Selke S, Zeh J, et al.: The acquisition of herpes simplex virus during pregnancy, *NEngi] Med*, 1997. 337:509-514.

[16] Brown ZA, Benedettij, Ashley R, et al.: Neonatal herpes simplex virus infection in relation to asymptomatic maternal infection at the time of labor, *N Engl J Med*.1991, 324:1247-1250.

[17] Koutsky LA, Stevens CE, Holmes KK, et al: Under-diagnosis of genital herpes by current clinical and viral-isolation procedures, *N Engl J Med*,1992. 326:1533-1539.

[18] Hutto C, Alvin A, Jacobs R, et al: Intrauterine herpes simplex virus infections, *Pediatr*, 1987. 110:97-102.

[19] Whitley R, Alvin A, Prober C, et al: Predictors of morbidity and mortality in neonates with herpes simplex virus infections: the National Institute of Allergy and Infectious Diseases Collaborative Antiviral Study Group, *N Engl J Med*, 1991. 324:450-460.

[20] Lindegren, M. L., L. J. Fehrs, S. C. Hadler, and A. R. Hinman. Update: rubella and congenital rubella syndrome, 1980–1990. *Epidemiol. Rev*. 1991. 13: 341–348.

[21] Miller, E., P. A. Tookey, P. Morgan-Capner, L. Hesketh, D. W. G. Brown, P. A. Wraight, J. E. Vurdien, G. Jones, and C. S. Peckham. Rubella surveillance to June 1994: third joint report from the PHLS and the National Congenital Rubella Surveillance Programme. *Communicable Dis. Rep*. 1994. 4:146–152.

[22] Galazka, A. Rubella in Europe. *Epidemiol. Infect*. 1991. 107:43–54.

[23] Miller, C. L.. Rubella in the developing world. Epidemiol. *Infect.* 1991, 107: 63–68.

[24] Schopfer K, Lawber E, Krech U. Congenital cytomegalovirus infection in newborn infants of mothers infected before pregnancy. *Archives of disease in childhood*, 1978, 53:536-9.

[25] Dehner LP, Askin FB. Cytomegalovirus endometritis: report of a case associated with spontaneous abortion. *Obstetrics and gynecology*, 1975, 45:211-214.

[26] Hanshaw JB. Congenital cytomegalovirus infection: a fifteen year perspective. *Journal of infectious diseases*, 1971, 123: 555-561.

[27] McCraken Jr GH et al. Congenital cytomegalic inclusion disease. A longitudinal study of 20 patients. *American journal of diseases of children*, 1969, 117:522-539.

[28] Priya K, Madhavan HN. Use of nested polymerase chain reaction (nPCR) for the detection of cytomegalovirus (CMV) in clinical specimens. *Indian J MedRes.* 2002;115:5–10.

[29] ohnson G, Nelson S, Petric M, Tellier R. Comprehensive PCR-based assay for detection and species identification of human herpes viruses. *J Clin Microbiol.* 2000; 38: 3274–3279.

[30] De Santis M, Cavaliere AF, Straface G, Caruso A. Rubella infection in pregnancy. *Reprod Toxicol*. 2006; 21(4): 390-398.

[31] Enders, G., and U. Nickerl. Rubella vaccination: antibody persistence for 14-17 years and immune status of women without and with a history of vaccination. *Immun. Infect.* 1988. 16:58-64

[32] Das S, Ramachandran VG, Arora R. Cytomegalovirus and rubella infection in children and pregnant mothers--a hospital based study. *J Commun Dis*. 2007;39(2):113-117.

[33] Fomda BA, Thokar MA, Farooq U, Sheikh A. Seroprevalence of rubella in pregnant women in Kashmir. *Indian J Pathol Microbiol.* 2004 ; 47(3): 435-437.

[34] Thapliyal N, Shukla PK, Kumar B, Upadhyay S, Jain GTORCH infection in women with bad obstetric history--a pilot study in Kumaon region. *Indian J Pathol Microbiol.* 2005;48(4):551-553.

[35] Odland JØ, Sergejeva IV, Ivaneev MD, Jensen IP, Stray-Pedersen B. Seropositivity of cytomegalovirus, parvovirus and rubella in pregnant women and recurrent aborters in

Leningrad County, Russia. *Acta Obstet Gynecol Scand.* 2001; 80(11):1025-1029. 36.CDC. Rubella among Hispanic adults-Kansas, 1998, and Nebraska, 1999. *MMWR* 2000;49:225-228.

[36] Muller CP, Kremer JR, Best JM, Dourado I, Triki H, Reef S; WHO Steering Committee for Measles and Rubella Reducing global disease burden of measles and rubella: report of the WHO Steering Committee on research related to measles and rubella vaccines and vaccination, 2005. *Vaccine.* 2007, 2; 25(1):1-9.

[37] Grangeot-Keros L. Rubella and pregnancy. *Pathol Biol.* 1992 ;40(7):706-710.

[38] Odland J, Sergejeva IV, Ivaneev MD. Seropositivity of cytomegalovirus,parvovirus and rubella in pregnant women and recurrent aborters in Leningrad country, Russia. *Acta Obstetricia Gynecol Scand.* 2001; 80:1025–1030.

[39] Panum Jensen L, Thorsen P, Jeune B. An epidemic of parvovirus B 19 in a population of 354 pregnant women: a study of sociodemographic and medical risk factors. *Br J Obstet Gynaecol.* 2000;107:637–643.

[40] Frenkel LM, Garratty EM, Shen JP. Clinical reactivation of herpes simplex virus type 2 infection in seropositive pregnant women with no history of genital herpes. *Ann Intern Med.* 1993; 118:414–418.

[41] Sifakis S, Koumantakis E, Koffa M. Detection of herpes simplex virus (HSV) in aborted material using the polymerase chain reaction technique. *Gynaecol Obstet Invest.* 1998;45:109–115.

[42] Arechavaleta-Velasco. Viral infection of the trophoblast: time to take a serious look at its role in abnormal implantation and placentation? *J of Reprod Immunol*, 2003, 55/113 F .

[43] .Gerard J N; Lynn C D; Deborah B. Histologic, Infectious, and Molecular Correlates of Idiopathic Spontaneous Abortion and Perinatal Mortality. *Diagnostic Molecular Pathology*. 2005, 14(3):152-158,.

[44] Aksakal F N, Maral I, Cirak M Y, Agun K. Rubella seroprevalence among women of childbearing age residing in a rural regions : Is there a need for Rubella vaccination in Turkey. *Jpn J Infect Dis*. 2007, 60;157-160.

[45] CDC. Control and Prevention of Rubella: Evaluation and Management of Suspected Outbreaks, Rubella in Pregnant Women, and Surveillance for Congenital Rubella Syndrome. MMWR *Recommendations and reports 50(RR12),1-23.*

[46] Okuda M, Yamanaka M, Takahashi T, Ishikawa H, Endoh M, Hirahara F. Positive rates for rubella antibody in pregnant women and benefit of post-partum vaccination in a Japanese perinatal center. *J Obstet Gynaecol Res*. 2008;34(2):168-173.

[47] Pereira L, Maidji E, McDonagh S, Genbacev O, Fisher S. Human cytomegalovirus transmission from the uterus to the placenta correlates with the presence of pathogenic bacteria and maternal immunity. *J Virol.* 2003 ;77(24):13301-13314

[48] Xu W, Sundqvist VA, Brytting M et al., Diagnosis of cytomegalovirus infection using polymerase chain reaction, virus isolation and serology. *Scand J Infect Dis.* 1993, 25/3:311-316.

[49] el-Sayed Zaki M, Goda H. Relevance of parvovirus B19, herpes simplex virus 2, and cytomegalovirus virologic markers in maternal serum for diagnosis of unexplained recurrent abortions. *Arch Pathol Lab Med.* 2007 ;131(6): 956-960.

In: Infectious Pregnancy Complications
Editors: Richard N. Canfield

ISBN: 978-1-60471-038-6

Chapter 5

Appendicitis during Pregnancy: A Serious Disease and a Diagnostic Problem

L. Penninga[*] and E.I. Penninga

Abstract

The incidence of appendicitis during pregnancy is equal to that in the normal population. However, during pregnancy appendicitis may occur with a variety of clinical presentations, thereby causing severe diagnostic difficulties, especially during the second half of gestation. As a result, appendicitis during pregnancy is associated with an increase in perforation rate, morbidity and mortality compared to that in the normal population. In addition, it may cause pre-term birth and/or fetal loss.

In this chapter we review diagnostic and treatment strategies and complications of appendicitis occuring during pregnancy

Keywords: pregnancy, appendicitis, infectious diseases

Introduction

Acute appendicitis is caused by inflammation of the vermiform apppendix and usually causes pain in the right lower abdominal quadrant, referred rebound tenderness, overlying muscle spasm and cutaneous hyperesthesia. The disease is common and occurs with an annual incidence of 0.25% in the normal population, and there is a lifetime risk for acute appendicitis of 7–9% (Rothrock). As appendicitis occurs with a high incidence in the second

[*] Corresponding author: Luit Penninga, M.D., Department of Surgery CTX, afsn. 2122, Copenhagen University Hospital, Rigshospitalet, Blegdamsvej 9, DK-2100 Copenhagen Ø, Denmark, Email: Penninga@dadlnet.dk, Tel: (+ 45) 35451875/ 35452122

and third decade of life, it also occurs frequently during pregnancy, and the incidence of appendicitis during pregnancy is equal to that in the non-pregnant population (Maslovitz).

Unfortunately, appendicitis during pregnancy is associated with an increase in morbidity and mortality compared to that in the normal population, and often causes diagnostic difficulties.

In this chapter we review history, incidence, diagnostic and treatment strategies of appendicitis during pregnancy. Furthermore, we discuss maternal morbidity and mortality and the possible consequences for the fetus.

History

Berengarius Carpus, professor of surgery in Bologna and Pavia, was the first to describe the appendix in the year 1522. He spoke of a certain 'additamentum' at the end of the caecum with a breadth less than the smallest finger of the hand and a length of three inches or thereabouts (McCarthy). In 1579, Fallopius was the first to compare the appendix with a worm, and during the following centuries the anatomy of the appendix was described in more detail (McCarthy). McBurney contributed in 1889 his classical sign of the diagnosis of appendicitis, and since the 1890s the history of appendicitis consists of refinement in treatment and diagnosis. The first case of appendicitis during pregnancy was described in the 1840s by Hancock (Hancock). A century ago, Balber wrote his paper in which he reported about 200 pregnancies complicated by appendicitis (Balber). In this group there was a maternal mortality of 24% and a fetal mortality rate of 40% (Balber). Currently, a few hundred articles are found dealing with appendicitis during pregnancy. Sir Zachary Cope once stated 'the diagnosis of appendicitis (in non-pregnant patients) is usually easy'; however, he added 'but there are difficulties which need to be discussed' (Beasley). Now we know that pregnancy certainly is one of those difficulties. Borgstein and colleagues have called acute appendicitis 'a clear-cut case in men, and a guessing game in young women' (Borgstein). And we can only add that appendicitis in pregnant women is a mystery wrapped in an enigma.

Incidence

Approximately 1 in 500 pregnancies is complicated by non-obstetric surgical problems (Jackson). Appendicitis is the most common non-obstetric surgical disease occuring during pregnancy, and it accounts for 25% of surgeries for non-obstetric complications in pregnancy, followed by cholecystitis and bowel obstruction (Andersen, Al-Mulhim, Dietrich). In the literature several studies describe the incidence of appendicitis during pregnancy: Maslovitz et al. reviewed 40,112 deliveries and found an incidence of appendicitis of 1/2,111 (Maslovitz); Babaknia et al. reviewed 503,496 deliveries and found an incidence of appendicitis of 1/1,500 (Babaknia); Tamir et al. reported an incidence of 1/1,400 in a review of 73,000 deliveries (Tamir); Gomez et al. found an incidence of 1/1,258 in a review of 76,608 deliveries (Gomez); Eryilmaz et al. described an incidence of 1/1,312 in a review of 31,480 deliveries (Eryilmaz); and, finally, Andersen et al. found an incidence of 1/766 pregnancies (Andersen). Some studies report that appendicitis occurs with equal frequency in each trimester of pregnancy, though others have found an overpresentation in the second trimester of pregnancy (Brown, Yilmaz). The perforation rate of appendicitis during pregnancy (43%) is much higher than that in the normal population (4–19%) (Tamir). This probably reflects the problems in diagnosing the disease, and maybe the reluctance to operate on pregnant patients. Of note, perforation of the appendix occurs twice as often in the third trimester (69%) compared to the first and second trimesters (Jackson).

Anatomical Appendiceal Displacement

In non-pregnant patients, classically the tenderness of acute appendicitis is localized over McBurney's point, until rupture and generalized peritonitis supervene. McBurney reports, '...I believe that in every case the seat of the greatest pain, determined by the pressure of one finger has been very exactly between an inch and a half and two inches from the anterior spinous process of the ilium on a straight line drawn from that process to the umbilicus. This may appear to be an affection of accuracy, but, so far as my experience goes this observation is correct' (McBurney, 1890). Displacement of the appendix during pregnancy from McBurney's point has been discussed in the literature: In 1932 Baer et al. performed radiological studies with barium enemas to confirm that during pregnancy anatomical displacement of the appendix occurs (Baer, Eryyilmaz). Bear's study showed that during the first trimester, the appendix had the same anatomical position as before pregnancy; however, at five months of pregnancy the appendix is placed at the iliac crest level, and rises above this level during the last trimester of pregnancy, which, according to Baer, might explain why some pregnant patients present with pain in the right upper quadrant (Baer, Eryilmaz). Seven decades later, Hodjati and colleagues performed a study in which they questioned Baer's statement that the appendix displaces during pregnancy (Hodjati). In their study, Hodjati et al. studied the position of the appendix in non-pregnant and pregnant patients undergoing appendectomy, and in pregnant patients undergoing caesarean section (Hodjati). This study showed that during surgery the appendix was located more than 8 cm from McBurney's point in 26% of the pregnant patients undergoing a ceasarean section, in 6% of the pregnant women undergoing appendectomy between 19 and 39 weeks of pregnancy and in 17% of non-pregnant patients undergoing appendectomy. From their study Hodjati concluded, opposite to Baer, that displacement of the appendix during pregnancy from McBurney's point is very limited (Baer, Hodjati).

Diagnostic Features

The most common symptoms of appendicitis during pregnancy are abdominal pain (100%), nausea (88%) and vomiting (83%). Diagnosis of appendicitis during pregnancy is difficult, because many of these classical symptoms are normal during pregnancy. In addition, some patients may lack symptoms and signs of appendicitis, and diagnosis may be delayed. In general, nausea and vomiting are unreliable symptoms during pregnancy; however, the occurrence of these symptoms after the first trimester of pregnancy warrants a thorough investigation (Maslovitz). Also, new-onset abdominal pain should be taken seriously. Abdominal pain due to appendicitis during pregnancy is often less characteristic compared to abdominal pain in non-pregnant patients with appendicitis. Generally, abdominal pain is less useful in the diagnosis of appendicitis during pregnancy than abdominal pain in non-pregnant patients with appendicitis. It has been stated that all patients with appendicitis during pregnancy had had pain in the right lower quadrant of the abdomen at some period of time. Approximately 70% of patients will have rebound, referring tenderness, which is not normally encountered during regular pregnancy. One study found that patients who presented with diffuse or periumbilical pain which later migrated to the right lower quadrant of the abdomen had a significantly higher chance to have appendicitis compared to those who had a normal appendix at operation (Andersen).

Interestingly, Kurtz et al. found that a positive Bryan's sign (abdominal pain caused by shifting a pregnant uterus to the right) was the most reliable sign of appendicitis during pregnancy (Kurtz). Rectal or pelvic pain may not be present due to enlargement of the uterus which displaces the appendix away from the rectum and pelvis (Dietrich). Perforation of the appendix should be suspected in patients where the pain changes from localized tenderness to pain with a more diffuse nature. Patients who present with back, flank or leg pain or leginfection during pregnancy might have a retrocoecal located inflammed appendix (Penninga). It is generally acknowledged that diagnosing appendicitis becomes more difficult as pregnancy enhances (Maslovitz, Tracy). During pregnancy the appendix moves away from the abdominal wall due to the growing uterus. This may decrease abdominal pain and referred rebound tenderness, and increase diagnostic difficulties. In addition the pregnant uterus prevents omental isolation of the inflammatory process (Tracy, Stone).

Infectious Signs and Laboratory Testing

Pregnancy is associated with a physiologic increase in maternal blood volume that diminishes the womens ability to demonstrate tachycardia and hypotension (Stone). Fever is not useful in diagnosing appendicitis, but an elevation in body temperature may predict perforation of the appendix (Maslovitz). During pregnancy leucocytosis may occur with an increase in neutrophils; however, neither an increase in leucocytes nor any other laboratory value has been found to be useful and reliable in diagnosing appendicitis during pregnancy (Stone, Tracy, Andersen).

Radiological Imaging

Radiological imaging might be beneficial in diagnosing appendicitis during pregnancy. Ultrasonography is the preferred imaging investigation during pregnancy (Melnick). The method is cheap and safe and it has a high specificity when a pathological appendix is found. Ultrasonography has been used in large series in non-pregnant patients with a sensitivity of

75% to 89% and a specificity of 86% to 100% (Borgstein). In addition, ultrasonography is the most accurate investigation to identify a periappendiceal abcess, however it is less sensitive in identifying a ruptured appendix (Dietrich). Ultrasonography is most accurate in the first and second trimester of pregnacy, and less accurate in the third trimester of pregancy due to the enlarged uterus.

Magnetic resonance imaging (MRI) is also used in diagnosing appendicitis during pregnancy. The method has a high sensitivity and specificity, and as ultrasonography has the advantage of non-ionizing radiation, and should therefore be considered safe. In addition, unenhanced focused single-detector helical CT scanning has also been used for diagnosing appendicitis during pregnancy. This method has the advantage of limited ionizing radition compared to normal CT scanning. Although there is limited data, than unenhanced focuse single-detector helical CT scanning was found to have the same sensitivity and specificity as ultrasonography, but at the moment has no established role in the diagnostics of appendicitis during pregnancy.

Treatment Strategy and Outcome

Early surgical treatment is of major importance to avoid the complications associated with perforation of the appendix. A 66% perforation rate has been reported when surgery is delayed by more than 24 hours compared to no perforations when surgical management is initiated within 24 hours after presentation (Tamir). Balber noticed this already in the beginning of the 20th century and he wrote 'The mortality of appendicitis complicating pregnancy is the mortality of delay' (Balber).

The 'early and aggressive' surgical treatment approach is also one of the reasons that appendicitis during pregnancy has a low diagnostic accuracy compared to the non-pregnant population. Twenty-five percent of the pregnant women who underwent surgery during pregnancy under the suspicion of appendicitis turn out to have a normal appendix, and in some studies even up to 50% turn out to have a normal appendix.

Pregnant patients with appendicitis can be operated on by both an open and laparoscopic approach (Al-Fozan, Carver). Possible benefits of laparoscopic surgery are decreased postoperative narcotic requirements, which might cause less fetal depression, fewer wound complications, decreased postoperative maternal hypoventilation and faster maternal recovery. Possible risks of laparoscopic surgery are premature labor (due to an increased intraabdominal pressure), decreased uterine bloodflow and uterine injury and the negative effects of a carbondioxide pneumoperitoneum (Neudecker). Several animal studies performed in the third trimester of pregnancy have shown that a carbondioxide pneumoperitoneum causes fetal acidosis and an increase in fetal heart rate and blood pressure; however, these effects seem not to be clinically significant (Hunter, Reynolds).

In general there has been a tendency to choose the open surgical approach as pregnancy advances. Lyass et al. showed nevertheless that the laparoscopic appendectomy approach is technically feasible in all trimesters of pregnancy and associated with the same known benefits of laparoscopic surgery that non-pregnant patients experience, and no maternal mortality and/or fetal loss was seen in their study (Lyass). In contrast to Lyass et al., McGory et al. found a significantly higher risk of fetal loss in patients undergoing laparoscopic appendectomy (7%) than in patients undergoing open appendectomy (3%) (McGory). During recent years, as laparoscopy has generally advanced, there has also been a trend towards more laparoscopic procedures than open procedures in patients with appendicitis during pregnancy. In patients with advanced gestation undergoing laparoscopic appendectomy it is recommended to perforate the peritoneum and to insert the first trochar under direct visualisation ('Hasson' technique) to avoid perforation of the enlarged uterus (Jackson). Alternatively, ultrasound guided trochar placement has been described to avoid uterus perforation (Jackson)

Maternal Morbidity and Mortality and Fetal Loss

Perforation of the appendix is a major risk factor for maternal morbidity. Yilmaz et al. found a significant difference between patients with a perforated and non-perforated appendix in the rate of complications (52% vs. 17%) (Yilmaz). Earlier reports have described maternal mortality due to appendicitis during pregnancy and some years ago a maternal mortality of about 4% was common, but fortunately, in the Western world, maternal mortality has almost disappeared during the past few years.

Uncomplicated appendectomy has a 3% to 5% fetal loss rate with minimal maternal mortality. However, perforation of the appendix is associated with a 20% to 37% fetal loss rate, which has been used to justify early surgical intervention. In addition to fetal loss, appendectomy in pregnant patients causes preterm early delivery in 7–45% of the patients. Preterm delivery occurs most frequently in the first postoperative week (Mazze). Risk factors associated with preterm labor are advanced gestational age, interval between symptom onset and operation, and white blood cell count (Yilmaz). Surprisingly, one study found a preterm early delivery rate of 10% in patients undergoing surgery but with a normal appendix, compared to 11% in patients with a complicated appendicitis. The authors explain this by the fact that many of the women who were found to have a normal appendix during surgery were suffering from another disease that might have initiated preterm delivery. Threatened preterm labor might be successfully managed with tocolytic therapy (Jackson). No prophylactic effect of tocolytic treatment has been reported, but tocolytic treatment should be considered perioperatively when signs of preterm labor are present (Jackson).

Conclusion

Appendicitis is the most common non-obstetric surgical disease occuring during pregnancy, and it accounts for 25% of surgeries for non-obstetric complications in pregnancy.

The most common symptoms of appendicitis during pregnancy are abdominal pain, nausea and vomiting. These symptoms are all unspecific in pregnant women, as they also occur in pregnant women without appendicitis. Furthermore, infectious signs and laboratory tests are also unreliable, which makes appendicitis during pregnancy a severe diagnostic problem, and diagnosing appendicitis becomes even more difficult as pregnancy enhances. Ultrasonography is the radiological investigation of choice, and may be helpful in diagnosing appendicitis.

Early surgical treatment is of highest importantance to avoid the risk of perforation, and the associated increased risk of morbidity, preterm delivery and fetal loss. Both open and laparoscopic surgical approaches can be used in pregnant patients. Appendectomy can be complicated by preterm delivery and fetal loss; however, the risk of not operating on suspected appendicitis is by far greater and justifies prompt surgery of any suspected appendicitis in pregnant patients.

Naturally, careful history, clinical and radiological investigation are still of major importance in diagnosing appendicitis during pregnancy.

References

Al-Fozan F, Tulandi T. Safety and risks of laparoscopy in pregnancy. *Curr Opin Obstet Gynecol* 2002;14:375-9

Al-Mulhim AA. Acute appendicitis in pregnancy: a review of 52 cases. *Int Surg* 1996;81: 295-7

Andersen B, Nielsen TF. Appendicitis in pregnancy: Diagnosis, management and complications. *Acta Obstet Gyn Scand* 1999;78:758-62

Andersson REB. Meta-analysis of the clinical and laboratory diagnosis of appendicitis. *Br J Surg* 2004;91:28-37

Baer JL, Reis RS, Arens RA. Appendicitis in pregnancy with changes of in position and axis of the normal appendix in pregnancy. *JAMA* 1932;16:1359-64

Balber EA. Perforative appendicitis complicating pregnancy. *JAMA* 1908;51:1310-13

Beasley SW. Can we improve diagnosis of acute appendicitis? *BMJ* 2000;321:907-8

Borgstein PJ, Gordijn RV, Eijsbouts QAJ, Cuesta MA. Acute appendicitis- a clear-cut case in men, a guessing game in young women, a prospective study on the role of laparoscopy. Surg Endosc 1997; 11:923-7

Carver TW, Antevil J, Egan JC, Brown CV. Appendectomy during early pregnancy: What is the preferred surgical approach? *Am Surg* 2005;71:809-812 Dietrich CS III, Hill CC, Hueman M. Surgical diseases presenting during pregnancy. *Surg Clin N Am* 2008; 88:403-19

Eryilmaz R, Sahin M, Bas G, Alimoglu O, Kaya B. Acute appendicitis during pregnancy. *Dig Surg* 2002;19:40-44

Hancock H. Disease of the appendix caeci cured by operation. *Lancet* 1848;2:380-1

Hee P, Vikstrup L. The diagnosis of appendicitis during pregnancy and maternal and fetal outcome after appendectomy. *Int J Gyn Obstet* 1999;65:129-35

Hodjati H, Kazerooni T. Location of the appendix in the gravid patient: a re-evaluation of the established concept. *Int J Gyn Obstet* 2003; 81:245-7

Horrowitz M, Gomez GA, Santieesteben R, Burkett G. Acute appendicitis during pregnancy. *Arch Surg* 1985;120:1362-7

Hunter JG, Swanstrom L, Thornburg K. Carbon dioxide pneumoperitoneum induces fetal acidosis in a pregnant ewe model. *Surg Endosc* 1995;9:272-9

Jackson H, Granger S, Price R, Rollins M, Earle D, Richardson W, Fanelli R. Diagnosis and laparoscopic treatment of surgical diseases during pregnancy: an evidence-based review. *Surg Endosc* 2008;22:1917-27

Kurtz RJ, Heimann TM. Comparison of open and laparoscopic treatment of acute appendicitis. *Am J Surg* 2001;182:211-4

Lyass S, Pikarsky A, Eissenberg VH, Eichalal U, Schenker JG, Reissman P. Is laparoscopic appendectomy safe in pregnant women? *Surg Endosc* 2001;15:377-9

Mahmoodian S. Appendicitis complicating pregnancy. *South Med* J 1992;85:19-24

Maslovitz S, Gutman G, Lessing JB, Kupferminc MJ, Gamzu R. The significance of clinical signs and blood indices for the diagnosis of appendicitis during pregnancy. *Gyn Obstet Invest* 2003;56:189-91

McCarthy AC. History of appendicitis vermiformis, its diseases and treatment. Lecture to the innominate society 1927. www.innominatesociety.com

Melnick DM, Wahl WD, Dalton VK. Management of general surgical problems in the pregnant patient. *Am J Surg* 2004;187:170-180

Mourad J, Elliot JP, Erickson L, Lisboa L. Appendicitis in pregnancy: new information that contradicts long-held clinical beliefs. *Am J Obstet Gyn* 2000;182:1027-9

Neudecker J, Sauerland S, Neugebauer E, Bergamaschi R, Bonjer HJ, Cuschieri A, Fuchs KH, Jacobi Ch, Jansen FW, Koivusalo AM, Lacy A, McMahon MJ, Millat B, Schwenk W. European association for endoscopic surgery clinical practice guideline on the pneumoperitoneum for laparoscopic surgery. *Surg Endosc* 2002; 16:1121-43

Penninga L, Wettergren A. Perforated appendicitis during near-term pregnancy causing necrotizing fasciitis of the lower extremity: a rare complication of a common disease. *Act Obstet Gyn Scand* 2006;85:1150-1

Reynolds JD, Booth JV, de la Fuente S, Punnahitananda S, McMahon RL, Hopkins MB, Eubanks WS. A review of laparoscopy for non-obstretic related surgery during pregnancy. *Curr Surg* 2003;60:164-73

Rothrock SG, Pagane J. Acute appendicitis in children: emergency department diagnosis and management. *Ann Emerg Med* 2000;36:39-51

Stone K. Acute abdominal emergencies associated with pregnancy. *Clin Obstet Gynecol* 2002;45:553-601

Tamir IL, Bongard FS, Klein SR. Acute appendicitis in the pregnant patient. *Am J Surg* 1990;160:571-5

Tracy M, Fletcher HS. Appendicitis in pregnancy. *Am Surg* 2000;66:555-9

Ueberrueck T, Koch A, Meyer L, Hinkel M, Gastinger I. Ninety-four appendectomies for suspected acute appendicitis during surgery. *World J Surg* 2004;28:508-11

Yilmaz HG, Akgun Y, Bac B, Celik Y. Acute appendicitis in pregnancy-risk factors associated with principal outcomes: a case control study. *Int J Surg* 2007;5:192-7

In: Infectious Pregnancy Complications
Editor: Richard N. Canfield
ISBN 978-1-60741-038-6

Chapter 6

Mediastinal End Subcutaneous Emphysema as a Complication of Labor

***Arkadiusz Praski*[*1], *Włodzimierz Kupis*[2], *Marek Florczak*[1] and *Małgorzata Szpetnar*[1]**
[1]SP ZOZ - Mińsk Mazowiecki, Szpital Powiatowy,
Oddział Ginekologiczno- Położniczy
[2]Instytut Gruźlicy i Chorób Płuc - Warszawa,
V Klinika Chirurgii

Abstract

Mediastinal emphysema and subcutaneous emphysema are rare complications of labor. We describe a case of mediastinal and subcutaneous emphysema observed in the II stage of labor, otherwise known as healthy primigravida. The diagnosis was confirmed clinically through X-ray, and endoscopic examination in District Hospital, as well as in the Clinical Department of Surgery. The etiology of this condition was not established. The mediastinal and subcutaneous emphysema disappeared spontaneously. It was confirmed within 3 months by a check-up.

Introduction

Pneumomediastinum is a presence of free air within the mediastinum, which often occur with subcutaneous emphysema – Hamman´s syndrom. It is a rare complication of labor (its incidence is said to be between 1 in 100,000 and 1 in 2,000 deliveries). The symptoms are noticed often after labor.

* E-mail: a-praski@wp.pl , a.praski@t-online.de

Objective

The aim of the study was to present a case of mediastinal and subcutaneous emphysema observed in the II stage of labor, otherwise known as healthy primigravida.

Description of the Case

A nulliparous white woman at 39 weeks gestation was presented with contractions. Her pregnancy was without complications, besides not large vaginal infections. During the admittance examination the patient was in good condition. Gynecological examination - delivery in stage Ia, FHR+/- 140/min.

After the spontaneous rupture of membranes at 11.40pm 02.03.2006 (Friday), came regular contractions and the delivery progress was spontaneous. The patient was transferred to the delivery room.

02.04.06 at 3:00 am the patient was in good condition – mobile, used a Sako- sack, and a delivery-ball. Gynecological examination took place on 02.04.06 at 4:05 am – her cervix was fully dilated, head presentation, engaged head in pelvic inlet, and regular contractions. The patient pushed in sitting position on the delivery bed as well as on the delivery ball.

Because of weak contractions, the labor was augmented with oxytocin (a flow 90ml/h) at 4:50 am. In the second stage of labor, the examination revealed right side facial swelling which enlarged during pushing.

On 02.04.06 (Saturday) at 5:00 am after incision of pudendum, a 3250g/54cm female infant was delivered. The Apgar scores were 8-9-10 at 1 and 5 minutes, respectively.

Because of an uncompleted placenta, we carried out curettage of uterine cavity, and then sutured the pudendum.

After the delivery, her obstetrical condition, temperature, pulse and blood pressure were normal. During the physical exam, observations affirmed massive swelling of right side of face with entire closure of eyelid, neck swelling and upper part of chest and massive blood extravasations on the skin of the face, neck and chest.

The Patient complained of breathing capacity and discomfort in the throat. After 30 minutes, there was a decrease of blood pressure to 70/45 mmHg and a pulse of 76/min was observed. Half a ampoule of Ephedrine s.c., 500ml infusion with electrolytes i.v. and oxygen (flow 7l/min) were ordered. The blood pressure increased to normal value, but the dyspnoea was still observed.

Digital palpation showed characteristic crepitation of moving air under the skin. After surgical and medical consultations and chest X-ray, the pneumomediastinum and subcutaneous emphysema was confirmed. Laboratory investigations were in normal value. During the physical exam, besides the swelling of the upper part of the body, a paresis of right leg was observed. All pathological symptoms receded gradually.

On 02.07.06 (Monday), the patient was transferred to University Surgical Clinic so that we could carry out a diagnostic treatment. In the clinic, we carried out an endoscopical, radiological, gynecological, neurological and laboratory diagnostics.

Gastroscopy: without pathology in upper part of gestational track.

Bronchoscopy: larynx, trachea, and bronchial tree without pathology.

Chest Tomography: the lungs without pathology. Lymph nodes were not enlarged. Pleural cavity was without pathology. In upper-front mediastinum – thymus. Big amount of air is situated in front and back of mediastinum. Many bubbles of air are visible in tissues of the neck and middle and upper part of the chest.

Gynecological Examination: without pathology.

Neurological Consultation: a paresis of right leg (a rehabilitation of right leg was ordered).

Laboratory investigations: in norm value.

The symptoms of emphysema receded gradually and the patient was transferred to county hospital. On 02.09.06 the patient left the hospital in good condition with recommendation of rehabilitation of right leg and a control gynecological examination. During control examination, 3 months after labor, the results were subjective, radiological, gynecological, neurological, and in labors without pathology.

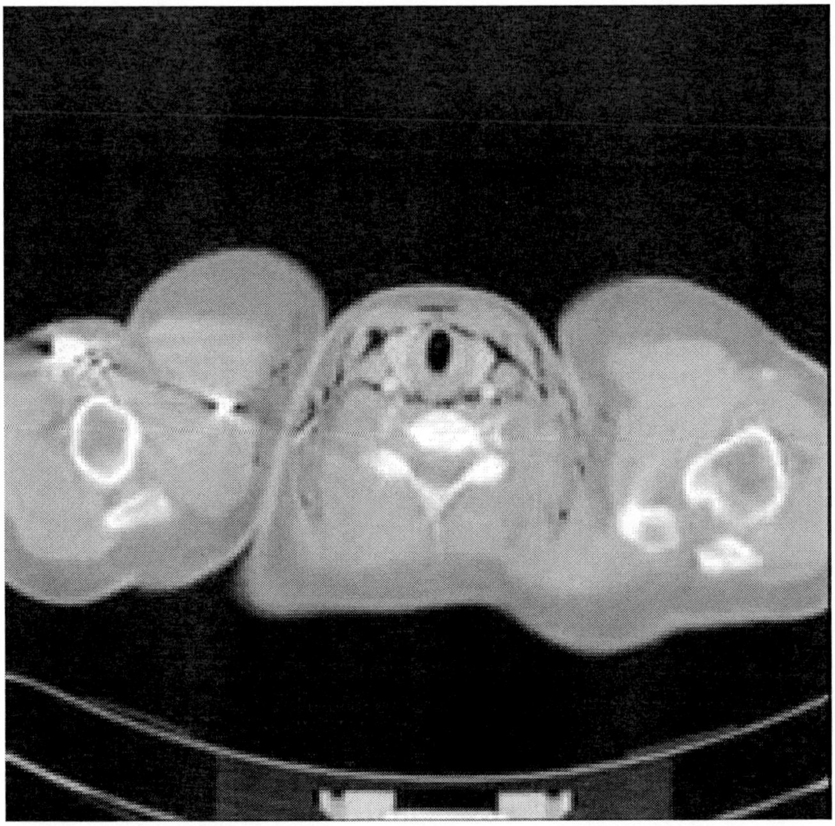

Picture 1. Tomogram of the neck showing subcutaneous emphysema.

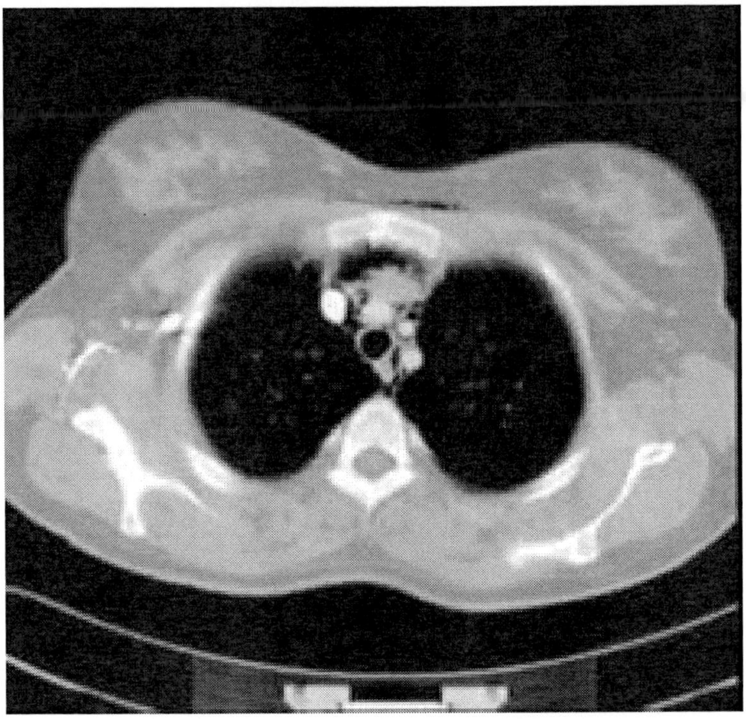

Picture 2. tomogram of the chest showing mediastinal end subcutaneous emphysema.

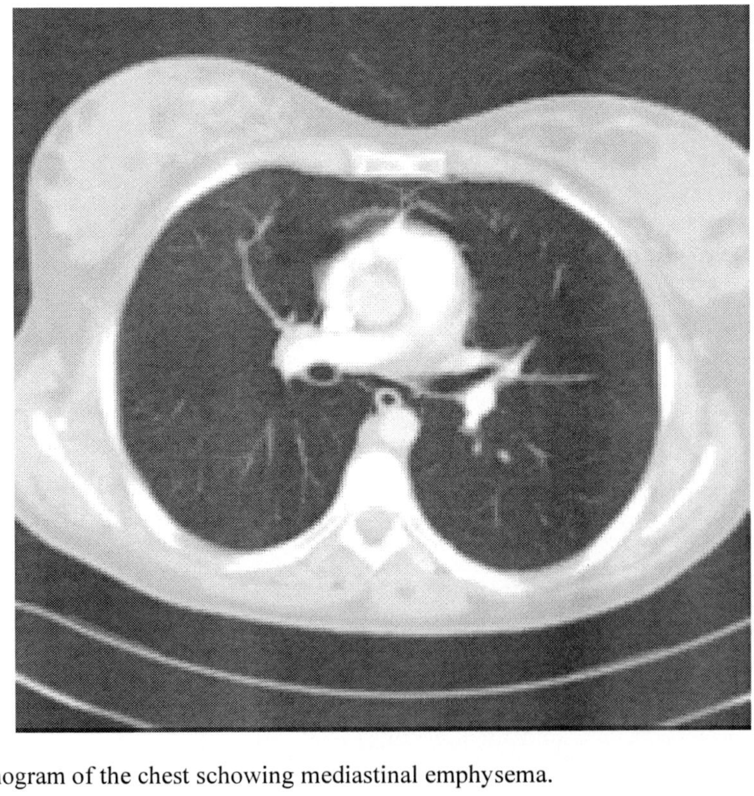

Picture 3. Tomogram of the chest schowing mediastinal emphysema.

Discussion

The first reports of pneumomediastinum and subcutaneous emphysema were publicized in "Observations" of L. Bourgeois. The first case of pneumomediastinum with subcutaneous emphysema as complication of labor was described by Simmons in 1783. Pneumomediastinum is defined in references as mild condition but four maternal deaths have been reported before 1908, by which during labor occurred pneumomediastinum [1,2,3]. Pneumomediastinum represents the presence of air or gas within the mediastinum. Pneumomediastinum can present with dyspnoea and substernal chest pain, subcutaneous and retroperitoneal emphysema, obliteration of cardiac dullness, cyanosis, engorged veins, tachycardia, shock with decrease of blood pressure, pneumothorax. Spontaneous pneumomediastinum can present by untypical symptoms such as jaw pain during labor.

Emphysema can be limited to mediastinum, but decreasing pressure can cause spread of emphysema along aorta and esophagus to retroperitoneal space or to superficial tissues of the neck and of the thorax and by these symptoms the diagnosis is not complicated. Occurrence of this disease can be limited just to mediastinum, without subcutaneous emphysema. In this case the diagnosis can be difficult [1,2,3,4,5,6]. Subcutaneous emphysema represents the presence of air in subcutaneous tissue. This symptom is also called Hamman's syndrome because it was first formally described by Louis Hamman in 1939 [2]. In advanced stages of emphysema, it can spread through the entire body with characteristic of swelling and crepitation, especially on head, neck, thorax and pudendal lips. If subcutaneous emphysema occurs on neck, we can suppose there are pneumomediastinum, since subcutaneous emphysema is one of the pneumomediastinum's symptom [1,2,4,6]. After Hamman, the causal mechanism depends on the transfer of air to mediastinum in four different ways: along superficial tissues of neck during injuries and or surgical procedures in throat-area, oral cavity-area or nasal sinuses-area, if trachea, bronchus or esophagus ruptures, from retroperitoneal space as a complication of procedures in kidneys area, or from interstitial tissue of lungs. Hamman considered that emphysema is a complication of injury or increasing of intra-alveolar pressure and spontaneous rupture of alveoli [2]. Other causes of Pneumomediastinum are perforation of trachea-wall, bronchus-wall or esophagus-wall during thorax injury, vomiting, (Boherhaave's syndrome), vomiting during pregnancy too, endoskopic procedures (esophagoscopy, bronchoscop), bronchitic asthma (status asthmaticus), intensive cough or intensive exercise by closed glottis: during lifting the weights, rectal tenesmus and pushing during labor [7]. During popular endoscopic procedures (laparoscopy) occurs emphysema because of difference of gas pressure between abdominal cavity and pleural cavity. Therefore, pressure-monitoring during laparoscopy is very significant [6]. Diagnostic of pneumomediastinum and subcutaneous emphysema involves usually radiograph-examination and endoscopic-examination. They should exclude the perforation of alimentary tract or respiratory tract and determinate the grade of extent of lesions. X-ray picture can show double contour of pleura of the left heart's margin. That picture should be differentiated with cardiac tamponade and induced by accumulation of fluid in pericardial sac. Thorax-CT can exclude pathology of respiratory tract which could be the cause of emphysema.. Without intensified symptoms, some authors propose to limit diagnostic examination to thorax x-ray with contrast medium in esophagus.

Pneumomediastinum and subcutaneus emphysema are seldom complications of labor. Just 200 cases of Pneumomediastinum with subcutaneous emphysema, as a complication of labor, would be described in world medical literature. Incidence of pneumomediastinum is said to be between 1 in 100 000 and 1 in 2000 deliveries. Appearance of pneumomediastinum during labor is connected with Valsalva manoeuvre which is carried out by the patient during pushing [2,8,9]. Some authors think that over half described cases of pneumomediastinum were connected with labor and probably were caused by repeated increase of intra-abdominal pressure[9].

Pneumomediastinum, as a complication of labor, occurred mainly by primiparas during prolonged or induced with oxytocin labor appears in the second stage of labor, although the symptoms were noticed after labor. Just in a few cases its appeared before and during the first stage of labor [8]. Pneumomediastinum, with subcutaneous emphysema, can create injury of the maxillary sinus. The symptoms are typically: oedema of face, neck and thorax [10]. Norwegians found, in world literature, one case of pneumomediastinum as a complication of epidural anesthesia in thoracic spine (Th5-Th6) as a result of penetration of catheter to pulmonary cavity. They stated however that epidural anesthesia in lumbal spine during labor causes not pneumomediastinum [11]. Presence of free air in subcutaneous tissue and mediastinum does not cause a real clinical consequence and doesn't required intensive treatment.

It is very essential to exclude causes of pneumomediastinum and subcutaneous emphysema, such as perforation of intestinal tract or respiratory tract. In case of large and increasing subcutaneous emphysema, we can decompress by puncturing subcutaneous tissue using needles with side entrances. We can incise and preparate subcutaneous spaces on neck and thorax. If symptoms of pneumomediastinum become dangerous, we should make decompression by mediastinostomy [4]. The treatment in most cases depends on relieving the symptoms to administrate pain relievers and sedatives, or oxygen [8]. In case of diagnostication of pneumomediastinum during labor it is recommended to shorten the second period of labor using forceps [5].

Conclusions

The pneumomediastinum with subcutaneous emphysema are seldom complications of labor, therefore we should take note of symptoms which can suggest the disease, carry out diagnostic that confirms pneumomediastinum, take into consideration the most common etiology and to monitor patient's condition. If patient's condition is stabile, we are confined to relieve the symptoms. If the symptoms increase and patient's condition gets worse, surgical treatment is necessary in a specialized hospital. The etiology of pneumomediastinum of our patient was not explained. The pneumomediastinum underwent spontaneous regression, which was confirmed by a check-up.

References

[1] Bending JJ. Spontaneous pneumothorax in pregnancy and labour. *Postgrad Med. J.* 1982, 58, 711-713.

[2] Hamman LV. Mediastinal emphysema. *JAMA.* 1945, 128, 1-6.

[3] Reeder SR. Subcutaneous emphysema, pneumomediastinum and pneumothorax in labor and delivery. *Am. J. Obstet. Gynecol.* 1986, 154, 487-489.

[4] Fibak J. Obrażenia klatki piersiowej. W: Chirurgia. Pod red. Fibaka J. Warszawa : *Wydawnictwo lekarskie PZWL*, 1996, 686-687.

[5] Karson EM., Saltzman D., Davis MR. Pneumomediastinum in Pregnancy: Two Case Reports and Review of the Literature, Pathophysiology, and Management. *Obstet. Gynecol.* 1984, 64, 39-43.

[6] Perko G., Fernandes A. Subcutaneous emphysema and Pneumothorax during laparoscopy for ectopic pregnancy removal. *Acta Anaesthesiol Scand.* 1977, 41, 792-4.

[7] Markiewicz R. Odma śródpiersia powikłana odmą podskórną w przebiegu stanu astmatycznego. *Wiad Lek.* 1988, 41, 572-575.

[8] Duffy B. Post Partum Pneumomediastinum. Anaesth Intensive Care. 2004, 32, 117-119.

[9] Kowalski MS. Odma podskórna jako powikłanie porodu. *Pol. Tyg. Lek.* 1955, 29, 1152-1153.

[10] Monksfield P., Whiteside O., Jaffe S., [et al.]. Pneumomediastinum, an unusual complication of facial trauma. *ENT Journal.* 2005, 05.

[11] Softeland E., Bergjord K. Pneumomediastinum in labour-probably not caused by a lumbar epidural anaesthesia. *Acta Anaesthesiol Scand.* 2004, 48, 123-125.

In: Infectious Pregnancy Complications
Editor: Richard N. Canfield

ISBN 978-1-60741-038-6

Chapter 7

Program for the Prevention of Infection-Related Premature Births: The Role of the *Lactobacilli* System and Vaginal pH

Erich Saling and Monika Dräger
Institute of Perinatal Medicine (charitable institute)
Vivantes-Clinic Berlin-Neukölln, Berlin, Germany

Abstract

Prevention of early preterm birth (<32 weeks of gestation) and of very-low-birth-weight infants (<1500 g) is one of the most urgent priorities of perinatal medicine. Ascending genital tract infection is an important preventable cause of early preterm birth. The protective effect of the *Lactobacillus* system and a low vaginal pH are important to maintain a normal microbial ecosystem in the lower genital tract and in the prevention of ascending intrauterine infections. Bacterial vaginosis, other changes in the microbial ecosystem and infections can lead to ascending intrauterine infection. They all often begin with a disturbance of this vaginal milieu—which we consider a precursor.

We recommend an assessment of the risk of preterm birth that includes obstetrical history, the early detection of warning signs (including screening for pre-infection states or overt infection by regular determinations of the vaginal pH) and, if indicated, the implementation of appropriate therapeutic measures.

Our prematurity prevention program includes measures taken by physicians and by midwives; "self-care" measures taken by the women themselves (preferably for all pregnant women); and additional special measures for women at risk.

The self-care measures for pregnant women are additional to regular prenatal care. They include information about risk factors and warning signs as well as regular measurement of the vaginal pH by the women themselves. With this self-care, the rate of premature births in the up-to-now published studies could be reduced. Most interesting are the results concerning preterm neonates at particularly high risk: In our experience the rate of very-low-birth-weight infants (<1500 g) was successfully reduced from 7.8%

in the immediate previous pregnancy to 1.3%. In Thuringia, the rate of infants born <32+0 weeks was reduced from 1.36 % to 0.94%. Several health insurance companies in Germany are currently offering and evaluating the self-care measures for their clients.

Further information can be found on:

- General information : http://www.saling-institut.de/eng/04infoph/01allg.html
- Prematurity Prevention Program: http://www.saling-institut.de/eng/04infoph/02programm.html
- Self-care measures: http://www.saling-institut.de/eng/04infoph/03selbst.html

Introduction

Preterm birth remains a major challenge, not only for perinatal medicine and the families of preterm neonates, but also for society as a whole. In particular, infants born before 32 weeks of gestation and/or with a birth weight lower than 1500g are at considerably higher risk of mortality and morbidity than infants born at term (see Figure 1 and Table 1).

Despite all of the progress in perinatal medicine, the rate of premature births is increasing. For example, in Germany, the rate of extremely preterm infants (less than 28 weeks) increased from 0.37% in 2001 to 0.56% in 2006 [9]. This is an increase of 51%. In the United States there was an increase from 1.81% in 1981 to 2.0% in 2004 for preterm births at less than 32 weeks [10]. An increased rate of multiple pregnancies due to assisted reproductive technologies and an increased maternal age are considered to be responsible for the rising rate of preterm births.

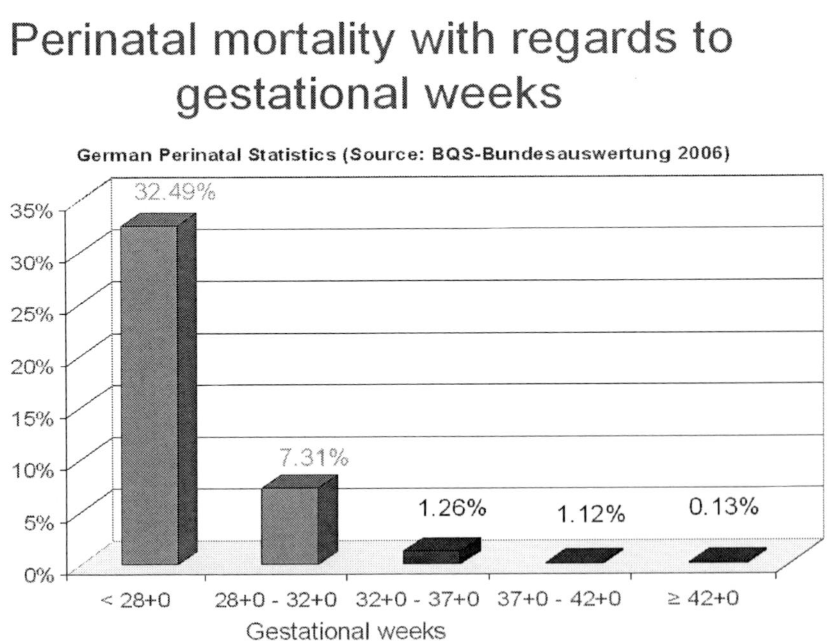

Figure 1. Perinatal mortality with regard to gestational weeks.

Table 1. Specific complications of preterm birth or low birth weight

1. *Perinatal morbidity and mortality*
   - respiratory distress syndrome
   - intraventricular hemorrhage
   - leucomalacia
   - necrotizing enterocolitis
   - infection [1, 2, 3]
2. *Long-term sequelae*
   - cerebral palsy
   - hearing defects
   - visual defects
   - epilepsy
   - neuro-developmental delay [4, 2, 6, 7]
   - subnormal weight
   - subnormal height
   - poor gross-motor function
   - poor adaptive functioning
   - behavioral problems
   - attention deficit disorder
   - learning disorders [2, 8]

Another problem that is particularly relevant for developing countries is the increased susceptibility of preterm neonates to infection. In addition, the financial burden of preterm birth is high. Recently, the Institute of Medicine of the National Academies of the United States estimated that the cost of preterm birth is $26 billion per year in the U.S. [11].

Causes of Premature Birth and Late Abortions

Late abortions and, in particular, very early preterm births should be considered together, because their etiology is often the same. But for simplicity of presentation, we will in most cases only use the term "preterm births".

"Indicated" versus "spontaneous" preterm birth: When discussing figures and causes of late abortions and preterm births, it is important to differentiate between "indicated" (for maternal or fetal indications) and so-called "spontaneous preterm birth." In the following we will only discuss the latter, as—although infections may also lead to complications for the mother, and therefore a termination of the pregnancy may be indicated—in most cases they will lead to a "spontaneous" preterm birth through premature labor and/or premature rupture of membranes.

Numerous causes of late abortions and preterm births have been identified. Roberto Romero and his colleagues introduced the term "preterm labor syndrome" and "preterm parturition syndrome" [12, 13, 14]. As causes, they list:

- infection/inflammation
- uterine ischemia/vascular disease
- cervical disease (primary or secondary)
- uterine overdistension
- abnormal allograft reaction
- allergic phenomenon
- abnormal endocrine function (untimely suspension of progesterone action)
- stress

The various patho-mechanisms initially follow different pathways, merge later on and cause changes in the cervix, leading to premature contractions and/or premature rupture of the membranes and finally to premature birth.

Regarding effective preventive measures, most of the preventable causes of preterm birth, particularly before 32 weeks, are found in patients with ascending genital tract infections. Therefore diagnostic and therapeutic strategies in this area are considered particularly important.

Treatment for less frequent causes of preterm birth is not as available and the chance of success is clearly lower than in the infection group. Furthermore, some problems are directly related to the causes resulting from genital tract infection.

We want to emphasize that smoking and abuse of other drugs (especially alcohol) are important preventable causes of preterm birth and low birth weight. Physicians should inform pregnant women about these risks and should encourage their patients to discontinue smoking, consuming alcohol or drug use.

Infection as Main Cause for Late Abortions and Early Premature Births

Infection plays an important role in preterm birth, particularly in births less than 32 weeks. Therefore, ascending genital tract infection represents a preventable cause of preterm birth. Confirmation of the role of ascending genital tract infection was found at the beginning of the 1980s when the operative Early Total Cervix Occlusion (ETCO) was introduced by us for patients with recurrent late abortions [15, 16]. This creates a complete barrier within the ascending area, and leads to remarkably good results (see also our contribution in Chapter 2 in this volume). Back in 1991 [17, 18] we were able to find evidence of infection in about three quarters of the infants with a birth weight of less than 2000g and 55% in cases of premature rupture of the membranes.

Subsequently, biochemical studies performed by Romero et al. [19] represented a major step forward in our understanding of the mechanisms by which infections lead to preterm birth. Another pioneering step which underlines how important it is to improve prevention of infections is the concept of the "fetal inflammatory response syndrome" [20]. It explains that fetal inflammation is linked to the onset of labor, and that the multi-systemic involvement in this condition can lead to fetal injury such as brain damage, which predisposes the subsequent development of cerebral palsy.

The association between infection and preterm birth has been confirmed by other investigators. If diagnosed early, infections can often be treated efficiently. In addition to ascending genital tract infections, such as Chlamydia trachomatis, and mycoplasmas, urinary tract infections should also be considered (and more rarely other infections). According to microbiological studies, infection may account for 25–40% of all preterm births, but this may represent an underestimation because, as Romero et al. [14] pointed out, infection is difficult to detect due to the limitations of standard microbiological techniques. But as infection is a major cause of inflammation, they refer to women belonging to an "inflammatory cluster" for cases with:

- proven infection,
- histological evidence of acute chorioamnionitis, or
- elevated pro-inflammatory cytokines in the amniotic fluid (AF).

In their overview article about preterm parturition syndrome, Romero et al. [14] give a list of evidence in support of a causal relationship between infection/inflammation and spontaneous preterm labor:

1. "intrauterine infection or systemic administration of microbial products to pregnant animals can result in spontaneous preterm labor and preterm birth;
2. extrauterine maternal infections, such as malaria, pyelonephritis, pneumonia, and periodontal disease, have been associated with preterm birth;
3. subclinical intrauterine infections are associated with preterm labor and preterm birth;
4. pregnant women with intra-amniotic infection or intrauterine inflammation (defined as an elevation of AF concentrations of cytokines and matrix degrading enzymes) in the mid-trimester are at risk of subsequent preterm birth;
5. antibiotic treatment of ascending intrauterine infections can prevent preterm birth in experimental models of chorioamnionitis; and
6. treatment of asymptomatic bacteriuria prevents preterm birth." [14, p. 19].

Ascending Genital and Intrauterine Infections

Most of the intrauterine infections are (at least in the beginning) subclinical in nature and cannot be detected without amniotic fluid analysis. As the amniotic fluid is normally sterile, any isolation of bacteria in the amniotic fluid is a pathological finding. According to Romero et al. [14] the frequency of microbial invasion of the amniotic cavity (MIAC) depends on the clinical presentation and gestational age: the rate of positive amniotic cultures is:

- 12.8% among women with preterm labor and intact membranes,
- 22% among women with preterm labor and intact membranes who deliver preterm,
- 32.4% among women with PPROM at admission,
- 75% among women with PPROM at the time of the onset of labor.

Also, MIAC is detected in up to 51% among those women presenting with the clinical picture of *cervical insufficiency* [21, 22]. We think this finding is particularly relevant to the discussion whether or not a cerclage or an ETCO is the appropriate measure for cases with recurrent preterm birth (please refer to our contribution in Chapter 2 in this volume).

The most common pathway for microorganisms to gain access to the amniotic cavity is *ascending from the vagina and the cervix*; however, other pathways such as haematogenous through the placenta, retrograde from the peritoneal cavity through the fallopian tube, and accidental introduction at the time of invasive procedures, are possible as well [14]. Evidence in support of ascending infection is that in twin gestations, in which a microbial invasion of the amniotic cavity (MIAC) is detected, the presenting sac is always involved, while the other amniotic cavity may not have MIAC [23].

Genital Infections

Many genital tract infections can lead to an increased rate of preterm birth as well as to increased morbidity of the mother and newborn (see Table 2).

Table 2. Urogenital infections and associated complications in pregnancy, after Martius [28]

Infection	Increased rate of preterm birth	Increased morbidity by infection of the mother	Increased morbidity by infection of the newborn
Bacterial vaginosis	yes	yes	unknown
Chlamydia trachomatis	yes	yes	yes
Streptococcus group B	unknown*	yes	yes
Neisseria gonorrhoea	yes	yes	yes
Trichomonas vaginalis	unknown	unknown	seldom
Mycoplasma hominis	unknown	unknown	unknown
Ureaplasma urealytikum	unknown	unknown	unknown
Urinary tract infection	yes	yes	no
Candida species	no	yes	yes

* Gibbs et al. [30] compared several studies concerning group B *Streptococci* and preterm delivery: Five of six studies demonstrated no significant association between colonization of the lower genital tract with group B *Streptococci* and preterm labor or preterm delivery. However, three of four studies found a significant relationship between colonization and preterm rupture of membranes. See also above the newer scientific findings from Donders [27] about the aerobic vaginitis.

The association between bacterial vaginosis and preterm birth is strong, as it is a risk factor for preterm delivery and premature rupture of membranes [24, 25]. However, bacterial vaginosis is asymptomatic in approximately 50% of patients [26]. Donders et al. [27]

supposed that a so-called "aerobic vaginitis" (which is associated with aerobic microorganisms, mainly group B *Streptococci* and *E. coli*) is as important as bacterial vaginosis. As in the case of bacterial vaginosis, the concentration of lactate is decreased (and therefore the vaginal pH increased). More investigation into that topic will be necessary.

Infections with *Candida* alone do not normally increase the risk of preterm birth, but they do affect the vaginal milieu and should therefore (also due to their morbidity for mother and child) be treated.

Other Infections

Maternal urinary tract infections or systemic infections can also lead to preterm birth. In countries with a high prevalence of serious infectious diseases, systemic infections, such as malaria, can play a more significant role in causing preterm birth than urogenital infections, see, for example, Kouam et al. [31]. Even periodontal disease has been associated with preterm birth [32, 33].

Role of *Lactobacilli*

For the prevention of ascending vaginal infection the "protective *Lactobacillus* system" plays a crucial role. The human vagina possesses an eco-system which under normal conditions provides a balance between physiologic *Lactobacilli* and pathogenic bacterial flora, ensuring protection against the spreading of pathogens, including ascending uterine infection. The importance of *Lactobacilli* for the normal vaginal milieu was in 1892 first described by Döderlein [34].

In an article of particular interest to us, Gregor Reid [35] described the role of *Lactobacilli* in preventing urogenital tract infections.

The following main functions of *Lactobacilli* are known (Figure 2):

- They produce acids, mainly lactic acid.
- They produce hydrogen peroxide (H_2O_2), which releases oxygen and has a disinfecting effect.
- These factors, combined with bacteriocines inhibit the growth of pathogens which are always present in the vagina.
- They produce biosurfactants, which cover the surface of the vaginal wall, thereby inhibiting the adhesion of pathogens.
- They produce coaggregation molecules which block the spread of pathogens.

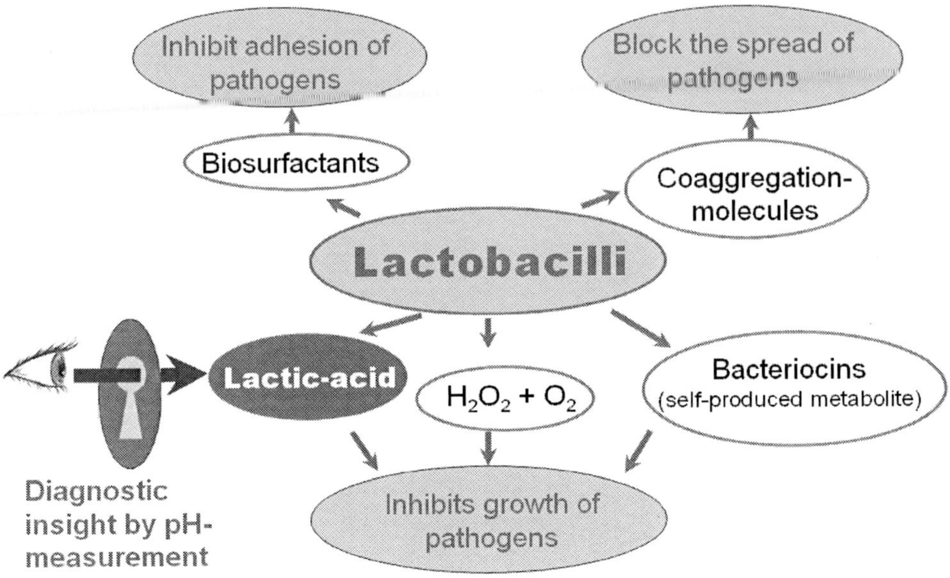

Figure 2. Protective vaginal bio-system.

Not every lactobacillus strain produces all the factors mentioned above. That is the reason why some strains are more effective against specific infections than others. For instance, women with H_2O_2-producing *Lactobacilli* run a lower risk of bacterial vaginosis than women whose *Lactobacilli* do not produce H_2O_2 [36]. Unfortunately, there are also some microorganisms, the growth of which is only marginally or not at all, inhibited by *Lactobacilli* (e.g., *Streptococci* and *Candida*).

However, we can assume that *Lactobacilli* are the main regulating factor of the vaginal milieu. Vaginal pH-measurement gives us an insight—like peering through a keyhole—into this protective bio-system. Vaginal pH-measurement was already used by Döderlein, in order to distinguish pathological from normal vaginal fluid [34].

Importance of pH Measurement

The importance of *Lactobacilli* and measurement of vaginal pH is illustrated for instance by the following evidence:

Ernest et al. [37] found out that the risk of premature rupture of the membranes before 37+0 weeks is three times higher when the vaginal pH is repeatedly above 4.5, compared to pregnant patients with pH ≤ 4.5.

From a retrospective evaluation, carried out by one of our co-workers, the following is revealed: The earlier in pregnancy the examined children were born, the more frequently the mothers had an increased vaginal pH when admitted to hospital. All 15 mothers (100%) of children with a gestational age lower than 32+0 weeks had increased pH values; as far as preterm birth between 32+0 weeks and 36+6weeks is concerned, the rate was still about 60%; when born mature only 43.5 % were affected [38]. It follows that ascending infections very frequently play a role concerning very early preterm birth, and that, in many of these cases the threat of preterm birth can be detected by measurement of increased pH-values.

In a prospective study, Hengst et al. [39] was able to show the practical importance of measuring the vaginal pH, which we recommend in routine prenatal care for the prevention of preterm birth. In a cohort of pregnant women with a normal course of pregnancy, who had increased pH values of > 4.5 and who had received no therapy for acidification, the number of preterm births amounted to 15.1%. On the other hand, the number was only 2.0% when an acidifying therapy with L. acidophilus preparations had been applied.

In an earlier evaluation, we also determined how many pregnant patients had normal vaginal pH values and how many had pathological values (≥ 4.7). In 67% of all the 695 evaluated cases, normal pH values were present; in 33%, the values were increased twice or more and 7% of these were permanently increased [40].

It is of particular interest to examine the success rate in normalizing the pH, in cases with increased vaginal pH values, by using L. acidophilus therapy. Success was achieved in 83% of 75 such patients, which represents an unexpectedly good result. This result was obtained when the duration of the therapy was 5 ± 3 days [40].

Normal Flora - Disturbed Milieu - Bacterial Vaginosis and other Infection

According to published data, a possible reason for the success of our Prematurity-Prevention Program is not the early detection of existing infections, but the early detection of their precursors, namely disturbances of the vaginal milieu (vaginal dysbiosis, see Figure 3):

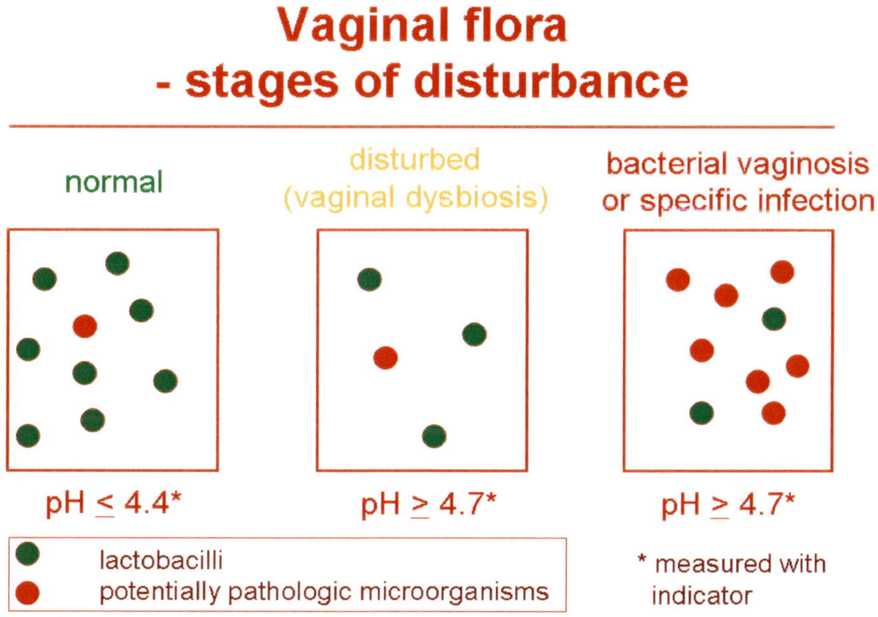

Figure 3. Vaginal flora—stages of disturbance.

Hillier et al. [41] diagnosed "an intermediate pattern" between normal flora and bacterial vaginosis—see the publication of Schröder in 1921 [42]—in 16% of the pregnant women examined, while 22% of the women had bacterial vaginosis, and 61% had normal flora. Of the women with such a "transitional stage" in the second trimester, in the third trimester about one-third still had this intermediate flora, in about one-third the flora was normal again, and about one-third developed a bacterial vaginosis. Hay et al. [43] found an association between an increased risk of loss of pregnancy, and an intermediate pattern as determined by Gram stain examination. Viehweg et al. [44] reported that an increased vaginal pH during the course of pregnancy is associated with an increased risk of preterm birth, even when the pH value stays within the normal range.

Our observations indicate that disturbances of the vaginal milieu can be detected by pH-measurement at regular intervals, before bacterial vaginosis develops [45]. In 24 pregnant patients who visited their physician because they had themselves detected an increased vaginal pH value, 33 diagnoses were made (we obtained this information from patients, rather than from the physicians, and therefore, this data should be interpreted taking this into account):

- 46% of the patients were told that they only had a disturbance of the vaginal milieu, and not yet a bacterial vaginosis.
- Bacterial vaginosis was diagnosed only in 4%.
- *Candida* was diagnosed in 33%, *Chlamydia* in 8%, and other bacteria in 8%.

Our Prematurity-Prevention Program

Overview

After having been engaged in the field of preterm birth prevention for more than 3 decades, we developed in 1989 a new "Prematurity-Prevention Program" which is based mainly on the ascending infection concept. The original part with its four stages is intended for physicians. The complete overview, because of its comprehensive content, is less suited for a detailed presentation within such a contribution. Therefore, we will limit our discussion to the essential part of this program (see Box 1). Some measures are explained below in the text. More details about the program and references are found on our homepage: *www.saling-institut.de.*

Box 1. Overview of the Prematurity Prevention Program

The first stage is based on a historical assessment. An increased risk for preterm birth is present in women who had two[3] or more previous late spontaneous abortions or very premature birth caused by infections or when no reason was detected. Our proposed therapeutic intervention is to use *Early Total Cervix-Occlusion* (see Chapter 2 in this volume) at about 12 weeks of gestation to create a *barrier* against the ascension of organisms.
The second stage of this process can be diagnosed in patients with a *disturbance of the vaginal milieu ("dysbiosis").* We consider this a "precursor"—which can be detected by simple pH-measurement at the introitus. "Dysbiosis" can be treated with *Lactobacillus acidophilus* preparations.
The third stage of increased risk includes cases *without symptoms of premature labor*, but in which a proven *bacterial vaginosis or another* vaginal infection is present. Other examples include *Chlamydia infection* of the cervical canal or urethra or *significant bacteriuria* (even asymptomatic *bacteriuria* has been known as a cause of preterm birth)[4]. In such cases, either local antimicrobial treatment or systemic treatment with antibiotics is recommended. The likelihood of success in these cases is high. In addition, in the last decade, an association has been reported between periodontal disease and preterm birth. However, it is still not clear enough, if treatment of this condition reduces the rate of preterm delivery (see below).
The fourth and most advanced stage involves cases with symptoms of preterm labor, such as preterm *uterine contractions* and/or critical ultrasonic findings of the *cervix*, such as a short cervix. In this stage, the likelihood of success is lower than in the previous stages.

Screening for Pre-Infection or Infection Signs

The main emphasis of our program lies in screening all pregnant women for signs of an altered microbial ecosystem, which leads to a change in pH. If such a program is not implemented early in gestation, then overt changes in the vaginal ecosystem or in the lower genital tract may develop. If this is the case, an opportunity for early intervention may have been lost. We assume that the unexpectedly high success rates in the reduction of preterm birth—achieved by our self-care measures—are based on the following new situation with its attendant opportunities: never before was it possible to detect the first disturbances of vaginal milieu in such an early stage and to start with therapeutic countermeasures so early (see also below under Self-Care Program). In cases where preterm birth occurs due to other reasons, the possibility of intervention and successful therapy are clearly not so good.

The measurement of the vaginal pH is particularly important. We have recommended this measure since 1989 [46, 18] for regular prenatal care. We are currently conducting a

[3] We sometimes recommend an ETCO after only one of these incidents; see our contribution about the ETCO in this volume.

[4] Screening for urinary tract infections is in many countries already part of routine care for pregnant women.

study in regards to regular prenatal care in Germany at the present time. According to our preliminary findings, about two-thirds of the physicians who returned the forms measure the vaginal pH of their patients regularly. An increase in the pH-value (≥ 4.2 if measured with pH-meter, > 4.4 if measured with indicator paper) 5 can be due to:

- *Disturbance* in the vaginal milieu (also called "dysbiosis"),
- *Bacterial vaginosis*. Diagnostic clinical criteria after Amsel [47] of bacterial vaginosis in addition to an increased pH-value (> 4.5) in vaginal fluid which are: thin, white, yellow, homogeneous discharge, fishy odor of the vaginal fluid (especially after the addition of 10% potassium hydroxide solution) and evidence of clue cells (three of these four criteria must be present to ensure the diagnosis).[6]
- *Aerobic vaginitis* as described and defined by Donders et al. [27] and
- other types of infection. If other infections are suspected, an appropriate examination should be carried out.

Treatment

The treatment will be performed according to the diagnosis. Here are the most common situations:

Disturbances of the Vaginal Milieu

Disturbances of the vaginal milieu (vaginal dysbiosis) without specific signs of bacterial vaginosis or specific infection should be treated with H_2O_2 producing lactobacillus preparations[7] for about seven days. For example the results of Hengst [39] show that pregnant

[5] *Devices for the measurement of the vaginal pH:* A simple and, if used for the examination of many patients, inexpensive way of measuring the pH is to use a small, portable pH-meter. Another alternative, a little more expensive, is the use of indicator strips which are introduced into the area of the introitus vaginae with the finger either before or after the vaginal examination and compared with the corresponding color scale. We made by far the best experiences, when using "Spezialindikator pH 4.0-7.0"; art-no. 1.09542 by Merck, Darmstadt (Germany), because reading is here especially easy and reliable. In the meantime, special disposable gloves with the indicator paper from Merck fixed on the index finger are available for use by the physician. The gloves are almost identical to the ones that we recommend for the patients (see below). The only difference is, that the indicator paper in the version for the physician is attached to the middle phalanx of the index finger, so that during vaginal examination the pH value will be measured automatically at the lower part of the vagina.

[6] In the context of clinical research the bacterial vaginosis is often diagnosed according to the criteria of Nugent [88]. But for diagnosis in the daily practice we consider the criteria according to Amsel as more practical and sufficient.

[7] Women with H_2O_2-producing lactobacilli have a lower risk of suffering from bacterial vaginosis than women whose lactobacilli do not produce H_2O_2 [36], therefore one should substitute the former strains of lacobacilli. But other factors are also important, for example whether or not the lactobacilli can adhere to the vaginal epithelial cells. Alvarez-Olmos and Oberhelman [49] demanded for clinical studies with probiotics: "Strain information should be reported with each clinical and microbiological study because even closely related probiotic strains may have different clinical effects." ([49], p. 1570). Although they discussed orally

women with elevated vaginal pH-values have a better outcome after treatment with lactobacillus preparations. According to our own evaluation [40] the pH-values could be normalized with *Lactobacillus acidophilus* therapy in 83 % of the pregnant patients within five days in the average ± three days (s).

Because lactobacillus therapy thus takes two to eight days, until the pH values normalize, additional local acidifying therapy might be indicated (e.g., lactic acid in the morning, and lactobacillus preparation in the evening). However, currently there is no scientific proof that this additional measure reduces the rate of preterm birth. Please note, that we recommend lactobacillus preparations only for vaginal dysbiosis and not for bacterial vaginosis (see below).

Bacterial Vaginosis

Bacterial vaginosis can be treated either locally or systemically with Metronidazol or with Clindamycin [50][8]. Up to now, there have been various studies with regard to treatment of bacterial vaginosis in pregnancy [51, 52, 53, 89]. Another therapeutic option might be local therapy with antiseptics. Friese et al. [54] compared octenidine dihydrochloride antiseptic solution with povidone-iodine vaginal suppositories and found that, in patients using octenidine hydrochloride, an improvement in symptoms was more frequent (75% vs. 65%) and restitution of *Lactobacilli* was significantly more common (46% vs. 29%). More research with this therapeutic option is neccessary; however, we sometimes recommend this option - particularly for cases with recurrent infections. However, after one meta-analysis from Leitich et al. [89] with regard to antibiotic treatment of BV in pregnancy, it seems that for women in *high risk populations* systemic treatment of longer duration is more recommendable. In the literature, there are controversial results concerning the success of treatment of bacterial vaginosis, and its effect on pregnancy outcome [55, 56, 57], see also Romero et al. [29]. This may partly be due to the heterogeneity of the study groups: Several meta-analyses concluded that the screening and treatment of bacterial vaginosis of combined low and high-risk populations did not reduce the risk of preterm birth [58], but a recent meta-analysis of Varma et al. [59] found a benefit in low risk populations. However, there may have also been little success, in cases when screening, diagnosis, and treatment took place rather late in the course of pregnancy. No studies have been published of cases where vaginal acidity was checked by pH-measurement so early in pregnancy and at such short intervals (allowing early treatment), as is the case for the pregnant women who participate in our Self-Care Program (see below). In addition to the gestational age at screening and treatment, Romero et al. [29] describe other reasons for the discrepant results: history of preterm birth, choice of antimicrobial agent and whether the diagnostic criteria for bacterial vaginosis optimally identify those at risk of infection-associated preterm birth.

---

supplemented probiotics, it may well be the case, that the same is true for vaginally supplemented lactobacilli. Much more research in this area is necessary.

[8] Please see also our discussion below with regards to the use of yoghurt or lactobacillus preparations for the treatment of bacterial vaginosis.

In several studies, women with bacterial vaginosis have been treated with lactobacillus preparations, for example [60, 61], with yoghurt [62] or with acid lactic gel [63]. Although these preparations have conferred some benefit and a reduction of bacterial vaginosis, we do not favor this, as Dennemark et al. [64] reported an improved pregnancy outcome for women treated with clindamycin vaginal cream than with lactobacillus preparations. Births less than 37 weeks had the following screening and treatment:

a) neither screening nor treatment: 15%
b) screening and treatment with lactobacillus 11,5 %
c) screening and treatment with clindamycin: 5,3 %

Also, the long-term benefit is uncertain. For example, Hallén et al. [61] treated women with bacterial vaginosis with H_2O_2 producing *Lactobacilli* versus placebo. In the treatment group, 16 out of 28 women had normal smears following treatment. There were no normal smears following treatment in the placebo group. However, after the next menstruation only 3 of the treated women were free from bacterial vaginosis. We therefore recommend *Lactobacilli* preparations only in cases with vaginal dysbiosis (see above). In the presence of bacterial vaginosis we recommend specific therapy with antibiotics, chemotherapeutics or disinfectants.

Specific Urogenital Infections

Specific urogenital infection (including asymptomatic bacteriuria) *in the absence of clinical signs of preterm labor or PROM* should be identified and treated with antibiotics effective against the causative organism. For patients with a clinically evident urogenital infection or with evidence of inflammation (e.g., CRP) *and who have symptoms of preterm labor*, systemic antibiotic therapy is often used. In addition, other interventions such as tocolysis, bed rest or progesterone may be appropriate according to the clinical circumstances. In women with preterm labor, antibiotics are used to prevent vertical transmission of group B streptococcus. However, in the absence of a specific infection, antibiotic administration should not be used in women with preterm labor and intact membranes. A recent study has suggested that fetuses exposed to antibiotics administered to women with preterm labor and intact membranes had an increased risk of cerebral palsy at the age of seven. Antibiotic administration to women with PROM is the standard of practice because it results in prolongation of pregnancy, and a reduction in the rate of infection-related complications, such as neonatal sepsis. However, long term follow-up of infants who received antibiotics does not demonstrate a benefit of such antibiotic administration [65, 66].

Systemic Infections

Systemic infections require specific therapy aimed at the nature of the infection and the causative organism. If *fever* is present, the use of indomethacin should be considered to prevent prostaglandin-related effects on the uterus (e.g., increase of uterine contractility and the induction of cervical ripening). Please note that this recommendation is only for systemic infections (such as influenza or pneumonia) and not for intrauterine infections. It is possible that this treatment could cause adverse events such as closure of the fetal ductus arteriosus and oligohydramnios. Therefore, the use of indomethacin is best reserved for women with a gestational age below 28–30 weeks, without intrauterine growth retardation and with a normal volume of amniotic fluid. Treatment with this agent should be restricted to 48 or maximum 72 h, see Di Renzo et al. [67].

Periodontal Disease

Periodontal disease has been associated with an increased risk of spontaneous preterm delivery [32]. However, it is less clear if treatment of this condition reduces the rate of preterm birth [33]. It is possible that periodontal disease is a marker for a host predisposed to elicit a robust inflammatory response rather than a specific mechanism of disease for preterm birth. Romero et al. [29] suggests that an inappropriate inflammatory response may be present in women with bacterial vaginosis and periodontal disease. It is possible that hyper-responsive individuals (hyper-responsive means that the patients mount a more severe inflammatory response to microbial products) are more likely to have periodontal disease and also infection-related preterm labor. Recent clinical trials suggest that periodontal treatment during pregnancy of women affected does not reduce the rate of preterm birth, for a review see [33]. Further research in this area is warranted.

Self-Care Program for Pregnant Women

The self-care measures for pregnant women represent the most important part of our Prematurity Prevention Program [68, 69, 70]. We recommend that pregnant patients monitor their vaginal pH twice a week from the beginning of the pregnancy using a CarePlan®VpH-test-glove which we developed in collaboration with a medical company. The indicator can be compared with a color chart to determine the pH value. If the pH is normal (4.4 or less), the indicator will turn yellow (see Figure 4).

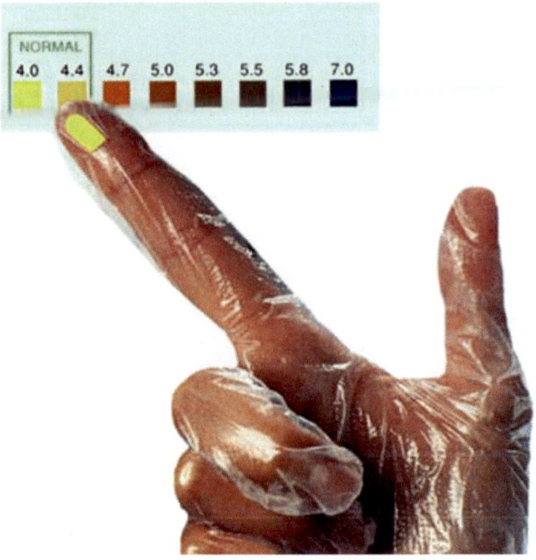

Figure 4. pH measurement: comparison with the color scale.

Twice weekly pH monitoring by the patient greatly reduces the intervals between measurements compared with the interval between visits with usual prenatal care. Frequent pH monitoring offers the possibility of early detection of symptoms and therefore, early intervention.

If a pH value of 4.7 or more is measured, the pregnant patient is advised to report the results to her physician as soon as possible, and if indicated, to start treatment. The test-glove packs also contain detailed information about the program such as the need to consult her physician if any of these signs are present:

- changes in vaginal discharge,
- burning and itching in the intimate regions,
- signs of urinary tract infection,
- cramping or pelvic pressure
- vaginal bleeding or spotting.

For more details, please see: http://www.saling-institut.de/eng/04infoph/03selbst.html

Results

The results of our program appear to justify the implementation of the self-assessment of vaginal pH by pregnant women and to demonstrate the efficacy of our Self-Care Program. The results have already been published in detail, e.g., [40, 69, 70]—here just the main figures are given:

Pre-Evaluation

In a study conducted in our department [71] in which 100 women measured their vaginal pH themselves using indicator paper, 91% of the measurements corresponded with the results obtained immediately afterwards by a physician with a pH-meter. In 9% of cases, the results were considered as false-positives; meaning that the indicator paper provided a value of the pH which was above that obtained with the pH meter, and that the latter was within normal range. There were no false-negative results, in other words, no pathological findings were missed. The false-positive findings are not considered by us a serious shortcoming because our emphasis is in detecting an abnormal milieu in the lower genital tract. It is also interesting to note that in about 70% of the patients who had increased pH-values measured both by indicator paper and by the pH-meter, we found evidence of pathogenous organisms in the vagina and/or the cervix, whereas when the pH values were within the normal range, the frequency of abnormal findings was only 8%.

Results from Our Self-Care Program

The full Self-Care Program was started in September 1993. The program was advertised in publications that are frequently read by pregnant women. Of the 1,715 women whose data have been evaluated, 595 were pregnant for the first time and 1,120 had been pregnant before. The obstetrical histories provided by women with previous pregnancies were particularly interesting. 46.4% had miscarriages and about 18.3% had infants < 2,500 g in the immediate previous pregnancy. Thus far, the participating women belong to a high-risk, rather than low-risk group. Additionally, according to the returned records, 60.8% of the patients reported events or diagnostic results in the current pregnancy which indicated higher risk of preterm birth. In women who had been pregnant before the index pregnancy, the assessment shows the following (see Figure 5):

- The rate of low birth weight infants (< 2500g) in those patients taking part in the Self-Care Program and who had been pregnant before was 6.2%, this means three times lower than that in the immediate previous pregnancy, which had been 18.3%.
- It is of special interest to note that the number of very low birth weight infants (< 1500g) was 1.3%: that is six times lower than in the immediate previous pregnancies, which had been 7.8%.
- The rate of extremely low-birth-weight infants (< 1000g) amounted to 0.9%, compared to 3.9% previously.

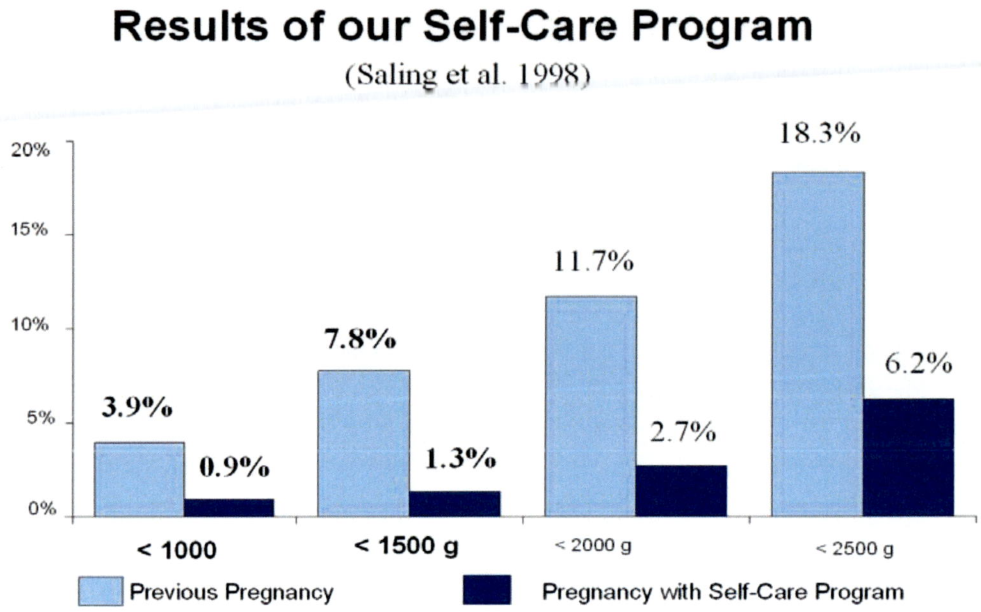

Figure 5. Results of our Self-Care Program, after Saling et al. [69].

Of the 111 women who had a preterm birth in the immediate previous pregnancy, only 20 (18%) had a preterm birth in the index pregnancy (< 37+0 weeks of gestation). Of the 38 women who had a preterm birth of < 32+0 weeks in the immediate previous pregnancy, only three (8%) had a similar outcome in the index pregnancy. Of the 22 women who had a preterm birth at < 28+0 weeks , there was no recurrence of preterm delivery.

Results from Other Places

Later Hoyme et al. [72] achieved similar encouraging results with our program in a prospective project undertaken in Erfurt, the capital of Thuringia, Germany. The results prompted the Government of Thuringia to employ our program. In the second half of the year 2000, the Self-Care Program was employed and the results were compared to those from the first six months of 2000 (before the program was implemented). In each half-year there were more than 8.000 births. The results represent a breakthrough, as most authors dealing with preterm birth have stated that in greater population areas the preterm birth rate had not changed at all during the previous decades, or that the rate had even increased.

In Thuringia the results were [73, 74, 75, 76, 77]:

- With regard to *gestational age*: the rate of infants born less than 32 weeks was 1.36% in the first half of the year 2000, and 0.94% in the second half. This is a significant reduction. [76, 77]
- With regard to *birth weight* (see Figure 6): the rate of infants born less than 1500g decreased significantly from 1.29% to 0.97%. In infants weighing less than 1000g, the rate decreased significantly from 0.61% to 0.38%. [75, 76, 77]

- In addition, the incidence of *premature rupture of membranes (PROM)* was significantly reduced. While in the first half of the year 2000, the frequency of PROM in cases where the infants were born with less than 32 weeks of gestation was 0.55% out of 7,870 deliveries it was significantly reduced in the second half of the year to 0.2% out of 8,406 deliveries (figures calculated by us according to the results from Hoyme et al. [74, 75])
- In the meantime, a series of observations have become available, which allow examination of the effect of the implementation of the Self Care program [76, 77]: After the Self Care program trial was completed, the preterm birth rate was monitored between 2002 and 2004. The rate of preterm birth after discontinuation of the Self Care program was as high as it was before the implementation of the program Figure 7 shows the numbers for children with a birth weight < 1000 g)

These observations provide confirmation of the efficacy of the program. We understand that these results do not derive from a randomized clinical trial. We consider the evidence rather persuasive and although we are personally of the opinion that such a randomized trial is not absolutely necessary, we think for the implementation of the program on an international level, it is now recommendable to perform one (see also the discussion below).

Based on these results, several *German health insurance companies* implemented our prenatal-care self-examination program as a pilot project at no cost. The companies started this project in December 2003: the official results are not available yet, but after first internal evaluations, they have reported significant savings. Siegmund-Schulze [78] from the Health insurance company KKH reported first results from two participating states (Bavaria and Lower Saxony).

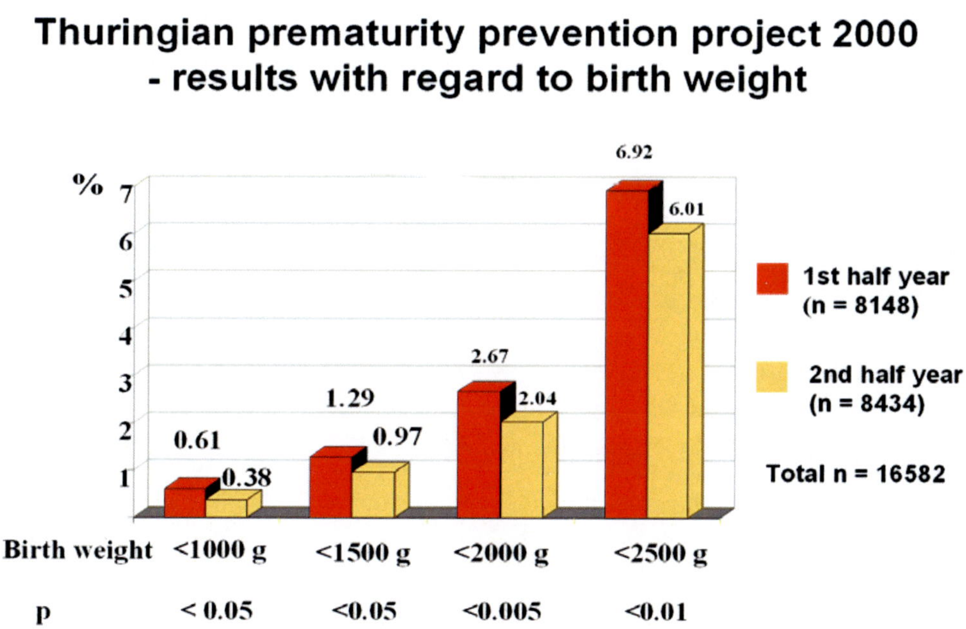

Figure 6. Thuringian prematurity prevention project 2000: Results with regard to birth weight, after Hoyme et al. [75, 76, 77].

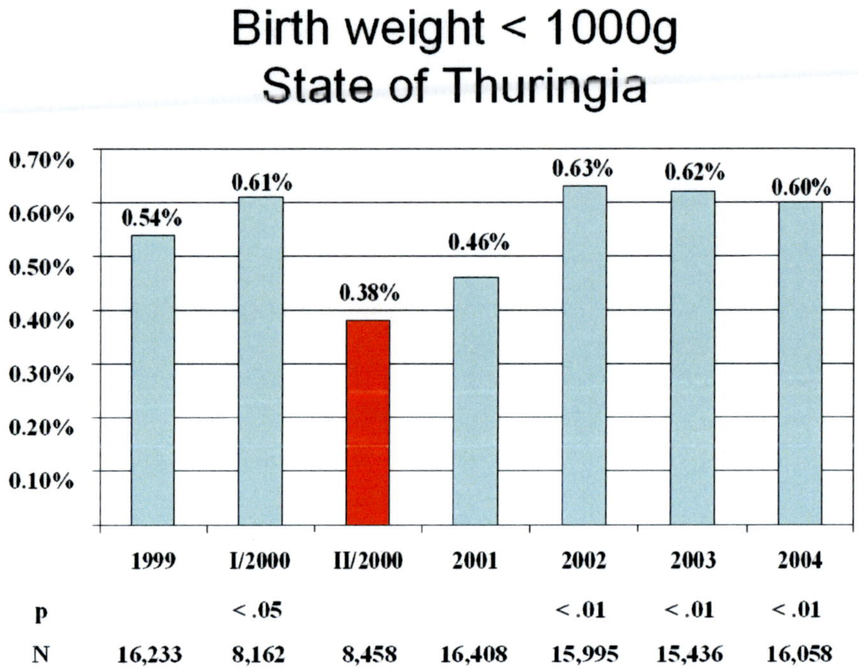

Figure 7. Secular trends in the rate of preterm birth before and after implementation of the Self Care program, after Hoyme et al. [76, 77].

All births from 2004–2006 of the participating health insurances served as a control group (n=57,273). Within the control group, the rate of very preterm births (< 32 weeks) was 0.86%. Of the 2,899 women insured with the health insurance KKH who took part in the self-care program and who returned their documentation forms, the rate of preterm births less than 32 weeks was 0.49%.

When to Start

Hübner confirmed the importance of early onset of pH self-measurement in pregnancy. She evaluated questionnaires from 607 pregnant women who participated in the "Thuringia Prematurity Prevention Campaign 2000" (Hübner, published in Hoyme and Saling [75]). Among women who started pH monitoring before 15+0 gw, the total rate of preterm births was 4.8%, and the rate of very early preterm births was 0%. In contrast, when women started pH monitoring at 15+0 weeks or later, there were 6.1% preterm births, and 0.9% very early preterm births.

Pregnancies with Increased Risk

Recurrent Late Abortions or Preterm Births

After one preterm birth, the risk of a recurrent preterm birth is increased [80, 81, 82]. Although the actual recurrence risk depends upon the etiology and the gestational age, the earlier in pregnancy the previous preterm birth occurred, the higher is the risk for recurrence. McManemy et al. [83] also found, that, in cases with two previous pregnancies, the risk is higher (21 %) if the sequence of previous pregnancies was term/preterm and lower (13%) if the sequence was preterm/term. After two preterm deliveries the risk of recurrence is about 40%—depending on the gestational age: 38% for two prior preterm deliveries between 32–36 weeks and 57% in cases with two prior deliveries between 21–31 weeks [83].

Particularly in cases with *two or more* late abortions (≥ 12+0 weeks) or early preterm births (<32+0 weeks) with either an infectious etiology or in the setting of premature rupture of membranes, we recommend an *Early Total Cervix Occlusion (ETCO)* as a preventive measure. Please note that the main reason for premature rupture of the membranes is ascending genital tract infection. The Total Cervix Occlusion (TCO) creates a complete barrier against ascending infections within the cervical canal (as opposed to cerclage). This operation is now an essential part of our Prematurity Prevention Program and also a widespread measure in Germany and is also performed in other German speaking countries. The ETCO is explained in detail in Chapter 2 in this volume.

Other measures concerning recurrent preterm birth, e.g., measurement of cervical length, fetal fibronectin or progesterone administration are the subject of debate in the literature [84, 85, 86, 14, 58].

Multiple Pregnancies

Another group with a higher risk of preterm birth is multiple pregnancies. It is noteworthy that our Self-Care Program enabled us to reduce the number of premature births in multiple pregnancies. In Thuringia the frequency of twins and triplets with birth weights less than 1,500g has been reduced from about 27% without the Self-Care Program to about 14% with the program and in the group low birth weight of less than 1000g from 11.6% to 2.0% [76].

G. Schulze reported a decrease in the rate of preterm birth in multiple pregnancies using operative ETCO. In 1990 Schulze began using ETCO in multiple pregnancies (regardless of whether or not there had been preterm births in the history) and in about 100 cases he was able to achieve a preterm birth rate of 17% as compared to a rate of 29% in cases without ETCO [87], a reduction of about 40%. We are convinced that this is an effective method to reduce the frequency of preterm birth in multiple pregnancies. Further research needs to be done to evaluate in which cases with multiple pregnancies screening for pre-infections and infections and pH monitoring is sufficient and which patients might benefit from an additional ETCO. (For details about the ETCO please see Chapter 2 in this volume.)

Other Prematurity Prevention Strategies

Research in the field of preterm birth prevention has yielded promising approaches such as:

- measurement of the cervical length,
- measurement of fetal fibronectin,
- Progesterone administration.

But there are still divergent results and different opinions in respect of the effectiveness of these methods which are often used in later stages of the process of preterm birth. It is also the case that both the measurement of cervical length and measurement of fetal fibronectin seem to be methods rather for risk assessment than actual screening methods. For a full discussion of current research in this area, we recommend studying the review publication of Romero et al. [14].

Other Diagnostic Measures

If one or more of the above-mentioned screening measures results in abnormal findings, then additional testing may be necessary such as:

- tests for bacterial vaginosis according to Amsel and/or Gram stain,
- neutrophil count,
- culture for microorganisms,
- other biochemical markers of inflammation, such as IL-6, IL-8.
- lavage of the lower uterine extra-amniotic space (egg-pole lavage)[9]
- amniocentesis for amniotic fluid examination, when the index of suspicion for infection is high.

Cascade of the Infectiological Prematurity Process

However, from our point of view, most of these above-mentioned interventions are implemented at later stages in the process of preterm birth. Romero et al. [14] point out there is a long preclinical stage between findings such as a short cervix or a positive fetal fibronectin and spontaneous preterm labor and/or preterm rupture of membranes (PROM). The same is true for intrauterine infection which can be clinically silent for weeks or months before the onset of preterm labor.

It is most likely that the process which leads to a premature birth initially starts with a disturbance of the vaginal milieu (see Figure 8). If the woman monitors her vaginal pH twice weekly from the beginning of pregnancy, it is possible to detect a very early stage of the

[9] See Saling [48] or www.saling-institute.org

process and treat her immediately with *Lactobacillus* preparations which could prevent further stages of the process. Never before has it been possible to detect it at such an early stage.

However, if the opportunity for early diagnosis and treatment is missed, the consequences are often a genital tract infection which can lead to an inflammatory process resulting in biochemical changes, cervical ripening, and a preterm birth (see Figure 8).

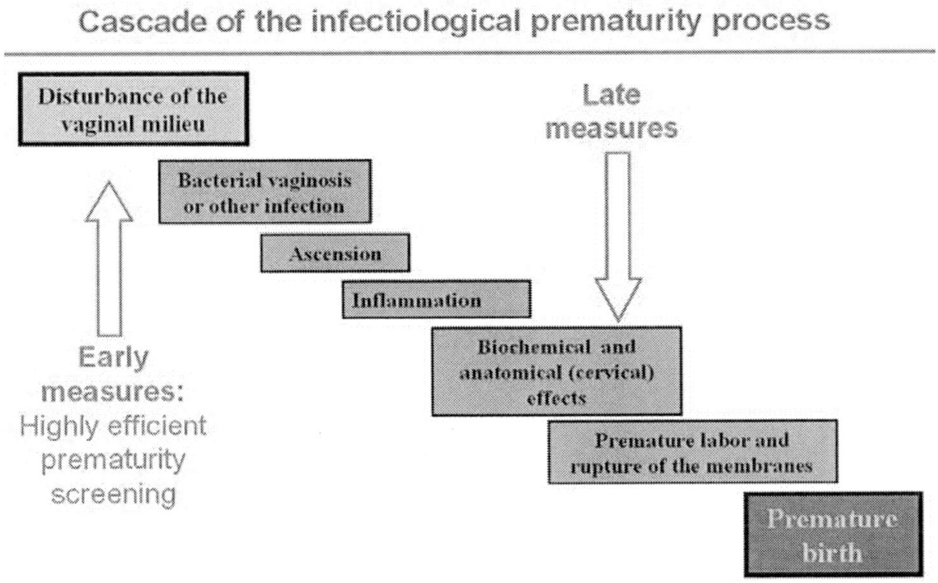

Figure 8. Cascade of the infection-related preterm parturition process.

Conclusion

Although the role of infection in the process of preterm birth has been well known for a long time, there is still a lot of research to be done—particularly in the area of preventing infection-related preterm births.

A main part of our Prematurity-Prevention Program focuses on the screening for, and treatment of, infections—particularly urogenital infections—and detecting disturbances in the vaginal milieu before an actual infection develops. This strategy takes into account the role of *Lactobacilli* in maintaining the vaginal milieu. In order to allow for the detection of these disturbances or infections even earlier, we developed the Self-Care Program for pregnant women.

Currently the Self-Care Program—as confirmed by our evaluation and subsequently by two prospective investigations by Hoyme et al. (see above)—seems to be an effective, easily implemented and inexpensive program for prevention of very early preterm birth. The explanation for the exceptionally positive results that we achieved may be that our prevention program—with cooperation of the pregnant patient—allows for the detection of very early disturbances of the vaginal ecosystem before any overt symptoms of infection—including bacterial vaginosis and aerobic vaginitis—are evident. This enables immediate therapeutic measures to be taken, leading to a rapid reestablishment of normal vaginal milieu, and may prevent some of the later stages of the process of preterm parturition.

We therefore recommend the Self-Care Program for *all* pregnant women. In countries where the circumstances do not permit the use of the self-care measures for all women, at the very least vaginal pH monitoring should be performed regularly by physicians or midwives. Other additional, more sophisticated measures may be necessary in special cases.

In Germany, the measurement of vaginal pH is developing into a standard measure in prenatal care:

- According to our first assessment of prenatal care in Germany, about two-thirds of the physicians who returned the forms measure the vaginal pH of their patients regularly, even though the measurement is not yet paid for by the health insurance providers as a routine prenatal care measure.
- In addition, the active participation of women in vaginal pH self monitoring is increasingly performed as part of prenatal care. In addition to the above-mentioned studies and model projects carried out by health insurance companies, it is now the case that, in 11 states out of 16 in Germany, a contract with regards to *Integrierte Versorgung* (integrated care) between two health insurance companies and the *Kassenärztliche Vereinigung* (Resident Doctors' Association) or the *Berufsverband der Frauenärzte* (Association of Gynecologists) has been implemented to improve the prevention of preterm births. This effort includes providing pH-test gloves and encouraging pregnant women to regularly monitor their vaginal pH.

Although randomized trials for the Self-Care Program are recommendable, we consider that the current evidence suggests that the program is effective. After the encouraging results described above and the studies performed by several health insurance companies, it seems difficult, if not impossible, that such a trial could be conducted in Germany. It may be possible that such trials could be conducted elsewhere. Indeed, in countries where either the measurement of vaginal pH by the physician and/or the self measurement by the patient is not yet widely performed, a randomized controlled trial could support the introduction of our program in these places. Additionally, it would at least give some women the chance to benefit from pH measurement (please refer to "Randomized Trials—Ethical Questions" in our contribution in Chapter 2 in this volume). Therefore, if individual scientists or study groups consider a randomized trial with pH measurement, we would welcome it and would support them with advice or assistance, if necessary.

Further Information

On www.saling-institute.org you can find detailed information about the Prematurity-Prevention Program, the Self-Care Program and the ETCO.

References

[1] Berkowitz GS, Papiernick E. (1993): Epidemiology of preterm birth. *Epidemiol. Rev.* 15 (2) 414-443.

[2] Hack M, Taylor HG, Klein N, Eiben R, Schatschneider C, Mercuri-Minich N (1994): School-age outcomes in children with birth weights under 750g. *N. Engl. J. Med.* 331: 753-759.

[3] Edwards WH, Little GA (1998): Outcome of the very-low-birth-weight baby: an American experience. In: Kurjak A: Textbook of perinatal medicine: a comprehensive guide to modern clinical perinatology. 1. *Perinatology.* Parthenon Publishin Group: S. 141-1152

[4] Saigal S, Rosenbaum P, Hattersley B, Milner R (1989): Decreased disability rate among 3-year-old survivors weighing 501 to 1000 grams at birth and born to residents of a geographically defined region from 1981 to 1984 compared with 1977 to 1980. *J. Pediatr.* 114: 839-846.

[5] Hack M, Wright LL, Shankaran S, Tyson JE, Horbar JD, Bauer CR, Younes N (1995): Very-low-birth-weight outcomes of the National Institute of Child Health and Human Development Neonatal Network, November 1989 to October 1990. *Am. J. Obstet. Gynecol.* 172: 457-464.

[6] Monset-Couchard M, de Bethmann O, Kastler B (1996): Mid- and long-term outcome of 89 premature infants weighing less than 1000 g at birth, all appropriate for gestational age. *Biol. Neonate* 70: 328-338.

[7] Wolke D, Meyer R (1994): Psychologische Langzeitbefunde bei sehr Frühgeborenen. *PerinatalMedizin* 6: 121-123.

[8] Wolke D (1998): Psychological development of prematurely born children. *Arch. Dis. child* 78: 567-570.

[9] Bundesgeschäftsstelle Qualitätssicherung (several years): BQS-Bundesauswertung http://www.bqs-outcome.de/

[10] Martin JA, Hamilton BE, Sutton PD, et al. (2005): Births: Final data for 2003. National vital statistics reports; vol 54 no 2. Hyattsville, MD: National Center for Health Statistics. 2005. Available at: http://www.cdc.gov/nchs/data/nvsr/nvsr54/nvsr54_02.pdf.

[11] Institute of Medicine of the National Academies (2007): Preterm Birth: Causes, Consequences, and Prevention. Richard E. Behrman and Adrienne Stith Butler, *Editors.* The National Academies Press, Washington, D.C. http://books.nap.edu/openbook.php?record_id=11622andpage=1.

[12] Romero R, Avila C, Brekus CA, Mazor M. (1990): The Role of Systemic and Intrauterine Infection in Preterm Parturition. In: Garfiel RE (ed.): *Uterine contractility,* 319-353.

[13] Romero R, Mazor M, Munoz H, Gomez R, Galasso M, Sherer DM (1994): The preterm labor syndrome. *Ann. N Y Acad. Sci.* 734: 414-429.

[14] Romero R, Espinoza J, Kusanovic JP, Gotsch F, Hassan S, Erez O, Chaiworapongsa T, Mazor M (2006b): The preterm parturition syndrome. *Br. J. Obstet. Gyneacol.* 113 (Suppl. 3): 17-42.

[15] Saling E (1981): Der frühe totale Muttermundverschluß zur Vermeidung habitueller Aborte und Frühgeburten. *Z Geburtshilfe Perinat* 185: 259-261.

[16] Saling E (1984): Prevention of habitual abortion and prematurity by early total occlusion of the external os uteri. *Eur. J. Obstet. Gynecol. Reprod. Biol.* 17: 165-170.

[17] Saling E, Brandt-Niebelschütz S, Schmitz C (1991): Vermeidung von Spätaborten und risikoreichen Frühgeburten—für die Routine geeignete Maßnahmen. *Z. Geburtshilfe Perinat.* 195: 209-221.

[18] Saling E (1991): Program for the Prevention of Prematurity. In: Hirsch HA: *Infection and Preterm Labor* (International Symposium Tübingen, 1990) Thieme, Stuttgart - New York.

[19] Romero R, Gomez R, Baumann P, Mazor M, Cotton D (1993): The role of the infection and cytokines in preterm parturition. In: Chwalisz K and Garfield RE: *Basic Mechanismus controlling term and preterm birth*; Ernst Schering Research Foundation, workshop 7; Springer, Berlin Heidelberg, New York: 197-240.

[20] Gomez R, Romero R, Ghezzi F, Yoon BH, Mazor M, Berry SM (1998): The fetal inflammatory response syndrome. *Am. J. Obstet. Gynecol.* 179: 194-202.

[21] Mays JK, Figueroa R, Shah J, Khakoo H, Kaminsky S, Tejani N (2000): Amniocentesis for selection before rescue cerclage. *Obstet Gynecol* 95: 652–655.

[22] Romero R, Gonzalez R, Sepulveda W, Brandt F, Ramirez M, Sorokin Y, Mazor M, Treadwell MC, Cotton DB (1992): Infection and labor. VIII. Microbial invasion of the amniotic cavity in patients with suspected cervical incompetence: prevalence and clinical significance. *Am. J. Obstet. Gynecol.* 167 (4 Pt 1): 1086-1091.

[23] Mazor M, Hershkovitz R, Ghezzi F, Maymon E, Horowitz S, Leiberman JR (1996): Intraamniotic infection in patients with preterm labor and twin pregnancies. *Acta Obstet Gynecol. Scand.* 75: 624–627.

[24] Martius J, Eschenbach DA (1990): The role of bacterial vaginosis as a cause of amniotic fluid infection, choriamnionitis and prematurity - a review. *Arch. Gynecol. Obstet.* 247: 1-13.

[25] Koumans EH, Kendrick JS, CDC Bacterial Vaginosis Working Group (2001): Preventing adverse sequelae of bacterial vaginosis: a public health program and research agenda. *Sex Transm Dis* 28 (5): 292-297.

[26] Eschenbach DA, Hillier S, Critchlow C, Stevens C, DeRouen T, Holmes KK (1988). Diagnosis and clinical manifestations of bacterial vaginosis. *Am. J. Obstet. Gynecol.* 158: 819-828.

[27] Donders G G G, Vereecken A, Bosmans E, Dekeersmaecker A, Salembier G, Spitz B (2002): Definition of a type of abnormal vaginal flora that is distinct from bacterial vaginosis: aerobic vaginitis. *Br. J. Obstet Gynecol.* 109: 34-43.

[28] Martius J (1998): Infektionen. In: Martius G, Rath W: Praxis der Frauenheilkunde, *Band 3: Geburtshilfe und Perinatologie*. Thieme Stuttgart, New York, S. 304-339.

[29] Romero R, Chairworapongsa T, Kuivaniemi H, Tromp G (2004): Bacterial vaginosis, the inflammatory response and the risk of preterm birth: A role for genetic epidemiology in the prevention of preterm birth. *Am. J. Obstet. Gynecol.* 190: 1509-19.

[30] Gibbs RS, Romero R, Hillier SL, Eschenbach DA, Sweet RL (1992): A review of premature birth and subclinical infection. *Am. J. Obstet. Gynecol.* 166: 1515-1528.

[31] Kouam L, Kamdom-Moyo J (1995): Frühgeburtenrate und perinatale Mortalität an der Universitätsfrauenklinik Yaoundé (Kamerun) von 1982-1992. Eine Analyse von 680 Fällen. *Z. Geburtshilfe Neonatol.* 199: 65-70.

[32] Offenbacher S, Beck JD, Lieff S, Slade G (1998): Role of periodontitis in systemic health: sponstaneous preterm birth. *J. Dent. Educ* 62 (19): 852-858.

[33] Xiong X, Buekens P, Fraser WD, Beck J, Offenbacher S (2006): Periodontal disease and adverse pregnancy outcomes: a systematic review. *Br. J. Obstet Gyn*ecol. 113:135–143.

[34] Döderlein A (1892): Das Scheidensekret und seine Bedeutung für das Puerperalfieber. Verlag von Eduard Besold, Leipzig.

[35] Reid G (2001): Probiotic agents to protect the urogenital tract against infection. *Am.* J. *Clin. Nutr.* 73 (suppl): 437S-443S.

[36] Hillier SL, Krohn MA, Klebanoff SJ, Eschenbach DA (1992a): The relationship of hydrogen peroxide producing lactobacilli to bacterial vaginosis and genital microflora in pregnant women. *Obstet. Gynecol.* 79 (3): 369-373.

[37] Ernest JM, Meis PJ, Moore ML, Swain M (1989): Vaginal pH: A marker of preterm premature rupture of the membranes. *Obstet. Gynecol.* 74: 734-737.

[38] Schumacher E (1999): Infektionsbezogene diagnostische Parameter bei Patientinnen mit Frühgeburtsymptomatik. Dissertation an der Freien Universität Berlin.

[39] Hengst P, Uhlig B, Bollmann R, Kokott Th (1992): Nutzen der vaginalen pH-Messung zur Frühgeburtsvermeidung. Ergebnisse einer prospektiven Studie. *Z Geburtshilfe Perinat* 196: 238-241.

[40] Saling E, Fuhr N, Placht A, Schumacher E (1995): Erste Ergebnisse der „Selbst-Vorsorge-Aktion von Schwangeren" zur Frühgeburtenvermeidung. *Arch. Gynecol. Obstet.* 257: 178-185.

[41] Hillier SL, Krohn MA, Nugent RP, Gibbs RS (1992b): Characteristics of three vaginal flora patterns assessed by Gram stain among pregnant women. *Am. J. Obstet. Gynecol.* 166: 938-944

[42] Schröder R (1921): Zur Pathogenese und Klinik des vaginalen Fluors. *Zentralbl. Gynakol.* 38: 1350-1361.

[43] Hay PE, Lamont RF, Taylor-Robinson D, Morgan DJ, Ison C, Pearson J (1994): Abnormal bacterial colonisation of the genital tract and subsequent preterm delivery and late miscarriage. *BMJ* 308: 295-298.

[44] Viehweg B, Junghans U, Stephan H, Voigt Th, Faber R (1997): Der Nutzen vaginaler pH-Messungen für die Erkennung potentieller Frühgeburten. *Zentralbl Gynakol* 119: 33-37.

[45] Saling E, Schreiber M (2005): Laktobazillen-Schutzsystem bei Schwangeren – effiziente Vermeidung von Frühgeburten durch Früherkennung von Störungen. *Z Geburtshilfe Neonatol.* 209 : 128-134.

[46] Saling E (1990b): Zusätzliche aktuelle Maßnahmen zur Vermeidung von Spätaborten und Frühgeburten. In: Dudenhausen JW, Saling E: Perinatale Medizin, Bd. XIII (14. Deutscher Kongreß für Perinatale Medizin, Berlin 3.-6.10.1989). Thieme, Stuttgart - New York.

[47] Amsel R, Totten PA, Spiegel CA, Chen KCS, Eschenbach D, Holmes KK (1983): Nonspecific vaginitis. *Am. J. Med.* 74: 14-22.

[48] Saling E (1992): Current Measures to Prevent Late Abortion or Prematurity. In: Saling, E.: *Perinatology. Nestlé Nutrition Workshop Series*, Vol. 26. Raven Press, New York.

[49] Alvarez-Olmos MI, Oberhelman RA (2001): Probiotic Agents and Infectious Diseases: A Modern Perspective on a Traditional Therapy. *Clin. Infect. Dis.* 32: 1567-1576.

[50] AWMF online (2008): Bakterielle Vaginose in Gynäkologie und Geburtshilfe. Arbeitsgemeinschaft der Wissenschaftlichen Medizinischen Fachgesellschaften Deutsche Gesellschaft für Gynäkologie und Geburtshilfe (DGGG), Arbeitsgemeinschaft Infektiologie und Infektionsimmunologie in der Gynäkologie und Geburtshilfe (AGII). http://www.uni-duesseldorf.de/AWMF/ll/015-028.htm(first published: 08/2001 last review: 06/2008).

[51] Lamont RF, Duncan SL, Mandal D, Basset P (2003): Intravaginal Clindamycin to reduce preterm birth in women with abnormal genital tract flora. *Obstet. Gynecol.* 101: 516-522.

[52] Leitich H, Brunbauer M, Bodner-Adler B, Kaider A, Egarter C, Husslein P (2003): Antibiotic treatment of bacterial vaginosis in pregnancy: A meta-analysis. *Am. J. Obstet. Gynecol.* 188: 752-758.

[53] Okun N, Gronau KA, Hannah ME (2005): Antibiotics for Bacterial Vaginosis or Trichomonas vaginalis in pregnancy: a systemic review. *Obstet. Gynecol.* 105: 857-868.

[54] Friese K, Neumann G, Siebert J, Harke HP, Kirschner W (2000): Vergleich zweier lokaler Antiseptika in der klinischen Anwendung bei bakteriell bedingten Vaginalinfektionen. Geburtsh. Frauenheilk. 60: 308-313

[55] Hauth JC, Goldenberg RL, Andrews WW, DuBard MB, Copper RL (1995): Reduced incidence of preterm delivery with metronidazole and erythromycin in women with bacterial vaginosis. *N. Engl. J. Med.* 333 (26): 1732-1736.

[56] Carey JC, Klebanoff MA Hauth JC et al. (2000): Metronidazole to prevent preterm delivery in pregnant women with asymptomatic bacterial vaginosis. *N. Engl. J. Med.* 342: 534-540.

[57] McDonald HM, O'Loughlin JA, Vigneswaran R, Jolley PT, Harvey JA, Bof A, McDonald PJ. (1997): Impact of metronidazole therapy on preterm birth in women with bacterial vaginosis flora (Gardnerella vaginalis): a randomised, placebo controlled trial. *Br. J. Obstet. Gynaecol.* Dec;104(12):1391-7.

[58] Varma R, Gupta JK, James DK, Kilby MD (2006a): Do screening-preventative interventions in asymptomatic pregnancies reduce the risk of preterm delivery – A critical appraisal of the literature. *Eur. J. Obstet. Gynecol. Reprod. Biol.* 127: 145-159.

[59] Varma R, Gupka JK (2006b): Antibiotic treatment of bacterial vaginosis in pregnancy: Multiple meta-analysis and dilemmas in interpretation. *Europ J. Obstet. Gynecol. Reprod. Biolog.* 124: 10-14.

[60] Parent D, Bossens M, Bayot D, Kirkpatrick C, Graf F, Wilkinson FE, Kaiser RR (1996): therapy of bacterial vaginosis using exogenously-applied Lactobacilli acidophili and a low dose of estriol: a placebo-controlles multicentric clinical trial. *Arzneimittelforschung* 46 (1): 68-73.

[61] Hallén A, Jarstrand C, Påhlson C (1992): Treatment of bacterial vaginosis with lactobacilli. *Sex Transm. Dis.* 19 (3): 146-148.

[62] Neri A, Sabah G, Samra Z (1993): Bacterial vaginosis in pregnancy treated with yoghurt. *Acta Obstet. Gynecol. Scand.* 72: 17-19.

[63] Andersch B, Lindell D, Dahlen I, Brandberg A (1990): Bacterial Vaginosis and the Effect of Intermittent Prophylaktic Treatment with an Acid Lactate Gel. *Gynecol. Obstet. Invest* 30: 114-119.

[64] Dennemark N, Meyer-Wilmes M, Schlüter R (1997): Screening and treatment of bacterial vaginosis in the early second trimester of pregnany: a sufficient measure for prevention of preterm deliveries? *Int. J. STD AIDS Vol 8 Supplement* 1: 38-40.

[65] Kenyon S, Pike K, Jones DR, Brocklehurst P, Marlow N, Salt A, Taylor DJ (2008a): Childhood outcomes after prescription of antibiotics to pregnant women with preterm rupture of the membranes: 7-year follow-up of the ORACLE I trial. *Lancet* 372 (9646): 1310-1308.

[66] Kenyon S, Pike K, Jones DR, Brocklehurst P, Marlow N, Salt A, Taylor DJ (2008b): Childhood outcomes after prescription of antibiotics to pregnant women with spontaneous preterm labor: 7-year follow-up of the ORACLE II trial. *Lancet* 372 (9646): 1319-1327.

[67] Di Renzo GC, Cutuli A, Liotta L, Burnelli L, Luzi G (2006): Management of preterm labor: pharmacological and non-pharmacological aspects. In: Kurjak A., Chervenak FA.: *Textbook of Perinatal Medicine.* Informa Healthcare, Second Edition 2006 pp. 1394-1400.

[68] Saling E (1998): Basic aspects of prematurity prevention and results achieved by a suitable, simple program. *J. Perinat. Med.* 26: 466-468.

[69] Saling E, Al-Taie T, Lüthje J, Masur W, Placht A (1998): Efficient and simple program including community-based activities for prevention of very small prematures. In: Kurjak A (ed.): *Textbook of Perinatal Medicine*. London, New York: 1337-1344.

[70] Saling E, Schreiber M, Al-Taie T (2001a): A simple, efficient and inexpensive program for preventing prematurity. *J. Perinat. Med.* 29: 199-211.

[71] Riedewald S, Hanifi-Afshar T, Saling E (1992): pH-Selbstmessung in der Vagina durch die Schwangere (im Vergleich zu Kontrollmessungen durch den Arzt) *Z. Geburtshilfe Perinat.* 196: 61-62.

[72] Hoyme UB, Grosch A, Roemer VM, Saling E (1998): Erste Resultate der Erfurter Frühgeburten-Vermeidungs-Aktion. *Z. Geburtshilfe Neonato.l* 202: 247-250.

[73] Hoyme UB, Möller U, Saling E (2002): Ergebnisse und mögliche Konsequenzen der Thüringer Frühgeburtenvermeidungsaktion 2000. *Geburtshilfe Frauenheilk.* 62: 257-263.

[74] Hoyme UB, Saling E (2004a): Effiziente Frühgeburtenvermeidung - Das Thüringer Modell. *Gynakol. Geburtshilfliche Rundsch.* 44 (1): 2-9.

[75] Hoyme UB, Saling E (2004b): Efficient prematurity prevention is possible by pH-self measurement and immediate therapy of threatening ascending infection. *Eur. J. Obstet. Gynecol. Reprod. Biol.* 115: 148-153.

[76] Hoyme UB, Schwalbe N, Saling E (2005a): Die Effizienz der Thüringer Frühgeburtenvermeidungsaktion 2000 wird durch die Perinatalstatistik der Jahre 2001 – 2003 bestätigt. *Geburtsh. Frauenheil.k* 65: 284-288.

[77] Hoyme UB, Schwalbe N, Saling E (2005b): Efficient Prematurity Prevention is possible by pH-self measurement and immediate therapy of threatening ascending infection. *J. Perinat. Med. 33 Suppl. 1 – Oral presentations.*

[78] Siegmund-Schultze E (2008): pH-Self-Assessment to Reduce the Risk of Preterm Birth. XXI. European Congress of Perinatal Medicine, Istanbul, Turkey, September 10 - 13, 2008. Oral presentation.

[79] BKK Landesverband Nordrhein-Westfalen, Presseservice (2008): "Hallo Baby" – Betriebskrankenkassen in NRW senken Frühgeburtenrate.http://www.bkk-nrw.de/service/presse/index.php?dbt_mode=viewandid=250 (07.02.2008).

[80] Bakketeig LS, Bergsjø P (1998): The epidemiology of preterm birth. In: Kurjak A (ed.): *Textbook of Perinatal Medicine*. London, New York: 1331-1336.

[81] Iams JD, Goldenberg RL, Mercer BM et al. (1998): The preterm prediction study: recurrence risk of spontaneous preterm birth. *Am. J. Obstet. Gynecol.* 178: 1035-1040.

[82] Mercer, Brian M. MD; Goldenberg, Robert L. MD et al. (1999): The Preterm Prediction Study: Effect of gestational age and cause of preterm birth on subsequent obstetric outcome. *Am. J. Obstet. Gynecol.* 181 (5, Part 1): 1216-1221.

[83] McManemy, J, Cooke, E, Amon E, Leet T (2007): Recurrence risk for preterm delivery. *Am. J. Obstet. Gynecol.* 196: 567.e1-567.e7.

[84] Mazaki-Tovi S, Romero R, Kusanovic JP, Erez O, Pineles BL, Gotsch F, Mittal P, Than NG, Espinoza J, Hassan S (2007): Recurrent Preterm Birth. *Semin. Perinatol.* 31: 142-158.

[85] Romero R (2007a): Prevention of spontaneous preterm birth: the role of sonographic cervical length in identifying patients who may benefit from progesterone treatment. *Ultrasound Obstet. Gynecol.* 30: 675-686.

[86] Romero R, Espinoza J, Erez O, Hassan S (2006a): The role of cervical cerclage in obstetric practice: Can the patient who could benefit from this procedure be identified? *Am. J. Obstet. Gynecol.* 194: 1-9.

[87] Schulze G (2008): [Results of Early Total Cervix Occlusion (ETCO) According to Saling in Multiple Pregnancies—a retrospective study of the period 1995-2005.] Ergebnisse des Frühen Totalen Muttermundverschlusses nach Saling (FTMV) bei Mehrlingsschwangerschaften—eine retrospektive Studie der Jahre 1995-2005 *Z. Geburtshilfe Neonatol.* 2008 212: 13-17.

[88] Nugent RP, Krohn MA, Hillier SL (1991): Reliability of diagnosing bacterial vaginosis is improved by a standardized method of gram stain interpretation. *J. Clin. Microbiol.* 29: 297-301

[89] Leitich, Harald; Brunbauer, Mathias; Bodner-Adler, Barbara; Kaider, Alexandra; Egarter, Christian; Husslein, Peter (2003): Antibiotic treatment of bacterial vaginosis in pregnancy: a meta-analysis. *Am. J. Obstet. Gynecol.*, 188, 3: 752–758.

Peer review by:
Prof. Roberto Romero, MD,
Hutzel Hospital,
Wayne State University, Perinatology Research Branch, Detroit

In: Infectious Pregnancy Complications
Editor: Richard N. Canfield

ISBN: 978-1-60471-038-6

Chapter 8

Challenges for the Management of HIV-Infected Pregnant Women in Resource Constrained Settings

***Stephen Mepham**[*a]**, Ruth Bland**[a,b] **and Marie-Louise Newell**[a,c]*

[a] Africa Centre for Health and Population Studies,
University of KwaZulu-Natal, South Africa.
[b] Division of Developmental Medicine, University of Glasgow, UK
[c]Centre for Paediatric Epidemiology and Biostatistics,
Institute of Child Health, UCL, London, UK

Abstract

Pregnant women are at significant risk of acquiring HIV, particularly in areas of high prevalence such as sub-Saharan Africa. HIV in pregnancy results in mother-to-child transmission (MTCT) rates of up to 35% in breast feeding populations as well as relative increases in antenatal death, spontaneous abortion, stillbirth, and low birth weight infants. The identification of HIV-infected women is crucial in the prevention of maternal and infant morbidity and mortality. Whilst most countries recommend 1st or 2nd trimester screening of pregnant women for HIV, the recognition that pregnant women are at risk of primary HIV infection has led to recommendations to repeat testing in the 3rd trimester or during delivery itself. In resource rich countries the use of combination highly active antiretroviral therapy (HAART), avoidance of breastfeeding, and caesarean section delivery has resulted in transmission rates of less than 2%. However, such preventive interventions have been associated with adverse consequences for women and their uninfected infants.

Effective interventions are difficult to implement in developing countries where breastfeeding is critical to infant survival and resources for costly drugs and surgical procedures are scarce. The health of HIV-infected pregnant women in these settings is

* Address all correspondence to:-Dr Stephen Mepham Email: smepham@africacentre.ac.za

further compounded by inter-current conditions, notably sexually transmitted infections, tuberculosis, anaemia, and malaria, which also require appropriate management.

A number of trials have shown the benefit of antiretrovirals alone in reducing mother-to-child transmission (MTCT) of HIV, with WHO recommendations for resource-poor settings potentially associated with significantly reduced perinatal and early post-partum transmission. However, women subsequently face a significant dilemma in the postpartum period where the benefits of breastfeeding but attached risks of HIV vertical transmission need to be balanced against the risk of gastroenteritis and malnutrition associated with replacement feeding and earlier cessation of breastfeeding. Recently evaluated strategies allowing safer breastfeeding include exclusive breastfeeding for six months and neonatal prophylaxis with either lamivudine or nevirapine. The use of prolonged maternal HAART during the breastfeeding period is currently under investigation.

Unfortunately many HIV-infected women remain undetected or fail to benefit from effective and affordable interventions as a result of inequitable access to health care. The greatest challenge of implementing Prevention of Mother-to-Child (PMTCT) interventions remains the provision of integrated, accountable healthcare systems with effective procedures of governance driven by strong leadership.

The Scale of the Problem

WHO estimated that by the end of 2007, 33.2 million (30.6 million-36.1 million) people were living with HIV, two-thirds in sub-Saharan Africa[1]. Over 2 million (1.9 million-2.4 million) are vertically infected children[1]. Pregnant women in sub-Saharan Africa are at significant risk of acquiring HIV with reported incidences of between 1.6 and 5.9 per 100 woman years[2-4]. In KwaZulu-Natal, South Africa, the incidence among women between 25-29 years old was estimated at 7.9 per 100 person-years[5], with prevalence at the first ANC visit of 37.7%[6].

HIV in pregnancy presents many challenges, including effects on pregnancy and pregnancy outcomes, detection, treatment, prevention of mother-to-child transmission (MTCT) of HIV, implementation of strategies to support optimal infant feeding, and interaction with other co-morbidities.

Untreated HIV in Pregnancy Leads to Poorer Maternal And Infant Outcomes

Early attempts to determine if there was a link between HIV infection *per se* and maternal and infant health proved difficult. A meta-analysis by Brocklehurst *et al*[7] in 1998 of 31 prospective observational cohort studies compared the pregnancy outcomes of HIV-infected and uninfected women from both resource rich and poor countries. Whilst HIV infected women appeared to have an increased risk of spontaneous abortion, stillbirth, low birth weight, and perinatal mortality, independent risk factors for poor outcomes such as drug abuse, numbers of sexual partners and sexually transmitted infections were mostly not allowed for (Table 1).

Table 1: Studies of Pregnancy Outcomes and Breastfeeding

Selected Studies	Sample size (Total)	Comparison	Event	Cohort 1	Cohort 2	Unadjusted Risk†/ Adjusted Risk‡ (CI)	P value
HIV and Pregnancy Outcomes (Observational Studies)							
Brocklehurst Meta-analysis[7]	-	HIV-infected v HIV un-infected pregnant women	Spontaneous Abortion	-	-	4.05† (2.75-5.96)	
	1936/28363		Still birth	3.7	2.9	3.91† (2.65-5.77)	
	1196/25053		Perinatal Mortality	3.9	0.4	1.79† (1.14-2.81)	
	3748/34399		Low Birth Weight (<2500g)	20.5	14.9	2.09† (1.86-2.35)	
Rollins *et al*[8]	1449/1401 (3465)	HIV-infected v HIV un-infected pregnant women	Antenatal death/spontaneous abortion/stillbirth	5.6	3.3	1.63‡	0.015
			Low Birth Weight (<2500g)	10.6	7.4	1.45‡	0.02
Safety of ARVs in Pregnancy (Observational Studies)							
European Cohort[135]	331/2092 (2423)	ZDV monotherapy v No ARVs	Prematurity	12.0	15.3	0.76† (0.53-1.09)	
			Low Birth Weight (< 2500g)	12.2	20.1	0.55† (0.39-0.79)	
			Injecting Drug use during pregnancy	15.4	38.4		
			CD4<200	19.0	12.2		
European /Swiss [60]	573/3024 (3920)	ZDV monotherapy v No ARVs	Prematurity	16.8	15.8	1.08† (0.84-1.38)	NS
Cotter *et al*[66]	492/507	ZDV monotherapy v any ARV combination	Low Birth Weight (<2500g)	14.9	16.2		NS
			Preterm Labour	23.9	29.6		<0.05
			Still Birth	0.6	0.4		NS
	134/373	Combination with PI v Combination without PI	Low Birth Weight (<2500g)	17.3	15.9	-	NS
			Still Birth	0	0.5	-	NS
			Preterm Labour	36.6	29.6	1.8‡ (1.1-3.0)	<0.05
			Preterm Labour (PIs <10 weeks)	-	-	2.2‡ (1.6-3.0)	0.0001

Table 1. (Continued)

Breastfeeding (Observational Studies)							
VTS[53]	(1372)	Exclusive BF/NVP (mother /child) v Mixed BF/NVP	Infant postnatal infection at 6 months in infants uninfected at 6 weeks.	4.04(2.29-5.76)	-		
BHITS Meta-analysis[99]	3025 (4085)	BF infants; HIV RNA PCR negative at 4wks	Meta-analysis of 9 trials. Cumulative infection rates of BF infants HIV RNA PCR negative at 4 wks.	3 months 1.6† 12 months 7.0† 6 months 4.2† 18 months 9.3 †			-
NVAZ dataset Taha *et al[100]*	1446 (2000)	BF infants	HIV-exposed but uninfected BF infants at 8wks. BF interval 24 months. Sd NVP at birth; ZDV 7days postpartum. Maternal sd-NVP. Cumulative infection rates at respective time points.	1.5-6 months 1.3/1.22† (CI 0.61-1.83) 6-12months 5.4/4.5† (CI 2.24—4.7) 12-18 months 9.8/ 3.48† (CI 2.24-4.70) 18-24 months 12.6/ 1.27† (CI 0.33-2.19)			-
Breastfeeding (Randomised controlled trial)			**Study Description**	**Intervention**	**Comparison**	**Reduction**	**Pvalue**
Kuhn *et al*[101]	481/477 (958)	EBF/4 month rapid wean v EBF/no rapid wean	Rapid weaning or continued BF (median 16 months). Infant HIV-free survival (HIV uninfected at 4 months)	83.9 (24 months)	80.7	0	0.27
	71/81 (958)		Infant mortality in those infected by 4 months	73.6(24mnth)	54.8	-18.8	0.007

In a more recent cohort study of HIV-infected and uninfected women conducted in the pre-HAART era in northern KwaZulu-Natal, South Africa[8], HIV-infected women had an increased risk of antenatal death, spontaneous abortion, stillbirth as well as a low birth weight (LBW; weight $<2500g$) infant. These infant outcome findings were supported by similar results from recent Tanzanian data[9]. Whilst LBW was significantly associated with infant acquisition of HIV (AOR 2.1, $p<0.01$) and early infant deaths before 6 weeks of age (AOR 8.3, $p<0.001$), maternal HIV was not an independent associated factor with early infant death *per se*. HIV was found to be a much weaker determinant of adverse maternal outcomes than anaemia and malaria in a Tanzanian study of over 1500 births[10]. The reasons for this are unclear although HIV may have contributed to the severity of both of these factors.

HIV Testing is increased By Comprehensive Counselling, PMTCT Availability, and Opt-Out Testing Strategies

The use of a single rapid HIV test at around 20 weeks gestation as recommended by the WHO[11] is a highly cost-effective screening test which should be offered as a minimum to all pregnant women. However, many women in low-resource parts of the world fail to benefit from this test[12]. Suggested reasons contributing to poor uptake of HIV testing include poverty and difficulty in accessing health care, late presentation to antenatal services, stigma, fear of obtaining a positive result and subsequent potential violence and ostracism at home, and lack of awareness of prevention of mother-to-child transmission (PMTCT) interventions[13-18]. In addition, the lack of health care infrastructure, irregular and insufficient supply of test kits, and inadequate numbers of health care professionals and counsellors also contributed[9, 12]. Addressing these issues is a significant challenge, although high test uptake has been demonstrated in some settings through the use of opt-out testing strategies, high quality counselling of pregnant women regarding testing benefits, increased availability of HIV testing services, promotion of PMTCT services to the public at all levels, and changing attitudes towards people living with HIV[19, 20].

Repeat Testing in Late Pregnancy May Be Important to Detect Primary HIV Infection

Routine HIV antibody tests remain negative for the first 4-5 weeks following acute infection[21]. Evidence is accumulating reporting infant perinatal infection arising from maternal HIV infection acquired during pregnancy[22-24]. Studies in Malawi[4] and Uganda[2] demonstrate the significantly increased risk of HIV acquisition during pregnancy with incidences of 5.98 and 7.9 per 100 person years respectively. This has highlighted the need to adopt enhanced testing strategies that will detect primary HIV infection (PHI) during pregnancy.

The detection of PHI is important for two reasons. Firstly, it allows early appropriate HIV clinical management with short term antiretroviral regimens for PMTCT prophylaxis, and secondly, early identification allows a longer potential duration of PMTCT antiretroviral therapy, reducing the risk of MTCT[25]. Given that a high maternal RNA viral load at the time of delivery acts as a major risk factor in transmission[26], it is likely that the MTCT rate will be increased during the high viral loads associated with PHI[27].

The diagnosis of HIV in developing countries is often dependant on a single use HIV test kit. A second test kit from a different manufacturer is conventionally used to confirm a first positive result (serial testing). However, in an approach endorsed by the WHO[28], some studies have shown that the detection of PHI may be improved if 2 rapid tests are used simultaneously on all women to also confirm a negative result (parallel testing)[21, 29]. Further, whilst modern laboratory based 3rd and 4th generation ELISAs (the latter including a p24 antigen) can reduce the window period to less than 2 weeks[30], a number of high and low-resource countries have introduced a 2-stage testing strategy which includes repeat testing in the third trimester [31, 32]. Some have even advocated providing rapid HIV testing to women of uncertain HIV status presenting in labour, an approach that has proved feasible and cost-effective in both a resource rich[33, 34] and resource poor environment[12].

In non-pregnant, HIV-antibody negative individuals other testing methodologies have been used to detect PHI notably nucleic acid amplification techniques (NAAT). The cost-effectiveness of NAAT is improved by pooling the serum of many individuals to screen for the presence of HIV RNA with a positive result then prompting individual testing of each sample. NAAT testing has proved cost effective in low seroprevalent areas[35], and has increased the case detection rate of acute infections by 6-8% in both high resource[36, 37] and low resource settings[21, 38]. Such alternative testing algorithms allows, in high prevalence and incidence settings, substantial numbers of PHIs to be detected, offering new opportunities for HIV prevention and treatment[21].

Mother to Child Transmission (MTCT) of HIV

Globally each year there are around 800,000 new paediatric HIV infections[39]. By 2 years of age around 35% of exposed infants can become infected with HIV, with transmission occurring in utero, during labour, and postpartum as a result of breastfeeding[40]. The risk of transmission increases with a low maternal CD4 count[41, 42], maternal high viral load[43-46], occurrence of sexually transmitted infections during pregnancy[47], prolonged rupture of membranes[47, 48], vaginal delivery (as opposed to caesarean section)[49, 50], breastfeeding duration[51, 52], mixed feeding[53, 54], and maternal mastitis[55, 56]. As antiretroviral regimens to reduce peripartum transmission have become widely available in high HIV prevalent areas, the reduction of transmission through breastfeeding is an urgent priority.

Antiretrovirals for Women in a Resource-Rich Setting

Highly successful interventions employed in developed countries including the use of HAART, elective caesarean sections, and the avoidance of breastfeeding, have reduced transmissions to under 2%[57]. Current US 2008 antiretroviral therapy (ART) guidelines for women requiring therapy for her own health (Table 2)[58] recommend commencing potent combination therapy consisting of 2 nucleoside reverse transcriptase inhibitors (NRTI) plus 1 non-nucleoside reverse transcriptase inhibitor (NNRTI) or protease inhibitor (PI). Because of its ability to cross the placenta, zidovudine (ZDV) has played a central role in most antiretroviral trials, and as such, should ideally form part of any treatment combination. The drug choices are the same as for non-pregnant individuals but with some caveats (Table 3).

A randomised controlled trial of 436 women showed that elective caesarean section at 38 weeks was associated with a reduced risk of MTCT at 6 weeks postpartum compared with vaginal delivery (1.8% versus 10.5%, OR 0.2(0.1-0.6), $p<0.001$)[49]. Current US guidelines (2008) recommend that the HIV plasma RNA viral load is rendered undetectable before delivery, and, despite the paucity of supportive evidence, advise women with viral loads over 1000 copies/ml to be scheduled for an elective caesarean section[58].

With these PMTCT strategies rates of less than 2% have been achieved (Table 4). Women requiring ARVs for their own health should be provided with the same antiretroviral options in conjunction with the avoidance of breastfeeding and the appropriate use of caesarean section (Table 2)[58].

ART Regimens Including Pis May Predispose to an Increased Risk of Preterm Delivery

Since 1998 combination ART, including protease inhibitors, has been associated with preterm labour, with European cohorts showing a link[59-62], although others from the United States showing no effect[63-65]. Drawing firm conclusions however has been difficult given the differences between the populations and methodological approaches[63] and the lack of controlling for the duration of PI use[63], prior preterm delivery and clinical stage/viral load[59-62], the latter 2 major risk factors for preterm delivery.

Table 2: Management Principles of Prevention of Mother to Child Transmission (PMTCT) of HIV-1

Resource Rich Settings (Modified from US PMTCT Guidelines 2008[58])			Resource Poor Settings (Modified from WHO Guidelines[40, 74])
Preconception and Antenatal		-Use of non teratogenic ARVs if planning pregnancy -Aim for maximal preconception viral suppression -Consider intrauterine/ intravaginal insemination in HIV discordant couples.	-Standard antenatal care (at least 4 visits) -Counselling: development of a birth plan, maternal and infant health and nutrition needs including breastfeeding, family planning and safe sexual practices -ART history including PMTCT interventions -Screening for anaemia, malaria, sexually transmitted infections (especially syphilis), HIV, tuberculosis -Iron/ folate/ multivitamin supplementation, impregnated bed net promotion/intermittent sulphadoxine-pyrimethamine -Immunization (especially tetanus).
		-Standard Antenatal Care, HIV Staging, ARV drug history -Baseline Bloods (CD4, HIV RNA Viral Load, Full blood count, renal and liver function), Baseline ARV resistance testing -Screen for HBV, HCV, rubella, syphilis -First trimester ultrasound to assess dates	
ARV	**For own Health purposes**	Criteria: CD4<350cells/ml; Viral load >100,000 copies/ml; Declining CD4 >100 cells/ml/year; symptomatic disease.	Criteria: CD4<200 cells/ml, or CD4<350 cells/ml PLUS Stage 3, or stage 4
		-Treatment: Immediate triple therapy (ZDV/another NRTI/NNRTI or PI), Avoid EFV, Avoid NVP if CD4>250 -Tailor to individual and resistance testing -Cotrimoxazole prophylaxis	-ZDV/3TC/NVP or PI or (less effective) triple NRTI Substitute EFV for NVP or a PI unless in 2nd/3rd trimester -Potential for suboptimal suppression in women receiving NNRTI who have had previous NVP PMTCT -Cotrimoxazole prophylaxis

Table 2. (Continued)

Resource Rich Settings (Modified from US PMTCT Guidelines 2008[58])			Resource Poor Settings (Modified from WHO Guidelines[40, 74])
	For PMTCT purposes	Initiation of HAART as above from 12 weeks gestation until end of delivery. Tailor to individual and resistance testing;	ZDV from 28 weeks until delivery. Contraindicated in significant maternal anaemia (<7g/L)
	Monitoring HIV RNA viral load response and toxicity	-4 weeks-1 log reduction; 24wks <400 copies/ml; 48wks <50 copies/ml. -Monitor monthly; If suboptimal suppression, consider resistance testing -Watch LFTs (PI, NVP, hepatic steatosis, lactic acidosis), FBC (ZDV)	Watch for hepatic dysfunction if NVP and CD4>250 cells/ml
Delivery		HIV RNA viral load 34-36wks >1000 copies/ml- arrange elective C/S at 38 weeks; If stopping ARVS postpartum, stop NNRTI 7 days before stopping other ARVs. Women of unknown HIV status: Rapid HIV test. If positive, intravenous ZDV and sd-NVP	Intrapartum maternal sd-NVP PLUS single dose ZDV/3TC
Postpartum/ Infant		-Infant feeding counselling with promotion of replacement feeding -6 weeks ZDV started within 6-12 hours -Immunisations -HIV RNA PCR 6 weeks -Infant Cotrimoxazole until shown to be HIV RNA PCR negative.	-Postpartum Maternal ZDV/3TC 7days; Infant sd-NVP PLUS ZDV 7days (28 days if maternal ART <4 weeks) -Infant feeding counseling detailing risks and benefits of different options. Support Exclusive Breastfeeding for 6 months (unless replacement feeding acceptable, feasible, sustainable, affordable, and safe before then) -Immunisations -HIV RNA PCR at 6 weeks -Infant Cotrimoxazole until shown to be PCR negative.

Table 3: Side effects of Antiretrovirals pertinent to pregnancy[58]

Nucleoside Reverse Transcriptase Inhibitors (NRTI)	
Anaemia	Zidovudine is associated with anaemia and neutropenia in women and infants[136]
Mitochondrial Toxicity	All NRTI drugs associated with neuropathy, myopathy, cardiomyopathy, pancreatitis, hepatic steatosis, and lactic acidosis. Combinations of d4T and 3TC[137], and d4T and ddI[138] have been particularly associated with severe life threatening lactic acidosis in pregnancy.
Non Nucleoside Reverse Transcriptase Inhibitors (NNRTI)	
Efavirenz (EFV) Induced Teratogenicity	EFV should be avoided in the first trimester due to significant fetal malformations in 3/20 monkeys in preclinical studies[139]. Use in the 2nd trimester may be considered if there are no other alternatives. Many clinicians would continue the drug if pregnancy has occurred whilst on EFV and the woman is into her 2nd trimester[58, 140].
Nevirapine (NVP)-Induced Hepatotoxicity	Women with a CD4 >250 cells/ml are at an increased risk of potentially life-threatening NVP-induced hepatotoxicity and rash. NVP should only be started in these circumstances when the benefits outweigh the risks in conjunction with frequent monitoring of liver function[141, 142].
Protease Inhibitors (PI), Entry inhibitors, and Integrase Inhibitors	
Hyperglycaemia	Whilst PIs may cause hyperglycaemia, there is no evidence that their use in pregnancy confers any additional risk[143].
No experience in pregnancy	PIs: Atazanavir, Darunavir, Fosamprenavir, Tipranavir; Entry inhibitors: Enfurvirtide and Maraviroc; Integrase inhibitor: Raltegravir[58].

Table 4: Studies of PMTCT Interventions

Selected Antiretroviral Studies	Sample size Arm/Arm (Total)	Comparison	Study Description	BF or RF	Intervention (95% CI; where listed)	Comparison (95% CI; where listed)	Reduction	P Value
Zidovudine monotherapy throughout pregnancy and delivery								
PACTG 076[136] (USA)	180/183	ZDV v placebo	From 14 wks antepartum, (iv) ZDV during delivery; 6 wks infant;	RF	8.3	25.5	67	0.001
Combination Antiretrovirals								
ANRS 075[64] (France)	445/899	ZDV/3TC v ZDV (historical control)	ZDV from 14 wks/3TC from 32 wks; infants 3TC 6 wks.	RF	1.6	6.8	76	<0.001
WITS, observational cohort[144]	710	ZDV	Observational study	RF	10.4(8.2-12.6)	Ref. Arm	-	-
	186/710	Dual Therapy v ZDV	Observational study	RF	3.8 (1.1-6.5)	10.4	OR 0.33	0.03
	250/710	HAART v ZDV	Observational study	RF	1.2 (0-2.5)	10.4	OR 0.15	0.002
Dorenbaum *[145]*	642/628	ZDV or Dual or HAART Plus NVP or placebo	Observational study. Maternal ARVs; NVP to mother and infant.	RF	1.4^{β}	1.6	0	NS
Short Course ARVs v Placebo								
5	192/197 (421)	ZDV v placebo	From 36 wks antenatal to intrapartum; 7 days ZDV postpartum (mother)	RF	18.0	27.5	35(0.05-0.60) 6 months MTCT Rate	0.027
RETRO CI[77] (Cote d'Ivoire)	140/140 (280)	ZDV v placebo	From 36 wks antepartum to intrapartum	BF	12.2(6.2-17.8)	21.7(14.0-28.8)	44 (4 wks MTCT Rate)	0.05
PETRA [78] (Tanzania, Uganda, South Africa)	475/371 (1797)	ZDV/3TC v placebo PETRA A	From 36 wks antepartum (mother); 1 wk infant, 1 wk postpartum (mother).	BF	5.7	15.3	63 (35-79) 6 wks MTCT Rate	0.001

Table 4. (Continued)

Selected Antiretroviral Studies	Sample size Arm/Arm (Total)	Comparison	Study Description	BF or RF	Intervention (95% CI; where listed)	Comparison (95% CI; where listed)	Reduction	P Value
	474/371 (1797)	ZDV/3TC v placebo PETRA B	Intrapartum (mother); 1 wk infant; 1 wk postpartum (mother).	BF	8.9	15.3	42(6-64) 6 wks MTCT Rate	0.016
	471/371 (1797)	ZDV/3TC v placebo PETRA C	Intrapartum	BF	14.2	15.3	0 (6 wks MTCT Rate)	NS
Selected Antiretroviral Studies	**Sample size** Arm/Arm (Total)	**Comparison**	**Study Description**	**BF or RF**	**Intervention** (95% CI; where listed)	**Comparison** (95% CI; where listed)	**Reduction**	**P value**
Longer Course versus Short Course								
PHPT-1[25] (Thailand)	419	ZDV: Long-Long arm	From 28 wks antepartum; 6 wks infant	RF	6.5(4.1-8.9)	Reference Arm	-	-
	350/419	ZDV: Long-Short arm	From 28 wks antepartum; 3 days infant	RF	4.7(2.4-7.0)	6.5(4.1-8.9)	28	NS
	345/419	ZDV: Short-Long arm	From 35 wks antepartum; 6 wks infant	RF	8.6(5.6-11.6)	6.5(4.1-8.9)	0	NS
	323/419	ZDV: Short-short arm	From 35 wks antepartum; 3 days infant[a]	RF	10.5(6.4-14.4)	6.5(4.1-8.9)	0	-
	1437 (all)	ZDV Pooled Analysis	(Long-Long PLUS Long-Short) v (Short-Long PLUS Short-Short). 6 Months MTCT Rate	RF	1.6(0.7-2.6)	5.1(3.2-7.0)	69	<0.001
Bhoopat *et al[79]* (Thailand)	23/27	ZDV (long) v ZDV (short)	ZDV 62-92 days antenatally v ZDV 14-35 days antenatally.HIV-1 detected in placental tissue	-	22	67	67	<0.02

Table 4. (Continued)

Selected	Sample	Comparison		BF or	Intervention	Comparison	Reduction	P

Antiretroviral Studies	size Arm/Arm (Total)		Study Description	RF	(95% CI; where listed)	(95% CI; where listed)		Value
Intrapartum Nevirapine								
HIVNET 012[80, 81] (Uganda)	308/310 (626)	sd-NVP v ZDV	200mg Intrapartum; 2mg/kg NVP infant within 72hours v Maternal ZDV 300 mg 3hrly until delivery; neonatal ZDV	BF	11.9(8.2-15.7)	21.3(16.4-26.2)	44 (8wks)	0.003
					15.7(11.5-19.8)	25.8(20.7-30.8)	39(18mnth MTCT rate)	0.0023
SAINT[82] (South Africa)	662/657 (1317)	Intrapartum Maternal/infant ZDV/3TC v Maternal/infant NVP	Intrapartum Maternal Multiple dose ZDV/3TC;Maternal/Infant ZDV/3TC 1 week v Intrapartum Maternal sd-NVP; Infant sd-NVP within 24-48 hours	BF	9.3(7.0-11.6)	12.3(9.7-15.0)	23 (8wks MTCT rate)	NS
Zidovudine combined with Nevirapine								
PHPT-2[83] (Thailand)	724/721 (1844)	ZDV/ NVP –NVP versus ZDV/NVP-Placebo versus ZDV/Placebo-Placebo$^{\delta}$	ZDV from 28 wks antepartum; NVP intrapartum (maternal); NVP (infant)	RF	1.1(0.3-2.2) NVP-NVP	6.3(3.8-8.9) Placebo/ placebo	83 (6mnths MTCT rate)	<0.001
Short course Neonatal prophylaxis								
NVAZ[90] (Malawi)	484/468 (1119)	NVP/ZDV v NVP	Single dose NVP at birth; ZDV for 7days postpartum	BF	15.3	20.9	27 (6wks MTCT rate)	0.03
Taha *et al[91]* (Malawi)	446/448 (894)	Maternal NVP; Neonatal NVP/ZDV v NVP alone	Maternal NVP; Single dose NVP at birth; ZDV for 7days postpartum	BF	16.3(12.7-19.8)	14.1(10.7-17.4)	0 (6 wks MTCT rate)	0.30

Table 4. (Continued)

Selected Antiretroviral Studies	Sample size Arm/Arm	Comparison	Study Description	BF or RF	Intervention (95% CI; where listed)	Comparison (95% CI; where listed)	Reduction	P Value

	(Total)							
Longer course Neonatal prophylaxis								
MASHI[97] (Botswana)	598/602 (1200)	BF/ZDV v RF	Maternal ZDV from 34 wks to intrapartum. Infant BF/ZDV,6 months or replacement feeding/ZDV,1 month	BF	9.0	5.6	0 (7 month cumulative MTCT rate)	0.04
	598/602 (1200)	BF/ZDV v RF	Maternal ZDV from 34 wks to intrapartum. Infant BF/ZDV,6 months or replacement feeding/ZDV,1 month	BF	15.1	13.9	0 (18 months death/HIV)	0.6
MITRA[103] (Tanzania)	398/264	Neonatal 3TC	Maternal ZDV/3TC from 36 wks to 7 days postpartum; Neonatal ZDV/3TC 7 days with/without 6 months 3TC	BF	8.5	15.5	45 (6 months death/HIV)	<0.001
SWEN[104] (multicentre)	977/1047	Neonatal 6 wks NVP v sd NVP	Intrapartum sd-NVP (maternal); neonatal sd-NVP or 6 weeks NVP	BF	5.1	6.3	19 (6 months MTCT rate)	0.16
PEPI[105] (Malawi)	1099/1088 (3016)	Neonatal NVP (long)/ZDV (short) v control	NVP 14 wks/ZDV 7days V Sd NVP/ZDV 7 days (control)	BF	5.2(3.9-7.0)	10.6(8.7-12.8)	51(9months MTCT rate)	<0.001
	1089/1088 (3016)	Neonatal NVP (long)/ZDV (long) v control	NVP 14 wks/ZDV 14 wks V Sd NVP/ZDV 7 days (control)	BF	6.4(4.9-8.3)	10.6(8.7-12.8)	45(9months MTCT rate)	0.002
SIMBA[106]	199/198 (413)	Neonatal 3TC v Neonatal NVP during BF period PLUS 4 weeks	Antepartum 36 weeks ZDV/ddI to1 wk post partum; Neonatal 3TC or NVP for BF PLUS 4 weeks.	BF	11.05	10.60	0 (6 months Total HIV/deaths)	NS

Table 4. (Continued)

Selected Antiretroviral Studies	Sample size Arm/Arm (Total)	Comparison	Study Description	BF or RF	Intervention (95% CI; where listed)	Comparison (95% CI; where listed)	Reduction	P Value

Postpartum maternal prophylaxis								
MITRA PLUS [108] Observational (Tanzania)	441 (total)	ZDV/3TC/NVP (NVP replaced by NLF[γ])	Maternal HAART from 34 wks to 6 months postpartum	BF	5.0 (6 months)	-	-	-

[α]PHPT-1 Short-Short arm was discontinued during the interim analysis (inferiority).
[β]Dorenbaum *et al* Trial terminated early- lower than expected transmission rates
[γ]MITRA PLUS Following the finding that women with higher CD4 counts have a higher risk of NVP-induced hepatotoxicity.
[δ]PHPT-2 Placebo-Placebo "Nevirapine" arm terminated during an interim analysis due to inferiority

3TC Lamivudine
BF Breastfeeding
HAART Highly Active Antiretroviral Therapy
NVP Nevirapine
RF Replacement Feeding
Sd-NVP Single Dose Nevirapine
ZDV Zidovudine

A 12 year, prospective, single centre American cohort study with a standardised protocol demonstrated that HIV-infected pregnant women treated with a PI-containing combination had an increased risk of preterm labour (<37 weeks) when compared to women using monotherapy or combination therapy without a PI[66] (Table 1). This finding was supported by results from a study of 227 women in London which found an association between preterm labour and PI-containing combinations only in those who had started their ARVs during their pregnancy (OR 3.5, CI 1.5-8, p=0.02)[67]. Another UK-based study showed an increased risk for women taking HAART *per se* (OR 1.51, CI 1.19-1.93, p=0.001) and not just PI-containing combinations[68]. However, although the benefits of HAART in reducing MTCT risk outweigh the potential adverse effects in most settings, PI-containing combinations should be started during pregnancy with some caution[66, 67], women counselled about potential risks[66, 67], with ZDV monotherapy combined with caesarean section remaining an alternative option for women receiving ART for prophylaxis purposes only[67].

One proposed mechanism that may explain the phenomenon of PI-induced premature delivery involves reversal of the TH1 to TH2 cytokine switch that naturally occurs during pregnancy. Immunosuppressive TH2 cytokines such as IL10 and IL4 are produced by the fetoplacental unit to reduce cell mediated activation and maintain the fetal "allograft". Antiretrovirals act to promote type 1 cytokines, such as IL2 and γ-interferon, which may benefit the control of HIV disease but which could harm the viability of a pregnancy[69, 70].

Antiretrovirals for Women in a Resource-Poor Setting

Many of the costly and complex interventions available in resource rich settings are inappropriate in a developing world setting. The complete avoidance of breastfeeding by HIV-infected women in many parts of the world exposes infants to risks including life-threatening infections[71] and malnutrition due to inadequate replacement feeding[72, 73]. WHO[74] ART recommendations for women requiring ART for their own health in developing countries tend to follow similar principles as for resource-rich settings (Table 2), although the absolute drug choices and the CD4 count at which they are started will vary locally according to cost and availability. However, for women requiring ART for PMTCT purposes, shorter, less expensive prophylactic regimens appropriate to a developing world setting have become available (Table 4).

1. Antepartum Arvs Alone Reduce Peripartum MTCT

Three early trials in a breastfeeding population, DITRAME[75, 76], RETRO-CI[77], and PETRA[78] demonstrated that ZDV or ZDV/lamivudine (3TC) given from 36 weeks was effective in reducing early HIV transmission at 6 weeks when compared to placebo. However, infants who were breastfed remained at risk of becoming infected and no significant difference was seen in the risk of MTCT[78] or infant death[76] at 18 months.

The subsequent PHPT-1 study[25] and that from Bhoopat et al[79] conducted in non-breastfeeding populations demonstrated that maternal ZDV starting at 28 weeks gestation was superior to those starting at 36 weeks gestation (1.6% versus 5.1%, p<0.001).

2. Intrapartum Nevirapine is Effective but Associated with NVP Resistance Mutations

In HIVNET 012[80] single dose nevirapine (sd-NVP) given to women at the onset of labour as well as to neonates (within 72 hours of birth) was shown to significantly reduce MTCT rates when compared to intrapartum maternal ZDV plus 7 days of neonatal oral ZDV (11.9% versus 21.3%). A significant difference remained through to 18 months, with a median of 9 months of breastfeeding for 99% of all infants. (15.7% versus 25.8%)[81]. The similar South African SAINT trial[82], which differed from HIVNET 012 by comparing maternal and neonate combined ZDV/3TC with maternal and neonate sd-NVP, showed equivalence between the two arms.

In formula-fed infants, the PHPT-2[83] trial demonstrated the superiority of combining maternal/infant NVP with maternal ZDV commencing at 28 weeks and infant oral ZDV for 1 week. The 6 week transmission rate of the arm receiving both maternal and infant NVP was lower than the placebo-placebo arm (1.9% v 6.3%), but statistically similar to the maternal NVP/infant placebo group (2.8%).

Subsequent analysis of the HIVNET 012 dataset showed that 19% (21/111) of women had developed NVP resistance (most commonly K103N) at 6-8 weeks[84] as had 46% (11/24) of evaluable infected infants (most commonly Y181C). These mutations became undetectable in all women and infants by 12-24 months. A meta-analysis of studies using sd-NVP found NVP resistance prevalence of 35.7% over 10 maternal treatment arms, and 52.6% in 7 infant treatment arms. This latter figure falls to 16.5% when combined with other antiretroviral[85]. An increased risk of virological failure appears to be present if NNRTI-containing HAART is started within 6 months of sd-NVP given for PMTCT purposes[86, 87] but not if the intervening period is longer than 6 months[86-88].

3. Nevirapine Resistance May Be Reduced By the Use of Antiretroviral "Tails" or Avoidance of Maternal Single Dose Nevirapine

NNRTI resistance following the use of sd-NVP occurs as result of prolonged sub-therapeutic levels resulting from its long half life. The provision of a simultaneous "tail" of shorter acting ARVs to provide additional viral suppression during this period leads to significantly fewer mutations. In one study the addition of a 3 day postpartum tail of ZDV/3TC to women receiving short-course ZDV/3TC and sd-NVP led to 4.3% (3/69, CI 0.9-12.2%) NVP mutations compared 38.1% (16/42, CI 23.6-54.4%) using short-course ZDV and sd-NVP without a postpartum tail[88]. In another study, NVP-resistance was less frequent in infants aged 6-8 weeks who had received sd-NVP plus ZDV and whose mothers had not received single dose NVP compared to infants who, along with their mothers, had received single dose NVP alone (4/15 (27%) versus 20/23 (87%), p<0.01) [89].

4. Additional Short Course Neonatal Prophylaxis Is Superior to Sd-NVP Alone

In a study from Malawi[90], infants of women presenting late to antenatal services (within 2 hours of delivery) who received 1 week of ZDV plus NVP were at significantly lower risk of becoming infected by 6-8 weeks than those who received NVP alone (15.3% versus 20.9%). In contrast, the addition of neonatal ZDV made no significant difference when intrapartum NVP was provided to both mother and child [91]. It is unclear why this study did not show an additional benefit of short course ZDV but it is speculated that ZDV may not have offered any additional inhibition over maximal neonatal concentrations of NVP.

Breastfeeding Interventions

Breastfeeding is crucial to the survival of infants in resource constrained environments[40, 71, 72, 92-95]. Its benefit is mediated through the transfer of passive immunity and nutrition[96], protection against infection (notably diarrhoea, pneumonia, neonatal sepsis, and otitis media), and also helps mothers space their pregnancies[40]. However, breastfeeding by HIV-infected mothers exposes infants to HIV[40].

Whilst many short course regimens result in a reduction in peripartum transmission assessed at 6 weeks, there is often either no improvement in the HIV-uninfected infant survival at 2 years as a result of infectious illness and malnutrition following rapid cessation of breastfeeding, or subsequent HIV infection through breastfeeding. The MASHI study[97], which randomised infants taking 1 month of oral ZDV to receive either breastfeeding or formula milk for 6 months, showed that whilst the formula arm resulted in fewer HIV infections at 7 months, the combined mortality and HIV infection between the arms at 18 months were similar (13.9% versus 15.1%, Table 4).

1. Exclusive Breastfeeding Reduces the Risk of Postpartum Vertical Transmission

Exclusive feeding means giving the infant breastmilk only, with no additional fluids or solids. The Vertical Transmission Study (VTS), conducted in a largely rural area of South Africa[53], was a non-randomised intervention study which examined postnatal HIV transmission among 1372 HIV-infected women, 1132 of whom initiated breastfeeding, mostly exclusive, after birth. The median duration of breastfeeding was 159 days. The estimated risk of acquisition of infection at 6 months of age in exclusively breastfed infants who were HIV-uninfected between 4 and 8 weeks was 4.04%. There was an almost 11-fold difference in postnatal risk between exclusively breastfed (EBF) infants and those who had received breast milk and solids; and a nearly two-fold difference between EBF infants and those who, at 12 weeks, had received breastmilk and formula milk (HR 1.82, 0.98-3.36, p=0.057).

2. Prolonged Breastfeeding Increases the Risk Of MTCT But Rapid Cessation of Breastfeeding May Be Associated with Increased Infant Mortality

Although it has been suggested that the highest risk of MTCT occurs during the early months of breastfeeding[98], the additional importance of late postnatal transmission was demonstrated by a meta-analysis of 9 trials which showed that 42% of infants with known timing of infection were infected through breastfeeding after 6 months[99]. A recent Malawian study[100] of 1256 breastfed infants known to be uninfected at age 6 weeks showed that 9.7% infants became infected by 24 months with the majority (87.4%) occurring as late infections after 6 months of age. Risk factors included high plasma and breast milk HIV RNA viral loads, and mastitis. These trials show that the risk of acquiring HIV continues for the duration of breastfeeding [100].

Recent studies suggest that policies of rapid cessation of breastfeeding at 6 months, when complementary feeds need to be introduced for all infants, may be associated with significant infant morbidities as well as incurring financial costs of milk-replacement provision and social costs of stigmatisation through the disclosure of HIV status[101]. A randomised trial in Zambia[101] compared HIV-infected women randomised to rapid weaning at 4 months with women who were supported to exclusively breastfeed for 6 months with cessation of breastfeeding when they thought appropriate after relevant counselling. In spite of the relatively long median duration of 16 months to cessation of breastfeeding in the group who exclusively breastfed, the study showed that the action of rapidly stopping breastfeeding HIV uninfected infants at 4 months did not improve infant HIV-free survival at 24 months. The difference may have been greater since only 69% of women in the rapid wean group had stopped by the end of 5 months with the rest continuing to breastfeed, increasing the number of HIV infected infants in that arm. WHO recommends that HIV-infected breastfeeding women should continue breastfeeding after 6 months unless an acceptable, feasible, affordable, sustainable, and safe (AFASS) alternative is available[102], with appropriate good quality counselling[51].

3. Longer Neonatal Prophylaxis Significantly Reduces the Risk of Postnatal Transmission Through Breastfeeding

A number of trials have investigated the principle of providing infants with a prolonged course of ZDV, 3TC, or NVP to cover the breastfeeding period[97, 103-106] (Table 4). Of these the PEPI trial[105], conducted in breastfeeding infants of mothers who had not received any MTCT interventions, showed that those infants receiving extended prophylaxis with NVP or NVP plus ZDV for 14 weeks showed significantly fewer MTCT at 9 months than the control group (5.2% versus 6.4% versus 10.6%). Whilst clearly effective and simple to implement, the risk of transmitting NVP or 3TC resistant virus to infants who become HIV-infected despite prophylaxis is of significant concern[107]. In addition, the costs of providing prolonged antiretrovirals at a programmatic level need to be addressed. Future studies are awaited, in particular the PROMISE study (NIH; extended NVP) and the PROMISE-PEP (ANRS; extended 3TC) in uninfected infants whose mothers receive antenatal and peripartum ART.

4. Post Partum Maternal Prophylaxis is Likely to Reduce the Risk of Postnatal Transmission in a Breastfeeding Population

The principle of providing up to 6 months of postpartum triple therapy to breastfeeding mothers to reduce the risk of postnatal transmission was demonstrated in the non-randomized, open-label, prospective MITRA PLUS study[108] and the similar Kisumu Breastfeeding Study (Kenya)[109], the former achieving 6 month MTCT rates of 5.0% (Table 4). Further information will come from two randomised trials evaluating the use of 6 months of maternal HAART for the prevention of postnatal transmission, the multicentre, sub-Saharan "Kesho Bora" trial[110] and the Breastfeeding, Antiretrovirals and Nutrition (BAN) study in Malawi[111].

Co-Morbidity with Malaria, Anaemia, and Tuberculosis Results in Poor Outcomes

With the burden of HIV in pregnancy occurring in sub-Saharan Africa, it is not surprising that there will be frequent overlap with other conditions which cause morbidity in pregnancy, notably malaria, anaemia, sexually transmitted infections, and tuberculosis (TB)[10].

Studies in areas of stable malaria transmission have demonstrated higher maternal HIV plasma RNA viral loads in dually infected women although it is unclear if this results in higher MTCT rates[112]. Infants are more likely to be of LBW, preterm birth, and intrauterine growth retardation than those infected with either pathogen alone. In addition, women have higher rates of clinical malaria, higher parasite counts, more anaemia, and reduced response to antimalarial therapy[112]. A recent meta-analysis demonstrated that the use of intermittent monthly sulphadoxine-pyrimethamine in HIV-infected women in their 1st or 2nd pregnancy not receiving cotrimoxazole resulted in less placental malaria (RR 0.34, CI 0.18-0.64) and higher birth weight (mean difference 112 g, CI 19-205g)[113-115]. Pregnant women in malarial areas are also advised to use impregnated bed nets.

Anaemia during pregnancy is common, particularly in resource poor countries. HIV-infected women have a higher prevalence of anaemia than HIV-uninfected women, especially with increasing immunosuppression[116, 117]. HIV may cause anaemia directly through disruption of haematopoiesis, through the host immune system cytokine response (anaemia of chronic disease), and through antiretroviral therapy, most notably ZDV[118]. As a result, the WHO recommends avoiding ZDV in women with a haemoglobin below 7g/L until the anaemia is corrected[74]. Anaemia may also be caused by nutritional deficiencies (iron, folate, and Vitamin A), parasitic infections (schistosomiasis and hookworm), and other chronic infections, and increases in severity as pregnancy progresses (up to 69% by the 3rd trimester)[119]. Conventional antenatal care provides iron, folate and multivitamin supplements as prophylaxis against anaemia. Severe HIV–associated anaemia has been managed with either blood transfusion or, in resource rich countries, erythropoietin alpha[120]. However mortality is increased with the use of the former, possibly secondary to transfusion related immunosuppression, and little experience exists with the latter in pregnancy[118]. Whilst anecdotal evidence exists implicating helminthic infections in adverse pregnancy outcomes and enhancing HIV-vertical transmission, they play a minor role in causing anaemia in HIV-infected pregnant women in developing countries[121, 122].

Nearly a million people acquire sexually transmitted infections (STI) including HIV every day[123]. HIV and STI's are intimately interlinked, having similar risk factors and with each potentiating the acquisition of the other. Concomitant genital ulcer disease, mostly herpes simplex virus type 2[124] and syphilis[125], has been attributed to an increased risk of HIV acquisition. In addition, symptomatic and asymptomatic shedding of herpes simplex type 2 increases HIV-1 viral loads[126]. Whilst initial trials of HSV-2 suppressive therapy with acyclovir seem ineffective at reducing HIV acquisition[127], it remains unclear if HSV suppression can delay HIV disease progression. Untreated, often asymptomatic, gonococcal and chlamydial infections results in pelvic inflammatory disease in up to 40% of women, 25% of which will result in infertility, as well as blindness in 4000 neonates every year as a result of neonatal opthalmia[123]. In a study of HIV-infected women, those co-infected with syphilis, but not other infections, had a significantly increased risk of stillbirth (OR 4.8; 95% CI 2.4-9.5)[128], in addition to the risk of congenital syphilis. All pregnant women should have on-site syphilis serology and screened for symptoms suggestive of an STI[123]. Appropriate diagnostics, targeted treatment, and contact tracing is ideal although a syndromic approach to management is often used in resource poor settings[123]. Antenatal clinics are an ideal opportunity in which to discuss and promote contraceptive choices, safe sexual practices, and family planning choices.

With nearly 9 million new cases and over 2 million deaths per year, TB is the second leading cause of infectious disease after HIV/AIDS[129]. TB accounted for 15% of maternal deaths in a prospective South African study of over 50,000 deliveries between 1996 and 1998, with a case fatality rate of 102.7 per 1000 in co-infected women, and an increased relative risk of 3.2 compared to HIV-uninfected individuals[130]. TB in pregnancy is often diagnosed in the postpartum period, possibly in part due to difficulty in diagnosis during pregnancy through the masking of weight loss and systemic symptoms, with an increased risk in those with CD4 counts <200 cells/ml and high viral load[131]. Women with a cough lasting longer than 2 weeks should receive a chest x-ray[74]. Commencement of TB treatment is complicated by potential ART drug interactions, notably with NVP or PIs, with efavirenz (EFV) based regimens being preferred in the 2nd and 3rd trimesters of pregnancy whilst ZDV/3TC/Abacavir (ABC), if available, offers an alternative option[74]. Children of women recently started on TB treatment should receive isoniazid or rifampicin/isoniazid prophylaxis for 6 or 3 months respectively. The optimal screening strategy of HIV-infected pregnant women, and the relative merits and timing of prophylaxis remains a matter of debate[131].

Effective Health-Care Systems are Crucial if Women are to Access Appropriate Treatment

Only an estimated 18% of pregnant women in low and middle-income countries received an HIV test in 2007, with 12% of HIV-infected women being assessed to determine appropriateness of antiretrovirals for her own health[1].

For PMTCT programmes to run effectively and sustainably, they need to be integrated within existing programmes rather than running independently in a vertical fashion[132]. Antenatal and obstetric services need to adopt the role of primary service provider of PMTCT services and work closely alongside counsellors, physicians, family planning services, and civil society representatives of people living with HIV. Investment in health information is required, in particular surveillance, monitoring and evaluation, to assess the effectiveness of their programme[133]. Only through the auditing of each step of a PMTCT programme, from the uptake of HIV testing, through the delivery of PMTCT, testing of exposed infants, and provision of specific HIV care, will a quality service be delivered[134].

PMTCT needs to be a key part of any national HIV plan, with government driven coordination of different departments, numerical targets, standard packages of care in line with international standards and investment made in appropriate infrastructure[133]. National governments need to train and retain medical staff as well as appropriate task-shifting to non-professional staff, whilst systems of procurement need to be strengthened to prevent drugs and other vital supplies running out of stock[133].

Summary

Mother-to-child transmission rates in resource-rich countries are exceptionally low with HAART, avoidance of breastfeeding, and appropriate use of elective caesarean section. Whilst ZDV monotherapy appears safe, evidence exists as the potential for HAART, and in particular those containing protease inhibitors, to cause preterm labour and pre-eclampsia.

Pregnant women are at significant risk of acquiring HIV, particularly if they live in areas of high prevalence such as sub-Saharan Africa. Undetected and untreated HIV not only leads to poorer maternal and infant outcomes *per se* but also runs a significant risk of MTCT. Additional inter-current common diseases of poverty such as malaria, tuberculosis, anaemia, sexually transmitted infections and malnutrition make the situation worse.

Whilst the benefits of exclusive breastfeeding are of paramount importance in infant survival, much remains to be clarified in maximising its advantages and minimising risk. Given the detrimental effects of rapid breastfeeding cessation in reducing infant survival, we do not know how long the transition period should be from breastmilk to replacement feed, or how infant nutrition should be optimised during this period. Despite the recent exciting strategies in postpartum maternal HAART and infant prophylaxis, further work needs to be done to clarify their role in reducing transmission as well as their potential for subsequent ARV resistance.

HIV-related maternal and infant morbidity and mortality requires the identification of high risk HIV-infected women during pregnancy to allow them to receive comprehensive nutritional support, appropriate antenatal care, and appropriate antiretroviral therapy. This can only be achieved in the context of integrated antenatal/PMTCT programmes with testing strategies able to detect primary HIV infection, and with surveillance systems able to track adverse pregnancy outcomes, MTCT rates, infant mortality rates, and monitor health system performance.

Despite the challenges ahead, there is cause to provide some cautious optimism. An increasing number of countries are providing combination antiretrovirals, with at least eight countries (Argentina, Belize, Botswana, Brazil, Jamaica, Russian Federation, Thailand, and Ukraine) exceeding the UN target of 40% PMTCT prophylaxis by 2005, and 3 countries in sub-Saharan Africa (Namibia, South Africa, and Swaziland) doubling their uptake between 2004 and 2006[133]. In the absence of an effective vaccine any time soon, HIV will only brought under control through robust health systems at national and local levels promoting effective methods of prevention.

References

[1] WHO. Towards Universal Access: Scaling up priority HIV/AIDS interventions in the health sector. *Progress Report* 2008. 2008.

[2] Gray, H. R, Li, X., Kigozi, G., Serwadda, D., Brahmbhatt, H., Wabwire-Mangen, F., Nalugoda, F., Kiddugavu, M., Sewankambo, N., Quinn, C. T, Reynolds, J. S, Wawer, J. M. Increased risk of incident HIV during pregnancy in Rakai, Uganda: a prospective study. *Lancet* 2005,366:1182-1188.

[3] Morrison, S. C, Wang, J., Pol VD, B., Padian, N., Salata, A. R, Richardson, A. B. Pregnancy and the risk of HIV-1 acquisition among women in Uganda and Zimbabwe. *AIDS* 2007,21:1027-1034.

[4] Taha, E. T, Dallabetta, A. G, Hoover, R. D, Chiphangwi, D. J, Mtimavalye, A. L, Liomba, N. G, Kumwenda, I. N, Miotti, G. P. Trends of HIV-1 and sexually transmitted diseases among pregnant and postpartum women in urban Malawi. *AIDS* 1998,12:197-203.

[5] Barnighausen, T., Tanser, F., Gqwede, Z., Mbizana, C., Herbst, K., Newell, L. M. High HIV incidence in a community with high HIV prevalence in rural South Africa: findings from a prospective population-based study. *AIDS* 2008,22:139-144.

[6] Rice, D. B, Batzing-Feigenbaum, J., Hosegood, V., Tanser, F., Hill, C., Barnighausen, T., Herbst, K., Welz, T., Newell, L. M. Population and antenatal-based HIV prevalence estimates in a high contracepting female population in rural South Africa. *BMC Public Health* 2007,7:160.

[7] 7. Brocklehurst, P., French, R. The association between maternal HIV infection and perinatal outcome: a systematic review of the literature and meta-analysis. *Br J Obstet Gynaecol* 1998,105:836-848.

[8] Rollins, C. N, Coovadia, M. H, Bland, M. R, Coutsoudis, A., Bennish, L. M, Patel, D., Newell, L. M. Pregnancy outcomes in HIV-infected and uninfected women in rural and urban South Africa. *J Acquir Immune Defic Syndr* 2007,44:321-328.

[9] Habib, A. N, Daltveit, K. A, Bergsjo, P., Shao, J., Oneko, O., Lie, T. R. Maternal HIV status and pregnancy outcomes in northeastern Tanzania: a registry-based study. *BJOG* 2008,115:616-624.

[10] Watson-Jones, D., Weiss, A. H, Changalucha, M. J, Todd, J., Gumodoka, B., Bulmer, J., Balira, R., Ross, D., Mugeye, K., Hayes, R., Mabey, D. Adverse birth outcomes in United Republic of Tanzania--impact and prevention of maternal risk factors. *Bull World Health Organ* 2007,85:9-18.

[11] WHO. Rapid HIV tests- Guidelines for use in HIV testing and counselling in resource constrained settings. 2004.

[12] Pai, P. N, Barick, R., Tulsky, P. J, Shivkumar, V. P, Cohan, D., Kalantri, S., Pai, M., Klein, B. M, Chhabra, S. Impact of round-the-clock, rapid oral fluid HIV testing of women in labor in rural India. *PLoS Med* 2008,5:e92.

[13] Samuel, M. N, Srijayanth, P., Dharmarajan, S., Bethel, J., Hook V, H., Jacob, M., Junankar, V., Chamberlin, J., Collins, D., Read, S. J. Acceptance of HIV-1 education & voluntary counselling/testing by & seroprevalence of HIV-1 among, pregnant women in rural south India. *Indian J Med Res* 2007,125:49-64.

[14] Kalichman, C. S, Simbayi, C. L. HIV testing attitudes, AIDS stigma, and voluntary HIV counselling and testing in a black township in Cape Town, South Africa. *Sex Transm Infect* 2003,79:442-447.

[15] Matovu, K. J, Gray, H. R, Makumbi, F., Wawer, J. M, Serwadda, D., Kigozi, G., Sewankambo, K. N, Nalugoda, F. Voluntary HIV counseling and testing acceptance, sexual risk behavior and HIV incidence in Rakai, Uganda. *AIDS* 2005,19:503-511.

[16] Pignatelli, S., Simpore, J., Pietra, V., Ouedraogo, L., Conombo, G., Saleri, N., Pizzocolo, C., Iaco D, G., Tall, F., Ouiminga, A., Carosi, G., Castelli, F. Factors predicting uptake of voluntary counselling and testing in a real-life setting in a mother-and-child center in Ouagadougou, Burkina Faso. *Trop Med Int Health* 2006,11:350-357.

[17] Bajunirwe, F., Muzoora, M. Barriers to the implementation of programs for the prevention of mother-to-child transmission of HIV: a cross-sectional survey in rural and urban Uganda. *AIDS Res Ther* 2005,2:10.

[18] Mkwanazi, B. N, Patel, D., Newell, L. M, Rollins, C. N, Coutsoudis, A., Coovadia, M. H, Bland, M. R. Rapid testing may not improve uptake of HIV testing and same day results in a rural South African community: a cohort study of 12,000 women. *PLoS ONE* 2008,3:e3501.

[19] Kilewo, C., Massawe, A., Lyamuya, E., Semali, I., Kalokola, F., Urassa, E., Giattas, M., Temu, F., Karlsson, K., Mhalu, F., Biberfeld, G. HIV counseling and testing of pregnant women in sub-Saharan Africa: experiences from a study on prevention of mother-to-child HIV-1 transmission in Dar es Salaam, Tanzania. *J Acquir Immune Defic Syndr* 2001,28:458-462.

[20] Creek, L. T, Ntumy, R., Seipone, K., Smith, M., Mogodi, M., Smit, M., Legwaila, K., Molokwane, I., Tebele, G., Mazhani, L., Shaffer, N., Kilmarx, H. P. Successful introduction of routine opt-out HIV testing in antenatal care in Botswana. *J Acquir Immune Defic Syndr* 2007,45:102-107.

[21] Fiscus, A. S, Pilcher, D. C, Miller, C. W, Powers, A. K, Hoffman, F. I, Price, M., Chilongozi, A. D, Mapanje, C., Krysiak, R., Gama, S., Martinson, E. F, Cohen, S. M. Rapid, real-time detection of acute HIV infection in patients in Africa. *J Infect Dis* 2007,195:416-424.

[22] McDonald, C., Lambert, J., Nayagam, D., Welz, T., Poulton, M., Aleksin, D., Welch, J. Why are children still being infected with HIV? Experiences in the prevention of mother-to-child transmission of HIV in south London. *Sex Transm Infect* 2007,83:59-63.

[23] Moses, E. S, Tosswill, J., Sudhanva, M., Poulton, M., Zuckerman, M. HIV-1 seroconversion during pregnancy resulting in vertical transmission. *J Clin Virol* 2008,41:152-153.

[24] Struik, S. S, Tudor-Williams, G., Taylor, P. G, Portsmouth, D. S, Foster, J. C, Walsh, C., Hanley, C., Walters, S., Smith, H. J, Lyall, H. Infant HIV infection despite "universal" antenatal testing. *Arch Dis Child* 2008,93:59-61.

[25] Lallemant, M., Jourdain, G., Coeur L, S., Kim, S., Koetsawang, S., Comeau, M. A, Phoolcharoen, W., Essex, M., McIntosh, K., Vithayasai, V. A trial of shortened zidovudine regimens to prevent mother-to-child transmission of human immunodeficiency virus type 1. Perinatal HIV Prevention Trial (Thailand) Investigators. *N Engl J Med* 2000,343:982-991.

[26] Newell, L. M. Current issues in the prevention of mother-to-child transmission of HIV-1 infection. *Trans R Soc Trop Med Hyg* 2006,100:1-5.

[27] Nesheim, S., Jamieson, J. D, Danner, P. S, Maupin, R., O'Sullivan, J. M, Cohen, H. M, Webber, P. M, Dennis, R., Bulterys, M. Primary human immunodeficiency virus infection during pregnancy detected by repeat testing. *Am J Obstet Gynecol* 2007,197:149 e141-145.

[28] 2WHO. Guidance on provider-initiated HIV testing and counselling in health facilities. *http://whqlibdoc.who.int/publications/2007/9789241595568_eng.pdf* 2007.

[29] Bhore, V. A, Sastry, J., Patke, D., Gupte, N., Bulakh, M. P, Lele, S., Karmarkar, A., Bharucha, E. K, Shrotri, A., Pisal, H., Suryawanshi, N., Tripathy, S., Risbud, R. A, Paranjape, S. R, Shankar, V. A, Kshirsagar, A., Phadke, A. M, Joshi, L. P, Brookmeyer, S. R, Bollinger, C. R, Jr. Sensitivity and specificity of rapid HIV testing of pregnant women in India. *Int J STD AIDS* 2003,14:37-41.

[30] Yeom, S. J, Jun, G., Chang, Y., Sohn, J. M, Yoo, S., Kim, E., Ryu, H. S, Kang, J. H, Kim, A. Y, Ahn, Y. S, Cha, E. J, Youn, T. S, Park, W. J. Evaluation of a new fourth generation enzyme-linked immunosorbent assay, the LG HIV Ag-Ab Plus, with a combined HIV p24 antigen and anti-HIV-1/2/O screening test. *J Virol Methods* 2006,137:292-297.

[31] Jamieson, J. D, Clark, J., Kourtis, P. A, Taylor, W. A, Lampe, A. M, Fowler, G. M, Mofenson, M. L. Recommendations for human immunodeficiency virus screening, prophylaxis, and treatment for pregnant women in the United States. *Am J Obstet Gynecol* 2007,197:S26-32.

[32] DOH SA. Policy and Guidelines for the Implementation of the PMTCT Programme. *http://www.doh.gov.za/docs/policy-f.html* 2008.

[33] Jamieson, J. D, Cohen, H. M, Maupin, R., Nesheim, S., Danner, P. S, Lampe, A. M, O'Sullivan, J. M, Webber, P. M, Wiener, J., Carter, J. R, Rivero, Y., Fowler, G. M, Bulterys, M. Rapid human immunodeficiency virus-1 testing on labor and delivery in 17 US hospitals: the MIRIAD experience. *Am J Obstet Gynecol* 2007,197:S72-82.

[34] Jamieson, J. D, O'Sullivan, J. M, Maupin, R., Cohen, M., Webber, P. M, Nesheim, S., Lampe, M., Garcia, P., Lindsay, M., Bulterys, M. The challenges of informed consent for rapid HIV testing in labor. *J Womens Health (Larchmt)* 2003,12:889-895.

[35] Pilcher, D. C, Fiscus, A. S, Nguyen, Q. T, Foust, E., Wolf, L., Williams, D., Ashby, R., O'Dowd, O. J, McPherson, T. J, Stalzer, B., Hightow, L., Miller, C. W, Eron, J. J, Jr., Cohen, S. M, Leone, A. P. Detection of acute infections during HIV testing in North Carolina. *N Engl J Med* 2005,352:1873-1883.

[36] Priddy, H. F, Pilcher, D. C, Moore, H. R, Tambe, P., Park, N. M, Fiscus, A. S, Feinberg, B. M, Rio d, C. Detection of acute HIV infections in an urban HIV counseling and testing population in the United States. *J Acquir Immune Defic Syndr* 2007,44:196-202.

[37] Truong, M. H, Grant, M. R, McFarland, W., Kellogg, T., Kent, C., Louie, B., Wong, E., Klausner, D. J. Routine surveillance for the detection of acute and recent HIV infections and transmission of antiretroviral resistance. *AIDS* 2006,20:2193-2197.

[38] Karim, S. S, Mlisana, K., Kharsany, B. A, Williamson, C., Baxter, C., Karim, A. Q. Utilizing nucleic acid amplification to identify acute HIV infection. *AIDS* 2007,21:653-655.

[39] Stringer, S. J, Chi, H. B. Extended nevirapine prophylaxis to prevent HIV transmission. *Lancet* 2008,372:267-269.

[40] WHO. HIV Transmission Through Breastfeeding - a Review of available evidence. *http://whqlibdoc.who.int/publications/2008/9789241596596_eng.pdf* 2007.

[41] HIV-infected pregnant women and vertical transmission in Europe since 1986. European collaborative study. *AIDS* 2001,15:761-770.

[42] Blanche, S., Rouzioux, C., Moscato, L. M, Veber, F., Mayaux, J. M, Jacomet, C., Tricoire, J., Deville, A., Vial, M., Firtion, G., al. e. A prospective study of infants born to women seropositive for human immunodeficiency virus type 1. HIV Infection in Newborns French Collaborative Study Group. *N Engl J Med* 1989,320:1643-1648.

[43] Borkowsky, W., Krasinski, K., Cao, Y., Ho, D., Pollack, H., Moore, T., Chen, H. S, Allen, M., Tao, T. P. Correlation of perinatal transmission of human immunodeficiency virus type 1 with maternal viremia and lymphocyte phenotypes. *J Pediatr* 1994,125:345-351.

[44] Jourdain, G., Mary, Y. J, Coeur, L. S, Ngo-Giang-Huong, N., Yuthavisuthi, P., Limtrakul, A., Traisathit, P., McIntosh, K., Lallemant, M. Risk factors for in utero or intrapartum mother-to-child transmission of human immunodeficiency virus type 1 in Thailand. *J Infect Dis* 2007,196:1629-1636.

[45] Sperling, S. R, Shapiro, E. D, Coombs, W. R, Todd, A. J, Herman, A. S, McSherry, D. G, O'Sullivan, J. M, Dyke V, B. R, Jimenez, E., Rouzioux, C., Flynn, M. P, Sullivan, L. J. Maternal viral load, zidovudine treatment, and the risk of transmission of human immunodeficiency virus type 1 from mother to infant. Pediatric AIDS Clinical Trials Group Protocol 076 Study Group. *N Engl J Med* 1996,335:1621-1629.

[46] Dickover, E. R, Garratty, M. E, Herman, A. S, Sim, S. M, Plaeger, S., Boyer, J. P, Keller, M., Deveikis, A., Stiehm, R. E, Bryson, J. Y. Identification of levels of maternal HIV-1 RNA associated with risk of perinatal transmission. Effect of maternal zidovudine treatment on viral load. *JAMA* 1996,275:599-605.

[47] Mandelbrot, L., Mayaux, J. M, Bongain, A., Berrebi, A., Moudoub-Jeanpetit, Y., Benifla, L. J, Ciraru-Vigneron, N., Chenadec L, J., Blanche, S., Delfraissy, F. J. Obstetric factors and mother-to-child transmission of human immunodeficiency virus type 1: the French perinatal cohorts. SEROGEST French Pediatric HIV Infection Study Group. *Am J Obstet Gynecol* 1996,175:661-667.

[48] Landesman, H. S, Kalish, A. L, Burns, N. D, Minkoff, H., Fox, E. H, Zorrilla, C., Garcia, P., Fowler, G. M, Mofenson, L., Tuomala, R. Obstetrical factors and the transmission of human immunodeficiency virus type 1 from mother to child. The Women and Infants Transmission Study. *N Engl J Med* 1996,334:1617-1623.

[49] Elective caesarean-section versus vaginal delivery in prevention of vertical HIV-1 transmission: a randomised clinical trial. The European Mode of Delivery Collaboration. *Lancet* 1999,353:1035-1039.

[50] The mode of delivery and the risk of vertical transmission of human immunodeficiency virus type 1--a meta-analysis of 15 prospective cohort studies. The International Perinatal HIV Group. *N Engl J Med* 1999,340:977-987.

[51] Rollins, C. N, Becquet, R., Bland, M. R, Coutsoudis, A., Coovadia, M. H, Newell, L. M. Infant feeding, HIV transmission and mortality at 18 months: the need for appropriate choices by mothers and prioritization within programmes. *Aids* 2008,22:2349-2357.

[52] Leroy, V., Newell, L. M, Dabis, F., Peckham, C., Perre Vd, P., Bulterys, M., Kind, C., Simonds, J. R, Wiktor, S., Msellati, P. International multicentre pooled analysis of late postnatal mother-to-child transmission of HIV-1 infection. Ghent International Working Group on Mother-to-Child Transmission of HIV. *Lancet* 1998,352:597-600.

[53] Coovadia, M. H, Rollins, C. N, Bland, M. R, Little, K., Coutsoudis, A., Bennish, L. M, Newell, L. M. Mother-to-child transmission of HIV-1 infection during exclusive breastfeeding in the first 6 months of life: an intervention cohort study. *Lancet* 2007,369:1107-1116.

[54] Coutsoudis, A., Pillay, K., Kuhn, L., Spooner, E., Tsai, Y. W, Coovadia, M. H. Method of feeding and transmission of HIV-1 from mothers to children by 15 months of age: prospective cohort study from Durban, South Africa. *AIDS* 2001,15:379-387.

[55] Bland, M. R, Becquet, R., Rollins, C. N, Coutsoudis, A., Coovadia, M. H, Newell, L. M. Breast health problems are rare in both HIV-infected and HIV-uninfected women who receive counseling and support for breast-feeding in South Africa. *Clin Infect Dis* 2007,45:1502-1510.

[56] Kourtis, P. A, Butera, S., Ibegbu, C., Beled, L., Duerr, A. Breast milk and HIV-1: vector of transmission or vehicle of protection? *Lancet Infect Dis* 2003,3:786-793.

[57] Kourtis, P. A, Lee, K. F, Abrams, J. E, Jamieson, J. D, Bulterys, M. Mother-to-child transmission of HIV-1: timing and implications for prevention. *Lancet Infect Dis* 2006,6:726-732.

[58] Public Health Service Task Force: Recommendations for Use of Antiretroviral Drugs in Pregnant HIV-Infected Women for Maternal Health and Interventions to Reduce Perinatal HIV Transmission in the United States. *http://AIDSinfo.nih.gov* 2008.

[59] Thorne, C., Patel, D., Newell, L. M. Increased risk of adverse pregnancy outcomes in HIV-infected women treated with highly active antiretroviral therapy in Europe. *AIDS* 2004,18:2337-2339.

[60] ECS. European Collaborative Study and the Swiss Mother and Child HIV Cohort Study. Combination antiretroviral therapy and duration of pregnancy. *AIDS* 2000,14:2913-2920.

[61] Lorenzi, P., Spicher, M. V, Laubereau, B., Hirschel, B., Kind, C., Rudin, C., Irion, O., Kaiser, L. Antiretroviral therapies in pregnancy: maternal, fetal and neonatal effects. Swiss HIV Cohort Study, the Swiss Collaborative HIV and Pregnancy Study, and the Swiss Neonatal HIV Study. *AIDS* 1998,12:F241-247.

[62] ECS. European Collbaorative Study. Exposure to antiretroviral therapy in utero or early life: the health of uninfected children born to HIV-infected women. *J Acquir Immune Defic Syndr* 2003,32:380-387.

[63] Tuomala, E. R, Shapiro, E. D, Mofenson, M. L, Bryson, Y., Culnane, M., Hughes, D. M, O'Sullivan, J. M, Scott, G., Stek, M. A, Wara, D., Bulterys, M. Antiretroviral therapy during pregnancy and the risk of an adverse outcome. *N Engl J Med* 2002,346:1863-1870.

[64] Mandelbrot, L., Landreau-Mascaro, A., Rekacewicz, C., Berrebi, A., Benifla, L. J, Burgard, M., Lachassine, E., Barret, B., Chaix, L. M, Bongain, A., Ciraru-Vigneron, N., Crenn-Hebert, C., Delfraissy, F. J, Rouzioux, C., Mayaux, J. M, Blanche, S. Lamivudine-zidovudine combination for prevention of maternal-infant transmission of HIV-1. *JAMA* 2001,285:2083-2093.

[65] Tuomala, E. R, Yawetz, S. Protease inhibitor use during pregnancy: is there an obstetrical risk? *J Infect Dis* 2006,193:1191-1194.

[66] Cotter, M. A, Garcia, G. A, Duthely, L. M, Luke, B., O'Sullivan, J. M. Is antiretroviral therapy during pregnancy associated with an increased risk of preterm delivery, low birth weight, or stillbirth? *J Infect Dis* 2006,193:1195-1201.

[67] Martin, F., Taylor, P. G. Increased rates of preterm delivery are associated with the initiation of highly active antiretrovial therapy during pregnancy: a single-center cohort study. *J Infect Dis* 2007,196:558-561.

[68] Townsend, L. C, Cortina-Borja, M., Peckham, S. C, Tookey, A. P. Antiretroviral therapy and premature delivery in diagnosed HIV-infected women in the United Kingdom and Ireland. *AIDS* 2007,21:1019-1026.

[69] Fiore, S., Newell, L. M, Trabattoni, D., Thorne, C., Gray, L., Savasi, V., Tibaldi, C., Ferrazzi, E., Clerici, M. Antiretroviral therapy-associated modulation of Th1 and Th2 immune responses in HIV-infected pregnant women. *J Reprod Immunol* 2006,70:143-150.

[70] Fiore, S., Ferrazzi, E., Newell, L. M, Trabattoni, D., Clerici, M. Protease inhibitor-associated increased risk of preterm delivery is an immunological complication of therapy. *J Infect Dis* 2007,195:914-916; author reply 916-917.

[71] Effect of breastfeeding on infant and child mortality due to infectious diseases in less developed countries: a pooled analysis. WHO Collaborative Study Team on the Role of Breastfeeding on the Prevention of Infant Mortality. *Lancet* 2000,355:451-455.
[72] WHO. Feeding the Non-Breastfed Child 6-24 Months of Age. *http://www.who.int/nutrition/publications/feeding_non_breastfed_child.pdf* 2004.
[73] Becquet, R., Leroy, V., Ekouevi, K. D, Viho, I., Castetbon, K., Fassinou, P., Dabis, F., Timite-Konan, M. Complementary feeding adequacy in relation to nutritional status among early weaned breastfed children who are born to HIV-infected mothers: ANRS 1201/1202 Ditrame Plus, Abidjan, Cote d'Ivoire. *Pediatrics* 2006,117:e701-710.
[74] WHO. Antiretroviral drugs for treating pregnant women and preventing HIV infection in infants: Towards Universal Access. Recommendations for a public health approach. *WHO Library Cataloguing-in-Publication Data* 2006.
[75] Dabis, F., Msellati, P., Meda, N., Welffens-Ekra, C., You, B., Manigart, O., Leroy, V., Simonon, A., Cartoux, M., Combe, P., Ouangre, A., Ramon, R., Ky-Zerbo, O., Montcho, C., Salamon, R., Rouzioux, C., Perre Vd, P., Mandelbrot, L. 6-month efficacy, tolerance, and acceptability of a short regimen of oral zidovudine to reduce vertical transmission of HIV in breastfed children in Cote d'Ivoire and Burkina Faso: a double-blind placebo-controlled multicentre trial. DITRAME Study Group. DIminution de la Transmission Mere-Enfant. *Lancet* 1999,353:786-792.
[76] Dabis, F., Elenga, N., Meda, N., Leroy, V., Viho, I., Manigart, O., Dequae-Merchadou, L., Msellati, P., Sombie, I. 18-Month mortality and perinatal exposure to zidovudine in West Africa. *AIDS* 2001,15:771-779.
[77] Wiktor, Z. S, Ekpini, E., Karon, M. J, Nkengasong, J., Maurice, C., Severin, T. S, Roels, H. T, Kouassi, K. M, Lackritz, M. E, Coulibaly, M. I, Greenberg, E. A. Short-course oral zidovudine for prevention of mother-to-child transmission of HIV-1 in Abidjan, Cote d'Ivoire: a randomised trial. *Lancet* 1999,353:781-785.
[78] Efficacy of three short-course regimens of zidovudine and lamivudine in preventing early and late transmission of HIV-1 from mother to child in Tanzania, South Africa, and Uganda (Petra study): a randomised, double-blind, placebo-controlled trial. *Lancet* 2002,359:1178-1186.
[79] Bhoopat, L., Khunamornpong, S., Lerdsrimongkol, P., Sirivatanapa, P., Sethavanich, S., Limtrakul, A., Gomutbuthra, V., Kajanavanich, S., Thorner, S. P, Bhoopat, T. Effectiveness of short-term and long-term zidovudine prophylaxis on detection of HIV-1 subtype E in human placenta and vertical transmission. *J Acquir Immune Defic Syndr* 2005,40:545-550.
[80] Guay, A. L, Musoke, P., Fleming, T., Bagenda, D., Allen, M., Nakabiito, C., Sherman, J., Bakaki, P., Ducar, C., Deseyve, M., Emel, L., Mirochnick, M., Fowler, G. M, Mofenson, L., Miotti, P., Dransfield, K., Bray, D., Mmiro, F., Jackson, B. J. Intrapartum and neonatal single-dose nevirapine compared with zidovudine for prevention of mother-to-child transmission of HIV-1 in Kampala, Uganda: HIVNET 012 randomised trial. *Lancet* 1999,354:795-802.
[81] Jackson, B. J, Musoke, P., Fleming, T., Guay, A. L, Bagenda, D., Allen, M., Nakabiito, C., Sherman, J., Bakaki, P., Owor, M., Ducar, C., Deseyve, M., Mwatha, A., Emel, L., Duefield, C., Mirochnick, M., Fowler, G. M, Mofenson, L., Miotti, P., Gigliotti, M.,

Bray, D., Mmiro, F. Intrapartum and neonatal single-dose nevirapine compared with zidovudine for prevention of mother-to-child transmission of HIV-1 in Kampala, Uganda: 18-month follow-up of the HIVNET 012 randomised trial. *Lancet* 2003,362:859-868.

[82] Moodley, D., Moodley, J., Coovadia, H., Gray, G., McIntyre, J., Hofmyer, J., Nikodem, C., Hall, D., Gigliotti, M., Robinson, P., Boshoff, L., Sullivan, L. J. A multicenter randomized controlled trial of nevirapine versus a combination of zidovudine and lamivudine to reduce intrapartum and early postpartum mother-to-child transmission of human immunodeficiency virus type 1. *J Infect Dis* 2003,187:725-735.

[83] Lallemant, M., Jourdain, G., Coeur L, S., Mary, Y. J, Ngo-Giang-Huong, N., Koetsawang, S., Kanshana, S., McIntosh, K., Thaineua, V. Single-dose perinatal nevirapine plus standard zidovudine to prevent mother-to-child transmission of HIV-1 in Thailand. *N Engl J Med* 2004,351:217-228.

[84] Eshleman, H. S, Mracna, M., Guay, A. L, Deseyve, M., Cunningham, S., Mirochnick, M., Musoke, P., Fleming, T., Fowler G, M., Mofenson, M. L, Mmiro, F., Jackson, B. J. Selection and fading of resistance mutations in women and infants receiving nevirapine to prevent HIV-1 vertical transmission (HIVNET 012). *AIDS* 2001,15:1951-1957.

[85] Arrive, E., Newell, L. M, Ekouevi, K. D, Chaix, L. M, Thiebaut, R., Masquelier, B., Leroy, V., Perre, V. P, Rouzioux, C., Dabis, F. Prevalence of resistance to nevirapine in mothers and children after single-dose exposure to prevent vertical transmission of HIV-1: a meta-analysis. *Int J Epidemiol* 2007,36:1009-1021.

[86] Chi, H. B, Sinkala, M., Stringer, M. E, Cantrell, A. R, Mtonga, V., Bulterys, M., Zulu, I., Kankasa, C., Wilfert, C., Weidle, J. P, Vermund, H. S, Stringer, S. J. Early clinical and immune response to NNRTI-based antiretroviral therapy among women with prior exposure to single-dose nevirapine. *AIDS* 2007,21:957-964.

[87] Lockman, S., Shapiro, L. R, Smeaton, M. L, Wester, C., Thior, I., Stevens, L., Chand, F., Makhema, J., Moffat, C., Asmelash, A., Ndase, P., Arimi, P., Widenfelt v, E., Mazhani, L., Novitsky, V., Lagakos, S., Essex, M. Response to antiretroviral therapy after a single, peripartum dose of nevirapine. *N Engl J Med* 2007,356:135-147.

[88] Coffie, A. P, Ekouevi, K. D, Chaix, L. M, Tonwe-Gold, B., Clarisse, B. A, Becquet, R., Viho, I., N'Dri-Yoman, T., Leroy, V., Abrams, J. E, Rouzioux, C., Dabis, F. Maternal 12-month response to antiretroviral therapy following prevention of mother-to-child transmission of HIV type 1, Ivory Coast, 2003-2006. *Clin Infect Dis* 2008,46:611-621.

[89] Eshleman, H. S, Hoover, R. D, Hudelson, E. S, Chen, S., Fiscus, A. S, Piwowar-Manning, E., Jackson, B. J, Kumwenda, I. N, Taha, E. T. Development of nevirapine resistance in infants is reduced by use of infant-only single-dose nevirapine plus zidovudine postexposure prophylaxis for the prevention of mother-to-child transmission of HIV-1. *J Infect Dis* 2006,193:479-481.

[90] Taha, E. T, Kumwenda, I. N, Gibbons, A., Broadhead, L. R, Fiscus, S., Lema, V., Liomba, G., Nkhoma, C., Miotti, G. P, Hoover, R. D. Short postexposure prophylaxis in newborn babies to reduce mother-to-child transmission of HIV-1: NVAZ randomised clinical trial. *Lancet* 2003,362:1171-1177.

[91] Taha, E. T, Kumwenda, I. N, Hoover, R. D, Fiscus, A. S, Kafulafula, G., Nkhoma, C., Nour, S., Chen, S., Liomba, G., Miotti, G. P, Broadhead, L. R. Nevirapine and

zidovudine at birth to reduce perinatal transmission of HIV in an African setting: a randomized controlled trial. *JAMA* 2004,292:202-209.

[92] Victora C. Infection and disease: the impact of early weaning. *Food Nutr Bull* 1996,17:390-396.

[93] Victora, G. C, Smith, G. P, Vaughan, P. J, Nobre, C. L, Lombardi, C., Teixeira, M. A, Fuchs, M. S, Moreira, B. L, Gigante, P. L, Barros, C. F. Evidence for protection by breast-feeding against infant deaths from infectious diseases in Brazil. *Lancet* 1987,2:319-322.

[94] 9Yoon, W. P, Black, E. R, Moulton, H. L, Becker, S. Effect of not breastfeeding on the risk of diarrheal and respiratory mortality in children under 2 years of age in Metro Cebu, The Philippines. *Am J Epidemiol* 1996,143:1142-1148.

[95] Jones, G., Steketee, W. R, Black, E. R, Bhutta, A. Z, Morris, S. S. How many child deaths can we prevent this year? *Lancet* 2003,362:65-71.

[96] Nicoll, A., Williams, A. Breast feeding. *Arch Dis Child* 2002,87:91-92.

[97] Thior, I., Lockman, S., Smeaton, M. L, Shapiro, L. R, Wester, C., Heymann, J. S, Gilbert, B. P, Stevens, L., Peter, T., Kim, S., Widenfelt v, E., Moffat, C., Ndase, P., Arimi, P., Kebaabetswe, P., Mazonde, P., Makhema, J., McIntosh, K., Novitsky, V., Lee, H. T, Marlink, R., Lagakos, S., Essex, M. Breastfeeding plus infant zidovudine prophylaxis for 6 months vs formula feeding plus infant zidovudine for 1 month to reduce mother-to-child HIV transmission in Botswana: a randomized trial: the Mashi Study. *JAMA* 2006,296:794-805.

[98] Miotti, G. P, Taha, E. T, Kumwenda, I. N, Broadhead, R., Mtimavalye, A. L, Hoeven Vd, L., Chiphangwi, D. J, Liomba, G., Biggar, J. R. HIV transmission through breastfeeding: a study in Malawi. *JAMA* 1999,282:744-749.

[99] Coutsoudis, A., Dabis, F., Fawzi, W., Gaillard, P., Haverkamp, G., Harris, R. D, Jackson, B. J, Leroy, V., Meda, N., Msellati, P., Newell, L. M, Nsuati, R., Read, S. J, Wiktor, S. Late postnatal transmission of HIV-1 in breast-fed children: an individual patient data meta-analysis. *J Infect Dis* 2004,189:2154-2166.

[100] Taha, E. T, Hoover, R. D, Kumwenda, I. N, Fiscus, A. S, Kafulafula, G., Nkhoma, C., Chen, S., Piwowar, E., Broadhead, L. R, Jackson, B. J, Miotti, G. P. Late postnatal transmission of HIV-1 and associated factors. *J Infect Dis* 2007,196:10-14.

[101] Kuhn, L., Aldrovandi, M. G, Sinkala, M., Kankasa, C., Semrau, K., Mwiya, M., Kasonde, P., Scott, N., Vwalika, C., Walter, J., Bulterys, M., Tsai, Y. W, Thea, M. D. Effects of early, abrupt weaning on HIV-free survival of children in Zambia. *N Engl J Med* 2008,359:130-141.

[102] WHO. HIV and Infant Feeding-Update. *http://whqlibdoc.who.int/publications/2007/9789241595964_eng.pdf* 2006.

[103] Kilewo, C., Karlsson, K., Massawe, A., Lyamuya, E., Swai, A., Mhalu, F., Biberfeld, G. Prevention of mother-to-child transmission of HIV-1 through breast-feeding by treating infants prophylactically with lamivudine in Dar es Salaam, Tanzania: the Mitra Study. *J Acquir Immune Defic Syndr* 2008,48:315-323.

[104] Bedri, A., Gudetta, B., Isehak, A., Kumbi, S., Lulseged, S., Mengistu, Y., Bhore, V. A, Bhosale, R., Varadhrajan, V., Gupte, N., Sastry, J., Suryavanshi, N., Tripathy, S., Mmiro, F., Mubiru, M., Onyango, C., Taylor, A., Musoke, P., Nakabiito, C., Abashawl,

A., Adamu, R., Antelman, G., Bollinger, C. R, Bright, P., Chaudhary, A. M, Coberly, J., Guay, L., Fowler, G. M, Gupta, A., Hassen, E., Jackson, B. J, Moulton, H. L, Nayak, U., Omer, B. S, Propper, L., Ram, M., Rexroad, V., Ruff, J. A, Shankar, A., Zwerski, S. Extended-dose nevirapine to 6 weeks of age for infants to prevent HIV transmission via breastfeeding in Ethiopia, India, and Uganda: an analysis of three randomised controlled trials. *Lancet* 2008,372:300-313.

[105] Kumwenda, I. N, Hoover, R. D, Mofenson, M. L, Thigpen, C. M, Kafulafula, G., Li, Q., Mipando, L., Nkanaunena, K., Mebrahtu, T., Bulterys, M., Fowler, G. M, Taha, E. T. Extended antiretroviral prophylaxis to reduce breast-milk HIV-1 transmission. *N Engl J Med* 2008,359:119-129.

[106] Vyankandondera, J, Luchters, S, Hassink, E. Reducing the risk of HIV-1 transmission from mother to infant through breastfeeding using antiretroviral prophylaxis in infants (SIMBA study). *2nd International AIDS Conference on HIV Pathogenesis and Treatment, Paris, France, 13-17 July 2003, Abstract LB7* 2003.

[107] Mofenson, M. L. Antiretroviral Prophylaxis to Reduce Breast Milk Transmission of HIV Type 1: New Data but Still Questions. *J Acquir Immune Defic Syndr* 2008,48:237-240.

[108] Kilewo C. Prevention of mother-to-child transmission of HIV-1 through breastfeeding by treating mothers prophylactically with triple antiretroviral therapy in Dar es Salaam, Tanzania - the MITRA PLUS study. *4th IAS Conference on HIV Pathogenesis, Treatment and Prevention: Abstract no. TUAX101* 2007.

[109] Thomas, T, Masaba, R, Ndivo, R. PMTCT of HIV-1 among breast-feeding women using HAART: the Kisumu Breastfeeding Study, Kisumu, Kenya, 2003-2007. *15th Conference on Retroviruses and Opportunistic Infections, Boston, MA, 3-6 February 2008, Abstract 45aLB* 2008.

[110] WHO. Impact of Highly Active Anti Retroviral Therapy during Pregnancy and Breastfeeding on Mother-To-Child-Transmission of HIV and Mother's Health: The Kesho Bora Study. *http://www.who.int/reproductive-health/stis/mtct.htm.*

[111] Kourtis, ADF, Hyde, L, Tien, HC, Chavula, C, Mumba, N, Magawa, N, Knight, R, Chasela, C, Horst vd, C, Team atBS. Diarrhea in Uninfected Infants of HIV-infected Mothers Who Stop Breastfeeding at 6 Months: The BAN Study Experience. *Fourteenth Conference on Retroviruses and Opportunistic Infections (CROI). 2007: Los Angeles* 2007.

[112] Cohen C. Prevention and treatment of malaria in HIV-infected patients. *South African Medical Journal* 2008,26:280-282.

[113] Kuile t, O. F, Eijk v, M. A, Filler, J. S. Effect of sulfadoxine-pyrimethamine resistance on the efficacy of intermittent preventive therapy for malaria control during pregnancy: a systematic review. *Jama* 2007,297:2603-2616.

[114] Mbaye, A., Richardson, K., Balajo, B., Dunyo, S., Shulman, C., Milligan, P., Greenwood, B., Walraven, G. A randomized, placebo-controlled trial of intermittent preventive treatment with sulphadoxine-pyrimethamine in Gambian multigravidae. *Trop Med Int Health* 2006,11:992-1002.

[115] Menendez, C., Bardaji, A., Sigauque, B., Romagosa, C., Sanz, S., Serra-Casas, E., Macete, E., Berenguera, A., David, C., Dobano, C., Naniche, D., Mayor, A., Ordi, J.,

Mandomando, I., Aponte, J. J, Mabunda, S., Alonso, L. P. A randomized placebo-controlled trial of intermittent preventive treatment in pregnant women in the context of insecticide treated nets delivered through the antenatal clinic. *PLoS ONE* 2008,3:e1934.

[116] Belperio, S. P, Rhew, C. D. Prevalence and outcomes of anemia in individuals with human immunodeficiency virus: a systematic review of the literature. *Am J Med* 2004,116 Suppl 7A:27S-43S.

[117] 117. Meda, N., Mandelbrot, L., Cartoux, M., Dao, B., Ouangre, A., Dabis, F. Anaemia during pregnancy in Burkina Faso, west Africa, 1995-96: prevalence and associated factors. DITRAME Study Group. *Bull World Health Organ* 1999,77:916-922.

[118] Buskin, E. S, Sullivan, S. P. Anemia and its treatment and outcomes in persons infected with human immunodeficiency virus. *Transfusion* 2004,44:826-832.

[119] Broek vd, R. N, Letsky, A. E. Etiology of anemia in pregnancy in south Malawi. *Am J Clin Nutr* 2000,72:247S-256S.

[120] Sullivan, P. Associations fo Anemia, treatments for anemia, and survival in patients with Human Immunodeficiency Virus Infection. *Journal of Infectious Diseases* 2002,185:S138-142.

[121] Gallagher, M., Malhotra, I., Mungai, L. P, Wamachi, N. A, Kioko, M. J, Ouma, H. J, Muchiri, E., King, L. C. The effects of maternal helminth and malaria infections on mother-to-child HIV transmission. *AIDS* 2005,19:1849-1855.

[122] Muhangi, L., Woodburn, P., Omara, M., Omoding, N., Kizito, D., Mpairwe, H., Nabulime, J., Ameke, C., Morison, A. L, Elliott, M. A. Associations between mild-to-moderate anaemia in pregnancy and helminth, malaria and HIV infection in Entebbe, Uganda. *Trans R Soc Trop Med Hyg* 2007,101:899-907.

[123] WHO. Global strategy for the prevention and control of sexually transmitted infections: 2006-2015: breaking the chain of transmission. *http://www.who.int/reproductive-health/publications/stisstrategy/stis_strategy.pdf* 2007.

[124] Abu-Raddad, J. L, Magaret, S. A, Celum, C., Wald, A., Longini, M. I, Jr., Self, G. S, Corey, L. Genital herpes has played a more important role than any other sexually transmitted infection in driving HIV prevalence in Africa. *PLoS ONE* 2008,3:e2230.

[125] Reynolds, J. S, Risbud, R. A, Shepherd, E. M, Rompalo, M. A, Ghate, V. M, Godbole, V. S, Joshi, N. S, Divekar, D. A, Gangakhedkar, R. R, Bollinger, C. R, Mehendale, M. S. High rates of syphilis among STI patients are contributing to the spread of HIV-1 in India. *Sex Transm Infect* 2006,82:121-126.

[126] Strick, B. L, Wald, A., Celum, C. Management of herpes simplex virus type 2 infection in HIV type 1-infected persons. *Clin Infect Dis* 2006,43:347-356.

[127] Watson-Jones, D., Weiss, A. H, Rusizoka, M., Changalucha, J., Baisley, K., Mugeye, K., Tanton, C., Ross, D., Everett, D., Clayton, T., Balira, R., Knight, L., Hambleton, I., Goff L, J., Belec, L., Hayes, R. Effect of herpes simplex suppression on incidence of HIV among women in Tanzania. *N Engl J Med* 2008,358:1560-1571.

[128] Temmerman, M., Plummer, A. F, Mirza, B. N, Ndinya-Achola, O. J, Wamola, A. I, Nagelkerke, N., Brunham, C. R, Piot, P. Infection with HIV as a risk factor for adverse obstetrical outcome. *AIDS* 1990,4:1087-1093.

[129] Dye, C. Global epidemiology of tuberculosis. *Lancet* 2006,367:938-940.

[130] Khan, M., Pillay, T., Moodley, M. J, Connolly, A. C. Maternal mortality associated with tuberculosis-HIV-1 co-infection in Durban, South Africa. *AIDS* 2001,15:1857-1863.

[131] Gupta, A., Nayak, U., Ram, M., Bhosale, R., Patil, S., Basavraj, A., Kakrani, A., Philip, S., Desai, D., Sastry, J., Bollinger, C. R. Postpartum tuberculosis incidence and mortality among HIV-infected women and their infants in Pune, India, 2002-2005. *Clin Infect Dis* 2007,45:241-249.

[132] Freedman, P. L, Waldman, J. R, Pinho d, H., Wirth, E. M, Chowdhury, M. A, Rosenfield, A. Transforming health systems to improve the lives of women and children. *Lancet* 2005,365:997-1000.

[133] WHO. Guidance on Global Scale-up of the Prevention of Mother-To-Child Transmission of HIV. In: *WHO Library Cataloguing-in-Publication Data*; 2007.

[134] Rollins, C. N, Dedicoat, M., Danaviah, S., Page, T., Bishop, K., Kleinschmidt, I., Coovadia, M. H, Cassol, A. S. Prevalence, incidence, and mother-to-child transmission of HIV-1 in rural South Africa. *Lancet* 2002,360:389.

[135] Is zidovudine therapy in pregnant HIV-infected women associated with gestational age and birthweight? The European Collaborative Study. *AIDS* 1999,13:119-124.

[136] Connor, M. E, Sperling, S. R, Gelber, R., Kiselev, P., Scott, G., O'Sullivan, J. M, VanDyke, R., Bey, M., Shearer, W., Jacobson, L. R, al. e. Reduction of maternal-infant transmission of human immunodeficiency virus type 1 with zidovudine treatment. Pediatric AIDS Clinical Trials Group Protocol 076 Study Group. *N Engl J Med* 1994,331:1173-1180.

[137] Luzzati, R., Bravo D, P., Perri D, G., Luzzani, A., Concia, E. Riboflavine and severe lactic acidosis. *Lancet* 1999,353:901-902.

[138] FDA. FDA/Bristol Myers Squibb Issues Caution For HIV Combination Therapy With Zerit and Videx in Pregnant Women. http://www.fda.gov/bbs/topics/answers/ns01063.html 2001.

[139] Nightingale, L. S. From the Food and Drug Administration. *JAMA* 1998,280:1472.

[140] Chersich, F. M, Urban, F. M, Venter, W. F, Wessels, T., Krause, A., Gray, E. G, Luchters, S., Viljoen, L. D. Efavirenz use during pregnancy and for women of child-bearing potential. *AIDS Res Ther* 2006,3:11.

[141] Lyons, F., Hopkins, S., Kelleher, B., McGeary, A., Sheehan, G., Geoghegan, J., Bergin, C., Mulcahy, M. F, McCormick, A. P. Maternal hepatotoxicity with nevirapine as part of combination antiretroviral therapy in pregnancy. *HIV Med* 2006,7:255-260.

[142] Baylor, S. M, Johann-Liang, R. Hepatotoxicity associated with nevirapine use. *J Acquir Immune Defic Syndr* 2004,35:538-539.

[143] Dinsmoor, J. M, Forrest, T. S. Lack of an effect of protease inhibitor use on glucose tolerance during pregnancy. *Infect Dis Obstet Gynecol* 2002,10:187-191.

[144] Cooper, R. E, Charurat, M., Mofenson, L., Hanson, C. I, Pitt, J., Diaz, C., Hayani, K., Handelsman, E., Smeriglio, V., Hoff, R., Blattner, W. Combination antiretroviral strategies for the treatment of pregnant HIV-1-infected women and prevention of perinatal HIV-1 transmission. *J Acquir Immune Defic Syndr* 2002,29:484-494.

[145] Dorenbaum, A., Cunningham, K. C, Gelber, D. R, Culnane, M., Mofenson, L., Britto, P., Rekacewicz, C., Newell, L. M, Delfraissy, F. J, Cunningham-Schrader, B., Mirochnick, M., Sullivan, L. J. Two-dose intrapartum/newborn nevirapine and standard antiretroviral therapy to reduce perinatal HIV transmission: a randomized trial. *JAMA* 2002,288:189-198.

In: Infectious Pregnancy Complications
Editor: Richard N. Canfield

ISBN 978-1-60741-038-6

Chapter 9

Impact of Materno-Placental Malaria, Anaemia and HIV Infection on Perinatal Outcome in Nigeria

***C. J. Uneke*[1], *I. Sunday-Adeoye*[2], *F. E. Iyare*[3], *O. G. Asiegbu*[2] and *D. D. Duhlinska*[4]**

[1]Department of Medical Microbiology/Parasitology,
Faculty of Clinical Medicine Ebonyi State University Abakaliki Nigeria
[2]Department of Obstetrics and Gynaecology,
Ebonyi State University Teaching Hospital Abakaliki Nigeria
[3]Department of Morbid Anatomy/Histopathology,
Faculty of Clinical Medicine Ebonyi State University Abakaliki Nigeria
[4]Applied Parasitology Unit, Department of Zoology,
Faculty of Natural Sciences University of Jos Nigeria

Abstract

Malaria, HIV infection and anaemia constitute major public health problems during pregnancy and are important factors associated with increased risk for adverse pregnancy outcomes. The objective of this study was to evaluate the impact of maternal and placental malaria, HIV infection and anaemia on perinatal outcome. Pregnant women were enrolled at labour ward (LW) at full pregnancy term at Ebonyi State University Teaching Hospital (EBSUTH), Abakaliki Nigeria. The study was conducted from November 2006 to November 2007. At childbirth, fetal length and head circumference, birth weight and placental weight were determined using standard techniques. Maternal peripheral, placental, and cord blood samples were obtained. Peripheral and placental malaria was detected using microscopy. Haemoglobin concentration (HbC), ABO blood group and genotype were performed using standard techniques. HIV infection was screened using ELISA and confirmed by Immunoblot analysis. Prevalence of malaria was 16.0% and *P. falciparum* was the only species identified. Individuals of younger age, primigravidae and those who never attended antenatal clinic (ANC) were more likely to have malaria. Prevalence of malaria significantly decreased with increase in HbC (χ^2=23.8, P<0.05). Individuals with HbAA genotype and those with blood group O had higher prevalence of malaria infection. Prevalence of HIV infection at childbirth was 3.6% and malaria prevalence was significantly higher among HIV-positive women (χ^2=13.3, P<0.05). Malaria infected women had a significantly higher proportion of LBW babies (P<0.05). A higher proportion of LBW was recorded among anemic women, primigravidae, those with HIV infection, blood group O and HbAA genotype and those who never attended ANC. Prevalence of placental malaria was 12.2%. Women with peripheral malaria infection had significantly higher proportion (54.2%) of placental infection than those without peripheral malaria infection (3.5%) (χ^2=94.4, P<0.05). A significantly higher proportion (33.3%) of malaria infected placentas had the lowest placental weight (0.4kg) (χ^2=6.99, P<0.05) and a higher proportion of babies born by mothers with malaria infected placenta had low birth weight (<2.5kg), lower fetal length and head circumference. Prevalence of fetal anaemia (cord HbC<12.5g/dl) was 65.6%. Babies of malaria infected, HIV-positive, and anaemic mothers had a higher proportion of FA. There is need to strengthen ANC services to ensure delivery of malaria, HIV and anaemia interventions within existing health systems, to reduce adverse perinatal outcome.

Introduction

Malaria in Pregnancy

Malaria during pregnancy is a serious problem in sub-Saharan Africa, affecting an estimated 24 million pregnant women (Steketee *et al.* 2001). Each year between 75,000 and 200,000 infant deaths are attributed to malaria infection in pregnancy globally (Steketee *et al.* 2001). Pregnancies in women living in malaria endemic regions particularly in sub-Saharan Africa are associated with a high frequency and density of *Plasmodium. falciparum* parasitaemia, with high rates of maternal morbidity including fever and severe anaemia, with abortion and stillbirth, and with high rates of placental malaria and consequently low birth weight in newborns caused by both prematurity and intrauterine growth retardation (Steketee *et al.* 2001; Garner and Gülmezoglu, 2001; Bouvier *et al.* 1997).

The clinical features of *P. falciparum* malaria in pregnancy depend to a large extent on the immune status of the woman, which in turn is determined by her previous exposure to malaria. In pregnant women with little or no pre-existing immunity, such as women from non-endemic areas or travelers to malarious areas, infection is associated with high risks of severe disease with maternal and perinatal mortality and the women are at particular risk of cerebral malaria, hypoglycemia, pulmonary edema and severe hemolytic anaemia (Shulman and Dorman, 2003). In malaria-endemic areas, where women have substantial acquired immunity, *P. falciparum* infection during pregnancy is often asymptomatic, thus the more transmission is intense and regular, the higher the prevalence of asymptomatic infections (Rogier *et al.* 2005), however the prevalence of clinical and asymptomatic malaria is highest in young women and those in their first and second pregnancies (McGregor, 1984). With successive pregnancies, women usually acquire a gravidity-dependent form of immunity, resulting in a decrease in both prevalence and severity of infection (Brabin, 1983). Hence, most studies suggest that malarial infection is more prevalent and intense in primigravid women than in multigravid women in areas endemic for malaria such as sub-Saharan Africa (McGregor, 1984; Shulman *et al.* 1996; Menendez, 1995; Nosten *et al.* 1991). In recent times however, there is increasing evidence indicating significant susceptibility in the multigravidae as well (Shulman *et al.* 2001).

One outstanding feature of P. falciparum malaria in pregnancy is the sequestration of infected RBC within the placenta and this causes premature delivery, low birth weight, and increased mortality in the newborn and anaemia in the mother. Parasitized RBC isolated from placentas have a unique adhesion property different from parasites collected from non-pregnant individuals (Beeson et al. 1999; Fried and Duffy, 1996). These parasites bound to CSA and failed to adhere to CD36, the critical host receptor for sequestration in microvasculature. The apparent dichotomy in adhesion to these receptors was selected to allow the parasite to sequester not to endothelium but in placenta, perhaps a site of reduced immunity. Indeed, CSA-binding parasites express PfEMP1 with a DBLγ domain that binds CSA and a non-CD36-binding CIDR1 (Buffet et al. 1999; Gamain et al. 2001). In contrast, CD36-adherent parasites express a PfEMP1 with a CD36-binding CIDR1 (Gamain et al. 2001).

Placental Malaria

The sequestration of malaria parasites in the placenta, known as placental malaria, is one of the major features of malaria during pregnancy. Its distribution in an infected gravid woman varies with the endemicity of malaria and acquired immunity (Okoko *et al.* 2002). In semi-immune women, the proportion of parasitized erythrocytes is often higher in the placental than in peripheral blood (Ibanesebhor and Okolo, 1992). The placental sequestration of *P. falciparum* results in the accumulation of parasitized erythrocytes in the intervillous space, infiltration by inflammatory cells and release of pro-inflammatory mediators (Fried *et al.* 1998), which cause pathologic alterations (Walter *et al.* 1982, Bulmer *et al.* 1993; Ordi *et al.* 1998). Histological abnormalities described in parasitized placenta show pathological changes that could reduce the area of syncytium exposed to maternal blood and, thus, impair materno-fetal exchanges (Walter *et al.* 1982, Bulmer *et al.* 1993). Likewise, considerable abnormality in intervillous spaces may jeopardize the nutritional function of the placenta, resulting in poor fetal outcome (Matteelli *et al.* 1997; Philippe and Walter, 1985).

Placental infection has been widely used as a standard indicator to characterize malaria infection in epidemiologic investigations. However, the pathogenesis of placental malaria is only partially understood, but it is clear that it leads to a distinct epidemiological pattern of malaria during pregnancy. It is necessary therefore, to understand the local events at the maternal-fetal interface which encompass immunological and pathological processes, because they relate to the epidemiological pattern of malaria in pregnancy in areas of both high and low malaria transmission (Brabin *et al.* 2004). Measuring malaria infection in the placenta is fairly non-technical, and a large proportion of women in developing countries are only seen at a late stage of pregnancy, it is therefore not surprising that placental infection is the only available information regarding their parasitological status (Cottrell *et al.* 2005).

Diagnosis of Placental Malaria

It is well established that accurate laboratory diagnosis of infections facilitates evidence-based management of patients and improvement of the specificity of treatment and other control measures. Accurate diagnosis of placental malaria in pregnancy is therefore very important for both operational and research purposes. This is because placental infection may be detected in the absence of peripheral blood parasitemia and may persist after initiation of antimalarial treatment (Sartelet *et al.* 1997). Because not all malaria-exposed pregnant women in areas of malaria endemicity suffer from placental malaria and its serious consequences, a number of studies have assessed the prevalence and risk factors of placental malaria in sub-Saharan Africa while others have attempted to elucidate protective immune responses against placental infection and/or immune pathogenesis. However, results from the various studies are often discordant, and one of the major factors in the discordance is that different techniques of sample collection and analysis were employed in different studies based on the differences in the definition of placental malaria (Othoro *et al.* 2006). Some studies based their definition on the presence of malaria parasite and/or pigments in blood smear from placental blood (Ismail *et al.* 2000; Mockenhaupt *et al.* 2006; Tako *et al.* 2005), others based their definition on histological findings (Menendez *et al.* 2000; Walter *et al.* 1981;), while some others based their definition on the use of histitidine-rich-protein-2 (HRP2) capture test (Leke *et al.* 1999; Mayengue *et al.* 2004; Singer *et al.* 2004) and polymerase chain reaction (PCR) (Kamwendo *et al.* 2002; Kassam *et al.* 2006; Singer *et al.* 2004).

Characteristics of Malaria Infected Placenta

The placenta is a complex, sophisticated organ with several important functions throughout gestation, with the primary purpose of providing sustenance for the developing fetus. The placenta is also a site for *P. falciparum* sequestration. Many hypotheses, based on a systemic or local failure of the immunological response to malaria, have been proposed to explain the 'preference' of the parasites for replication in the placenta and some of these hypothesis have been reviewed (Matteelli *et al.* 1997). Histologically, placental malaria is characterized by the presence of parasites and leucocytes within the intervillous spaces, pigment within macrophages, fibrin deposits and trophoblasts, proliferation of cytotrophoblastic cells and thickening of the trophoblastic basement membrane (Matteelli *et al.* 1997). In Haut-Ogooue, Gabon, malarial brown pigment was observed in all cases of placental malaria examined and was characterized by ultrastructural features and occurred in perivillous deposits of fibrinoid, in macrophages, or free in intervillous spaces (Walter *et al.* 1982). Furthermore, excessive perivillous fibrinoid deposits were a constant histologic finding and were usually associated with syncytiotrophoblastic necrosis or ultrastructural damage such as partial microvilli loss, filamentous material accumulation in intracytoplasmic vacuoles, and "podocytelike" cytoplasmic projections on the basal surface (Walter *et al.* 1982). It is at these sites the trophoblastic basal lamina was usually thickened.

Effects of Malaria on Maternal Health

Although pregnant women in endemic areas have higher rates of parasitemia and parasite density compared with non-pregnant women, infection is largely asymptomatic because some degree of pre-existing immunity is retained during pregnancy (Dorman and Shulman, 2000). However, even malaria-immune women are susceptible to placental malaria (Tako *et al.* 2005). Because so many parasites become sequestered within the placenta, peripheral blood smears often fail to detect evidence of infection. The resulting lack of appropriate or timely treatment may lead to adverse pregnancy outcome including severe anaemia, which is the main maternal consequence of malaria and the mechanism by which malaria causes maternal death in endemic areas (Dorman and Shulman, 2000). Apart from an effect through anaemia, malaria may contribute to maternal mortality by increasing the risk and severity of obstetric conditions such as pre-eclampsia/eclampsia and postpartum hemorrhage (Brabin and Johnson, 2005). The mechanisms by which malaria causes anaemia are understood, but its relationship with obstetric factors is not and evaluating the link between malaria, obstetric disorders, and maternal death has been recommended (Etard *et al.* 2003). The effects of placental malaria on maternal health can better be understood when considered in relation with various maternal parameters including maternal age, parity, peripheral malaria infection, anaemia, and HIV infection.

Maternal Age

A number of studies conducted in parts of sub-Saharan Africa have reported a significant association between maternal age and malaria infection during pregnancy (Bouyou-Akotet *et al.* 2003; Rogerson *et al.* 2000). In a study conducted in Blantyre, Malawi, after stratifying by gravidity, associations between age and parasite prevalence were reportedly stronger than those between gravidity and prevalence after stratifying by age (Rogerson *et al.* 2000). It was noted that under conditions of low-to-moderate transmission, pregnancy-specific immunity is slow to develop, and that age-related immunity may influence malaria prevalence in childbearing years (Rogerson *et al.* 2000). Studies have shown that young women of child-bearing age may be more susceptible than older women to malaria because they are still in the process of acquiring natural immunity to malaria (Shi *et al.* 1995).

Parity

The relationship between placental malaria and parity is well established. Many recent studies conducted in sub-Saharan Africa have found the prevalence of placental malaria to be higher in primigravidae than multigravidae (Cottrell *et al.* 2005; Okoko *et al.* 2002). These observations are consistent with the findings of earlier studies in malaria-endemic regions where, among several factors, parity independently influenced the placental malaria prevalence rate (McGregor, 1984). The risk of placental malaria among the primigravidae in southwestern Burkina Faso, was two fold that of multigravidae (Cottrell *et al.* 2005). In the Gambia, it was observed that primigravidae had a four-fold risk of having placental malaria compared to the multigravidae and the severest form of placental parasitization occurred in a higher proportion of the primigravidae than in the multigravidae (Okoko *et al.* 2002).

Peripheral Malaria Infection

The relationship between maternal peripheral parasitemia and placental malaria has been evaluated in some parts of sub-Saharan Africa. However, whether placental infection reflects the existence of peripheral infection over a short period preceding the delivery or whether it is related to infection at any other moment during the whole course of pregnancy has never been rigorously studied.

Two studies have shown some relation between a late infection and positivity of placental smears or presence of pigment (Watkinson and Rushton, 1983; McGready *et al.* 2004), but it has been argued that a single measure can hardly reflect the entire history of infection during pregnancy.

Therefore in Burkina Faso the relationship between placental infection and peripheral infection at different periods of pregnancy was investigated using data collected during a randomized trial of malaria prophylaxis in pregnant women (Cottrell *et al.* 2005). In the study, the occurrence of peripheral parasitemia at the beginning and at the end of pregnancy were significantly related to placental infection, whereas peripheral parasitemia in the middle of pregnancy was not (Cottrell *et al.* 2005). This suggests that a peripheral parasitemia at the beginning of pregnancy may persist within the placenta throughout gestation, with possibly more severe consequences on the placenta and the newborn, than a later infection.

Maternal Anaemia

It is well established that anaemia is the most common consequence of *P. falciparum* malaria infection. In sub-Saharan Africa, it is estimated that between 200,000 and 500,000 pregnant women develop severe anaemia as a result of malaria (Guyatt and Snow , 2001), and *P. falciparum* malaria in pregnancy is also known to be the primary cause of up to 10,000 maternal anaemia-related deaths in sub-Saharan Africa annually (WHO, 1992). However, there have been conflicting reports from parts of sub-Saharan Africa on the relationship between placental malaria and maternal anaemia. An earlier report from the Ubangi district of Zaire, noted that malarious placentas had no consistent relationship to maternal anaemia (Anagos *et al.* 1986).

More recently, in southwestern Cameroon, the prevalence of anaemia was significantly higher in mothers whose placental biopsy were free of malaria parasites than in those whose placental samples had malaria parasites (Achidi *et al.* 2005). On the contrary, in Yaoundé,

Cameroon, maternal anaemia and placental malaria were associated in all gravidity and age groups, with maternal anaemia higher among women with placental malaria than those without placental malaria (Tako *et al.* 2005). The reason for this variation is not immediately clear, but it may not be unconnected with the complex and multifactorial etiology of anaemia in pregnancy in sub-Saharan Africa (Fleming, 1988).

In most areas of malaria endemicity, many other causes of anaemia have been identified, including both nutritional (iron, folate and protein deficiency) and non-nutritional factors (hook worms and haemoglobinopathies) (Fleming, 1989) and increasingly HIV infection (Antelman *et al.* 2000). Since many of the causes of anaemia occur concurrently in pregnancy and no hallmarks of malaria anaemia have been identified, it is difficult to evaluate the contribution made to anaemia in pregnancy by placental malaria infection (Matteelli *et al.* 1994). However, apart from its significant contribution to maternal mortality and to both maternal and fetal morbidity, anaemia in pregnancy is a risk factor for infant iron deficiency anaemia (Colomer *et al.* 1990) that, if left uncorrected, can be associated with adverse behavioral and cognitive development (Nokes *et al.* 1998).

Placental Malaria and Perinatal Outcome

Although malaria in pregnancy is a major factor associated with adverse perinatal outcome, the link between malaria and perinatal morbidity/mortality is less clear in areas with stable endemic malaria where pregnant women have acquired immunity (van Geertruyden *et al.* 2004). However, placental malaria is recognized as a common complication of malaria in pregnancy in areas of stable transmission and as a consequence serious health problems arise for the mother and especially her baby. Placenta results are more sensitive than peripheral blood for detecting maternal infection, and are more accurate in predicting fetal morbidity (Nyirjesy *et al.* 1993).

Low Birth Weight

In sub-Saharan Africa the rate of low birth weight (LBW) (i.e.,<2.5kg) newborns is high, and malaria is known to be an important contributor to the 3.5 million LBW babies born annually in the sub-region (Brabin, 1997). Malaria is thought to reduce birth weight through a combination of systemic and local effects. Although malaria may affect birth weight through malaria-induced anaemia, malaria also may reduce birth weight through placental infection (Okoko *et al.* 2002).

In this case, parasites either directly cause a mechanical compromise of placental circulation or indirectly interfere with placental functions and/or induce pathological lesions (Galbraith *et al.* 1980). Despite the prevalence of placental infections for women of all gravidities, ranging from 5% to 52%, the risk of LBW associated with infection was relatively consistent, with babies born to mothers with an infected placenta being twice as likely to be of LBW than those born to mothers with an uninfected placenta (Guyatt and Snow, 2004). It is important to state that there is still no agreement on which are the main mechanisms that mediate reductions in birth weight in placental malaria (Menendez *et al.* 2000).

Neonatal Anthropometric Parameters

Neonatal anthropometric parameters such as neonatal length, head circumference as well as placental weight have been related to placental malaria. In southeastern Tanzania, chronic malaria infection of the placenta was associated with significant reductions in mean head circumference, neonatal length, and body index (weight/length^2), whereas past infections were associated with reduced mean length at birth only (Menendez *et al.* 2000). In the Ubangi district of Zaire, malarious placentas had no consistent relationship with neonatal length or head circumference (Anagos *et al.* 1986). The reduction in the length and head circumference of the newborns associated with chronic infections probably indicate a prolonged effect on fetal nutrition, which was suggested in other studies (Meuris *et al.* 1993). Similarly, it has also been suggested that the reduction in the body mass index may reflect the severity and duration of fetal malnutrition (Menendez *et al.* 2000).

Two earlier studies that evaluated the relationship between placental malaria and placental weight in Haut-Ogooue and Franceville, both in Gabon indicated that the mean weight of term placentas with malarial changes was significantly less than that of placentas without such changes (Walter *et al.* 1982; Gazin *et al.* 1994).

Fetal Anaemia

The prevalence of fetal anaemia defined as cord hemoglobin level <12.5g/dl is reportedly very high in sub-Saharan Africa. Interestingly, a link was established between fetal anaemia and maternal malaria infection. The contributory role of placental malaria to fetal anaemia has been evaluated in a number of studies with varying results.

In southern Malawi, a higher prevalence of fetal anaemia occurred with increasing peripheral *P. falciparum* parasite density and geometric mean placental parasite densities were higher in babies with fetal anaemia than in those without it (Brabin *et al.* 2004). On the contrary, Abrams *et al.* (2005) noted from their study in Blantyre, Malawi, mean cord hemoglobin levels did not differ between malaria-infected and uninfected women, in addition, malarial disease severity, including peripheral and placental parasite density, stage of disease, and deposition of fibrin and malaria pigment in placental monocytes, had no effect on cord hemoglobin level.

In Kisumu, Kenya, although children born to mothers with detectable *P. falciparum* parasitemia on a peripheral blood film at delivery had a lower mean cord hemoglobin level at birth compared with children born to mothers free of parasitemia at delivery, no association was found between malaria infection of the placenta and mean cord hemoglobin level at birth, or at any age thereafter (McElroy *et al.* 1999). It was however noted that the lack of an association between placental parasitemia and cord hemoglobin level in the study may have been due to the exclusion of LBW infants. This is because the LBW associated with placental parasitemia in earlier studies may have accounted for the detection of reduced hemoglobin values in children born to mothers with placental parasitemia.

Perinatal Mortality

Placental malaria and its effects on perinatal mortality (fetal or infant deaths from 28th week of pregnancy up to the seventh day after birth), have been investigated in various parts of sub-Saharan Africa. The impact of placental malaria on perinatal death (stillbirth and early neonatal death) is still under debate and conflicting results have been obtained from various studies that investigated the relationship between them. Newman *et al.* (2003) reported a seven-fold increased risk of stillbirth in association with placental parasitaemia in areas with unstable malaria transmission in Ethiopia. McGregor *et al.* (McGregor *et al.* 1983) observed some seasonal differences in stillbirth rates, with the lowest rate occurring during the three months of the late dry season when placental malaria prevalence was low. Conversely, in a more recent study, Okoko *et al.* (2002) also in the Gambia, observed a two-fold increased risk of stillbirth among mothers with malaria-infected placenta and noted that placental malaria infection was independently associated with a higher risk of delivering stillbirths in the population studied.

On the contrary, no statistical association was detected between stillbirth and placental malaria in Zaire (Anagos *et al.* 1986). Similarly in rural Malawi, placental malaria infection was not found to be significantly associated with stillbirth or with early neonatal death, either with birth weight excluded or in models including only LBW or only normal birth weight (NBW) infants (McDermott *et al.* 1996).

Malaria and HIV Coinfection in Pregnancy

The effects of human immunodeficiency virus (HIV) on maternal health have been superimposed on that of malaria in the malaria-endemic regions particularly the sub-Saharan Africa (ter Kuile *et al.* 2004). Concerning the global HIV epidemic, the sub-Saharan Africa remains by far the worst-affected region with 25.4 million people living with HIV (Just under two thirds, i.e. 64% of all people living with HIV) (WHO, 2004). The HIV/AIDS epidemic is affecting the females most severely and because heterosexual transmission is predominant in the sub-region, women of reproductive age make up almost 57% of adults living with HIV, accounting for up to 80% of the world's HIV-infected women (WHO, 2004; Dabis and Ekpini, 2002; De Cock, 2000), and the prevalence rates sometimes exceeding 40% among pregnant women in the sub-region (UNAIDS, 2001). Because of the high prevalence of HIV and malaria in sub-Saharan Africa, co-infections are common. Initial studies conducted among children and adults failed to show a consistent pattern of a biologic or clinical interaction between malaria and HIV infection Chandramohan and Greenwood, 1998; French Gilks, 2000; Rowland-Jones and Lohman, 2002), the two diseases were however, identified to critically intersect in pregnancy and have serious consequences in pregnant women, their fetuses, and infants (ter Kuile *et al.* 2004; Ticconi *et al.* 2003). Although there is now accumulating evidence for an effect of HIV-1 infection in adults and children on malaria (French *et al.* 2001; Whitworth *et al.* 2000; Francesconi *et al.* 2001), the effect of HIV on malaria in pregnancy is much more pronounced as HIV appeared to impair a pregnant woman's ability to control malaria parasitemia, resulting in more frequent and higher density parasitemia than in HIV-uninfected pregnant women (Steketee *et al.* 1996; Ticconi *et al.* 2003).

Approximately one million pregnancies per year are thought to be complicated by coinfection with malaria and HIV in sub-Saharan Africa, because the two diseases are known to critically intersect in pregnancy and have serious consequences in pregnant women, their fetuses, and infants (ter Kuile *et al.* 2004). HIV infection has been associated with an increased prevalence and density of malaria in pregnancy in a number of studies in sub-Saharan Africa, also, in most studies, the prevalence of placental malaria infection was also found to be significantly more prevalent in HIV-positive compared with HIV-negative mothers (ter Kuile *et al.* 2004; Ladner *et al*, 2002; Verhoeff *et al.* 1999).

Interactions in Pregnancy

Pregnant women have specific risks of complications from both malaria and HIV infection. Many women are exposed to both infections; in 11 of the 43 sub-Saharan African countries with malaria at least 10%of pregnant women attending antenatal clinics are HIV infected (WHO 2004). The symptoms and complications of malaria during pregnancy differ with the intensity of malaria transmission and thus with the level of pre-existing immunity already acquired by the pregnant woman. Each year in malaria endemic areas of tropical Africa an estimated 25 million women become pregnant. In these areas, most adult women have developed sufficient immunity such that, even during pregnancy, *P.falciparum* infection does not usually result in fever or other clinical symptoms. However, particularly during their first or second pregnancy, women are highly vulnerable to the adverse consequences of malaria: maternal anaemia, placental malaria and low birth weight infants due to preterm delivery and intrauterine growth retardation (IUGR). For pregnant women in areas of unstable malaria, the risk of developing severe malaria is 2-3 times higher than for non-pregnant women (WHO 2004). In addition, in these areas, malaria may result in low birth weight infants, spontaneous abortion or neonatal death. The health of women in malaria-endemic areas is further affected by HIV. Women in Africa are being infected at an earlier age than men and at present in sub-Saharan Africa there are, on average,13 HIV-positive women for every 10 HIV-positive men. HIV has become one of the major causes of maternal mortality in many resource-constrained settings (Mc Inytre, 2003; Bicego *et al.* 2002). It has an impact on obstetrical causes of maternal mortality by increasing the risk of pregnancy complications such as anaemia, post-partum haemorrhage and puerperal sepsis. Furthermore, in the absence of interventions about a third of infants born to HIV-infected women will become infected with the virus.

The Effect of HIV on Malaria during Pregnancy

A meta-analysis of studies on co-infection in pregnancy (ter Kuile *et al.* 2004) demonstrates that HIV infection impairs the ability of pregnant women to control *P. falciparum* infection. They are more likely to develop clinical and placental malaria, more often have detectable malaria parasitaemia and have higher malaria parasite densities. Most women in their first or second pregnancy are at higher risk of severe or complicated malaria than during subsequent pregnancies. However, this protective effect is diminished in HIV-infected women who, irrespective of the number of pregnancies, remain susceptible to the negative consequences of malaria infection. Hence,in the presence of HIV infection, the malaria-associated risks in pregnant women who have had two or more pregnancies are comparable to the malaria-associated risks during the first or second pregnancy in women without HIV infection.

Anaemia can result from infection with malaria or HIV and during pregnancy contributes to higher levels of maternal morbidity and mortality as well as low birth weight infants. Studies from western Kenya (Ayisi *et al.* 2003) describe a synergistic interaction between malaria and HIV such that pregnant women with dual infection are at a significantly greater risk of anaemia than women with malaria or HIV infection alone. The increased risk of anaemia that occurs in co-infected pregnant women may be due to the higher parasite densities and longer duration of malaria infection that occurs in HIV-infected pregnant women. Studies on cellular and humoral responses to malaria suggest that the increased susceptibility of HIV-infected pregnant women to malaria is due to modifications in systemic and placental immunologic parameters (ter Kuile *et al.* 2004).

Estimating the Magnitude of the Impact of HIV on the Burden of Malaria in Pregnancy

The impact of HIV on the burden of malaria during pregnancy can be estimated using data on the prevalence of HIV among pregnant women, and on the HIV-associated increased risk of malaria during pregnancy. In areas with stable malaria in Africa, approximately 25 million pregnant women are exposed each year to the disease. Of these women, at least 10.5 million develop malaria in the second or third trimester. It can be estimated that in 2003,the proportion of malaria infections during pregnancy attributable to HIV was 4.2%(range 3.8%-4.6%), based on an HIV prevalence among pregnant women in sub-Saharan Africa of 7.5%(range 6.9%-8.3%)in 2003.Using this data, it can be calculated that in 2003 the HIV epidemic resulted in an additional 440 000 (range 399 000 –483 000) malaria cases during pregnancy in Africa (ter Kuile *et al.* 2004).

Impact of Co-Infection with Malaria and HIV on Pregnancy Outcome

P. falciparum malaria during pregnancy, can lead to parasite sequestration in the maternal placental vascular space, with consequent maternal anaemia, abortion, stillbirth, fetal distress, prematurity, low birthweight, congenital malaria and neonatal or maternal death

(Brabin, 1983; Greenwood, 1989; Brabin, 1991). The risk of these adverse pregnancy outcomes is further increased with HIV co-infection (Ticconi *et al.* 2003; Ayisi *et al.* 2004). As a result, a considerable proportion of infants exposed in utero to both placental malaria and maternal HIV infection have an increased risk for postneonatal death three to eightfold higher than infants born to mothers with either infection alone (Bloland *et al.* 1995; Ayisi, *et al.* 2003). Whether the dual infection with maternal malaria and HIV increases the risk of mother-to-child transmission (MTCT) of HIV or congenital malaria, is yet to be unequivocally established, as studies examining these relationships have inconsistent findings and a wide range of unanswered questions (Ticconi *et al.* 2003; Brahmbhatt *et al.* 2003; Inion, *et al.* 2003; Ayisi *et al.* 2004; Villamor, *et al.* 2005).

Compared to women with either malaria or HIV infection, women who are co-infected have a higher risk of preterm birth and intrauterine growth retardation and are therefore more likely to have low birth weight infants. Reports suggest that there is no consistent effect of maternal HIV on congenital malaria (Steketee *et al.* 1996). In addition, whether dual exposure to both placental malaria and HIV increases the risk of infant mortality compared with infants born to HIV-infected women without placental infection is not clear; data from studies in Malawi (Bloland *et al.* 1995) and studies from southern Malawi (Verhoeff., 2004) have reported conflicting results. Maternal HIV infection induces pathological changes in the placenta that potentially could interfere with the materno-fetal transfer of antibodies. However, the mechanism of this process and whether a decreased transfer of antibodies to some malaria antigens has an impact on increased susceptibility to malaria in infants is not known.

Malaria and ABO Blood Group

Attempts have been made to determine the significance of particular ABO phenotypes to disease susceptibility such as *P. falciparum* malaria. Although the relationship between blood group and susceptibility to malaria has been studied by several researchers, results have been contradictory and unable to establish an unequivocal link between ABO blood groups and the incidence of malaria parasitemia (Facer and Brown 1979, Martin *et al.*1979, Montoya *et al.* 1994, Gupta and Chowdhuri 1980), malaria antibody levels (Akinboye and Ogunrinade 1987, Thakur and Verma 1992), or the rate of repeat attacks of malaria (Singh *et al.* 1995). However the virulence of *P. falciparum* has been associated with the capacity of the infected RBC to adhere to endothelial cells and to uninfected RBCs, a process known as rosetting which has been linked to the occurrence of severe malaria i.e., cerebral malaria and anaemia (Carlson *et al.* 1990, Rowe *et al.* 1995). And previous studies have implicated the ABO blood group type in rosetting (Rowe *et al.* 1995, Udomsangpetch 1993) and strain-specific blood group preferences for rosette formation have been described previously (Carlson and Wahlgren 1992).

Evidence from some of the studies reviewed clearly established that parasitized erythrocytes form rosettes more readily with red blood cells of either A, B or AB blood groups than with those belonging to blood group O (Udomsangpetch *et al.* 1989,1993, Carlson and Wahlgren 1992, Rowe *et al.* 1995, Barragan *et al.* 2000). Also, it is well established that this parasite-triggered red blood cell rosette formation is associated with the severity of clinical disease (Rowe *et al.* 1995) and with the development of cerebral malaria (Treutiger *et al.* 1992, Chotivanich *et al.* 1998). This may explain why severe malaria, lower haemoglobin levels, jaundice or central nervous system symptoms were relatively more frequent in individuals in the non-O blood groups as was observed in Zimbabwe (Fischer and Boone 1998). Although evidence abound that rosetting potential which is influenced by the ABO blood group, is related to the severity of clinical disease in malaria, but it remains unclear whether rosetting itself is important in pathogenesis or is simply a marker for some other factor which mediates the disease process.

Malaria and Haemoglobin Genotype

Epidemiological and clinical studies have indicated that malaria susceptibility and severity are influenced by hemoglobin genotype with hemoglobin (Hb) AS individuals having a selective advantage in malarial environments. Thus the high frequency of HbAS in human populations has been attributed to the decreased malarial morbidity and mortality experienced by HbAS heterozygotes (Friedman, 1987). However, the precise mechanism by which the sickle cell trait (genotype HbAS) confers a high degree of resistance to severe and complicated malaria remains unknown (Pasvol *et al.* 1978). Furthermore, the extent of the influence of hemoglobin genotype on the susceptibility and severity of malaria in pregnancy is yet to be clearly established.

To some extent it almost certainly relates to the peculiar physical or biochemical properties of HbAS red blood cells: invasion, growth, and development of Plasmodium falciparum parasites are all reduced in such cells under physiological conditions in vitro (Friedman, 1987; Pasvol *et al.* 1978), and parasite-infected HbAS red blood cells also tend to sickle, a process that may result in their premature destruction by the spleen (Luzzato *et al.* 1970; Roth *et al.* 1978; Shear *et al.* 1993). Nevertheless, while such factors appear to be important, recent observations suggest that the mechanism might also involve an immune component. For example, in a study conducted in Gambia, it was found that the immune recognition of *P.falciparum* infected red blood cells was enhanced in HbAS children (Marsh *et al.* 1989), and up-regulation of malaria-specific cell-mediated immune responses has also been observed in HbAS individuals in Sudan (Abu-Zeid *et al.* 1992; Bayoumi *et al.* 1990). While potentially important, such observations could represent epi-phenomena, rather than proximate effects of the HbAS red cell phenotype. Establishing whether or not immune processes are involved may prove useful in learning about malaria protection more generally.

The mechanism by which HbAS protects against malaria has been the subject of speculation for more than 50 years. While to some extent it probably relates to the physical characteristics of HbAS erythrocytes, a number of studies suggest that HbAS may also enhance the acquisition of natural immunity (Guggenmoos *et al.* 1981; Cornille-Brogger *et al.* 1979); however, establishing this relationship is difficult because immunity to malaria is hard to measure.

Relevance of the Research

Despite the severe public health burden of malaria, HIV infection and anaemia particularly on both maternal and neonatal health, they are all preventable. This study would therefore provide comprehensive population-based scientific data that have policy relevance on strategies to address these major health burdens in pregnancy in Nigeria and other parts of the sub-Saharan Africa with similar setting. It would also provide information that will promote policy change required for:

(1) The recognition that malaria, anaemia, and HIV-infection in pregnancy are significant health problems in Nigeria.
(2) Creating the awareness of the availability and feasibility of cost-effective preventive and control strategies.

Project Aim and Specific Objectives

The aim of this study is to provide epidemiologic data leading to the development of practical, affordable, and innovative approaches to reduce the burden of maternal malaria, anaemia, and HIV infection and their impact on pregnant women and on pregnancy outcome in resource-limited settings. Because of the paucity of comprehensive population-based data, the formulation of policies that would transform into effective and sustainable maternal malaria and HIV-infection intervention/control programs for women of child-bearing age, is still an enormous challenge to health policy-makers in this part of the globe.

The specific objectives are:

1. To determine at childbirth the prevalence of maternal/placental malaria, anaemia and HIV infection and their relationship with; (a) Birth weight, (b) Placental weight, (c) Fetal anaemia, (d) Maternal ABO blood group, (e) Maternal Haemoglobin genotype, (f) Socio-demographic parameters, (g) Obstetrics history, (h) Antenatal clinic visits, (i) Use of insecticide treated bed nets (ITNs).
2. To evaluate the association of placental malaria infection with; (a) Placental weight, (b) Neonatal birthweight, (c) Maternal peripheral malaria infection, (d) Neonatal length, (e) Neonatal head circumference.

Materials and Methods

Study Area

This study was conducted in Abakaliki the capital of Ebonyi State in South Eastern Nigeria (Figure 4), from July 2005 to November 2006 and an additional study from February 2007 to April 2007. Ebonyi state is bounded on the west by Enugu while its North and South share boundaries with Benue and Abia State respectively. It is located in the lower belt of

Nigeria. The major river is the Ebonyi River, which is a tributary of Cross-river. The study area is defined by longitude 8°6'6''E and latitude 6°22'28''N, elevated at 380ft above sea level, the vegetation characteristic is that of the tropical rain forest with an average annual rainfall of about 1,600mm and an average atmospheric temperature of 29.5°C (Ebonyi State Ministry of Lands and Survey, 2003). There are two distinct seasons, the wet and the dry seasons, the former takes place between April and October, while the latter occurs from November to March. Malaria transmission in the area is perennial but usually at the peak towards the end of the rainy season. The study was done at the Ebonyi State University Teaching Hospital (EBSUTH), Abakaliki. Apart from being the largest health facility in the area, the choice of the hospital was because it serves as referral centre for gynaecological services in Ebonyi State. As a result of the free maternal health care services rendered by the EBSUTH courtesy of the Ebonyi State Government, the hospital enjoys large patronage from almost all the local government areas of Ebonyi State.

Ethical Considerations

The study protocol was approved by Infectious Diseases Research Division, Department of Medical Microbiology/Parasitology, Faculty of Clinical Medicine, Ebonyi State University, Abakaliki, Nigeria. Ethical clearance was obtained from the Ethical/Medical Advisory committees of the EBSUTH, Abakaliki. The approval was on the agreement that patient anonymity must be maintained, good laboratory practice/quality control ensured, and that every finding would be treated with utmost confidentiality and for the purpose of this research only. All work was performed according to the international guidelines for human experimentation in clinical research (World Medical Association Declaration of Helsinki, 2000).

Study Population/Sampling Technique

Pregnant women were enrolled at labour ward (LW) at full pregnancy term at Ebonyi State University Teaching Hospital (EBSUTH), Abakaliki Nigeria. The study was conducted from November 2006 to November 2007.

Screening at the Labour Ward

The study population comprised of 300 women at full pregnancy term. A Pregnant woman was eligible for participation in the study if she met the following study inclusion criteria:

(i) attended the antenatal clinic at EBSUTH,
(ii) had an uncomplicated singleton pregnancy $\geq$ 32 weeks' gestation (based on the fundal height estimation),

(iii) reside in Abakaliki or neighbouring local government areas, and
(iv) had no known underlying chronic illness.

Following informed consent, a structured questionnaire was administered to each participant shortly before child birth to obtain information on socio-demographic, health, and obstetric factors including parity, use of insecticide treated bednets ITNs and antimalaria chemoprophylaxis-intake compliance and number of antenatal clinic visits during pregnancy. At delivery, about 5ml of the maternal peripheral blood, umbilical cord blood, and placental blood samples were obtained using a sterile needle and syringe and placed in ethylyn-diammine tetra-acetic acid (EDTA) bottle. The placenta of each subject was also collected as soon as it was voided into a transparent sterile plastic container and thereafter preserved for further analysis using formalin.

Placenta blood was collected into EDTA by incising the cleaned maternal surface of the placenta and aspirating blood welling from the incision. The cord blood was obtained from the newborns' side of the umbilical cord veins by venepuncture technique. Information was obtained on the delivery outcome including; baby's sex and mode of delivery. The baby birthweight (Kg) and weight of placenta (Kg) were determined using an electronic weighing balance. The fetal length and fetal head circumference were determined using a measuring tape. All neonatal parameters including birth weight, fetal length, head circumference, and placental weight were assessed immediately after child birth.

The maternal blood sample obtained from each subject was analysed for malaria parasite infection (using both Giemsa stined blood smear microscopic technique and Rapid diagnostic test Kits), haemoglobin concentration, packed cell volume, ABO blood group, haemoglobin genotype and HIV infection. The placental blood sample was analysed for malaria parasite, while the cord blood was analysed for haemoglobin concentration.

Strategies to Keep Variables Constant

Because of the possibility of the existence of potential variables which could serve as confounding factors in this study, a number of strategies were adopted to eliminate or keep these variables constant through out the study. Such variables include (a). Varying skills of gynaecologists and obstetricians, (b). Presence of maternal underlying disease conditions, (c) Wide gap in the socio-economic status of subjects, (d). Advanced HIV disease, (e). Other anaemia causing conditions, (f). Variations in the methods of sample collection, (g). Variations in the laboratory procedures. The strategies adopted to eliminate or keep these variables constant include the following:

(i) Well established maternal care and fetal delivery procedures generally stipulated by the authorities of the hospital were adopted by all the gynaecologists and obstetricians who participated in this work.
(ii) As indicated in the study inclusion criteria, all pregnant women with known or established underlying disease condition were excluded from the study.

(iii) There was no very wide gap among the subject socio-economically. Because of the free maternal care services offered by the hospital, majority of the subjects fall within the middle and low income category.
(iv) All the subjects with advanced HIV disease were excluded from this study
(v) To eliminate to a great extent other causes of anaemia, apparently healthy women were enrolled into the study. The subject enrolment was done with the assistance of a gynaecologist who examined each subject before inclusion into the study. None of the patients enrolled presented symptoms of causes of anaemia such as tuberculosis, urinary schistosomiasis, and hookworm infection; although no laboratory screening was done to confirm this. No laboratory screening was done to assess nutritional anaemia, but it was ensured that any subject clearly presenting with symptoms of nutritional anaemia was excluded from the study.
(vi) Same sampling methods were used in the collection of all samples. Any sample that was poorly collected was excluded.
(vii) Same laboratory procedures were used for sample analysis. All samples were analysed within one hour of collection. Any sample that could not be analysed within this stipulated period was excluded.

Laboratory Analysis

In this phase of the study conducted at the Labour Ward, the maternal blood sample obtained from each subject was analysed for malaria parasite infection (using both Giemsa stained blood smear microscopic technique), haemoglobin concentration, packed cell volume, ABO blood group, haemoglobin genotype and HIV infection. The placental blood sample was analysed for malaria parasite, while the cord blood was analysed for haemoglobin concentration and packed cell volume.

Malaria Parasite Microscopy Technique

Giemsa-stained thick and thin blood films were performed and the Plus System was used for the determination of parasite density as previously outlined (WHO, 1991).

Determination of Haemoglobin Concentration (HBC) and Packed Cell Volume PCV)

The haemoglobin (Hb) concentration was determined using the cyanmethaemoglobin method described previously (Dacie and Lewis, 1994); reading was done using a Spectrophotometer (Bayer RA 50). While the packed cell volume (PCV) was determined using the hematocrit technique (Dacie and Lewis, 1994). The WHO definition of anaemia in pregnancy i.e., haemoglobin concentration Hb<11g/dl (WHO, 1992), and fetal anaemia defined by Hb<12.5 g/dl (Brabin *et al.* 2004; le Cessie *et al.* 2002) were adopted in this investigation.

Determination of Haemoglobin Genotype

The hemoglobin genotype was determined by the Hemoglobin electrophoresis technique at alkaline pH using cellulose acetate membrane (CAM) as described previously (Schneider, 1974; Wild and Bain, 2004). Haemoglobin solutions (haemolysates) were prepared by lysing packed cell in Triton-X 100 or EDTA and these were applied to cellulose acetate by an applicator that gives a discrete line. Tris-EDTA-borate buffer pH 8.4 was used and the electrophoresis was run at 350v for 25mins.The sample plates were then stained simultaneously using ponceaus stain in trichloro acetic acid solution. Excess stain was removed by washing in acetic acid solution and the plates were left to dry; the samples appeared as discrete red binds on a white background.

Determination of ABO Blood Group

The ABO blood grouping test was performed using the slide method as outlined previously (Dacie and Lewis, 1994), with commercially available reagents which produced strong agglutination within 1-2 minutes (Murex Diagnostics, Inc. Dartford, UK).

Data and Statistical Analysis

The Chi-Square test was used in the analysis of all data in the tables in which association between variables or parameters were assessed in accordance with a number of similar earlier studies in other parts of sub-Saharan Africa (Steketee *et al.* 1996c; Verhoeff *et al.* 1999; Van Eijk *et al.* 2001; Okoko *et al.* 2002). The choice of the chi-square if because it is an effective statistical analysis tool for the comparison or analysis of differences in prevalence rates, proportions or linear trend (Steketee *et al.* 1996c; Verhoeff *et al.* 1999). In this study, a P value of < 0.05 was considered statistically significant. The calculated chi-square value of each parameter investigated at the appropriate degree of freedom denoted by n —1, is indicated at the tables. This was compared with the tabulated chi-square values at 0.05 level of probability to ascertain if the trend was statistically significant or not.

Results

Demographic Parameters and Characteristics of Women Studied

A total of 300 women at full pregnancy term were studied during childbirth in the Phase 2 of this research, and of these, 278(92.7%) had spontaneous vaginal delivery (SVD), 19(6.3%) had caesarean section (CS), while 3(1.0%) had vaccum extractor (ventouse).

Information was available on the babies born by only 226 of the mothers and resulted to 231 babies, comprised of 119(51.5%) males and 112(48.5%) females. A total of 219 babies

(116 males and 103 females) were singleton, 6 sets of twins (3 sets of females and 3 sets of male and female), and a set of triplet (2 males and 1 female).

Information on the babies of the remaining 74 mothers could not be obtained due to logistic problems encountered at the labour ward during the study. The distribution of subjects according to demography and obstetrics data is summarized in Table 1.

Table 1. Demographic/obstetrics data of women studied during delivery at childbirth

Parameter	Number(%) of subjects
Age	
15-19	1(3.7)
20-24	72(24.0)
25-29	106(35.3)
30-34	76(25.3)
35-39	26(8.7)
≥ 40	9(3.0)
Total	300
Parity	
Primiparous	89(29.7)
Multiparous	211(70.3)
Total	300
Occupation	
Students	28(11.8)
Civil Servants	72(30.3)
Housewives	44(18.5)
Business	69(30.0)
Farmer	25(10.5)
Total	238
Antenatal visits	
None	89(27.7)
≤ 4	46 (18.7)
5-9	81(27.0)
≥10	74(24.7)
Total	300
ITNs Possession	
Yes	17(15.7)
No	283(94.3)
Total	300
Educational Level	
None	32(13.4)
Primary	75(31.5)
Secondary	73(30.7)
Tertiary	58(24.4)
Total	238

The prevalence of malaria infection, HIV infection and haematological characteristics of the women studied is summarized in Table 2. The average age of the women at childbirth was 28 years and age ranged from 15-43 years. Up to 29.7% were primiparous with a greater number in civil service (30.3%).

Table 2. Prevalence of malaria infection, HIV infection and haematological characteristics of women studied at childbirth in the labour ward

Parameters	Number (%) of subjects
Malaria infection (microscopy)	
Infected	48(16.0)
Uninfected	252(84.0)
Total	300
Malaria parasitemia	
1-10 parasites per 100 thick film fields	
('+' or 4-40 parasites per mm3)	11(22.9)
11-100 parasites per 100 thick film fields	
('++' or 41-400 parasites per mm3).	37(77.1)
Total	48
Packed Cell Volume	
<24	2(1.1)
25-29	12(6.7)
30-34	23(12.8)
35-39	29(16.1)
≥ 40	114(63.3)
Total	180
Haemoglobin Concentration	
< 7.0	2(1.1)
7.0- 8.9	7(3.8)
Haemoglobin Concentration	
9.0-10.9	22(12.2)
≥ 11	149(82.8)
Total	180
HIV Status	
Positive	8(3.6)
Negative	217(96.4)
Total	225
Blood group	
A	40(19.2)
B	34(16.3)
AB	4(1.9)
O	118(56.7)
Total	208
Genotype	
AS	80(38.5)
AA	128(61.5)
Total	208

Among the subjects, 27.7% did not visit the antenatal clinic while 24.7% visited the antenatal clinic up to ten times during pregnancy. Results indicated that 13.4% of the women had no formal education while 24.4% got to tertiary level of education but only 17(15.7%) of the subjects possessed insecticide treated bednets (Table 1). Eight (3.6%) of the women were HIV positive, while a total of 118(56.7) and 80(38.5%) had blood group O and HbAS genotype respectively. Results showed that up to 149(82.8%) of the subjects had HbC values equal or greater 11g/dl (Table 2).

According to the criteria of this investigation malaria parasite were found in the peripheral blood of 48(16.0%) women. Of the 48 women infected by malaria parasite, 1-10 parasites per 100 thick film fields were recorded in 11(22.9) while 11-100 parasites per 100 thick film fields were recorded in the remaining 37(77.1%) (Table 2).

Demographic Parameters and Characteristics of Babies Studied

The characteristics of neonates and placentas of subjects studied at childbirth are summarized in Table 3. Of the 300 babies delivered, a total of 52 (22.5%) had low birth weight (LBW)($\leq$ 2.5kg) while 36(15.6%) had birthweight greater than 3.5kg.

A majority of the babies (68.7%) had HbC values less than 13.5g/dl. A total of 30(14.0%) of the placentas weighed less or equal to 0.4Kg and malaria parasites were found in 34(12.2%) of placental blood samples (Table 3).

Table 3. Characteristics of neonates and placentas of women studied at childbirth in the labour ward of EBSUTH, Abakaliki, Nigeria

Parameters	Number (%) of subjects
Neonatal Sex	
Female	116(38.7)
Male	184(61.3)
Total	300
Neonatal Birthweight (Kg)	
≤ 2.5	52(22.5)
2.6-3.5	189 (60.2)
≥ 3.6	36(15.6)
Total	231
Neonatal PCV (%)	
< 25	42(20.2)
25 – 34	58(27.9)
35 – 44	58(27.9)
45 – 54	25(12.0)
≥55	16(7.7)
Total	208

Table 3. (Continued)

Parameters	Number (%) of subjects
Neonatal HbC (g/dl)	
<12.5	139(65.6)
≥12.5	73(84.4)
Total	212
Placental Weight (Kg)	
≤ 0.4	30(14.0)
0.5 - 0.7	164(76.6)
≥0.8	20(9.3)
Total	214
Placental Malaria	
Infected	34(12.2)
Uninfected	244(87.8)
Total	278

The Prevalence of Malaria Infection in Relation to Maternal Age, Parity, ANC Attendance and HIV Infection

According to the criteria of this investigation malaria parasite were found in the peripheral blood of 48(16.0%) women. Of the 48 women infected by malaria parasite, 1-10 parasites per 100 thick film fields were recorded in 11(22.9) while 11-100 parasites per 100 thick film fields were recorded in the remaining 37(77.1%). The prevalence of malaria infection in relation to maternal age, parity ANC attendance and HIV infection among the women at childbirth is summarized in Table 4.

Individuals of age group 20-24 years had the highest prevalence of maternal malaria (20.8%) while the least was recorded among those older than 39years (11.1%), but there was no significant difference in the trend (χ^2=2.02, df =4, P>0.05). Malaria infection was more frequent among the primigravidae (18.0%), than the multigravidae (15.2%) but there was no significant difference in the trend (χ^2=0.17, df=1, P>0.05). Women who did not attend antenatal clinic (ANC) during pregnancy and those who attended ANC less than 5 times were more likely to have malaria infection, although the difference was not statistically significant (χ^2=3.79, df=3, P>0.05) (Table 4).

The prevalence of malaria infection was higher (16.3%), among individuals who did not have insecticide treated bednets (ITNs) than among those who had (11.8%) but the difference was not statistically significant (χ^2=1.33, df=1, P>0.05). Result showed that the prevalence of HIV infection was 3.6% and HIV-positive women had higher prevalence of malaria infection than the HIV-negative women (37.5% versus 14.3%), the difference was statistically significant (χ^2 =13.3, df=1, P<0.05). The prevalence of malaria infection decreased with increase in HbC and the difference was statistically significant (χ^2=23.8, df=3, P<0.05) (Table 4).

Table 4. Prevalence of malaria infection in relation to demographic/obstetrics data, HIV infection and haemoglobin concentration among women at childbirth in, Abakaliki.

Parameter	Number Examined	Number(%)with Malaria Infection	Statistical Analysis χ^2 test P value	Statistical Difference
Age				
≤ 19	11	2(18.2)	2.02 P>0.05	No
20-24	72	15(20.8)		
25-29	106	16(15.1)		
30-34	78	11(14.5)		
35-39	26	8(11.5)		
≥ 40	9	1(11.1)		
Total	300	48(16.0)		
Parity				
Primigravidae	89	16(18.0)	0.17 P>0.05	No
Multigravidae	211	32(15.2)		
Total	300	48(16.0)		
Antenatal Visits				
None	35	6(17.1)	3.79 P>0.05	No
≤ 4	71	15(21.1)		
5 – 9	86	11(12.8)		
≥ 10	45	4(8.9)		
Total	237	36(15.2)		
HIV Status				
Positive	8	3(37.5)	13.3 P<0.05	Yes
Negative	217	32(14.3)		
Total	225	35(15.6)		
HbC (g/dl)				
<7.0	2	2(100)	23.8 P<0.05	Yes
7.0-8.9	7	3(42.9)		
9.0-10.9	22	7(31.8)		
≥ 11	149	28(18.8)		
Total	180	40(22.2)		
ITNs Possession				
Yes	17	2(11.8)	1.33 P>0.05	No
No	283	46(16.3)		
Total	300	48(16.0)		

Prevalence Peripheral Malaria in relation to Maternal Demographic and Haematological Parameters

Individuals of age group 20-24 years had the highest prevalence of maternal malaria (20.8%) while the least was recorded among those older than 39years (11.1%), but there was no significant difference in the trend ($\chi2$=2.02, df =4, P>0.05) (Table 5). Those whose occupation was farming were significantly more infected with malaria parasite (32.0%), than individuals of other occupations ($\chi2=12.9$, df=6, $P<0.05$) (Table 5). Women, who had no formal education recorded the highest prevalence of malaria infection (28.1%) though, statistically there was no significant difference ($\chi2=2.69$,df=3, $P>0.05$).

Individuals with HbAA genotype were more infected with malaria parasite than those with HbAS genotype (17.9% versus 12.5%) but the difference was not statistically significant ($\chi2=1.11$, df=1,$P>0.05$).

The highest prevalence of malaria infection was recorded among women with blood group O (19.5%) followed by those of blood group A (15.4%), there was also no significant difference in the trend ($\chi2 =1.55$, df=3, $P>0.05$) (Table 5). The prevalence of malaria infection decreased with increase in HbC and the difference was statistically significant ($\chi2=23.8$, df=3, $P<0.05$) (Table 5).

Table 5. Prevalence of malaria infection in relation to demographic/obstetrics data, and haematological parameters among women at childbirth.

Parameter	Number Examined	Number(%)with Malaria Infection	Statistical Analysis χ^2 test *P* value	Statistical Difference
Occupation				
Students	28	5(17.9)	12.9 P<0.05	Yes
Civil Servants	72	9(12.5)		
Housewives	44	8(18.2)		
Business	69	14(20.3)		
Farmers	25	8(32.0)		
Total	238	44(18.5)		
Educational Level				
None	32	9(28.1)	2.69 P>0.05	No
Primary	75	12(16.0)		
Secondary	73	13(17.8)		
Tertiary	58	9(15.3)		
Total	238	43(18.1)		
Genotype				
AA	128	23(17.9)	1.11 P>0.05	No
AS	80	10(12.5)		
Total	208	33(15.9)		
Blood Group				
A	52	8(15.4)	1.55 P>0.05	No
B	34	5(14.7)		
AB	4	0(0)		
O	118	23(19.5)		
Total	208	36(17.3)		

Prevalence Maternal Peripheral Malaria, HIV Infection and Parity in relation to Neonatal Birthweight

The results of the association of neonatal birth weight with maternal malaria infection, HIV infection, parity and ANC attendance are summarized in Table 6. A higher proportion of malaria infected women (21.6%) had babies with low birth weight compared to women without malaria infection (18.8%). Statistical analysis using chi-square showed no significant difference in the trend (χ^2=1.81, df=1, P>0.05). Anaemic women (with HbC <11.0g/dl) had a higher proportion of low birth weight babies (20.0%) than the non-anaemic women (16.4%) but the difference was not statistically significant (χ^2=0.53, df=1, P>0.05). The frequency of low birth weight was higher among the primigravidae (29.9%) than among the multigravidae (12.6%), and the difference was statistically significant (χ^2=9.92, df=1, P<0.05) (Table 6).

Table 6. Association of neonatal birthweight with maternal malaria infection, demographic/obstetrics data, HIV infection and haemoglobin concentration among women at childbirth in Abakaliki, Nigeria

Maternal Parameters	Neonatal Birthweight(Kg) (%)			Overall	Mean	Statistical Analysis		
	< 2.5	≥2.5-3.5	3.6	Total	Birthweight (kg)	χ2 test	*P value*	*Statistical Difference*
Malaria Infection								
Infected	8(21.6)	26(70.3)	3(8.1)	37	2.37	1.81	*P>0.05*	No
Uninfected	34(18.8)	115(63.5)	32(17.7)	181	2.94			
Total	42	141	35	218				
HIV Status								
Positive	1(25.0)	3(75.0)	0(0.0)	4	2.58	0.75	*P>0.05*	No
Negative	30(16.5)	122(67.0)	30(16.5)	182	2.98			
Total	31	125	30	186				
Parity								
Primigravidae	20(29.9)	42(62.7)	5(7.5)	67	2.75	9.92	*P<0.05*	Yes
Multigravidae	20(12.6)	119(74.8)	20(12.6)	159	3.03			
Total	40	161	25	226				
Antenatal Visits								
None	4(25.0)	9(56.3)	3(18.8)	16	2.80	7.51	*P>0.05*	No
1-4	12(21.4)	39(69.6)	5(8.9)	56	2.85			
5-9	7(9.2)	58(76.3)	11(14.5)	76	3.04			
≥ 10	2(8.3)	19(79.2)	3(12.5)	24	3.22			
Total	25	125	22	172				

The HIV positive women had higher proportion of LBW babies (25.0%) compared to the HIV negative women (16.5%), but there was no statistically significant difference in the trend (χ^2=0.75, df=1, P>0.05). The highest proportion of LBW occurred among women who never attended the ANC during pregnancy (25.0%) and the least among those who attended up to ten times (8.3%), statistically there was no significant difference in the trend (χ^2=7.51, df=3, P>0.05).

Association of Neonatal Birthweight and Haematological Parameters

The Women with blood group O recorded the highest proportion of LBW (23.4%) followed by those of the blood group A (14.0%), statistically however, no significant difference was observed in the trend (χ^2=6.56,df=3, P>0.05). The proportion of LBW was higher among those with HbAA genotype (17.4%) than those with HbAS genotype (12.0%). The difference in the trend was not statistically significant (χ^2=3.54,df=3, P>0.05) (Table 7).

Table 7. Association of neonatal birth weight and haematological parameters among women at childbirth in Abakaliki, Nigeria

Maternal Parameters	Neonatal Birthweight(Kg)(%)			Overal l	Mean		Statistical Analysis	
	< 2.5	2.5-3.5	≥ 3.6	Total	Birthweight (kg)	χ2 test	*P value*	*Statistical Difference*
Haemoglobin concentration								
<11.0g/dl	5(20.0)	16(64.3)	4(16.0)	25	3.04	0.53	*P>0.05*	No
≥11.0g/dl	19(16.4)	83(71.6)	14(12.1)	116	2.97			
Total	24	99	18	141				
Blood Group								
A	6(14.0)	30(69.8)	7(16.3)	43	3.04	6.56	*P>0.05*	No
B	2(6.5)	25(80.6)	4(12.9)	31	3.09			
AB	0(0.0)	2(100.0)	0(0.0)	2	2.85			
O	25(28.0)	68(63.6)	14(13.1)	107	2.98			
Total	33	125	25	183				
Genotype								
AS	9(12.0)	59(78.7)	7(9.3)	75	2.97	3.54	*P>0.05*	No
AA	19(17.4)	72(66.1)	18(16.5)	109	2.98			
Total	28	131	25	184				

Prevalence Placental Malaria in Relation to Maternal Peripheral Malaria, Placental Weight, Neonatal Birthweight and Anthropometric Parameters

A total of 278 placental blood samples were available for study, and of these, 34(12.2%) had malaria parasites of between 1-10 parasites per 100 thick film fields. Placental weight was determined for 214 placental samples. Neonatal birthweight was determined for 231 babies while the fetal length and fetal head circumference were determined for 195 and 190 babies respectively (Table 8).

Table 8. Association of placental malaria with maternal malaria, placental weight and fetal parameters in Abakaliki, south-eastern Nigeria

Parameter	Number Examined	Number (%) with Infected placenta	Statistical Analysis .		
			χ2 test	*P value*	*Statistical Difference*
Maternal Malaria Infection					
Infected	48	26(54.2)	94.4	*P<0.05*	Yes
Uninfected	230	28(3.5)			
Total	278	34(12.2)			
Placental Weight (Kg)					
≤ 0.4	30	10 (33.3)	6.99	*P<0.05*	Yes
0.5-0.7	164	21(12.8)			
≥ 0.8	20	3(15.0)			
Total	214	34(15.9)			
Birthweight (Kg)					
<2.5	52	8(15.4)	0.031	*P>0.05*	No
2.6- 3.5	139	20(14.4)			
≥ 3.6	36	5(13.9)			
Total	231	33(14.3)			
Fetal length (cm)					
≤ 45	29	4(13.8)	1.31	*P>0.05*	No
46-50	131	15(11.5)			
≥51	35	2(5.7)			
Total	195	21(10.8)			
Fetal head circumference (cm)					
<35	51	6(11.8)	0.04	*P>0.05*	No
≥ 35	139	15(10.8)			
Total	190	21(11.1)			

The association of placental malaria infection with placental weight, neonatal birthweight, maternal malaria infection, fetal length and fetal head circumference is summarized Table 8. Results showed that of the total of 214 placental sample of which the weight was determined, 34(15.9%) had malaria parasite infection with a higher proportion (33.3%) of malaria infected placentas having placental weight equal or less than 0.4kg. There was a statistical significant difference in the trend (χ^2=6.99, df=2, P<0.05). A higher proportion of babies born by mothers with malaria infected placenta had LBW (15.4%), but statistical analysis showed no significant difference in the trend (χ^2=0.031, df=3, P>0.05) (Table 8). Women with peripheral malaria infection had significantly higher proportion (54.2%) of placental malaria infection than those without peripheral malaria infection (3.5%) (χ^2=94.4, df=1, P<0.05). When placental malaria was related to fetal length and fetal head circumference, a higher proportion of infected placenta was associated with lower fetal length and lower fetal head circumference although no significant difference was observed in the fetal length (χ^2=1.31, df=2, P>0.05) and fetal head circumference (χ^2=0.04, df=1, P>0.05) (Table 8).

Prevalence Maternal Peripheral Malaria, Parity, HIV Infection and Haemoglobin levels in relation to Neonatal (Fetal) Anaemia

The association of fetal haemoglobin concentration with maternal malaria infection, parity and HIV infection is summarized in Table 9. The prevalence of fetal anaemia was 65.6%. The primigravidae had slightly higher proportion of babies with fetal anaemia (67.5%) than the multigravidae (65.0%), the difference was also not statistically significant (χ^2 =0.09, df=1, P>0.05). Women with peripheral malaria infection had babies with higher proportion of fetal anaemia (72.2%) compared with the uninfected women (64.2%), but the difference was not statistically significant (χ^2 =1.97, df=1, P>0.05). Fetal anaemia prevalence was higher among babies born by anemic women (82.6%) than those of the non-anemic women (63.5%) but the difference was not statistically significant (χ^2 =3.32, df=1, P<0.05). The prevalence of fetal anaemia was higher among babies born by the HIV-positive women (83.3%) than those of the HIV-negative women (65.0%). Statistical analysis showed no significant difference in the trend (χ^2 =0.86, df=1, P>0.05) (Table 9).

Table 9. Association of fetal haemoglobin concentration (HbC) with maternal malaria Infection, anaemia and HIV infection among women at childbirth in the Abakaliki-Nigeria

Maternal Parameters	Fetal HbC (g/dl) .		Overall		Statistical Analysis .	
	No.(%) <12.5	No.(%) ≥ 12.5	Total	χ2 test	*P value*	*Statistical Difference*
Parity						
Primigravidae	33(67.5)	16(32.7)	49	0.09	*P>0.05*	No
Multigravidae	106(65.0)	57(35.0)	163			
Total	139(65.6)	73(84.4)	212			
Malaria Infection						
Infected	26(72.2)	10(27.8)	36	1.97	*P>0.05*	No
Uninfected	113(64.2)	63(35.8)	176			
Total	139(65.6)	73(84.4)	212			
HbC						
<11g/dl	19(82.6	4(17.4)	23	3.32	*P>0.05*	No
≥11g/dl	120(63.5)	69(36.5)	189			
Total	139(65.6)	73(84.4)	212			
HIV Status						
Positive	5(83.3)	1(16.7)	6	0.86	*P>0.05*	No
Negative	134(65.5)	72(35.0)	206			
Total	139(65.6)	73(84.4)	212			

Discussion

Effects of Malaria and HIV Infection on Maternal Parameters at Childbirth and on Birthweight

Malaria and Age

Individuals of the ≤19 years and 20-24 years age categories were more infected with malaria infection than other age groups categories, although the difference in the trend was not statistically significant. This observation supported previous findings from eastern Sudan (Adam *et al.* 2005) and in Kigali, Rwanda (Lander *et al.* 2002) which indicated that age was not significantly associated with malaria during pregnancy. In contrast however, a number of earlier studies reported a significant association between maternal age and malaria infection during pregnancy (Bouyou-Akotet *et al.* 2003; Rogerson *et al.* 2000). In a study conducted in Blantyre, Malawi, after stratifying by gravidity, associations between age and parasite prevalence were reportedly stronger than those between gravidity and prevalence after stratifying by age (Rogerson *et al.* 2000). The reason for the occurrence of these age-related differences in malaria prevalence may probably be related to host or environmental factors.

Malaria and Parity

The prevalence of malaria infection was higher among the primigravidae than the multigravidae, although the difference in the trend was not statistically significant. This finding is consistent with reports from other parts of the sub-Saharan Africa which have consistently indicated that primigravidae are more susceptible to malaria infection than the multigravidae probably because immune suppression is more marked in primigravidae and the protective immunity acquired through malaria infection during the first pregnancy, appears to reduce susceptibility in subsequent pregnancies (Mockenhaupt *et al.* 2000).

Malaria and HIV Infection

The women with HIV infection had a higher prevalence of malaria infection than those without HIV infection and the difference was statistically significant. Similar findings were reported in a number of sub-Saharan African countries including Malawi (Steketee *et al.* 1996), Zimbabwe (Ticconi *et al.* 2003), Kenya (van Eijk *et al.* 2003), and Rwanda (Lander *et al.* 2002). The reason for the higher prevalence of malaria infection among the HIV positive individuals may be due to the impairment of the ability of pregnant women to control *P. falciparum* infection, which was earlier demonstrated (ter Kuile *et al.* 2004), and the interference with the maintenance of immune recognition of malaria by HIV infection in pregnancy (van Eijk *et al.* 2003).

Malaria and Anaemia

In this study, anaemic women had higher prevalence of malaria infection than non-anaemic women. This was consistent with reports from a number of sub-Saharan African countries which indicated that the prevalence of anaemia was consistently higher among pregnant women infected with malaria parasites than those uninfected (Adam *et al.* 2005; Mockenhaupt *et al.* 2006). Individuals with no insecticide treated bed nets and those who never visited the ANC or attended ANC less than 5 times during pregnancy also had higher prevalence of malaria infection. In Kenya (Wabwire-Mangen *et al.* 1989) and Burkina Faso (Parise *et al.* 2003), similar results were reported.

These findings underscore the importance of ANC attendance during pregnancy. It has been demonstrated that substantial reductions in maternal malaria, anaemia, and LBW have been achieved by intervention programs, including the use of ITNs, preventive intermittent treatment and chemoprophylaxis administered at the ANC (Parise *et al.* 2003; Wabwire-Mangen *et al.* 1989). Interventions also exist for maternal anaemia (e.g., good nutrition, iron and folate supplementation, and hookworm treatment) and these have been provided through antenatal care programs. In fact, studies from sub-Saharan Africa have suggest that between 25% and 90% of these adverse events might be prevented by full implementation of existing interventions at the ANC (Miaffo *et al.* 2004).

Low Birth Weight in Relation to Maternal Malaria and Parity

In this study, statistical analysis showed that low birth weight (LBW) was associated with maternal malaria infection, although babies born by infected mothers had a lower mean birth weight and higher prevalence of LBW compared to the uninfected mothers. This indicates that other factors aside from malaria could also be playing major roles in the determination of low birth weight in the study population. The prevalence of LBW was higher among babies born by primigravidae than the multigravidae and the difference was statistically significant ($P<0.05$). This is consistent with the findings from similar studies conducted in south-western Cameroon (Mockenhaupt *et al.* 2006), and Zanzibar, Tanzania (Matteelli *et al.* 1996). Primigravidae have been shown to be more predisposed to have LBW babies than the multigravidae and the risk is even higher when malaria infection is present (Okoko et al. 2002). Because falciparum malaria during pregnancy has been recognized as an important determinant of low birth weight (Brabin, 1991), a number of randomized controlled trials of preventive antimalarial measures during pregnancy have confirmed this causal effect by showing that preventing malaria increases birth weight (Menendez *et al.* 1994). Therefore, the prevention of malaria in pregnancy and, thus, of malaria-attributable low birth weight should increase the survival of young babies.

Low Birth Weight and Anaemia

Shulman *et al.*(2001) established that the major adverse effect of malaria in pregnancy on the mother is anaemia and that in malarious areas, malaria and anaemia are likely to act together to reduce birth weight but their independent effects are difficult to distinguish. In this study however, the prevalence of LBW was considerably higher among women who were anaemic than the non-anaemic women. In a similar study conducted in Papua New Guinea to examine the separate contribution of anaemia or malaria to low birthweight (Brabin and Piper, 1997), it was observed that there was a trend towards increased low birthweight with decreasing haemoglobin levels. Furthermore, in another related study

(Msolla and Kinabo, 1997), it was showed that there was a positive correlation (r = 0.76; P = 0.01) between Hb concentration and weight of the infants at birth and the mean birth weight of the infants born to anaemic subjects was significantly lower compared to that of infants born to non-anaemic subjects. These previous observations in addition to those of this present study, suggest that anaemia had some influence on the birth weight of the infant. Therefore the treatment of anaemia in pregnancy is most likely to improve birthweight. However in an attempt to quantitate the separate effects of anaemia- and malaria-attributable low birth weight, Brabin and Piper (1997) concluded that, in malarious areas, malaria was a more important risk factor for low birth weight than was anaemia.

Low Birth Weight and HIV Infection

Interestingly, the prevalence of LBW was considerably higher among the HIV positive women than the HIV negative women in this present study, although the difference was not statistically significant ($P>0.05$). This is similar to the findings in northern Zimbabwe (Ticconi *et al.* 2003), where HIV infection was independently associated with increased risk of low birth weight (OR = 3.16, 95% CI: 1.80-5.54) and very low birth weight (OR = 10.74, 95% CI: 2.12-54.41). Furthermore, in Kigali, Rwanda, it was observed that the frequencies of low birthweight, prematurity, and intrauterine growth retardation were higher in infants born to HIV positive women than to HIV negative women (Castetbon *et al.* 1999). In yet another study conducted in Kigali, Rwanda, low birth weight was significantly more frequent in full-term infants born to HIV-positive mothers than to HIV-negative mothers (Leroy *et al.* 1994). These results underscore the need for nutritional surveillance and dietary counseling, hoping to improve the prognosis of pregnancy in HIV positive women, regardless of other therapeutic interventions.

Low Birth Weight and ANC Attendance

It was noted in this study that a very high proportion of LBW occurred among babies born by women who did not attend the antenatal clinic and the prevalence of LBW reduced with increase in the number of antenatal clinic visits. This finding clearly demonstrates the efficacy of antimalarial chemoprophylaxis and haematenics which are usually administered during ANC in the prevention of malaria and anaemia and improvement of neonatal birth weight. Despite the non statistically significant difference observed in the trend, this finding supported earlier reports from The Gambia where the birth weight of children born to women who received chemoprophylaxis was increased by an average of 153 g (Menendez *et al.* 1994). In another related study the administration of chemoprophylaxis led to a reduction in the prevalence of low birth weight babies and to an increase in the median birth weight and the perinatal mortality rate was lower, although not significantly so, among the babies of women who had received chemoprophylaxis (Greenwood *et al.* 1994).

Furthermore in a study in rural Malawi (Steketee *et al.* 1996), it was noted that the use of an effective antimalarial was protective against LBW through its effect on reducing placental and umbilical cord blood malaria infection. The study concluded that effective prevention of malaria in pregnant women in malaria-endemic settings may reduce the likelihood of LBW by 5-14%, and may reduce the amount of preventable LBW by more than 30%. Therefore, when evaluating antenatal care programs, health policy makers must consider providing an effective preventive drug as a means to prevent low birth weight and its consequences.

The Relationship between Maternal Malaria, Demographic Parameters, ABO Blood Group, Genotype and Birth Weight at Childbirth

Malaria and Demographic Parameters

Although lower literacy level and younger age were more predisposing factors to malaria infection in this study, the differences in the trend were however not statistically significant. However, occupation was significantly associated with malaria infection but the reason for this outcome was somewhat obscure. Previous findings from eastern Sudan (Adam *et al.* 2005) and Kigali, Rwanda (Lander *et al.* 2002) had indicated that age was not significantly associated with malaria during pregnancy and the report of an investigation from Zanzibar, Tanzania, showed no apparent relationship between malaria and socio-demographic parameters including occupation (Matteelli *et al.* 1994).

Malaria and Genotype

The prevalence of malaria infection in this study was higher among individuals with HbAA genotype than those with HbAS genotype but the difference was not statistically significant (P>0.05). Although studies that investigated this relationship between malaria and haemoglobin genotypes in pregnancy are essentially lacking, malaria has been shown to be consistently higher in non-pregnant individuals with HbAA genotype compared to those with HbAS (Eteng, 2002). The sickle cell trait (HbAS) has been shown to confers a high degree of resistance to severe and complicated malaria (Aluoch, 1997; Aidoo, 2002), but the mechanisms by which the hemoglobin genotype HbAS protect against severe malaria are not fully understood. The greater susceptibility of HbAA individuals to *P. falciparum* malaria and the enhanced severity of an attack in this group may be due to low red cell membrane resistance to the invading parasite and a non-hypoxic environment within the red cell which enhances its development (Eteng, 2002). Furthermore, results from a study that evaluated the immune basis for malaria protection by the sickle cell trait in Kenya suggested that malaria protection by HbAS involves the enhancement of not only innate but also of acquired immunity to the parasite and indicated that a better understanding of the underlying mechanism might yield important insights into both these processes (Williams *et al.* 2005).

Malaria and ABO Blood Group

The highest prevalence of malaria infection in the present investigation was recorded among women with blood group O. Studies evaluating the relationship between malaria and ABO blood group during pregnancy are also essentially lacking. The only current study related to this was the evaluation of the ABO phenotypes and malaria outcomes in mothers and babies in The Gambia (Loscertales and Brabin, 2006). In that study, blood group O was associated with an increased prevalence of active placental infection in primiparae and with a reduced risk of placental malaria in multiparae. Placental parasitaemia was observed to occur at least twice as frequently in primiparae but only among blood group O women. More systematic studies are urgently needed to further elucidate this.

Low Birth Weight in Relation to Blood Group and Genotype

In this investigation maternal malaria infection was not significantly associated with birth weight, although infected mothers had a higher proportion of low birthweight (LBW) babies than the uninfected mothers. Similarly, none of the haematological parameters investigated indicated any significant association with birthweight. The proportion of LBW babies were higher among anaemic women, those with blood group O and individuals of the HbAA genotype. The reason for this outcome could not be clearly ascertained, however it is interesting to note that individuals who belong to these categories had higher prevalence of malaria infection. Therefore these results suggest that maternal malaria may be the major determining factor to LBW in this study and that the haematological parameters may have played only a secondary role in the LBW observed. Falciparum malaria during pregnancy has long been recognized as an important determinant of low birth weight (Brabin, 1991; Menendez *et al.* 1995) and a number of randomized controlled trials of preventive antimalarial measures during pregnancy have confirmed this causal effect by showing that preventing malaria increases birth weight (Cot *et al.* 1995; Menendez *et al.* 1994).

Placental Malaria and Its Relationship with Perinatal Outcome

Prevalence of Placental Malaria

Placental infection measured by placental smear at delivery has been described as a standard indicator, which is widely used to characterize malaria infection in pregnant women (Cottrell *et al.* 2005). Using this technique, a placental *P. falciparum* malaria prevalence of 12.2% was obtained in this study. Placental malaria prevalence results from various parts of sub-Saharan Africa have been discordant, and one of the major factors in the discordance is that different techniques of diagnosis of employed based on the differences in the definition of placental malaria (Othoro *et al.* 2006). Using the placental blood smear microscopy, placental malaria prevalence rates of 9.5%,18.5%,19.9%, and 37.1% were obtained in Senegal (N'Dao *et al.* 2006), Sierra Leone (Morgan, 1994), Cameroon (Tako *et al.* 2005), and Gambia (Okoko *et al.* 2002) respectively.

These results indicate that placental malaria is still unacceptably high in the sub-Saharan Africa and calls for the intensified efforts in malaria control in pregnancy. The importance of effective control measures cannot be overstated because apart from the adverse perinatal outcomes associated with placental malaria, some studies also suggest that children born to mothers with placental malaria are at a high risk of acquiring larger numbers of *P. falciparum* infections in the first 2 years of life compared to infants born to women without placental malaria (Van Eijk *et al.* 2003). Furthermore, it was reported that placental malaria infection diminished the development of antibody responses to malarial epitopes in the first year of life, the age at which most of the severe malaria-associated morbidity occurs in areas of holoendemicity (McElroy *et al.* 1999).

Placental Malaria and Maternal Peripheral Malaria

In this study maternal peripheral malaria infection was significantly associated with placental malaria (P<0.05). This is consistent with a report from Burkina Faso, where a strong correlation was found between placental infection and peripheral infection at the end of pregnancy (Cottrell *et al.* 2005). The authors suggested that peripheral parasitemia at the end of pregnancy is a very strong risk factor for placental infection (a five fold increase), thus confirming the importance of late maternal malaria infection which was noted in another study (Leke *et al.* 1999). Interestingly, up to 3.5% of the mothers without detectable peripheral parasitemia had placental infection in this present study. In Ghana, roughly half of the women with microscopically proven placental parasitemia had a negative peripheral blood film; it was thus suggested that a negative peripheral blood film in pregnant women in endemic areas is hardly informative (Mockenhaupt *et al.* 2006). This finding underscores the importance of assessment of placental malaria, because placental infection may be detected in the absence of peripheral blood parasitemia and may persist after initiation of antimalarial treatment *et al.* (Sartelet *et al.* 1997).

Placental Malaria and Its Relationship with Placental Weight, Fetal Length and Head Circumference

The least placental weight was found to be significantly associated with the highest proportion of placental malaria infection (P<0.05) in this present study. Two earlier studies that evaluated the relationship between placental malaria and placental weight in Haut-Ogooue and Franceville, both in Gabon indicated that the mean weight of term placentas with malarial changes was significantly less than that of placentas without such changes (Gazin *et al.* 1994; Walter *et al.* 1982). Similarly, LBW, lower fetal length and lower fetal head circumference were also associated with higher proportion of malaria infected placenta in this study, although the differences were not statistically significant.

It was noted that despite the prevalence of placental infections for women of all gravidities, ranging from 5% to 52% in sub-Saharan Africa, the risk of LBW associated with infection was relatively consistent, with babies born to mothers with an infected placenta being twice as likely to be of LBW than those born to mothers with an uninfected placenta (Guyatt and Snow, 2004). In southeastern Tanzania, chronic malaria infection of the placenta was associated with significant reductions in mean head circumference, neonatal length, and body index (weight/length^2), whereas past infections were associated with reduced mean length at birth only (Tako *et al.* 2005), but in the Ubangi district of Zaire, malarious placentas had no consistent relationship with neonatal length or head circumference (Anagnos *et al.* 1986). The reduction in the length and head circumference of the newborns associated with chronic infections probably indicate a prolonged effect on fetal nutrition, caused by *P. falciparum* placental parasitization suggested in other studies (Barros *et al.* 1992).These findings were not surprising because, maternal *P. falciparum* malaria was already found to be strongly associated with placental malaria which adversely affects birth weight and fetal anthropometric parameters, thought to be mediated through placental insufficiency, leading to preterm delivery (PTD) and intrauterine growth retardation (IUGR) (Le Hesran *et al.* 1997).

Placental Malaria and Low Birthweight

The processes by which placental malaria leads to LBW and lower fetal anthropometric parameters remain unclear, though it has been suggested that IUGR and PTD associated with maternal malaria could play contributory roles (Kasumba *et al.* 2000; Okoko *et al.* 2002). Many hypotheses, based on a systemic or local failure of the immunological response to malaria, have been proposed to explain the 'preference' of the parasites for replication in the placenta but the exact mechanisms leading to placental changes and determining the observed impairment of materno-foetal exchange are incompletely understood (Matteelli *et al.* 1997). However it has been suggested that parasites are unlikely to be directly responsible for the placental pathology, but leucocytes, through the production of non-chemotactic cytokines, might be associated with the thickening of the trophoblastic basement membrane, and might cause a mechanical blockage of oxygen and nutrient transport across the placenta (Matteelli *et al.* 1997). Thus, the high frequency of adverse perinatal outcomes including prematures, hypotrophic neonates and still-births in the malarial population associated with *P. falciparum* placental infection is explained by the intervillous macrophages, which decrease the maternal blood output and the perivillous excess of fibrin which reduces the materno-fetal exchanges (Philippe and Walter, 1985). These may explain why placental malaria was associated with the reduced placental weight, LBW and lower fetal anthropometric parameters observed in this study.

Epidemiological evidence has shown that the assessment of the impact of malaria on the outcome of pregnancy is complicated because the greatest incidence of infection occurs during the second trimester, and placental and peripheral blood parasitaemia may have resolved by the time of delivery (Brabin, 1983). This may have accounted for the absence of a significant effect of placental malaria on the birthweight observed in this study even though the LBW babies recorded slightly higher proportion of infected placenta. Nevertheless the importance of the assessment of placental malaria cannot be overstated. This is to enable adequate care and monitoring of infants born by mothers with placental malaria, since these infants may be at an increased risk of anaemia, increased malaria prevalence rates, and mortality, during their first year of life (Brabin 1983; Kasumba *et al.* 2000).

It is important to state that a major limitation of this study was the use of placental smear as the technique to diagnose placental malaria. Although the use of placental smear is reasonably diagnostic, the possibility of under-estimation may not be ruled out completely. This is because it has been demonstrated that placental blood film is less sensitive than placental histology (Menendez *et al.* 2000; Mockenhaupt *et al.* 2006).

Placental histology is thus the "gold standard" for the diagnosis of malaria at delivery, but it is relatively costly and labor-intensive and, hence, is frequently not available in most settings of malaria endemic developing countries. However, the use of histological diagnosis of placental malaria in epidemiological studies will allow more detailed characterization of the burden of morbidity attributable to malaria in pregnancy. This is advocated in future studies.

Effects of Maternal Malaria, Anaemia and HIV Infection on Fetal Haemoglobin Levels

Prevalence of Fetal Anaemia

A high level of fetal anaemia (65.6%) defined by cord blood Hb<12.5g/dl, was observed in this study. This was consistent with an earlier report which indicated that the prevalence of fetal anaemia was high in developing countries particularly in malarious areas (Brabin, 1992). In two separate studies conducted in Southern Malawi, a fetal anaemia prevalence of 23.4% (Brabin *et al.* 2004) and 23.3% (Ie Cessie *et al.* 2002) were recorded, while in Maputo Mozambique, up to 93% of newborns were found to have fetal anaemia (Bergstrom *et al.* 1993). These findings were contrary to those obtained from developed countries where it was shown that anaemia in newborns is rare, regardless of maternal status, and furthermore, normal neonatal haemoglobin levels in these populations are higher than adult levels (Erdem *et al.* 2002). In most parts of the sub-Saharan Africa where malaria is endemic, cord haemoglobin levels have been described as lower-than-expected, and it was hypothesized to result from fetal immune activation to maternal malarial antigens (Brabin, 1992). Thus it was suggested that exposure of the fetus to malaria antigens due to damage of the placental barrier may make the newborn more susceptible to immunologically mediated hemolysis or to dyserythropoiesis (Brabin, 1992).

Fetal Anaemia and Maternal Malaria

In this study, the prevalence of fetal anaemia was higher among babies born by malaria infected mothers compared to those of the uninfected mothers, although the difference was not statistically significant ($P>0.05$). This was in conformity with findings from a study conducted in Kisumu, Kenya, where children born to mothers with detectable *P. falciparum* parasitemia on a peripheral blood film at delivery had a lower mean Hb level at birth compared with children born to mothers free of parasitemia at delivery (McElroy *et al.* 1999). Similarly in southern Malawi, a higher prevalence of fetal anaemia occurred with increasing peripheral *P. falciparum* parasite density (p=0.03) and geometric mean placental parasite densities were higher in babies with fetal anaemia than in those without (3331 vs 2152 parasites/microl, p=0.07) (Brabin *et al.* 2004).

On the contrary, Abrams *et al.* (2005) noted from their study in Blantyre, Malawi, that, though malaria was associated with a reduction in maternal haemoglobin (10.8 g/dL vs. 12.1 g/dL, $p < 0.001$), no reduction in cord haemoglobin and no significant relationship between maternal and cord haemoglobin levels were found. According to their report, cord blood markers of haematological and hypoxic statuses did not differ between malaria-infected and uninfected women. This lack of consistency in the findings from various studies may be explained on the basis of the fact that malaria in pregnancy varies with transmission intensity, access to treatment, coverage and quality of antenatal services, and drug resistance, among others (Ie Cessie *et al.* 2002). Variations in these factors may account for the differences in the relationship between maternal malaria and fetal anaemia. Furthermore, the etiology of fetal anaemia is complex and multifactorial and so maternal malaria could either play a major or minor role depending on local epidemiological situation (Brabin, 1992).

Fetal Anaemia and Maternal Anaemia

Maternal anaemia was not significantly associated with fetal anaemia ($P<0.05$) in this study, which suggests that maternal anaemia at childbirth might not play a central role in the development of fetal anaemia. On the contrary, in Southern Malawi, maternal Hb at delivery < 8 g/dl (AOR 1.61, 1.10-2.42) or <11 g/dl (AOR 1.60, 1.10-2.31) was found to be a major factor associated with fetal anaemia (Brabin, 1992). And in an assessment of nutritional anaemia in pregnant Beninese women and its consequences on the haematological profile of the newborn, haemoglobin concentration was significantly lower in babies born of mothers with Fe-deficient anaemia than in babies born of Fe-sufficient mothers (Hercberg *et al.* 1987). These findings were however, not consistent with the results from a similar study conducted in Blantyre, Malawi, where cord haemoglobin values were not correlated to maternal haemoglobin concentration (Abrams *et al.* 2005). The reason for this was not clear but authors noted that the high cord haemoglobin levels observed may relate to the high rates of antimalarial usage and iron supplementation in the Malawian women studied, which might provide a protective effect.

Furthermore it was argued that the maintenance of cord haemoglobin levels despite the presence of maternal anaemia appeared to suggest that the fetus has developed mechanisms to preferentially obtain sufficient iron and produce adequate amounts of red cells, since it was long shown that iron is transported unidirectionally from mother to foetus across a concentration gradient, and thus stores should be preferentially preserved in the fetus (Abrams *et al.* 2005). However, mounting evidence indicates that maternal iron deficiency in pregnancy reduces fetal iron stores, perhaps well into the first year of life and this deserves further exploration because of the tendency of infants to develop iron deficiency anaemia and because of the documented adverse consequences of this condition on infant development (Allen, 2000). Therefore because of a wide range of unanswered questions about the mechanisms involved in the relationship between maternal anaemia and fetal anaemia, further studies using molecular biological tools are urgently needed to properly elucidate this in the sub-Saharan Africa.

Fetal Anaemia and HIV Infection

In this present study, the prevalence of fetal anaemia was considerably higher among babies born by the HIV-positive mothers compared to those of the HIV-negative mothers. Although there is paucity of published data on the relationship between maternal HIV infection and fetal anaemia in sub-Saharan Africa, an available report from Western Kenya, indicated that maternal infection with HIV was a major risk factor to fetal and infant anaemia not only directly, through mother-to-child transmission of HIV, but also indirectly, as suggested by the finding that infant anaemia was worse in HIV-uninfected infants when born to HIV-seropositive mothers compared with those born to HIV-seronegative mothers (van Eijk *et al.* 2002).

A major limitation was the inability to evaluate other potential causes of fetal anaemia including blood loss (through obstetrical causes and internal hemorrhage) and red blood cell destruction (through intrinsic and extrinsic causes). This may have affected adequate assessment of the effects of maternal malaria, HIV infection and anaemia on the fetal anaemia. The inclusion of these factors in future studies is advocated. Another limitation worth mentioning was the use of microscopy technique for the screening of maternal malaria. Although this method is arguably the "gold standard", it is important to note that the possibility of under-diagnosis cannot be completely ruled out. However, because of the public health significance of fetal anaemia and other adverse perinatal outcomes associated with maternal malaria, anaemia and HIV infection in pregnancy, the importance of effective interventional effort cannot be overstated. Interventions should aim to reduce fetal anaemia by improving malaria, HIV infection and anaemia control and treatment in pregnancy and by addressing the determinants of pre-term delivery as this may also affect fetal haemoglobin levels (Brabin *et al.* 2004). It has been suggested that improving antimalarial control and iron supplementation throughout pregnancy should have direct effects on reducing fetal and infant anaemia and improving child development and survival (Draper, 1996). Antiretroviral regimens can also improve the health of HIV-positive pregnant women and reduce fetal anaemia. The WHO guidelines currently recommend highly active antiretroviral therapy (HAART) using the combination of nevirapine, lamivudine,and either stavudine or zidovudine for HIV-infected pregnant women with clinical or laboratory evidence of immunosuppression (WHO, 2004).

Public Health Considerations

Importance of Antenatal Clinics

Despite the concerted efforts by various countries of the sub-Saharan Africa to control the scourge of maternal HIV infection and malaria, there is yet to be any significant reduction of the burden in the sub-region (WHO, 2005). Making motherhood safer still remains an enormous challenge in this part of the world, thereby making the need for a more pragmatic approach to interventional efforts absolutely imperative. In most part of the developing world, maternal and child health services are the most accessible health services in many communities including Nigeria (WHO, 1993). The free maternal health care services offered at the antenatal clinics of Ebonyi State government hospitals has resulted into unprecedented attendance by pregnant women. This development has contributed in the improvement of maternal health in this part of Nigeria. The ANC clinics have served as the main entry point for prevention and care services for pregnant women and their children, and they also served as a good link to other health services for families and communities.

In sub-Saharan Africa, antenatal care utilization is relatively high as more pregnant women are encouraged to avail themselves with the antenatal care services offered (Parise *et al.* 2003). Hence, reproductive health services, and antenatal care services in particular, could serve as the pivotal entry point for simultaneous delivery of interventions for the prevention and control of malaria and HIV in pregnant women and their neonates with linkages to the community, child health, HIV counseling and testing, treatment, care and support services, family planning and other services for tuberculosis and sexually transmitted infections (WHO, 2005). Partnerships and collaboration among maternal and child health, malaria, HIV and other programs are a prerequisite for joint planning and implementation of effective integrated services (WHO, 2002).

Strategies for Malaria Prevention Programs for Pregnant Women

In spite of these challenges efforts are continuously being made to develop new and effective strategies for malaria prevention programs for pregnant African women. A prospective evaluation of malaria prevention in pregnant women in rural Malawi conducted by Steketee *et al.* (1996d) (The Mangochi Malaria Research Project -MMRP), contributed to establishing new criteria for policy and program development for malaria prevention in pregnancy. The principle findings of the MMRP include: (1) populations at risk of the adverse consequences of malaria in pregnancy include women with low parity, women infected with human immunodeficiency virus, pregnancy during the high malaria transmission season, and the use of a malaria drug that is suboptimally efficacious; (2) the estimated maximum benefits of an antimalarial intervention that clears placental and umbilical cord parasitemia are a 5-12% reduction of low birth weight (LBW), an approximately 35% reduction in the risk of LBW for risks that are actually preventable once a woman has become pregnant (e.g., risks such as infectious disease or poor nutrition during gestation), and a 3-5% reduction in the rate of infant mortality; (3) the intervention must be capable of rendering the woman malaria parasite free, including clearance of parasites from the placental vascular space and umbilical cord blood; (4) other diseases adversely affect pregnancy outcome and, while the control of malaria in pregnancy may not warrant independent programming, if coupled with prevention programs to provide a range of antenatal services, the incremental costs of malaria control may prove to be highly cost-effective; and (5) the choice of a regimen must balance intervention efficacy with safety, availability, affordability, and simplicity of delivery, and several antimalarials may meet these criteria.

Treatment and Management of Malaria and HIV Co-Infection in Pregnancy

The importance of a complete overhaul of the existing health system in most areas with HIV and malaria endemicity, to make it more result oriented cannot be overemphasized. The recognition of the immunologic, infectious, and drug-drug interactions in malarial and HIV coinfection is essential for safe and effective treatment and prevention of malaria, during pregnancy. However, low adherence and poor-quality drugs are important factors that must be addressed because they decrease the effectiveness of both antiretroviral and antimalarial drugs and may further hamper treatment outcome in pregnant women with the coinfection (WHO, 2005).

In the face of the mounting evidence of the relative failure of many antimalarial and antiretroviral drugs in most parts of sub-Saharan Africa, the WHO will undoubtedly continue to revise and put forward new guidelines for the treatment of malaria and HIV infection during pregnancy that are operationally feasible in the sub-region (Brentlinger *et al.* 2006; Okereke, 1999). The choice of a regimen must balance intervention efficacy with safety, availability, affordability, and simplicity of delivery. Since pregnant women have increased specific risks of complications from both malaria and HIV infection, the financial and human resource constraints of health systems in countries most affected by malaria and HIV, and the shared determinants of vulnerability for both diseases, indicate the need for integration of preventive and curative services for malaria and HIV and strengthening the health systems that deliver these services (WHO, 2005). This is important because the implementation of the current WHO guidelines is burdened by the notorious problems complicating health service delivery in the developing world particularly in the African continent: the logistical challenges of reaching remote regions, resource scarcity, lack of infrastructure, inadequate treatment, continuing poverty, and armed conflict (Prual *et al.* 2002; Steketee *et al.* 1996d).

It is well established that women in Africa use prenatal care extensively when it is available and accessible. Prenatal health services are a critical place to offer routine provider-initiated HIV testing and counselling and to follow this up with prevention of MTCT interventions according to national policy for those who test positive, coupled with entry to ART programs for those sick and in need of immediate therapy. These services, therefore, need to be strengthened to ensure the delivery of the WHO-recommended antenatal care, which includes a minimum package of interventions for the prevention of both malaria and HIV (WHO, 2005; Prual *et al.* 2002).

This opportunity must be used to implement evidence-based malaria and HIV infection control actions with appropriate and realistic goals. A potentially effective malaria and HIV treatment content for prenatal care adapted to the context of developing countries especially in sub-Saharan Africa must be developed as well as careful monitoring for drug resistance. Furthermore, there is an urgent need to improve access of rural women to ANC services in the sub-Saharan Africa where they can obtain antiretroviral and antimalarial drugs free or at affordable costs, either through increasing the number of rural health centres or establishing functioning outreach services. The distribution of insecticide-treated bed nets need to become implemented on a large scale as this would reduce the incidence of malaria further and would benefit both HIV positive and HIV-negative pregnant women (Prual et al., 2002; Steketee et al., 1996d). Better application of these malaria and HIV interventions could markedly reduce the maternal and infant mortality burden of these diseases and will save many lives.

References

Abrams, E.T., Kwiek, J.J., Mwapasa, V., Kamwendo, D.D., Tadesse, E., Lema, V.M., Molyneux, M.E., Rogerson, S.J. and Meshnick, S.R. (2005). Malaria during pregnancy and foetal haematological status in Blantyre, Malawi. *Malaria Journal* 4:39.

Abu-Zeid, Y.A., Abdulhadi, N.H.,Theander, T.G., Hviid, L., Saeed, B.O. (1992). Seasonal changes in cell mediated immune responses to soluble Plasmodium falciparum antigens in children with haemoglobin AA and haemoglobin AS. *Transactions of the Royal Society of Tropical Medicine and Hygiene* 86:20-22.

Achidi, E.A., Kuoh, A.J., Minang, J.T. (2005). Malaria infection in pregnancy and its effects on hemoglobin levels in women from a malaria endemic area of Fako Division, South West Province, Cameroon. *Journal of Obstetrics and Gynaecology* 25:235-240.

Adam, I., Khamis, A.H. and Elbashir, M.I. (2005). Prevalence and risk factors for *Plasmodium falciparum* malaria in pregnant women of eastern Sudan. *Malaria Journal* 4:18.

Adegnika, A.A., Verweij, J.J., Agnandji, S.T., Chai, S.K., Breitling, L.P., Ramharter, M., Frolich, M., Issifou, S., Kremsner, P.G. and Yazdanbakhsh, M. (2006). Microscopic and sub-microscopic *Plasmodium falciparum* infection, but not inflammation caused by infection, is associated with low birth weight. *American Journal of Tropical Medicine and Hygiene* 75(5):798-803.

Aidoo, M., Terlouw, D.J., Kolczak, M.S, McElroy, P.D. and ter Kuile, F.O. (2002). Protective effects of the sickle cell gene against malaria morbidity and mortality. *Lancet* 359: 1311–1312.

Akinboye, D.O. and Ogunrinade, A.F. (1987). Malaria and loaisis among blood donors at Ibadan, Nigeria. *Transactions of the Royal Society of Tropical Medicine and Hygiene* 81: 398–399.

Allen, L.H. (2000). Anaemia and iron deficiency: effects on pregnancy outcome. *American Journal of Clinical Nutrition* 71: 1280S-1284S.

Allen, L.H. (1997). Pregnancy and iron deficiency: unresolved issues. *Nutrition Review* 55: 91–101.

Aluoch, J.R. (1997). Higher resistance to Plasmodium falciparum infection in patients with homozygous sickle cell disease in western Kenya. *Tropical Medicine and International Health 2*:568-571. Anagnos, D., Lanoie, L.O., Palmieri, J.R., Ziefer, A. and Connor, D.H. (1986). Effects of placental malaria on mothers and neonates from Zaire. *Zournal du Parasitenkd* 72:57-64.

Anorlu, R.I., Odum, C.U. and Essien, E.E. (2001). Asymptomatic malaria parasitaemia in pregnant women at booking in a primary health care facility in a periurban community in Lagos, Nigeria. *African Journal of Medicine and Science* 30:39- 41.

Antelman, G., Msamanga, G.I. and Spiegelman, D. (2000). Nutritional factors and infectious disease contribute to anaemia among pregnant women with human immunodeficiency virus in Tanzania. *Journal of Nutrition* 130:1950-1957.

Ayisi, J.G., van Eijk, A.M., Newman, R.D., ter Kuile, F.O. and Shi, Y.P. (2000). Risk factors for HIV infection among asymptomatic pregnant women attending an antenatal clinic in western Kenya. *International Journal of STD and AIDS* 11:393-401.

Ayisi, J.G., van Eijk, A.M., Newman, R.D., ter Kuile, F.O. and Shi, Y.P., Yang, C., Kolczak, M.S., Otieno, J.A., Misore, A.O., Kager, P.A., Lal, R.B., Steketee, R.W. and Nahlen, B.L. (2004). Maternal malaria infection and perinatal HIV transmission in a malarious area of western Kenya. *Emerging Infectious Diseases* 10: 643–652.

Ayisi, J.G., van Eijk, A.M., ter Kuile, F.O. and Shi, Y.P., Yang, C., Kolczak, M.S., Otieno, J.A., Misore, A.O., Kager, P.A., Lal, R.B., Steketee, R.W. and Nahlen, B.L. (2004). The effect of dual infection with HIV and malaria on pregnancy outcome in western Kenya. *AIDS* 2003; 17: 585–594.

Ayoya, M.A., Spiekermann-Brouwer, G.M. and Traore, A.K. (2006). Determinants of anaemia among pregnant women in Mali. *Food and Nutrition Bulletin* 27:3-11.

Barragan, A., Kremsner, P.G., Wahlgren, M. and Carlson, J. (2000). Blood group A antigen is a coreceptor in *Plasmodium falciparum* rosetting. *Infection and Immunology* 68: 2971-2975.

Barros, F.C., Huttly, S.R.A., Victora, C.G., Kirkwood, B.R. and Vaughan, J.P. (1992). Comparison of the causes and consequences of prematurity and intrauterine growth retardation: longitudinal study in southern Brazil. *Pediatrics* 90:238-244.

Bayoumi, R.A., Abu-Zeid, Y.A., Abdulhadi, N.H., Saeed, B.O. and Theander, T.G. (1990). Cell-mediated immune responses to Plasmodium falciparum puri .ed soluble antigens in sickle-cell trait subjects. *Immunology Letter* 25:243-249.

Bergstrom, S., Fernandes, A., Schwalbach, J., Perez, O. and Miyar, R. (1993). Materno-fetal transmission of pregnancy malaria: an immunoparasitological study on 202 parturients in Maputo. *Gynecology and Obstetrics Investigations* 35:103-107.

Bicego, G., Boerma, J.T. and Ronsmans, C. (2002). The effect of AIDS on maternal mortality in Malawi and Zimbabwe. *.AIDS* 16:1078-1081.

Bloland, P.B., Wirima, J.J., Steketee, R.W., Chilima, B., Hightower, A. and Breman, J.G. (1995). Maternal HIV infection and infant mortality in Malawi: evidence for increased mortality due to placental malaria infection. *AIDS* 9: 721–726.

Bouvier, P., Breslow, N., Doumbo, O., Robert, C.F., Picquet, M., Mauris, A., Dolo, A., Dembele, H.K., Delley, V. and Rougement, A. (1997). Seasonality, malaria, and impact of pophylaxis in a West African village II. Effect on birthweight. *American Journal of Tropical Medicine and Hygiene* 56:384-389.

Bouyou-Akotet, M.K., Ionete-Collard, D.E., Mabika-Manfoumbi, M., Kendjo, E., Matsiegui, P.B. and Mavoungou, E. (2003). Prevalence of *Plasmodium falciparum* infection in pregnant women in Gabon. *Malaria Journal* 2:18. Brabin, B. (1992). Fetal anaemia in malarious areas:its causes and significance. *Annals of Tropical Paediatrics* 12:303-310.

Brabin, B. and Piper, C. (1997). Anaemia- and malaria-attributable low birthweight in two populations in Papua New Guinea. *Annals of Human Biology* 24:547-555.

Brabin, B.J., Ginny, M., Sapau, J., Galme, K. and Paino, J. (1990). Consequences of maternal anaemia on outcome of pregnancy in a malaria endemic area in Papua New Guinea. *Annals of Tropical Medicine and Parasitology* 84(1):11-24.

Brabin, B.J. and Johnson, P.M. (2005). Placental malaria and pre-eclampsia through the looking glass backwards? *Journal of Reproductive Immunology* 65:1-15.

Brabin, B.J., Kalanda, B.F., Verhoeff, F.H., Chimsuku, L.H. and Broadhead, R.L. (2004). Risk factors for fetal anaemia in a malarious area of Malawi. *Annals of Tropical Paediatrics* 24:311-321.

Brabin, B.J., Romagosa, C. and Abdelgalil, S. (2004). The sick placenta-the role of malaria. *Placenta* 25:359-378.

Brabin, B.J. (1983). An analysis of malaria in pregnancy in Africa. *Bulletin of the World Health Organization* 61:1005-1016.

Brabin, B.J. (1997). Malaria in pregnancy: current issues. *Africa Health* 19:19-20.

Brabin, B.J. (1991). The risks and severity of malaria in pregnant women: Applied field in malaria reports, no. 1. TDR/FIELD-MAL/1. WHO. Geneva.

Brahmbhatt, H., Kigozi, G., Wabwire-Mangen, F., Serwadda, D., Sewankambo, N., Lutalo, T., Wawer, MJ., Abramowsky, C., Sullivan, D. and Gray, R. (2003). The effects of placental malaria on mother-to-child HIV transmission in Rakai, Uganda. *AIDS* 17:2539–2541.

Brentlinger, P.E., Behrens, C.B., Micek, M.A. (2006). Challenges in the concurrent management of malaria and HIV in pregnancy in sub-Saharan Africa. *Lancet Infectious Diseases* 6: 100-111.

Bruce-Chwatt, L.T. (1980). Essential Malariology. London, William Heinemann Medical Books Ltd. 354p.

Bulmer, J.N., Rasheed, F.N., Francis, N., Morrison, L. and Greenwood, B.M. (1993). Placental malaria. I. Pathological classification. *Histopathology* 22:211-218.

Camacho, J. (1992). Serum erythropoietin levels in anaemic patients with advanced human immunodeficiency virus infection. *British Journal of Haematolology* 82: 608–614.

Carlson, J. and Wahlgren, M. (1992). *Plasmodium falciparum* erythrocyte rosetting is mediated by promiscuous lectin-like interactions. *Journal of Experimental Medicine* 176: 1311-1317.

Carlson, J., Helmby, H., Hill, A.V.S., Brewster, D., Greenwood, B.M. and Wahlgren, M. (1993). Human cerebral malaria: association with erythrocyte rosetting and lack of anti-rosetting antibodies. *Lancet* 336:1457–1460.

Castetbon, K., Ladner, J. and Leroy, V. (1999). Low birthweight in infants born to African HIV-infected women: relationship with maternal body weight during pregnancy: Pregnancy and HIV Study Group (EGE). *Journal of Tropical Pediatrics* 45(3):152-157.

Chandramohan, D. and Greenwood, B.M. (1998). Is there an interaction between human immunodeficiency virus and *Plasmodium falciparum*? *International Journal of Epidemiology* 27: 296–301.

Colomer, J., Colomer, C. and Gutierrez, D. (1990). Anaemia during pregnancy as a risk factor for infant iron deficiency: report from the Valencia Anaemia cohort (VIAC) Study. *Paedeatrics Perinatal Epidemiology* 4:196-204.

Cornille-Brogger, R., Fleming, A.F., Kagan, I., Matsushima, T. and Molineaux, L. (1979). Abnormal haemoglobins in the Sudan savanna of Nigeria.II. Immunological response to malaria in normals and subjects with sickle cell trait. *Annals Tropical Medicine Parasitolology* 73:173-183.

Cot, M. and Deloron, P. (2003). Malaria prevention strategies. *British Medical Bulletin* 67: 137-48.

Cot, M., Le Hesran, J.Y and Miailhes, P. (1995). Increase of birth weight following chemoprophylaxis during the first pregnancy: results of a randomised trial in Cameroon. *American Journal of Tropical Medicine and Hygiene53*:581–585.

Cottrell, G., Mary, J.Y., Barro, D. and Cot, M. (2005). Is malarial placental infection related to peripheral infection at any time of pregnancy? *American Journal Tropical Medicine and Hygiene* 73:1112-1118.

Dabis, F. and Ekpini, E.R. (2002). HIV-1/AIDS and maternal and child health in Africa. *Lancet* 359: 2097–2104.

Dacie, J.V. and Lewis, SM. (1994). Practical Haematology. 8 th edition. Edinburgh, Churchill Livingstone, 720p.

Davis, B.R. and Zauli, G. (1995). Effect of human immunodeficiency virus infection on haematopoiesis. *Baillieres Clinical Haematolology* 8: 113–130.

De Cock, K.M., Fowler, M.G., Mercier, E., de Vincenzi, I., Saba, J., Hoff, E., Alnwick, D.J., Rogers, M. and Shaffer, N. (2000). Prevention of mother-to-child HIV transmission in resource-poor countries: translating research into policy and practice. *Journal of American Medical Association* 283: 1175–1182.

Diagne, N., Rogier, C., Cisse, B. and Trape, J.F. (1997). Incidence of clinical malaria in pregnant women exposed to intense perennial transmission. *Transactions of the Royal Society of Tropical Medicine and Hygiene* 91:166-170.

Dicko, A., Mantel, C. and Aly Thera, M. (2003). Risk factors for malaria infection and anaemia for pregnant women in the Sahel area of Bandiagara, Mali. *Acta Tropica* 2003; 89:17-23.

Djibo, A., Cenac, A. (2000). Congenital malaria. Parasitological and serological studies in Niamey Niger. *Sante*10:183-187.

Dorman, E. and Shulman, C. (2000). Malaria in pregnancy. *Current Obstetrics and Gynecology* 10:183-189.

Draper, A. (1996). Child development and iron deficiency. Early action is critical for healthy mental, physical and social development. The Oxford Brief. International Nutritional Anaemia Consultative Group. Washington DC: ILSI Human Nutrition Institute. 358p.

Ebonyi State Ministry of Lands and Survey (2003). Geography and Planning Unit, Abakaliki, Ebonyi State.

Erdem, A., Erdem, M., Arslan, M., Yazici, G., Eskandari, R. and Himmetoglu, O. (2002). The effect of maternal anaemia and iron deficiency on fetal erythropoiesis: comparison between serum erythropoietin, haemoglobin and ferritin levels in mothers and newborns. *Journal of Materno-Fetal and Neonatal Medicine* 11:329-332.

Etard, J.F., Kodio, B. and Ronsmans, C. (2003). Seasonal variation in direct obstetric mortality in rural Senegal: role of malaria? *American Journal of Tropical Medicine and Hygiene* 68:503-504.

Eteng, M.U. (2002). Effect of Plasmodium falciparum parasitaemia on some aematological parameters in adolescent and adult Nigerian HbAA and HbAS blood genotypes. *Central African Journal of Med*icine 48:129-132.

Facer, C.A. and Brown, J. (1979). ABO blood groups and falciparum malaria. *Transactions of the Royal Society of Tropical Medicine and Hygiene* 73: 599-600.

Fievet, N., Cot, M., Chougnet, C., Maubert, B., Bickii, J., Dubois, B., Lehesran, J.Y., Frobert, Y., Migot, F., Romain, F., Verhave, JP., Louis, F. and Deloron, P. (1995). Malaria and pregnancy in Cameroonian primigravidae, humoral and cellular immune responses to *Plasmodium falciparum* blood-stage antigens *American Journal of Tropical Medicine and Hygiene* 53:612- 617.

Fleming, A.F. (1989). Joint Meeting of the Royal College of Obstetricians and Gynaecologists and the Royal Society of Tropical Medicine and Hygiene Manson House, London, 10 November 1988, Tropical obstetrics and gynaecology. 1. Anaemia in pregnancy in tropical Africa. *Transactions of the Royal Society of Tropical Medicine and Hygiene* 83:441-448.

Francesconi, P., Fabiani, M., Dente, M.G., Lukwiya, M., Okwey, R., Ouma, J., Ochakachon, R., Cian, F. and Declich. S. (2001). HIV, malaria parasites, and acute febrile episodes in Ugandan adults: a case control study. *AIDS* 2001; 15: 2445–2450.

French, N. and Gilks, C.F. (2000). Royal Society of Tropical Medicine and Hygiene Meeting at Manson House, London, March 18, 1999. Fresh from the field: some controversies in tropical medicine and hygiene. HIV and malaria, do they interact? *Transactions of the Royal Society of Tropical Medicine and Hygiene* 94: 233–237.

French, N., Nakiyingi, J., Lugada, E., Watera, C., Whitworth, J.A. and Gilks, C.F. (2001). Increasing rates of malarial fever with deteriorating immune status in HIV-1- infected Ugandan adults. *AIDS* 15: 899–906.

Fried, M., Muga, R.O., Misore, A.O. and Duffy, P.E. (1998). Malaria elicits type 1 cytokines in the human placenta: IFN-gamma and TNFalpha associated with pregnancy outcomes. *Journal of Immunology* 160:2523-2530.

Fried, M. and Nossten, F. (1998). Maternal antibodies block malaria. Nature 395:851-852.

Friedman, M.J. (1978). Erythrocytic mechanism of sickle cell resistance to malaria. *Proceedings of the National Academy of Science USA* 75:1994-1997.

Fuchs, D. (1993). Association between immune activation, changes of iron metabolism and anaemia in patients with HIV infection. *European Journal of Haematolology* 50: 90–94.

Galbraith, R.M., Fox, H., His, B., Galbraith, G.M.P., Bray, R.S. and Faulk, W.P. (1980). The human materno-fetal relationship in malaria. II. Histological, ultrastructural and immunopathological studies of the placenta. *Transactions of the Royal Society of Tropical Medicine and Hygiene* 74:61-72.

Garin, Y.J., Blot, P., Walter, P., Pinon, J.M. and Vernes, A. (1985). Malarial infection of the placenta. Parasitologic, clinical and immunologic aspects. *Archives of French Pediatrics* 42:917-920.

Garner, P. and Gülmezoglu, A. (2001). Prevention versus treatment for malaria in pregnant women Cochrane Review. In: *The CochraneLibrary* Issue 3 Oxford: Update Software.

Gazin, P.P., Compaore, M.P., Hutin, Y. and Molez, J.F. (1994). Placental infections with *Plasmodium* in an endemic zone: risk factors. *Bulletin of Soceity of Patholological Exot* 87: 97-100.

Geelhoed, D.W., Visser, L.E., Addae, V., Asare, K., Schagen van Leeuwen, J.H. and van Roosmalen, J. (2001). Malaria prophylaxis and the reduction of anaemia at childbirth. *International Journal of Gynaecology and Obstetrics* 74(2): 133-138.

Gilles, H. M. (1993). The malaria parasites. *In*: Bruce-Chwatt's Essential Malariology. H.M. Gilles H. M. and D.A. Warrell D.A. London, Heinneman Publishers. pp. 12-34.

Greenwalt, TJ. (1997). A short history of transfusion medicine. *Transfusion* 37, 550-563.

Greenwood, A.M., Menendez, C. and Todd, J. (1994). The distribution of birth weights in Gambian women who received malaria chemoprophylaxis during their first pregnancy and in control women. *Transactions of the Royal Society of Tropical Medicine and Hygiene* 88:311-312.

Greenwood, B.M., Greenwood, A.M., Snow, R.W., Byass, P., Bennett, S. and Hatib- N'Jie, A.B. (1989). The effects of malaria chemoprophylaxis given by traditional birth attendants on the course and outcome of pregnancy. *Transactions of the Royal Society of Tropical Medicine and Hygiene* 83:589-594.

Guggenmoos-Holzmann, I., Bienzle, U. and Luzzatto, L. (1981). *Plasmodium falciparum* malaria and human red cells.II.Red cell genetic traits and resistance against malaria. *International Journal of Epidemiology* 10:16-22.

Gupta, M. and Chowdhuri, A.N.R. (1980). Relationship between ABO blood groups and Malaria. *Bulletin of the World Health Organization* 58: 913-915.

Guyatt, H.L. and Snow, R.W. (2004). Impact of Malaria during Pregnancy on Low Birth Weight in Sub-Saharan Africa. *Clinical and Microbiological Review* 17:760-9.

Guyatt, H.L. and Snow, R.W. (2001). The epidemiology and burden of *Plasmodium falciparum*-related anaemia among pregnant women in sub-Saharan Africa. *American Journal of Tropical Medicine and Hygiene* 64:36-44.

Harvey, P.W., Dexter, P.B. and Darnton-Hill I. (2000). The impact of consuming iron from non-food sources on iron status in developing countries. *Public Health Nutrition.* 3: 375-383.

Hercberg, S., Galan, P., Chauliac, M., Masse-Raimbault, A.M., Devanlay, M. and Bileoma, S. (1987). Nutritional anaemia in pregnant Beninese women: consequences on the haematological profile of the newborn. *British Journal of Nutrition* 57:185-193.

Ibanesebhor, S.E. and Okolo, A.A. (1992). Placental malaria and pregnancy outcome. *International Journal of Gynaecology and Obstetrics* 37:247-252.

Inion, I., Mwanyumba, F., Gaillard, P., Chohan, V., Verhofstede, C., Claeys, P., Mandaliya, K., van Marck, E. and Temmerman, M. (2003). Placental malaria and perinatal transmission of human immu-nodeficiency virus type 1. *Journal of Infectious Diseases* 188: 1675–1678.

Ismail, M.R., Ordi, J. and Menendez, C. (20002). Placental pathology in malaria: a histological, immunohistochemical, and quantitative study. Hum Pathol. 31:85-93.

Johnson, P.H. and Hopkinson, D.A. (1992). Detection of ABO blood group polymorphism by denaturing gradient gel electrophoresis. *Human Molecular Genetics* 1:341-344.

Kamwendo, D.D., Dzinjalamala, F.K. and Snounou, G. (2002). *Plasmodium falciparum* PCR detection and genotyping of isolates from peripheral, placental, and cord blood of pregnant Malawian women and their infants. *Transactions of the Royal Society of Tropical Medicine and Hygiene* 96:145-149.

Kassam, S.N., Nesbitt, S., Hunt, L.P., Oster, N., Soothill, P. and Sergi, C. (2006). Pregnancy outcomes in women with or without placental malaria infection. *International Journal of Gynaecology and Obstetrics* 93:225-232.

Kasumba, I.N., Nalunkuma, A.J., Mujuzi, G., Kitaka, F.S., Byaruhanga, R., Okong, P. and Egwang TG. (2000). Low birthweight associated with maternal anaemia and *Plasmodium falciparum* infection during pregnancy, in a peri-urban/urban area of low endemicity in Uganda. *Annals of Tropical Medicine and Parasitology* 94: 7–13.

Kwiatkowski, D.P. (2005). How Malaria Has Affected the Human Genome and What Human Genetics Can Teach Us about Malaria. *American Journal of Human Genetics* 77:171–190.

Lander, J., Leroy, V., Simonon, A., Karita, E., Bogaerats, J., Clercq, A.D., Van de Perre. P. and Dabis, F. (2002). HIV infection, malaria, and pregnancy: a Prospective cohort study in Kigali, Rwanda. *American Journal of Tropical Medicine and Hygiene 66:*56-60.

Le Cessie, S., Verhoeff, F.H., Mengistie, G., Kazembe, P., Broadhead, R. and Brabin, B.J. (2002). Changes in haemoglobin levels in infants in Malawi: effect of low birth weight and fetal anaemia. *Archives of Diseasea of Children-Fetal and Neonatal Edition* 86:F182-F187.

Le Hesran, J.Y., Cot, M. and Personne, P. (1997). Maternal placental infection with *Plasmodium falciparum* and malaria morbidity during the first 2 years of life. *American Journal of Epidemiology* 146:826-831.

Leke, R.F., Djokam, R.R., Mbu, R., Leke, R.J., Fogako, J.,Megnekou, R., Metenou, S., Sama, G., Zhou, Y., Cadigan, T., Parra, M. and Taylor, D.W. (1999).

Detection of the *Plasmodium falciparum* antigen histidine-rich protein 2 in blood of pregnant women:implications for diagnosing placental malaria. *Journal of Clinical Microbiology* 37:2992-2996.

Leroy, V., Ladner, J. and Nyiraziraje, M. (1992). Effect of HIV-1 infection on pregnancy outcome in women in Kigali, Rwanda, 1992-1994. Pregnancy and HIV Study Group. *AIDS* 1998; 12:643- 650.

Loscertales, M.P. and Brabin, B.J. (2006). ABO phenotypes and malaria related outcomes in mothers and babies in The Gambia: a role for histo-blood groups in placental malaria? *Malar Journal* 17:5:72.

Luzzatto, L., Nwachuku-Jarrett, E.S. and Reddy, S. (1970). Increased sickling of parasitised erythrocytes as mechanism of resistance against malaria in the sickle-cell trait. *Lancet* 1:319-321.

Madrigal, L. (1989). Hemoglobin genotype, fertility, and the malaria hypothesis. *Human Biology* 61(3):311-325.

Mangochi Malaria Research Project (MMRP) (1993). Malaria prevention in pregnancy: the effects of treatment and chemoprophylaxis on placental malaria infection, low birth weight, and fetal, infant, and child survival. U.S. Agency for International Development in conjunction with Centers for Disease Control and Prevention, Atlanta, Ga; 753p.

Mankhambo, L., Kanjala, M., Rudman, S., Lema, V. and Rogerson, S. (2002). Evaluation of the OptiMAL rapid antigen test and species-specific PCR to detect placental *Plasmodiu falciparum* infection at delivery. *Journal of Clinical Microbiology* 40:155-158.

Marsh, K., Otoo, L., Hayes, R.J., Carson, D.C. and Greenwood, B.M. (1989). Antibodies to blood stage antigens of Plasmodium falciparum in rural Gambians and their relation to protection against infection. *Transactions of the Royal Society of Tropical Medicine and Hygiene* 83:293-203.

Martin, S.K., Miller, L.H., Hicks, C.U., David-West, A., Ugbode, C. and Deane, M. (1979). Frequency of blood group antigens in Nigerian children with falciparum malaria. *Transactions of the Royal Society of Tropical Medicine and Hygiene* 73: 216-218.

Matteelli, A., Caligaris, S., Castelli, F. and Carosi, G. (1979). The placenta and malaria. *Annals of Tropical Medicine and Parasitology* 91: 803-810.

Matteelli, A., Donato, F., Shein, A., Muchi, J.A., Abass, A.K., Mariani, M., Leopardi, O., Maxwell, C.A. and Carosi, G. (1996). Malarial infection and birthweight in urban Zanzibar, Tanzania. *Annals of Tropical Medicine and Parasitology* 90(2):125-134.

Matteelli, A., Donato, F., Shein, A., Muchi, JA., Leopardi, O., Astori, L. and Carosi, G. (1994). Malaria and anaemia in pregnant women in urban Zanzibar, Tanzania. *Annals of Tropical Medicine and Parasitology* 88:475-483.

Mayengue, P.I., Rieth, H. and Khattab, A. (2004). Submicroscopic *Plasmodium Falciparum* infections and multiplicity of infection in matched peripheral, placental and umbilical cord blood samples from Gabonese women. *Tropical Medicine and International Health* 9:949-958.

Mc Inytre, J. (2003). .Mothers infected with HIV.Reducing maternal death and disability during pregnancy. *British Medical Bulletin* 67:127-135.

McCormick, MC. (1985). The contribution of low birth weight to infant mortality and childhood mortality. *New England Journal of Medicine* 312: 82-90.

McDermott, J.M., Wirima, J.J., Steketee, R.W., Breman, J.G. and Heymann, D.L. (1996). The effect of placental malaria infection on perinatal mortality in rural Malawi. *American Journal of Tropical Medicine and Hygiene* 55:61-65.

McElroy, P.D., Lal, A.A., Hawley, W.A., Bloland, P.B., Kuile, F.O., Oloo, A.J., Harlow, S.D., Lin, X. and Nahlen. B.L. (1999). Analysis of repeated hemoglobin measures in full-term, normal birth weight Kenyan children between birth and four years of age. III. The Asemobo Bay Cohort Project. *American Journal of Tropical Medicine and Hygiene* 61:932-940.

McGready, R., Davison, B.B. and Stepniewska, K. (2004). The effects of *Plasmodium falciparum* and *P. vivax* infections on placental histopathology in an area of low malaria transmission. *American Journal of Tropical Medicine and Hygiene* 70:398-407.

McGregor, I.A., Wilson, M.E. and Billewicz, W.Z. (1983). Malaria infection of the placenta in the Gambia,West Africa: its incidence and relationship of stillbirth, birthweight, and placental weight. *Transactions of the Royal Society of Tropical Medicine and Hygiene* 1983;77:232-44.

McGregor, I.A. (1984). Epidemiology, malaria, and pregnancy. *American Journal of Tropical Medicine and Hygiene* 1984; 33: 517-225.

Meeusen, E.N., Bischof, R.J. and Lee, C.S. (2001). Comparative T-cell responses during pregnancy in large animals and humans. *American Journal of Reproductive Immunology* 46:169-179.

Menendez, C., Ordi, J., Ismail, M.R., Ventura, P.J., Aponte, J.J., Kahigwa, E., Font, F. and Alonso, P.L. (2000). The Impact of placental malaria on gestational age and birth weight. *American Journal of Tropical Medicine and Hygiene* 81:1740-1745.

Menendez, C., Todd, J. and Alonso, P.L. (1994). Malaria chemoprophylaxis, infection of the placenta and birthweight in Gambian primigravidae. *American Journal of Tropical Medicine and Hygiene* 97:244-248.

Menendez, C. (1995). Malaria during pregnancy: a priority area of malaria research and control. *Parasitol Today* 11: 178–183.

Meuris, S., Piko, B.B., Eerens, P., Vanbellinghen, A.M., Dramaix, M. and Hennart, P. (1993). Gestational malaria: assessment of its consequences on fetal growth. *American Journal of Tropical Medicine and Hygiene* 48:603-609.

Miaffo, C., Some, F. and Kouyate, B. (2004). .Malaria and anaemia prevention in pregnant women of rural Burkina Faso. *BMC Pregnancy Childbirth* 2004; 4:18.

Mockenhaupt, F., Ulmen, U., von Gaertner, C., Bedu-Addo, G. and Bienzle, U. (2002). Diagnosis of placental malaria. *Journal of Clinical Microbiology* 40: 306-308.

Mockenhaupt, F.P., Bedu-Addo, G., von Gaertner, C., Boye, R., Fricke, K., Hanniba,l I., Karakaya, F., Schaller, M., Ulmen, U., Acquah, P.A., Dietz, E., Eggelte, T.A. and Bienzle U. (2006). Detection and clinical manifestation of placental malaria in southern Ghana. *Malaria Journal* 5:119.

Mockenhaupt, F.P., Rong, B. and Gunther, M. (2000). Anaemia in pregnant Ghanaian women: importance of malaria, iron deficiency and haemoglobinopathies *Transactions of the Royal Society of Tropical Medicine and Hygiene* 94:477- 483.

Mockenhaupt, F.P., Rong, B., Till, H., Eggelte, T.A., Beck, S., Gyasi-Sarpong, C., Thompson, W.N. and Bienzle, U. (2000). Submicroscopic *Plasmodium falciparum* infections in pregnancy in Ghana.*Tropical Medicine and International Health* 5:167-173.

Montoya, F., Restrepo, M., Montoya, A.E. and Rojas, W. (1994). Blood groups and malaria. *Revista do Instituto Medicinale Tropicale Sao Paulo* 1994; 36, 33-38.

Moore, R.D. (1999). Human immunodeficiency virus infection, anaemia, and survival. *Clinical Infectious Diseases* 29: 44–49.

Morgan, H.G. (1994). Placental malaria and low birthweight neonates in urban Sierra Leone. *Annals of Tropical Medicine and Parasitolology* 88:575-80.

Motulsky, A.G. (1964). Hereditary red cell traits and malaria. *American Journal of Tropical Medicine and Hygiene* 13: 147-158.

Msolla, M.J. and Kinabo, J.L.(1997). Prevalence of anaemia in pregnant women during the last trimester. *International Journal Food Science and Nutrition* 48:265-270.

Nair, L.S. and Nair, A.S. (1993). Effects of malaria infection on pregnancy. *Indian Journal of Malariology* 30:207-214.

National Population Commission Abakaliki (2006). Census figures for Ebonyi State.

N'Dao, C.T., N'Diaye, J.L., Gaye, A. and Le Hesran, J.Y. (2006). Placental malaria and pregnancy outcome in a peri urban area in Senega. *Review Epidemiological Sante Publique* 54:149-156.

Newman, R., Parise, M., Slutsker, L., Nahlen, B. and Steketee, R. (2003). Safety, efficacy and determinants of effectiveness of antimalarial drugs during pregnancy: implications for prevention programmes in *Plasmodium falciparum*-endemic sub-Saharan Africa. *Tropical Medicine and International Health* 8: 488–506.

Nokes, C., van den Bosch, C. and Bundy, D.A.P. (1998). The effects of iron deficiency and anaemia on mental and motor performance, educational achievement and behaviour in children: an annotated bibliography. Washington, DC: International Nutritional Anaemia Consultative Group. 704p.

Nosten, F., Ter Kuile, FO., Maelankirri, L., Decludt, B. and White, N.J. (1991). Malaria during pregnancy in an area of unstable endemicity. *Transactions of the Royal Society of Tropical Medicine and Hygiene* 1991; 85:424- 429.

Nyirjesy, P., Kavasya, T., Axelrod, P. and Fischer, P.R (1993). Malaria during pregnancy: neonatal morbidity and mortality and the efficacy of chloroquine chemoprophylaxis. *Clinical Infectious Diseases* 16:127-132.

O'hUigin, C., Sato, A. and Klein, J. (1997). Evidence for convergent evolution of A and B blood group antigens in primates. *Human Genetics* 101: 141-148.

Okereke, C.S. (1999). Management of HIV-infected pregnant patients in malaria-endemic areas: therapeutic and safety considerations in concomitant use of antiretroviral and antimalarial agents. *Clinical Therapy* 21:1456-1496.

Okoko, B.J., Ota, M.O., Yamuah, L.K., Idiong, D., Mkpanam, S.N., Avieka, A., Banya, W.A. and Osinusi K. (2002). Influence of placental malaria infection on foetal outcome in the Gambia: twenty years after Ian McGregor. *Journal of Health Population and Nutrition* 20: 4–11.

Onyenekwe, C.C., Arinola, O.G., Meludu, S.C., Salimonu, L.S., Adewale, I.F. and Obisesan, A.K. (2004). Malaria parasitaemia and *Plasmodium falciparum* specific-IgG in maternal peripheral, placental and cord circulaton. *Journal of Vector Borne Diseases* 41: 72-75.

Ordi, J., Ismail, M.R. and Ventura, P.J. (1998). Massive chronic intervillositis of the placenta associated with malaria infection. *American Journal of Surgical Pathology* 22: 1006-1011.

Othoro, C., Moore, J.M., Wannemuehler, K., Nahlen, B.L., Otieno, J., Slutsker, L., Lal, A.A. and Shi, Y.P. (2006). Evaluation of various methods of maternal placental blood collection for immunology studies. *Clinical Vaccine Immunology* 13:568-574.

Parise, M.E., Lewis, L.S. and Ayisi, J.G. (2003). A rapid assessment approach for public health decision-making related to the prevention of malaria during pregnancy. *Bulletin of the World Health Organization* 81:316-323.

Parry, E.H.O. (1978). Principles of Medicine in Africa. London, Oxford University Press, 690p.

Pasvol, G.,Weatherall, D.J. and Wilson, R.J. (1978). Cellular mechanism for the protective effect of haemoglobin S against *P.falciparum* malaria. *Nature* 274:701-703.

Philippe, E., Walter, P. (1985). Placental lesions in malaria. *Archives of French Pediatrics* 42 (2): 921-923.

Prual, A., De Bernis, L., El Joud, D.O. (2002). Potential role of prenatal care in reducing maternal and perinatal mortality in sub-Saharan Africa. *Journal of Gynecology. Obstetetrics and Biology of Reproduction* 31: 90-99.

Riley, E.M., Hviid, L. and Theander, TG. (1994). Malaria. *In:* F. Kierszenbaum (editor). Parasitic Infections and the Immune System., NewYork; Academic Press; pp.119-143.

Riley, E.M., Schneider, G., Sambou, I. and Greenwood, B.M. (1989). Suppression of cell-mediated immune responses to malaria antigens in pregnant Gambian women *American Journal of Tropical Medicine and Hygiene* 40:141-144.

Rogerson, S.J., Mkundika, P. and Kanjala, M.K. (2003). Diagnosis of Plasmodium falciparum malaria at delivery: comparison of blood film preparation methods and of blood films with histology. *Journal Clinical Microbiology* 41:1370-1374.

Rogerson, S.J., Van den Broek, N.R., Chaluluka, E., Qongwane, C., Mhango, C.G. and Molyneux, M.E. (2000). Malaria and anaemia in antenatal women in Blantyre, Malawi: a twelve-month survey. *American Journal of Tropical Medicine and Hygiene* 62:335-340.

Roth, E.F. Jr., Friedman, M., Ueda, Y.,Tellez, I. and Trager, W. (1978). Sickling rates of human AS red cells infected in vitro with *Plasmodium falciparum* malaria. *Science* 202:650-652.

Rowe, A., Obeiro, J., Newbold, C.I. and Marsh, K. (1995). *Plasmodium falciparum* rosetting is associated with malaria severity in Kenya. *Infection and Immunology* 63:2323–2326.

Rowland-Jones, S.L. and Lohman, B. (2002). Interactions between malaria and HIV infection-an emerging public health problem? *Microbes and Infection* 4: 1265–1270.

Santos, S.E.B., Salzano, F.M., Franco, M.H.L.P. and Freitas, M.J.M. (1998). Mobility, genetic markers, susceptibility to malaria and race mixture in Manaus, Brazil. *Journal of Human Evolution* 12: 373-381.

Sartelet, H., Milko-Sartelet, I., Garraud, O. and Picot, S. (1979). *Plasmodium falciparum* persists in the placenta after three days' treatment with quinine. *Transactions of the Royal Society of Tropical Medicine and Hygiene* 91:431.

Schneider, R.G. (1974). Identification of hemoglobin by electrophoresis. *In:* R.M. Schmidt, T.H.J. Huisman, H. Lehmann (editors). The detection of hemoglobinopathies. Cleveland, OH: CRC Press, pp.1- 11.

Service, M.W. (1996) Medical Entomology for students. Chapman and Hall UK, pp. 36-53.

Shear, H.L., Roth, E.F. Jr., Fabry, M.E., Costantini, F.D. and Pachnis, A. (1993). Transgenic mice expressing human sickle hemoglobin are partially resistant to rodent malaria. *Blood* 81:222-226.

Shi, Y.P., Sayed, U. and Qari, S.H. (1995). Natural immune response to the C-terminal 19-kilodalton domain of *Plasmodium falciparum* merozoite surface protein 1. *Infection and Immunology* 64: 2716-23.

Shulman, C.E., Marshall, T. and Dorman, E.K. (2001). Malaria in pregnancy: adverse effects on haemoglobin levels and birthweight in primigravidae and multigravidae. *Tropical Medicine and International Health* 6:770-778.

Shulman, C.E. and Dorman, E.K. (2003). Importance and prevention of malaria in pregnancy. *Transactions of the Royal Society of Tropical Medicine and Hygiene* 97(1):30-35.

Rogier, C., Fusai, T., Pradines, B. and Trape, J.F. (2005). Evaluating malaria attributable morbidity in endemic areas. *Review Epidemiological Sante Publique* 53(3):299-309.

Shulman, C.E., Graham, W.J., Jilo, H., Lowe, B.S., New, L., Obiero, J., Snow, R.W. and Marsh, K. (1996). Malaria is an important cause of anaemia in primigravidae: evidence from a district hospital in coastal Kenya. *Transactions of the Royal Society of Tropical Medicine and Hygiene* 90: 535–539.

Shulman, C.E., Marshall, T., Dorman, E.K., Bulmer, J.N., Cutts, F., Peshu, N. and Marsh, K. (2001). Malaria in pregnancy: adverse effects on haemoglobin levels and birthweight in primigravidae. *Tropical Medicine and International Health* 6: 770-778.

Singer, L.M., Newman, R.D., Diarra, A., Moran, A.C., Huber, C.S., Stennies, G., Sirima, S.B., Konate, A., Yameogo, M., Sawadogo, R., Barnwell, J.W. and Parise. M.E. (2004). Evaluation of a malaria rapid diagnostic test for assessing the burden of malaria during pregnancy. *American Journal of Tropical Medicine and Hygiene* 70: 481-485.

Singh, N., Shukla, M.M., Uniyal, V.P. and Sharma, V.P. (1995). ABO blood groups among malaria cases from district Mandla, Madhya Pradesh. *Indian Journal Malariology* 32:59-63.

Steketee, R.W., Nahlen, B.L., Parise, M.E. and Menendez, C. (2001). The burden of malaria in pregnancy in malaria-endemic areas. *American Journal of Tropical Medicine and Hygiene* 64:28-35.

Steketee, R.W., Wirima, J.J. and Hightower, A.W. (1996a). The effect of malaria and malaria prevention in pregnancy on offspring birthweight, prematurity, and intrauterine growth retardation in rural Malawi. *American Journal of Tropical Medicine and Hygiene* 55:33-41.

Steketee, R.W., Wirima, J.J., Slutsker, L., Breman, J.G. and Heymann, D.L. (1996b). Comparability of treatment groups and risk factors for parasitemia at the first antenatal clinic visit in a study of malaria treatment and prevention in pregnancy in rural Malawi. *American Journal of Tropical Medicine and Hygiene* 55: 17-23.

Steketee, R.W., Wirima, J.J., Bloland, P.B., Chilima, B., Mermin, J.H., Chitsulo, L, and Breman, J.G. (1996c). Impairment of a pregnant woman's acquired ability to limit *Plasmodium falciparum* by infection with human immunodeficiency virus type-1. *American Journal of Tropical Medicine and Hygiene 55:* 42–49.

Steketee RW, Wirima JJ, Campbell CC. (1996d). Developing effective strategies for malaria prevention programs for pregnant African women. *American Journal of Tropical Medicine and Hygiene.* 55(1): 95-100.

Steketee, R.W. (2003). Pregnancy, nutrition and parasitic diseases. *Journal of Nutrition* 133:1661S-1667S.

Tako, E.A., Zhou, A., Lohoue, J., Leke, R., Taylor, D.W. and Leke, R.F. (2005). Risk factors for placental malaria and its effect on pregnancy outcome in Yaoundé, Cameroon. *American Journal of Tropical Medicine and Hygiene* 72:236-242.

ter Kuile, F.O., Parise, M.E., Verhoeff, F.H., Udhayakumar, V., Newman, R.D., van Eijk, A.M., Rogerson, S.J. and Steketee, R.W. The burden of co-infection with human immunoideficiency virus type 1 and malaria in pregnant women in sub-Saharan Africa. *American Journal of Tropical Medicine and Hygiene* 71: 41-54.

Thakur, A. and Verma, I.C. (1992). Malaria and ABO blood groups. *Indian Journal of Malariology* 29: 241–244.

Ticconi, C., Mapfumo, M., Dorrucci, M., Naha, N., Tarira, E., Pietropolli, A. and Rezza, G. (2003). Effect of maternal HIV and malaria infection on pregnancy and perinatal outcome in Zimbnabwe. *Journal of Acquired Immune Deficiency Syndrome* 34: 289-294.

Udomsangpetch, R., Todd, J., Carlson, J. and Greenwood, B.M. (1993). The effects of hemoglobin genotype and ABO blood group on the formation of rosettes by *Plasmodium falciparu*m-infected red blood cells. *American Journal of Tropical Medicine and Hygiene* 48: 149-153.

Udomsangpetch, R., Wählin, B., Carlson, J., Berzins, K., Torii, M., Aikawa, M., Perlmann P, and Wahlgren, M. (1989). *Plasmodium falciparu*m-infected erythrocytes form spontaneous eryth-rocyte rosettes. *Journal of Medicine* 169: 1835-1840.

UNAIDS (2001). Global HIV/AIDS epidemic update. Geneva, UNAIDS/World Health Organization. 891p.

van den Broek, N.R., White, S.A. and Neilson, J.P. (1998). The relationship between asymptomatic human immunodeficiency virus infection and the prevalence and severity of anaemia in pregnant Malawian women *American Journal of Tropical Medicine and Hygiene* 59:1004-1007.

Van Dongen, P.W. and Van't Hof, M.A. (1982). Sickle cell trait malaria and anaemia in Zambian pregnant women *Transactions of the Royal Society of Tropical Medicine and Hygiene* 16:58-62.

van Eijk, A.M., Ayisi, J.G., ter Kuile, F.O., Misore, A.O., Otieno, J.A. and Kolczak, M.S. (2002) Malaria and human immunodeficiency virus infection as risk factors for anaemia in infants in Kisumu, western Kenya. *American Journal of Tropical Medicine and Hygiene* 67:44-53.

Van Eijk, A., Slutsker, I., and ter Kuile, F.O. (2003a). Placental malaria is associated with increased risk of parasitemia during infancy. *American Journal of Tropical Medicine and Hygiene* 69:315-326.

van Eijk, A.M., Ayisi, J.G., ter Kuile, F.O., Misore, A.O., Otieno, J.A. and Rosen, D.H. (2003b). HIV increases the risk of malaria in women of all gravidities in Kisumu, Kenya. AIDS. 2003; 17:595-603.

Van Geertruyden, J.P., Ntakirutimana, D. and Erhart, A. (2005). Malaria infection among pregnant women attending antenatal clinics in six Rwandan districts. *Tropical Medicine and International Health* 10:681-8.

van Geertruyden JP, Thomas F, Erhart A, D'Alessandro U. (2004). The contribution of malaria in pregnancy to perinatal mortality *American Journal of Tropical Medicine and Hygiene* 71:35-40.

Verhoeff, F.H., Brabin, B.J., Chimsuku, L., Kazembe, P., Russell, W.B. and Broadhead, R.L. (1998). An evaluation of the effects of inter-mittent sulfadoxine-pyrimethamine treatment in pregnancy on parasite clearance and risk of low birth weight in rural Malawi. *Ann Trop Med Parasitol 92:* 41–150.

Verhoeff, F.H., Brabin, B.J., Hart, C.A., Chimsuku, L., Kazembe, P. and Broadhead, R.(1999). Increased prevalence of malaria in HIV infected pregnant women and its implications for malaria control. *Tropical Medicine and International Health* 4:5-12.

Verhoeff, F.H. (2004). Post-neonatal infant mortality in Malawi:the importance of maternal health. *Annals of Tropical Paediatrics:International Child Health* 24 (2):161-169.

Villamor, E., Msamanga, G., Aboud, S., Urassa, W., Hunter, D.J. and Fawzi, W.W. Adverse perinatal outcomes of HIV-1-infected women in relation to malaria parasitemia in maternal and umbilical cord blood. *American Journal of Tropical Medicine and Hygiene* 73: 694-697.

Wabwire-Mangen, F., Shiff, C.J. and Vlahov, D. (1989). Immunological effects of HIV-1 infection on the humoral response to malaria in an African population. *American Journal of Tropical Medicine and Hygiene* 41:504-511.

Walter, P., Garin, J.F., Blot, P. and Philippe, E. (1981). The placenta and malaria. A morphologic, parasitologic and clinical study. *Journal of Gynecolology, Obstetrics and Biology of Reproduction (Paris)*10:535 42.

Walter, P.R., Garin, Y. and Blot, P. (1982). Placental pathologic changes in malaria. A histologic and ultrastructural study. *American Journal of Pathology* 109: 330-342.

Watkinson, M. and Rushton, D.I. (1983). Plasmodial pigmentation of placenta and outcome of pregnancy in West African mothers. *British Medical Journal (Clinical Research Edition)* 287: 251-254.

Weatherall, D.J., Miller, L.H., Baruch, D.I., Marsh, K., Doumbo, O.K., Casals-Pascual, C. and Roberts, D.J. (2002). Malaria and the red cell. *Hematology American Society of Hematolology Education Program* 35-57.

Whitworth, J., Morgan, D., Quigley, M., Smith, A., Mayanja, B., Eotu, H., Omoding, N., Okongo, M., Malamba, S. and Ojwiya, A. (2000). Effect of HIV-1 and increasing immunosuppression on malaria parasitaemia and clinical episodes in adults in rural Uganda: a cohort study. *Lancet* 2000; 356: 1051–1056.

Wild, B.J. and Bain, B.J. (2004). Detection and quantitation of normal and variant haemoglobins: and analytical review. *Annals of Clinical Biochemistry* 41: 355-369.

Williams, T.N., Mwangi, T.W., Roberts, D.J., Alexander, N.D., Weatherall, D.J., Wambua, S., Kortok, M., Snow, R.W. and Marsh, K. (2005). An immune basis for malaria protection by the sickle cell trait. *PLoS Medicine 2*(5): e128.

Williams, T.N., Mwangi, T.W., Roberts, D.J., Alexander, N.D., Weatherall, D.J., Wambua, S., Kortok, M., Snow, R.W. and Marsh, K. (2005). An immune basis for malaria protection by the sickle cell trait. *PLoS Med*icine 2(5):e128.

World Health Organization. (1989). WHO Report of the African Regional Consultation on Control of Anaemia in Pregnancy. Document AFR/MCH/86, AFR/NUT/104. Brazzaville, Congo, 489p.

World Health Organization. (1992). World malaria situation, 1990. *Weekly Epidemiological Record* 67: 161-167.

World Health Organization. (1991). Basic Malaria Microscopy. Learner's Guide. Geneva, 1991.

World Health Organization (1992). The Prevalence of Anaemia in Women: A Tabulation of Available Information. WHO/MCH/MSM/92.2. Geneva, 602p.

World Health Organization. (1993). A global strategy for malaria control. World Health Organization, Geneva, pp. 1-26.

World Health Organization. (1997). World malaria situation in 1994. *Weekly Epidemiological Record* 72: 285-290.

World Health Organization. (2000). Expert Committee on Malaria. WHO Technical Report Series. Geneva. 892: i-v.

World Health Organization (2000). Severe falciparum malaria. *Transactions of the Royal Society of Tropical Medicine and Hygiene*, 94 (Suppl 1): 1-90.

World Health Organization (2002). Strategic framework for malaria control during pregnancy in the WHO African Region. Geneva, 902p.

World Health Organization. (2004). AIDS epidemic update. Geneva: UNAIDS/WHO. Geneva, 203p.

World Health Organization (2005). Malaria and HIV interactions and their implications for public health policy. Report of a Technical Consultation on Malaria and HIV Interactions and Public Health Policy Implications 2004. Geneva, 145p.

World Medical Association Declaration of Helsinki (WMADH) (2005). Ethical principles for medical research involving human subjects. World Medical Association, 2000. Available at *http://www.wma.net/e/policy/b3.htm.* Accessed June 15, 2006.

In: Infectious Pregnancy Complications
Editor: Richard N. Canfield

ISBN 978-1-60741-038-6

Chapter 10

Toxoplasma gondii and Pregnancy: Priorities for Diagnostics of Congenital Infection

Alessandra Sensini[*]
Microbiology Section and S. Maria della Misericordia General Hospital
Department of Experimental Medicine and Biochemical Sciences
University of Perugia, Perugia, Italy

Abstract

Toxoplasmosis is a disease of considerable public health impact. As the transmission, occurrence and phenotype of this disease are influenced in a complex way by host genetics, immunity, behavior and by the agent characteristics, prevention is not simple. Primary toxoplasmosis is a relatively benign disease usually acquired by ingestion of food contaminated by a protozoan parasite with a complex life cycle. However, in the case of primary infection during pregnancy, the parasite can be transmitted to the fetus, causing visual or neurological impairment or even death. The main risk factors for toxoplasmosis in pregnant women are unsanitary feeding habits, poor immune system, contact with cats, contact with soil, pregnancy, number of births, older age, race, travelling outside the country, drinking beverages prepared with unboiled water, consumption of municipal or uncontrolled water and *T. gondii* strain virulence. The severity of congenital *T. gondii* infection underlines the need for a precise diagnosis of acute infection during pregnancy. The microbiological diagnosis is primarily based upon serological tests, since the recovery of the parasite from biological samples is often unpractical due to its particular life cycle. Infection in the mother or congenital infection in the child are usually asymptomatic and can only be detected by serological screening for *Toxoplasma* specific antibodies. The search for specific IgM has been widely used for this purpose, but their possible early disappearance or persistence over time limits their meaning. This has led to the search of additional serological biomarkers which include

[*] Email: sensini@unipg.it

the detection of specific IgA, IgE and IgG avidity. Identifying acute infection through repeated antenatal tests facilitates fetal diagnosis through polymerase chain reaction amplification of DNA in amniotic fluid and ultrasonography to monitor fetal development. Eventually, the presence of IgM and IgA antibodies and/or persistence of IgG at one year of life in neonatal serum samples confirm congenital infection. As prenatal treatment of women and postnatal treatment of infants are hampered by the lack of proven efficacy, prenatal serological screening, although a matter of debate, should be considered in a constructive approach to better monitor and reduce the impact of toxoplasmosis on pregnant women and their newborn infants.

1. The Protozoan

T. gondii, an obligate intracellular protozoan of the phylum Apicomplexa, is a ubiquitous parasite that occurs in most areas of the world. It is capable of infecting an unusually wide range of hosts and many different host cells [1]. Intermediate hosts are probably all warm-blooded animals including most livestock, and humans. Definitive hosts are members of the family Felidae, for example domestic cats. There are three infectious stages of *T. gondii*: the tachyzoites (in groups or clones), the bradyzoites (in tissue cysts), and the sporozoites (in oocysts). These stages are linked in a complex life cycle [2].

1.1. Tachyzoites

The term "tachyzoite" (ταχύς = speedy in Greek) was coined by Frenkel [3] to describe the stage that rapidly multiplied in any cell of the intermediate host and in nonintestinal epithelial cells of the definitive host. The term "tachyzoite" replaces the previously used term "trophozoite" (τρέφω = feeding in Greek). The tachyzoite is often crescent shaped, approximately 2-4 μm wide and 4-8 μm long, with a pointed anterior (conoidal) end and a rounded posterior end. Tachyzoites enter all nucleated host cells by actively penetrating through the host cell plasmalemma or by phagocytosis [4-9]. After entering the host cell, the tachyzoite becomes ovoid and is surrounded by a parasitophorous vacuole, which appears to be derived from both the parasite and the host cell. Tachyzoites multiply asexually within the host cell by repeated endodyogeny and cause the host cell death, with rapid invasion of neighboring cells. By the dissemination via the bloodstream many tissues, including the CNS, eye, skeletal and heart muscle, and placenta, can be infected. The tachyzoites are responsible of the strong inflammatory response and tissue destruction and, therefore, causes clinical manifestation of the disease. Tachyzoites are transformed into bradyzoites under the pressure of the immune response to form cysts.

1.2. Bradyzoites and Tissue Cysts

The term "bradyzoite" (βραδύς = slow in Greek) was also coined by Frenkel [3] to describe the organism multiplying slowly and persisting for the life of the host within a tissue cyst. Tissue cysts grow and remain intracellular as the bradyzoites divide by endodyogeny [10]. Tissue cysts vary in size; young tissue cysts may be as small as 5 μm in diameter and contain only two bradyzoites, while older ones may contain hundreds of organisms. Although tissue cysts may develop in visceral organs, including the lungs, liver, and kidneys, they are more prevalent in the neural and muscular tissues, including the brain, eyes, and skeletal and cardiac muscles. Intact tissue cysts probably do not cause any harm and can persist for the life of the host without causing a host inflammatory response. Bradyzoites differ structurally only slightly from tachyzoites and express stage-specific molecules. Bradyzoites can be released from cysts and transformed back into tachyzoites. In immunocompetent host the immune response limits the diffusion of the parasite, allows the closure of the cyst, and this phenomenon could explain the persistence of specific antibodies for many years. In immunocompromised patients the impaired mechanism of control of the diffusion causes the recrudescence of infection, which can produce severe clinical manifestations. Cysts represent infective stages for intermediate and definite hosts.

1.3. Enteroepithelial Stages

Cats shed oocysts after ingesting any of the three infectious stages of *T. gondii*, i.e., tachyzoites, bradyzoites, and sporozoites. After the ingestion of tissue cysts, the cyst wall is dissolved by proteolytic enzymes in the stomach and small intestine. The released bradyzoites penetrate the epithelial cells of the small intestine, undergo several rounds of division and differentiate to microgametocytes and macrogametocytes. The gametocytes fuse to form a "zygote". After fertilization, an oocyst wall is formed around the parasite. Infected epithelial cells rupture and discharge oocysts into the intestinal lumen. Several million of oocysts are shed in the feces of cats for 7-21 days.

1.4. Oocysts

Unsporulated oocysts are subspherical to spherical and are 10 by 12 μm in diameter. Sporulation occurs outside the cat within 1 to 21 days of excretion depending upon aeration and temperature. Sporulation takes place in 2 to 3 days at 24°C, 5 to 8 days at 15°C, and 14 to 21 at 11°C [11]. Oocysts do not sporulate below 4°C or above 37°C [12]. Each oocyst contains two ellipsoidal sporocysts. Sporocysts measure 6 by 8 μm. Each sporocyst contains four sporozoites. As the sporulation continues, the sporoblasts elongate and sporocysts are formed. Four sporozoites are formed in each sporocyst [13]. The oocysts can remain infective in soil and probably water for up to 1 year, depending on ambient temperature and humidity. After ingestion the sporozoites differentiate into the rapidly dividing tachyzoites, which establish the acute infection.

1.5. Genotypes

T. gondii has a highly clonal population structure [14-16], despite the opportunity for genetic recombination in the feline definitive host. Population genetic analysis based on restriction fragment length polymorphism indicates that *T. gondii* consists of only three clonal lineages, designated types I, II and III, which occur in both animals and humans [15] and may have different pathogenicity [17,18]. Type I is highly virulent in murine infections, whereas type II and III strains are relatively less virulent [19]. There is no evidence that the difference in virulence observed in mice will correlate with similar infections in humans. Types I, II, and III are the archetypal lineages that predominate in Europe and North America [15,20,21]. Non archetypal strains with atypical genotypes are more frequent in other geographical areas, such as Africa and South America. To investigate the genetic diversity of *T. gondii*, Ajzenberg *et al.* [22] analysed parasite strains isolated from remote geographical regions by multilocus microsatellite sequencing and phylogenetic analysis, and suggested that the global *T. gondii* population is highly diversified and not characteristic of a clonal organism. The hypothesis was formulated that *T. gondii* presents a complex population structure with a mix of clonal and sexual propagation as a function of the environmental conditions. The comparison between domestic strains data on one hand and wild strains data on the other hand is in favour of more frequent sexual recombinations in wild environment even though *Toxoplasma* subpopulation in human and domestic animals is largely clonal [22,23]. There is no clear correlation between strain genotype and human disease. Congenital infections are commonly associated with type II strains in France and the United States [15,24,25], but they were found to be associated with atypical or type I genotypes in Colombia [26]) and Brazil [27]. Type I and unusual genotypes have been associated with acquired ocular toxoplasmosis [28-32]. Severe cases of toxoplasmosis, especially in remote regions of French Guiana [33] and Suriname [34] due to atypical genotypes in immunocompetent hosts have been reported. Recently, serological typing has been applied in association with multiplex PCR in congenitally infected infants from Poland [35]. A different serotyping was used for examining serum samples collected from chronically infected pregnant women in Europe and in Colombia [36], and for symptomatic and asymptomatic infections in Europe and South America [37]. The results confirmed a geographical distribution of the different genotypes, independently of clinical status, and arised a question about the role played by the parasitic load and host factors in determining the clinical manifestations.

2. Epidemiology

2.1. Transmission

The infection can be acquired by three primary routes: ingestion of tissue cysts in undercooked infected meat; ingestion of food or water contaminated with sporulated oocysts shed in the feces of an infected cat; and congenitally, across the placenta from the mother to the fetus when she is infected through one of the previous two routes during pregnancy [38].

The comparative importance of the first two routes to pregnant women can vary from one report to another, depending on hygiene, customs and socio-economic status. Blood transfusion and organ transplantation from seropositive donors to recipients are also possible ways of acquiring toxoplasmosis. Direct human-to-human transmission other than from mother to fetus has not been recorded. Transmission during breastfeeding was suspected in one reported case [39]. There is no biological test that can distinguish infections due to oocysts eliminated by cats from tissue cysts ingested from infected meat. Therefore, epidemiological surveys examining risk factors in infected and non-infected persons remain the most useful way to assessing the relative importance of different sources of *T. gondii* infection in humans [40,41]. The risk factors have been classified as related to demographic, biological and behavioral characteristics [42] and are listed in Table 1.

Table 1. Risk factors for *T. gondii* infection

Risk factors	Comments	References
Demographic		
Age	Increase with age due to the increasing exposure to *T. gondii*	41,43,44,45,46,47
Gender	No significant differences in the prevalence between males and females	46, 48, 49, 50, 51
Residency	Key role of the climate and reported differences between native and from abroad women in the some countries	52, 53, 54, 55
Biological		
Pregnancy	Down regulation of the cellular immune response	56
Number of births	Increased parity probably associated with increased age	52, 53, 57
Genetic predisposition	Homogeneous and heterogeneous profile of the disease in monozygotic and dizygotic twins, respectively. Different frequency of some HLA antigens in different clinical status. Association between clinical outcomes of congenital toxoplasmosis and polymorphisms of two genes involved in ocular disease	58, 59, 60, 61
Immunodeficiency	Reactivation of latent chronic infection	62,63, 64, 65, 66
Strain virulence	No clear correlation between genotype and pathogenicity	36,37
Behavioral		
Contacts with cats	Conflicting results	67,68, 69, 70, 50, 71, 41
Contacts with soil	Important role suggested	72, 73, 40, 43, 45
Contaminated food	Ingestion of tissue cysts in infected meat major source of infection for humans. Consumption of undercooked and cured meat the principal risk factor	1, 43, 41, 74, 57, 75, 76, 77, 78, 79
Untreated water	Contamination of the drinking water supply with oocysts	80, 81, 82, 83, 84, 85, 86

2.2. Prevalence

The seroprevalence of infection varies greatly with geographical areas. The reasons for differences in the prevalence of toxoplasmosis in different countries have been attributed to different causes; for instance, high prevalence of infection in Europe has been related to a preference for eating raw or undercooked meat, while high prevalence in Central America and other developing countries has been attributed to the low socio-economic status [86,87] and frequency of stray cats in a climate favoring survival of oocysts. Also, infection is more common in warm climates and at lower altitudes than in cold, dry climates and mountainous regions [88-91]. The prevalence of *T. gondii* antibodies has been steadily falling in various countries in the past few decades [92-95]. A significant decrease of the seroprevalence has been observed also in our area: in 1985 the percentage of seropositivity was 44% in pregnant women older than 35 years, and fell to 22% in 2006 in the same age group of pregnant women (unpublished results). The reasons of this widely observed phenomenon are probably linked to a better knowledge of risk factors for the acquisition of the infection, changes in the food habits, increased consumption of frozen meat, and improved hygienic measures. The decrease of seroprevalence implies, however, an increase of susceptible childbearing age women with possible effects on the burden of congenital infection.

3. *T. gondii* Infection and Pregnancy

Congenital infection of *T. gondii* from an infected mother to her fetus was the first form of transmission to be recognized [96]. Transmission to the fetus occurs predominantly in case of primary infection of the mother during pregnancy, as a consequence of maternal parasitemia. The parasites are present in the blood stream during the acute stage of both subclinical and symptomatic infections and before the appearance of specific antibodies. The delay between initial infection and occurrence of parasitemia is not known [38]. Placental infection is an obligatory event between maternal and fetal infection in all vertically transmitted infections, including *T. gondii* congenital infection. After placental infection, the parasite enters the fetal circulation and infects the fetus. When primary infection occurs during pregnancy, the parasite is transmitted to the fetus in approximately 40% of cases, but the frequency of congenital transmission varies considerably according to the time during gestation that the mother became infected [97]. Frequency of transmission and severity of disease are inversely related. When fetal infection occurs early in gestation (first and second trimester), it can result in miscarriage or severe fetopathy. Fetal infection in the third trimester usually results in asymptomatic newborn, which is at risk to develop chorioretinitis during the first 2 decades of life [91].

4. Diagnosis

Ideally the diagnosis of congenital infection by *T. gondii* should be achieved by examining all the subjects involved. The diagnostic approaches are tailored to the type of patient (mother, fetus and newborn) and are based on the knowledge of the complex life cycle of the parasite and of the immune response of the host. Three factors must be kept in mind and are crucial for a reliable diagnosis: 1) the optimal schedule of the test performance; 2) the optimal test in that clinical context; 3) the optimal laboratory for such test (Table 2). The confirmatory tests and the definitive diagnosis should be carried out by experienced reference laboratories, participating in external quality control and aware of the opportunities and pitfalls of diagnostic tests.

Table 2. Schedules, tests and laboratories in the diagnosis of congenital infection: a practical guideline.

Who	When	What	Where
Pregnant woman	Onset of pregnancy	IgG and IgM detection	Clinical non-reference laboratory
Seronegative	Monthly monitoring last test after delivery	IgG and IgM detection	Clinical non-reference laboratory
IgG+IgM−	No need for further controls, unless immunocompromised		
IgG−IgM+	2-3 weeks apart	IgG and IgM detection	Clinical non-reference laboratory
IgG+IgM+	2-3 weeks apart	IgG, IgM, IgA, IgG avidity	Reference laboratory
Fetus	Prenatal diagnosis: after 18th week, 4-6 weeks after onset of infection	PCR on amniotic fluid	Reference laboratory
Neonate	At birth	- IgG, IgM, IgA, IgG avidity - Test in parallel maternal and neonatal IgG by WB - PCR on blood, CSF and urine in the case of suspected infection and/or clinical signs	Reference laboratory
IgG+IgM+ and/or IgA+	After 10 days	IgG, IgM, IgA, IgG avidity	Reference laboratory
IgG+IgM−	At 1-2-3 months	Test in parallel maternal andneonatal IgG by WB	Reference laboratory
IgG+IgM−	Follow-up until 1 year	IgG and IgM	Clinical non-reference laboratory

+,-, refers to the presence or absence of antibodies, respectively. WB=western blotting

4.1. Maternal Infection

Most cases of primary *Toxoplasma* infection in children and adults (including pregnant women) are asymptomatic and self-limited. When symptomatic infection does occur the only clinical findings may be focal lymphadenopathy, most often involving a single site around the head and neck. Less commonly, acute infection is accompanied by a mononucleosis-like syndrome characterized by fever, malaise, sore throat, headache and an atypical lymphocytosis on peripheral blood smear. Very infrequently, myocarditis, polymyositis, pneumonitis, hepatitis, or encephalitis can arise in otherwise healthy individuals [91].

In absence of specific symptoms, serologic tests to determine specific antibodies are the first-line method of diagnosis and are used to establish whether a pregnant woman has been infected and, if so, when it happened, recently or in the past. An approved guideline for the interpretation has been edited by NCCLS in 2004 [98]. However, these tests generate several false-positive and false-negative results, mostly for IgM and IgA antibodies, making the diagnosis of primary infection a challenging situation [99]. Ideally, the serological tests should be performed immediately before or at the onset of pregnancy. However, the frequency of testing varies widely, according to the national health policy adopted in different countries. A screening program is mandatory in some countries (monthly in France and in each trimester in Austria) and the *Toxoplasma* antibodies test is monthly offered free of charge to seronegative pregnant women in Italy, but most of European countries do not recommend screening. Testing for specific IgG and IgM is the only approach to determine the serological status of the pregnant woman. Successive tests and the conclusive diagnosis will depend on these first results.

4.1.1. Serological Patterns

Absence of Specific Antibodies (IgG Negative and IgM Negative)

This indicates that the woman has never been infected and is at risk of acquiring primary infection. The optimal time to perform the test is at the beginning of the pregnancy, in order to give appropriate information on how to avoid the exposure to the parasite. All clinical laboratories, including non reference laboratories, are normally able to detect IgG and IgM. When the seroconversion occurs, the diagnosis of primary infection is confirmed. However, only a regular serological follow-up allows checking for antibodies appearance. Maternal monitoring is usually stopped in the third trimester or just before delivery. However, the infection could be acquired at the very end of pregnancy with the mother still seronegative at delivery. The percentage of transmission from mother to fetus is more than 70% in this period [97] and the newborn will be infected without clinical manifestation at birth. For this reason a serological control after delivery should be counseled.

Presence of IgG in the Absence of IgM (IgG Positive and IgM Negative)

The detection of IgG without IgM defines the classical serologic pattern of past infection. The right time for the test is, also in this case, at the beginning of the pregnancy, because an immunocompetent pregnant woman with serologically demonstrated chronic (or latent) infection at the onset of pregnancy is considered not at risk of giving birth to a neonate with congenital infection [38]. In the third trimester, a negative IgM titer most probably reflects past infection, but does not exclude an acute infection early in pregnancy. It can occur rarely and in some patients exhibiting a rapid decline in their IgM titers. Few cases of infected offspring from previously immune mothers have been published [100-105], although regarded as exceptions. Interestingly, in some cases, IgA antibodies were also present. Since these immunoglobulins are produced during the digestive phase of the acute infection, it was suggested that reinfection was probably linked to accidental ingestion of oocysts from a different or particularly virulent strain after maternal contact with kittens. In rare case, congenital infections have occurred in newborns from immunocompromised mothers, i.e. those with AIDS or in treatment with immunosuppressive drugs, including corticosteroids [106,107].

Presence of IgM in the Absence of IgG (IgG Negative and IgM Positive)

IgM antibodies are characteristic markers of acute infection. They appear at the onset of infection and persist for variable periods, but their time-dependent detection is strictly influenced by the level of sensitivity of the test. Numerous commercial products are available. In immunocompetent subjects, IgG production follows IgM production at different times, according to the diagnostic methods. When IgG antibodies are detected, the diagnosis of primary infection is confirmed. The development of the *Toxoplasma*-specific IgG antibody response occurs within the first 8 weeks after infection, after which time IgG levels are maintained at a high level, with or without declining IgM antibodies [108,109]. Some pregnant women can show persistent positivity only for IgM, and during the serologic follow-up IgG may not be observed. These "natural" IgM antibodies are believed to react with toxoplasmic antigens in the absence of infection. Natural antibodies are prevalently of the IgM class [110], or occasionally of the IgG class [111] and vary greatly on electrophoretic examination [112]. They are rarely found in newborns and children younger than six months. In pregnant women they can be present for the whole gestation [113] or for a limited period [114]. In these cases, because of the slow increase of IgG titers observed with conventional ELISA, it is advisable to employ additional tests with the use of whole parasite as antigen, such as dye test, indirect immunofluorescence assay or agglutination [115]. A sudden IgM seropositivity in the course of pregnancy alerts the physician, who starts therapeutic treatment before the confirmation of the infection (seroconversion) in an attempt to prevent transmission to the fetus. However, it should be considered that early therapeutic treatment, particularly with pyrimethamine and sulfadiazine, can block the production of IgG (our own unpublished results). In this case, the serologic pattern may remain unchanged and the primary infection is confirmed by the increased production of antibodies at the stop of the therapy.

Presence of IgG and IgM Antibodies (IgG Positive and IgM Positive)

One most challenging situation is when IgG and IgM are positive and the serologic status before pregnancy is unknown. In this serological scenario, "the earlier in pregnancy the sample is taken, the easier the interpretation of results" [116]. The collection of a second serum sample after 3 weeks is recommended, but meaningful differences in IgG and IgM titers are rarely observed. IgG titers can show a great variability among individuals and even the high titer, as IgG titer ≥300 IU/ml at dye test, cannot be used as a diagnostic criterion for recent primary infection because of its low sensitivity [117]. IgM positivity can be interpreted as: 1) a true-positive result in recently acquired infection; 2) a true-positive result in past infection; 3) a false-positive result [118]. Many commercial products for IgM detection have been extensively studied and compared for sensitivity and specificity [119-122], but since there is no accepted "gold standard", parameters of test accuracy are poorly defined. The specificity and positive predictive value of new assays are directly related to the prevalence of negative and positive samples, respectively, as detected by the reference test. Therefore, the selection of sera used for evaluation markedly influences the accuracy of the test [108].

Several groups of investigators are working to find specific antigens and to produce recombinant antigens to improve the performance of IgM assay [123-132]. IgM can be detected for a long period after the acute infection and therefore a true-positive result cannot discriminate between acute, recent and past infection. Timing the onset of the infection is crucial in pregnant women, especially because postconceptional acquisition represents a risk for the fetus. For this purpose, other diagnostic tools can be utilized, such as IgA and IgG avidity detection. Because IgA antibodies are the main effectors of local immunity, and because *Toxoplasma* usually enters the human body via the mouth, this isotype could theoretically serve as reliable marker. IgA antibodies appear shortly after IgM and persist for some months (usually 6-7) after the onset of infection. IgA-ISAGA is the more sensitive assay [133-136]. However, IgA have been detected for more than a year in some subjects and were never detected in a small percentage of acute infections [137]. Therefore, a negative IgA result does not exclude an acute infection and a positive IgA result does not necessarily indicate an acute infection [138].

IgE antibody detection has been proposed to define the stage of infection [139-142], because they are only found in serum samples of patients with acute infection and the duration of seropositivity is shorter than that of IgM and IgA. EIA and ISAGA tests have been used for determination, but these preparations are home-made and applied only in few reference centers. However, Foudrinier *et al.* showed limited (few months) IgE seropositivity in 85.7% of asymptomatic seroconverters and long persistence (several months) at very high titer in 100% of seroconverters with overt toxoplasmosis. Furthermore, IgE emerged concomitantly with the increase of IgG during reactivation [143].

Since its introduction [144,145], many studies have been published on the use of IgG avidity test to discriminate between recently acquired and past infections by employing natural [146,147] or recombinant antigens [148] and adapted to automated systems [138,149,150]. The functional affinity of specific IgG antibodies is initially low after primary antigenic challenge and increased during subsequent weeks and months by antigen-driven B-cell selection. Protein-denaturing reagents, including urea, are used to dissociate the antibody-antigen complex. The avidity value is determined by using the ratios of antibody titration curves of urea-treated and untreated samples. The maturation of IgG avidity has been studied monitoring subjects with seroconversion or with typical clinical manifestations: high-avidity results exclude *Toxoplasma* infection in the last 3-5 months. The length of time of conversion from low- to high-avidity antibodies depends on the method used. There are relatively few commercial tests and in-house tests lack both interest and interlaboratory reproducibility [151]. Examination of the literature demonstrated an important heterogeneity in the type of assay used, the calculation of the avidity, the cut-off above which avidity was considered to be elevated, and the delay since infection after which indices are expected to be high (116). In pregnant women a high-avidity test is highly predictive of past infection if performed in the first trimester. Low- or borderline-IgG-avidity antibodies are known to persist for months to more than a year and, for this reason, are not reliable for the diagnosis of recently acquired infection. Furthermore, it has been suggested that antibiotic treatment can modify the maturation of IgG avidity with contradictory findings [150,152-154]. Recently,

Lefevre-Pettazzoni et al demonstrated that the rate of increase in the avidity ratio was lower if infection occurred late in pregnancy and higher if the delay to spiramycin treatment was long [155].

4.2. Fetal Infection

The only way to demonstrate the transmission from mother to the fetus is to search for the presence of the parasite in fetal fluids, amniotic fluid or fetal blood. The isolation of *T. gondii* is performed by inoculation of the biological samples into mice or cell culture [1]. Mice are injected intraperitoneally or subcutaneously with amniotic fluid or whole fetal blood. The mice are bled before and 3-6 weeks after inoculation. Antibody detection and demonstration of brain cysts are proof of infection [156]. After cell culture inoculation the parasite is demonstrated by indirect IFA in monolayers within 3-6 days. Cell culture method has shown less sensitivity with respect to the mice inoculation [157]. Overall, these methods appear complex, expensive and relatively insensitive [158].

Polymerase chain reaction (PCR) on amniotic fluid is currently the most used molecular method for prenatal diagnosis of toxoplasmosis. In clinical practice, amniocentesis has essentially replaced cordocentesis followed by culture and serological analysis of fetal blood, because of its inherently lower risk of fetal loss and higher sensitivity [38]. PCR techniques for detection of *T. gondii* DNA in amniotic fluid or other samples are not standardized, and there is no consensus on the best protocol to use. Recently, a commercial PCR proficiency test became available. Sensitivity can be influenced by the gene target. In fact, the sensitivity of the PCR is enhanced if the target sequence exists in specie-specific multicopies. The most used sequence is the 35-fold repetitive gene B1 [159]. A variety of primers have been used for amplification, including nested PCR. Other target sequence used was the single copy gene P30, which encodes for the surface antigen SAG1, and the 18S ribosomal DNA. AF146527, a 529-bp sequence specific for *T. gondii* and 200 to 300-fold repetitive has been identified in 2000 [160]. The last technologic updating of the PCR is real time PCR, which reduces contamination risks, ensures specificity, and suppresses the cumbersome processing of gels and Southern blots. Furthermore, it enables rapid detection of amplification products and quantitative study, allowing determination of parasite count and its correlation with clinical symptoms and impact of treatment [161].

The optimal time to collect amniotic fluid for DNA is at 18 weeks of pregnancy or later. Amniotic fluid obtained before have not been studied; in addition, the procedure done early in gestation is associated with a higher risk to the fetus and likely less useful [162]. Furthermore, the collection should be performed at least 4 weeks after the presumptive onset of infection, taking into account the parasitemic stage in the infected mother and the delay in the parasite transmission. Amniotic fluid examination by PCR should be considered for pregnant women who (1) have serological test results diagnostic or highly suggestive of an infection acquired during pregnancy or shortly before conception; (2) have evidence of fetal damage by ultrasonographic examination; or (3) are significantly immunosuppressed and thus at risk of reactivation of their latent infection (with the exception of women with AIDS) [162]. Initially, sensitivity of PCR was close to 100% [163], but then Romand et al. [164]

reported an overall sensitivity of 64%, a negative predictive value of 88%, whereas specificity and positive predictive value reached 100%. Sensitivity varied according to gestational age and was statistically higher in case of maternal infection between 17 and 21 weeks of pregnancy. A prospective cohort study from the European Multicentre Study on Congenital Toxoplasmosis confirmed that the sensitivity of PCR diagnosis increased with gestational age at maternal seroconversion, but there was no evidence that sensitivity was significantly influenced by treatment or the timing of amniocentesis [165]. However, a positive PCR test is only suggestive of fetal infection, but it does not give any information about the clinical conditions of the fetus. The challenge is to find prognostic marker of the severity of fetal infection.

Romand et al., using real time PCR, demonstrated that maternal infections before 20 weeks of gestation with a parasitic load greater than 100 parasites/mL of AF have the highest risk of severe fetal outcome [166]. Our experience is different (unpublished results). From 1993 to 2007 117 amniotic fluid samples were assayed by nested PCR targeting B1 gene in our laboratory. Negative results were obtained from 110 samples (94%) and no congenital infection was reported in this group. Positive results were found in 7 cases (6%), 3 of whom resulted in non infected neonates, proved by serological follow up until 1 year of life. All positive samples were confirmed by a second PCR test. The first case referred to an immunocompetent seropositive woman before pregnancy and the other two were treated with pyrimethamine-sulfadiazine after PCR test positive. Low parasitic load or eradication by specific treatment could explain these findings. In conclusion, it appears that a negative PCR results in amniotic fluid does not rule out infection in the fetus and ultrasound examination should be performed each month following a negative PCR result on amniocentesis, because congenital infection with extensive involvement and hydrocephalus have occurred in the setting of a negative PCR assay result [167].

4.3. Neonatal Infection

The outcome of the congenital infection is depending by several factors: the virulence of the strain, the number of the organisms transmitted from the mother to the fetus, the time during pregnancy when the infection occurred, and the developmental maturity of the infant's immune system. Congenital *T. gondii* infection may occur in one of four forms: (1) a neonatal disease; (2) a disease (severe or mild) occurring in the first months of life; (3) sequelae or relapse of a previously undiagnosed infection during infancy, childhood, or adolescence; (4) a subclinical infection [38]. Clinical manifestations in newborns with congenital toxoplasmosis vary and can develop at different times before and after birth. Most infected newborns are asymptomatic at birth (70-90%) and classic triad of chorioretinitis, intracranial calcifications and hydrocephalus is found in less than 10% of infected neonates. When present, clinical manifestations are mainly non-specific and may include: a maculopapular rash, generalized lymphadenopathy, hepatomegaly, splenomegaly, hyperbilirubinemia, anemia, and thrombocytopenia. Chorioretinitis is the most prevalent consequence. Due to the above discussed arguments, the diagnosis of congenital *T. gondii* infection is far more complicated than the diagnosis of the acquired infection. However, it must be achieved as soon as possible after birth in order to plan a possible treatment and clinical follow up.

4.3.1. Serological Patterns

Absence of Specific Antibodies (IgG Negative and IgM Negative)

A negative serologic pattern can be a transitory phenomenon in congenital toxoplasmosis as a consequence of maternal and neonatal treatment, particularly when the maternal infection had occurred during the first two trimesters of pregnancy [168,169]. In this case, the initial diagnosis of congenital toxoplasmosis must not be questioned and the treatment and routine monitoring must be continued. Frequently, the transitory negativization is followed by a serologic rebound, more often after the cessation of therapy. The raise of antibody titers has not been associated with increased risk for the child and additional course of treatment and more ophthalmologic surveillance is apparently not warranted [170].

Presence of IgM in the Absence of IgG (IgG Negative and IgM Positive)

In congenital infection, detection of IgM but not IgA can occur at birth in the case of very late maternal infection during pregnancy, as discussed above. IgA and IgG are usually detected in subsequent serum samples. In the case of IgM and/or IgA detection in the neonate, the test should be repeated about 10 days after birth, because of relatively brief half-life of these antibodies, in order to exclude contaminating maternal antibodies [118].

Presence of IgG in the Absence of IgM (IgG Positive and IgM Negative)

At birth, the detection of IgG antibodies without any other serologic marker is indicative of: 1) congenital infection after maternal infection in the first or second trimester of pregnancy; 2) infection of neonates whose mothers have been treated during pregnancy; 3) non infection. In the case of early maternal acquisition, the newborn could be at the end of the sub-acute stage of infection, at the time at which the production of IgM and IgA has already occurred. In the case of maternal infection in the second trimester, IgA can be detected in the absence of IgM because of longer persistence of IgA than IgM, contrary to what happens in adults. It is advisable, however, to test serum samples of the newborn for detection of IgA, given the higher sensitivity of this class of immunoglobulins as a marker of the congenital infection [171-174]. A poor performance of IgM and IgA tests in the newborns, particularly in case of maternal seroconversion in early pregnancy, has been recently demonstrated. Furthermore, prenatal treatment with pyrimethamine-sulphonamide did not significantly reduce IgM or IgA sensitivity [175]. In the case of IgA detection in the neonate, the test should be repeated about 10 days after birth in order to exclude contaminating maternal antibodies [118].

In the case of suspected maternal infection and consequent therapeutic treatment, the fetal immune response can be blocked or retarded with the consequent delay in the production of predictive serologic markers. Persistence or increase of IgG antibodies in the first year of life remains the most reliable way of diagnosing congenital infection, but this procedure is time consuming. If only IgG antibodies are detected, it is crucial to distinguish if they are of maternal origin and passively transmitted or *de novo* synthesized by the congenitally infected fetus.

To compare antibody reactivity in mother and child, the immunoblotting method has been successfully employed for diagnosis of congenital toxoplasmosis [176]. Immunoblot combines electrophoresis of toxoplasmic antigens under denaturating conditions and a specific antibody test. The study of *T. gondii* antigens by western blotting allowed the determination of immunodominant antigens as well as stage-specific antigens to be utilized in serologic assays [177-179]. The strain-specific antigenic differences found explain the different electrophoretic patterns occurring among different subjects [180]. The definition of positivity is based on at least one IgG-reactive antigen present in the sample from the child and absent in the corresponding sample from the mother. A moderate variability has been observed among studies. However, the method is not standardized and antigen preparation, gel conditions, dilutions of patient sera and sources of secondary antibody are not defined, as yet. Nevertheless, some applications are semiautomated by a computer program, which makes the reading of the intensity of the bands easier and gives greater reproducibility. Best results in terms of sensitivity have been obtained when the method has been used for detection not only of IgG, but also of IgM and IgA antibodies and in combination with standard methods. Chumpitazi *et al.* evaluated the immunoblot method in comparison with the other conventional tests, including mouse inoculation and *in vitro* culture of the parasite, for prenatal, at-birth, and after-birth diagnosis of congenital toxoplasmosis. They concluded that for at-birth diagnosis, the immunoblot study of IgG, IgM and IgA antibodies reached a sensitivity of 92.6% with a specificity of 89.1%. The analysis of the electrophoretic bands showed antibodies directed against antigens with high and low molecular weights (from 18,000 to 185,000 kDa), but most of them were in the 18,000 to 135,000 range [181]. Gross *et al.* focalized their attention on IgG detection, reporting a sensitivity of 82.4%, a specificity of 93.00%, a positive predictive value of 73.7%, and a negative predictive value of 95.7%. The immunodominant *Toxoplasma* antigen SAG1/P30 was not preferentially recognized in child serum samples. In nearly all cases of congenital infection, the child developed IgG antibodies against at least two antigens and all of the IgG-reactive antigens were consistently larger than 30 kDa. The authors suggested collecting two samples, at birth and 4 to 6 weeks later, to confirm the diagnosis [182].

In a collaborative study for postnatal diagnosis of congenital infection, Pinon *et al.* compared immunoblotting and enzyme-linked immunofiltration assay (ELIFA) and standard methods for IgG, IgM, and IgA detection in the first year of life. In the case of treatment *in utero* and after one-year treatment of the child with pyrimethamine and sulfonamides, congenital infection was unidentified. In these individuals, immunologic markers were detected only when treatment was withdrawn, owing to a rebound of anti-*Toxoplasma* antibodies [183]. Combinating commercial western blot assays with conventional serologic analysis at birth and within the first 3 months, 94% of congenital infections were detected [184]. A two-dimensional immunoblotting method to improve the differentiation of mother and child immunoglobulin G profiles has been proposed [185]. To improve the early serologic diagnosis of toxoplasmosis in children at risk of congenital infection, recombinant antigens, epitopes carried by fragments of *T. gondii* MIC2, MIC3, MIC4, M2AP, AMA1, and SAG1 gene products, were assayed by enzyme immunoassays (Rec-ELISAs) with serum samples from 104 infants born to mothers with primary *T. gondii* infection acquired during pregnancy. Recombinant antigens preferentially reacted with IgG antibodies from infected infants compared to uninfected subjects (P < 0.0001), indicating that sera from infected children recognized a more diverse repertoire of antigens than sera transferred over the placenta from the mothers. Furthermore, infected newborns primarily produce IgG2 and IgG3 against recombinant antigens, whereas the maternally transferred antibodies were primarily IgG1 [186].

Presence of IgG and IgM Antibodies (IgG Positive and IgM Positive)

IgM detection in newborn serum samples is indicative of congenital infection. However, the test should be repeated 10 days after birth to exclude contaminating maternal antibodies. The ISAGA is more sensitive than the EIA in defining congenital infection. This serologic pattern presumes maternal infection acquired in the third trimester, if IgA are also detected, or in the last month of pregnancy, if IgA are still not present.

IgE antibodies were found in serum samples of congenitally infected newborns, but their sensitivity is lower than IgM and IgA [187]. Emergence of specific IgE during postnatal treatment is considered a sign of poor adherence or inadequate dosing [143]. Nevertheless, simultaneous measurement of IgM, IgA and IgE improved diagnostic yield. As for IgM and IgA, a positive test should be repeated about 10 days after birth to exclude contaminating maternal antibodies.

IgG avidity is generally not evaluated in the neonates, because it is similar to that of their mothers. However, it has been recently observed that, in the absence of maternofetal transmission, the avidity index remained stable until the disappearance of passively transmitted maternal antibodies. On the contrary, IgG avidity index showed a significant increase in congenitally infected children. In addition, long therapy with pyrimethamine-sulfonamide, as opposed to treatment with spiramycin alone, was found to slow down the progression of avidity index [154]. A delayed maturation of IgG avidity in congenital toxoplasmosis has been reported by Buffolano *et al.* The authors demonstrated the feasibility to perform the test on antibodies eluted from dried blood spots (Guthrie cards), allowing to individuate at birth maternal primary infection during the second or third trimester of gestation, and retrospectively evaluate the risk of congenital infection when suspicion of congenital infection arises during late infancy [188].

4.3.2. T. gondii Detection

Due to *T. gondii* particular life cycle, the recovery of the parasite is often impracticable. However, in order to improve the diagnosis of congenital infection, isolation technique and PCR can be added to serological tests. As above mentioned, placental infection is an obligatory event between maternal and fetal infection in all vertically transmitted infections, including *T. gondii* congenital infection. The placenta examination by PCR and mouse inoculation increased the sensitivity of the diagnosis at birth from 60% (serological tests only) to 75% (both serological diagnosis and placenta analysis) [189]. However, the infection can remain localized in the placenta without transmission to the fetus and a positive PCR test or isolation does not necessarily mean congenital infection. We observed a PCR positive placenta in a non infected newborn (unpublished results). PCR examination of peripheral blood, cerebrospinal fluid, and urine should be performed in any newborn suspected to have congenital infection [91].

Conclusion

Congenital toxoplasmosis is a dramatic, but, in theory, preventable disease, since the risk factors, at least in Europe, has been identified. The prevention programs should be addressed to seronegative pregnant women at risk of acquiring primary infection during gestation. Due to the asymptomatic course of infection, serological screening at the onset of pregnancy is the only effective way to identify these women. Even though health education programs are lacking in many countries, pregnant women should be advised by their obstetricians and primary-care providers on how to avoid the exposure to *T. gondii*. Systematic serological follow up allows to verify the efficacy of the prevention measures and to find out seroconversion. The recent debate about the effectiveness of prenatal treatment to reduce the transmission of infection from mother to the fetus and/or fetal damage and of postnatal treatment to prevent sequelae has questioned the serological screening [190-193]. However, until there is further clarification on this subject, this approach should be considered to better monitor and reduce the impact of toxoplasmosis on pregnant women and their newborn infants. Finally, the identification of maternal, fetal and neonatal infection should be based on the awareness of the priorities for a reliable diagnosis: optimal schedule to test, optimal test, and optimal laboratory. The benefits derived from this strategy have been undoubtedly demonstrated by Liesenfeld *et al.*, who reported a decrease of unnecessary abortions in about 50% of women for whom positive IgM had been reported by outside laboratories, when confirmatory tests had been carried out in a reference laboratory and communication of the results and their correct interpretation had been given to the patient's physician by an expert [194].

References

[1] Dubey, J. P. and Beattie C. P. (1988). Toxoplasmosis of animals and man. Boca Raton, Fla: CRC Press, Inc.

[2] Dubey, JP, Lindsay, DS, Spee, CA. Structures of *Toxoplasma gondii* tachyzoites, bradyzoites, and sporozoites and biology and development of tissue cysts. *Clin. Microbiol. Rev.* 1998, 11, 267-299.

[3] Frenkel, JK. *Toxoplasma* in and around us. *BioScience* 1973, 23, 343-352.

[4] Bonhomme, A, Pingret, L, Pinon, JM. Review: *Toxoplasma gondii* cellular invasion. *Parassitologia* 1992, 54, 31-43.

[5] Dubremetz, JF, Swartzman, JD. Subcellular organelles of *Toxoplasma gondii* and host cell invasion. *Res. Immunol.* 1993, 144, 31-33.

[6] Joiner, K. Cell entry by *Toxoplasma gondii*: all paths do not lead to success. *Res. Immunol.* 1993, 144, 34-48.

[7] Morisaki, JH, Heuser, JE, Sibley, LD. Invasion of *Toxoplasma gondii* occurs by active penetration of the host cell. *J. Cell Sci.* 1995, 108, 2457-2464.

[8] Sibley, LD. Invasion of vertebrate cells by *Toxoplasma gondii*. *Trends Cell. Biol.* 1995, 5, 129-132.

[9] Werk, R. How does *Toxoplasma gondii* enter host cells. *Rev. Infect. Dis.* 1985, 7, 449-457.

[10] Ferguson, DJP, Hutchison, WM. An ultrastructural study of the early development and tissue cyst formation of *Toxoplasma gondii* in the brains of mice. *Parasitol. Res.* 1987, 73, 483-49.

[11] Frenkel, JK, Dubey, JP, Miller, NL. *Toxoplasma gondii* in cats: fecal stages identified as coccidian oocysts. *Science* 1970, 167, 893-896.

[12] Dubey, JP, Miller, NL, Frenkel, JK. Characterization of the new fecal form of *Toxoplasma gondii*. *J. Parasitol.* 1970, 56, 447-456.

[13] Ferguson, DJP, Birch-Andersen, A, Siim, JC, Hutchison, WM. Ultrastructural studies on the sporulation of oocysts of *Toxoplasma gondii*. I. Development of the zygote and formation of sporoblasts. *Acta Pathol. Microbiol. Scand.* 1979, Sect. B 87, 171-181.

[14] Dardé, ML, Bouteille, B, Pestre-Alexandre, M. Isoenzyme analysis of 35 *Toxoplasma gondii* isolates and the biological and epidemiological implications. *J. Parasitol.* 1992, 78, 786-794.

[15] Howe, DK, Sibley, LD. *Toxoplasma gondii* comprises three clonal lineages: correlation of parasite genotype with human disease. *J. Infect. Dis.* 1995, 172, 1561-1566.

[16] Sibley, LD, Boothroyd, JC. Virulent strains of *Toxoplasma gondii* comprise a single clonal lineage. *Nature* (London) 1992, 359, 82-85.

[17] Grigg, ME, Bonnefoy, S, Hehl, AB, Suzuki, Y, Boothroid, JC. Success and virulence in Toxoplasma as the result of sexual recombination between two distinct ancestries. *Science* 2001, 294, 161-165.

[18] Su, C, Howe, DK, Dubey, JP, Ajioka, JW, Sibley, LD. Identification of quantitative trait loci controlling acute virulence in *Toxoplasma gondii*. *Proc. Natl. Acad. Sci.* 2002, 99, 10753-10758.

[19] Sibley, LD, Mordue, DG, Su, C, Robben, PM, Howe, DK. Genetic approaches to studying virulence and pathogenesis in *Toxoplasma gondii Philos. Trans. R. Soc. Lond.* 2002, 357, 81-88.

[20] Ajzenberg, D, Bañuls, AL, Tibayrenc, M, Dardé, ML. Microsatellite analysis of *Toxoplasma gondii* shows considerable polymorphism structured into two main clonal groups. *Int. J. Parasitol.* 2002, 32, 27-38.

[21] Dardé, ML, Bouteille, B, Peste-Alexandre, M.. Isoenzyme analysis of 35 *Toxoplasma gondii* isolates and the biological and epidemiological implications. *J. Parasitol.* 1992, 78, 786-794.

[22] Ajzenberg, D, Banuls, AL, Su, C, Dumetre, A, Demar, M, Carme, B, Dardé, ML. Genetic diversity, clonality and sexuality in *Toxoplasma gondii*. *Int. J. Parasitol*. 2004, 34, 1185-1196.

[23] Lehmann, T, Marcet, PL, Graham, DH, Dahl, ER, Dubey, JP. Globalization and the population structure of *Toxoplasma gondii*. *Proc. Natl. Acad. Sci. USA* 2006, 103:11423-11428.

[24] Ajzenberg, D, Cogné, N, Paris, L, Bessieres, H, Thulliez, P, Filisetti, D, Pelloux, H, Marty, P, Dardé, ML. Genotype of 86 *Toxoplasma gondii* isolates associated with human congenital toxoplasmosis and correlation with clinical findings. *J. Infect. Dis.* 2002, 186, 684-689.

[25] Howe, DK, Honoré, S, Derouin, F, Sibley, LD. Determination of genotypes of *Toxoplasma gondii* strains isolated from patients with toxoplasmosis. *J. Clin. Microbiol.* 1997, 35, 1411-1414.

[26] Gallego, C, Castaño, JC, Giraldo, A, Ajzenberg, D, Dardé, ML, Gómez, JE. Molecular and biological characterization of the CIBMUQ/HDC strain, a reference strain for Colombian *Toxoplasma gondii. Biomedica* 2004, 24, 282-290.

[27] Ferreira, AM, Victor, RW, Gazzinelli, RT, Melo, MN. Genetic analysis of natural recombinant Brazilian *Toxoplasma gondii* strains by multilocus PCR-RFLP. *Infect. Genet. Evol.* 2006, 6, 22-31.

[28] Grigg, ME, Ganatra, J, Boothroyd, JC, Margolis, TP. Unusual abundance of atypical strains associated with human ocular toxoplasmosis. *J. Infect. Dis.* 2001, 184, 633-639.

[29] Khan, A, Jordan, C, Muccioli, C, Vallochi, AL, Rizzo, LV, Belfort, R Jr,. Vitor, RW, Silveira, C, Sibley, LD. Genetic divergence of *Toxoplasma gondii* strains associated with ocular toxoplasmosis. *Brazil. Emerg. Infect. Dis.* 2006, 12, 942-949.

[30] Lin, A, Shin, EH, Kim, TY, Park, JH, Guk, SM, Chai, JY. Genetic characteristics of the Korean isolate KI-1 of *Toxoplasma gondii. Korean J. Parasitol.* 2005, 43, 27-32.

[31] Switaj, K, Master, A, Borkowski, PK, Skrzypczak, M, Wojciechowicz, J, Zaborowski, P. Association of ocular toxoplasmosis with type I *Toxoplasma gondii* strains: direct genotyping from peripheral blood samples. *J. Clin. Microbiol.* 2006, 44, 4262-4264.

[32] Vallochi, AL, Muccioli, C, Martins, MC, Silveira, C, Belfort, R Jr, Rizzo, LV. The genotype of *Toxoplasma gondii* causing ocular toxoplasmosis in humans in Brazil. *Am. J. Opthalmol.* 2005, 139, 350-351.

[33] Carme, B, Bissuel, F, Ajzenberg, D, Bouyne, R, Aznar, C, Demar, M,. Bichat, S, Louvel, D, Bourbigot, AM, Peneau, C, Neron, P, Dardé, ML. Severe acquired toxoplasmosis in immunocompetent adult patients in French Guiana. *J. Clin. Microbiol.* 2002, 40, 4037-4044.

[34] Demar, M, Ajzenberg, D, Maubon, D, Djossou, F, Panchoe, D, Punwasi, W, Valery, N, Peneau, C, Daigre, JL, Aznar, C, Cottrelle, B, Terzan, L, Dardé, ML, Carme, B. Fatal outbreak of human toxoplasmosis along the Maroni River: epidemiological, clinical and parasitological aspects. *Clin. Infect. Dis.* 2007, 45, e88-e95.

[35] Nowakowska, D, Colón, I, Remington, JS, Grigg, M, Golab, E, Wilczynski, J, Sibley, LD. Genotyping of *Toxoplasma gondii* by multiplex PCR and peptide-based serological testing of samples from infants in Poland diagnosed with congenital toxoplasmosis. *J. Clin. Microbiol.* 2006, 44, 1382-1389.

[36] Peyron, F, Lobry, J, Musset, K, Ferrandiz, J, Gomez-Marin, JE, Petersen, E, Meroni, V, Rausher, B, Mercier, C, Picot, S, Cesbron-Delauw, MF. Serotyping of *Toxoplasma gondii* in chronically infected pregnant women: predominance of type II in Europe and types I and III in Colombia (South America). *Microbes Infect.* 2006, 8, 2333-2340.

[37] Morisset, S, Peyron, F, Lobry, JR, Garweg, J, Ferrandiz, J, Musset, K, Gomez-Marin, JE, de la Torre, A, Demar, M, Carme, B, Mercier, C, Garin, JF, Cesbron-Delauw, MF. Serotyping of *Toxoplasma gondii*: striking homogeneous pattern between symptomatic and asymptomatic infections within Europe and South America. *Microbes Infect.* 2008, 10, 742-747.

[38] Remington, JS, McLeod, R, Thulliez, P, Desmonts, G. (2006) Toxoplasmosis, pp. 947-1091. *In* J. S. Remington and J. O. Klein (ed.), Infectious diseases of the fetus and newborn infant, 6th ed. W. B. Saunders Company, Philadelphia, Pa.

[39] Bonametti, AM, Passos, JN, Koga de Silva, EM, Macedo, ZS. Probable transmission of acute toxoplasmosis through breast-feeding. *J. Trop. Pediatr.* 1997, 43, 116.

[40] Dubey, JP. Sources of *Toxoplasma gondii* infection in pregnancy. Until rates of congenital toxoplasmosis fall, control measures are essential. *Br. Med. J.* 2000, 321, 127-128.

[41] Cook, AJ, Gilbert, RE, Buffolano, W, Zufferey, J, Petersen, E, Jenum, PA, Foulon, W, Semprini, AE, Dunn, DT. Sources of *toxoplasma* infection in pregnant women: European multicentre case-control study. European Research Network on Congenital Toxoplasmosis. *Br. Med. J.* 2000, 321, 142-147.

[42] Elsheikha, HM. Congenital toxoplasmosis: priorities for further health promotion action. *Public Health* 2008, 122, 335-353.

[43] Nash, JQ, Chissel, S, Jones, J, Warburton, F, Verlander, NQ. Risk factors for toxoplasmosis in pregnant women in Kent, United Kingdom. *Epidemiol. Infect.* 2005, 133, 475-483.

[44] Ertug, S, Okyay, P, Turkmen, M, Yuksel, H. Seroprevalence and risk factors for *Toxoplasma gondii* infection among pregnant women in Aydin province. *Turkey, BMC Public Health* 2005, 5, 66.

[45] Asthana, SP, Macpherson, CN, Weiss, SH, Stephens, R, Denny, TN, Sharma, RN, Dubey, JP. Seroprevalence of *Toxoplasma gondii* in pregnant women and cats in Grenada, West Indies. *J. Parasitol.* 2006, 92, 644-645.

[46] Fiedler, K, Hulsse, C, Straube, W, Briese, V. Toxoplasmosis antibody seroprevalence in Mecklenburg-Western Pomerania. *Zentralbl. Gynakol.* 1999, 121, 239-243.

[47] Hung, CC, Fan, CK, Su, KE, Sung, FC, Chiou, HY, Gil, V, da Conceicao dos Reis Ferreira, M, de Carvalho, JM, Cruz, C, Lin, JK, Tseng, LF, Sao, KY, Chang, WC, Lan, SH, Chou, SH. Serological screening and toxoplasmosis exposure factors among pregnant women in the Democratic Republic of Sao Tome and Principe. *Trans. R. Soc. Trop. Med. Hyg.* 2007, 101, 134-139.

[48] Fan, CK, Su, KE, Chung, WC, Tsai, YJ, Chiol, HY, Lin, CF, Su, CT, Chao, PH. Seroepidemiology of *Toxoplasma gondii* infection among Atayal aborigines and local animals in Naon-ao district, Ilan county and Jen-ai district, Nan-tou county, Taiwan. *Kaohsiung J. Med. Sci.* 1998, 14, 762-769.

[49] de la Rosa, M, Bolivar, J, Perez, HA. *Toxoplasma gondii* infection in Amerindians of Venezuelan Amazon, *Medicina* 1999, 59, 759–762.

[50] Taylor, MR, Lennon, B, Holland, CV, Cafferkey, M. Community study of *Toxoplasma* antibodies in urban and rural schoolchildren aged 4 to 18 years. *Arch. Dis. Child.* 1997, 77, 406–409.

[51] Zamorano, G, Contreras, MC, Villalobos, S, Sandoval, L, Salinas, P. Seroepidemiological survey of human toxoplasmosis in Osorno, region X, Chile, 1998, *Bol. Chil. Parasitol.* 1999, 54, 33–36.

[52] Jenum, PA, Kapperud, G, Stray-Pedersen, B, Melby, KK, Eskild, A, Eng, J. Prevalence of *Toxoplasma gondii* specific immunoglobulin G antibodies among pregnant women in Norway, *Epidemiol. Infect.* 1998, 120, 87–92.

[53] Jenum, PA, Stray-Pedersen, B, Melby, KK, Kapperud, G, Whitelaw, A, Eskild, A, Eng, J. Incidence of *Toxoplasma gondii* infection in 35,940 pregnant women in Norway and pregnancy outcome for infected women. *J. Clin. Microbiol.* 1998, 36, 2900–2906.

[54] Beattie, CP. The ecology of toxoplasmosis, *Ecol. Dis.* 1982, 1, 13–20.

[55] Ashburn, D. (1992) History and general epidemiology, pp 1-25. In: D.O. Ho-Yen and A.W.L. Joss, Editors, Human Toxoplasmosis, Oxford Medical Publications, Oxford.

[56] Smith, L. Foodborne infections during pregnancy. *J. Food Protection* 1999, 62, 818–829.

[57] Birgisdottir, A, Asbjornsdottir, H, Cook, E, Gislason, D, Jansson, C, Olafsson, I, Gislason, T, Jogi, R, Thjodleifsson, B. Seroprevalence of *Toxoplasma gondii* in Sweden, Estonia and Iceland, *Scand. J. Infect. Dis.* 2006, 38, 625–631.

[58] Peyron, F, Ateba, AB, Wallon, M, Kodjikian, L, Binquet, C, Fleury, J, Garweg, JG. Congenital toxoplasmosis in twins: a report of fourteen consecutive cases and a comparison with published data. *Pediatr. Infect. Dis. J.* 2000, 22, 695-701.

[59] Mack, G, Johnson, JJ, Roberts, F; Roberts, CW, Estes, RG, David, C, Grumet, FC, Mc Leod, R. HLA-class II genes modify outcome of *Toxoplasma gondii* infection. *Int. J. Parasitol.* 1999, 29, 1351–1358.

[60] Meenken, C, Rothova, A, de Waal, LP, van der Horst, AR, Mesman, BJ, Kijlstra, A. HLA typing in congenital toxoplasmosis. *Br. J. Ophthalmol.* 1995, 79, 494–497.

[61] Jamieson, SE, de Roubaix, LA, Cortina-Borja, M, Kuan, Tan H, *et al.* Genetic and epigenetic factors at COL2A1 and ABCA4 influence clinical outcome in congenital toxoplasmosis. PLoS ONE 2008, 3, e2285.

[62] Djurkovic-Djakovic, O. Toxoplasmosis and immunosuppression, *Srpski Arhiv Za Celokupno Lekarstvo* 1998, 126, 197–203.

[63] Gulesci, E, Otkun, MT. Investigation of anti-*Toxoplasma* antibodies in patients with hematological malignancy. *Turkiye Parazitol. Derg.* 2005, 29, 85-88.

[64] Galvan Ramirez, ML, Valdez Alvarado, V, Vargas Gutierrez, G, Jimenez Gonzalez, O, Garcia Cosio, C, Vielma Sandoval, M. Prevalence of IgG and IgM anti-*Toxoplasma* antibodies in patients with HIV and acquired immunodeficiency syndrome (AIDS), *Rev. Soc. Bras. Med. Trop.* 1997, 30, 465–467.

[65] Kasper, LH, Buzoni-Gatel, D. Some opportunistic parasitic infections in AIDS: candidiasis, pneumocystosis, cryptosporidiosis, toxoplasmosis, *Parasitol. Today* 1998, 14, 150–160.

[66] Simpore, J, Savadogo, A, Ilboudo, D, Nadambega, MC, Esposito, M, Yara, J, Pignatelli, S, Pietra, V, Musumeci, S. *Toxoplasma gondii*, HCV, and HBV seroprevalence and co-infection among HIV-positive and -negative pregnant women in Burkina Faso. *J. Med. Virol.* 2006, 78, 730–733.

[67] Garcia, L, Navarro, IT, Ogawa, L, de Oliveira, RC, Kobilka, E. Seroprevalence, epidemiology and ocular evaluation of human toxoplasmosis in the rural zone Jauguapita (Parana) Brazil. *Rev. Panam. Salud Publica* 1999, 6, 157–163.

[68] Ulmanen, I, Leinikki, P. The role of pet cats in the seroepidemiology of toxoplasmosis. *Scand. J. Infect. Dis.* 1975, 7, 67–71.

[69] Price, JH. *Toxoplasma* infection in an urban community. *Br. Med. J.* 1969, 4, 141–143.

[70] Kapperud, G, Jenum, PA, Stray-Pedersen, B, Melby, KK, Eskild, A, Eng, J. Risk factors for *Toxoplasma gondii* infection in pregnancy: results of a prospective case-control study in Norway. *Am. J. Epidemiol.* 1996, 144, 405–412.

[71] Weigel, RM, Dubey, JP, Dyer, D, Siegel, AM. Risk factors for infection with *Toxoplasma gondii* for residents and workers on swine farms in Illinois. *Am. J. Trop. Med. Hygiene* 1999, 60, 793–798.

[72] Weigel, RM, Dubey, JP, Siegel, AM, Kitron, UD, Mannelli, A, Mitchell, MA. *et al.* Risk factors for transmission of *Toxoplasma gondii* on swine farms in Illinois, *J. Parasitol.* 1995, 81, 736–741.

[73] Alvarado-Esquivel, C, Sifuentes-Alvarez, A, Narro-Duarte, SG, Estrada-Martinez, S, Diaz-Garcia, JH, Liesenfeld, O, Martinez Garcia, SA, Canales-Molina, A. Seroepidemiology of *Toxoplasma gondii* infection in pregnant women in a public hospital in northern Mexico, *BMC Infect. Dis.* 2006, 6, 113.

[74] Choi, WY, Nam, HW, Kwak, NH, Huh, W, Kim, YR, Kang, MW, Cho, SY, Dubey, JP. Foodborne outbreaks of human toxoplasmosis. *J. Infect. Dis.* 1997, 175, 1280–1282.

[75] Konishi, E, Takahashi, J. Some epidemiological aspects of *Toxoplasma* infections in a population of farmers in Japan. *Int. J. Epidemiol.* 1987, 16, 277–281.

[76] Palicka, P, Slaba, H, Zitek, K. Active control of congenital toxoplasmosis in the population. *Cent. Eur. J. Public Health* 1998, 6, 265–268.

[77] Warnekulasuriya, R, Johnson, JD, Holliman, RE. Detection of *Toxoplasma* gondii in cured meats. *Int. J. Food Microbiol.* 1998, 45, 211–215.

[78] Lunden, A, Uggla, A. Infectivity of *Toxoplasma gondii* in mutton following curing, smoking, freezing or microwave cooking. *Int. J. Food Microbiol.* 1992, 15, 357–363.

[79] Buffolano, W, Gilbert, RE, Holland, FJ, Fratta, D, Palumbo, F, Ades, AE. Risk factors for recent *Toxoplasma* infection in pregnant women in Naples. *Epidemiol. Infect.* 1996, 116, 347–351.

[80] Aramini, JJ, Stephen, C, Dubey, JP, Engelstoft, C, Schwantje, H, Ribble, CS. Potential contamination of drinking water with *Toxoplasma gondii* oocysts. *Epidemiol. Infect.* 1999, 122, 305–315.

[81] Sroka, J, Wojcik-Fatla, A, Dutkiewicz, J. Occurrence of *Toxoplasma gondii* in water from wells located on farms. *Ann. Agric. Environ. Med.* 2006, 13, 169–175.

[82] Lopez-Castillo, CA, Diaz-Ramirez, J, Gomez-Marin, JE. Risk factors for *Toxoplasma gondii* infection in pregnant women in Armenia, Colombia. *Rev. Salud Publica (Bogota)* 2005, 7, 180–190.

[83] Ertug, S, Okyay, P, Turkmen, M, Yuksel, H. Seroprevalence and risk factors for *Toxoplasma* infection among pregnant women in Aydin province, Turkey. *BMC Public Health* 2005, 5, 66.

[84] Bowie, WR, King, AS, Werker, DH, Isaac-Renton, JL, Bell, A, Enq, SB, Marion, SA. Outbreak of toxoplasmosis associated with municipal drinking water. Lancet 1997, 350, 173-177.

[85] Bahia-Oliveira, LM, Jones, JL, Azevedo-Silva, J, Alves, CC, Orefice, F, Addiss, DG. Highly endemic, waterborne toxoplasmosis in north Rio de Janeiro state. *Brazil. Emerg. Infect. Dis.* 2003;9:55-62.

[86] Francisco Fde, M, de Souza, SL, Gennari, SM, Pinheiro, SR, Muradian, V, Soares, RM. Seroprevalence of toxoplasmosis in a low-income community in the Sao Paulo municipality, SP, Brazil. *Rev. Inst .Med. Trop. Sao Paulo* 2006, 48, 167–170.

[87] Petersen, E, Pollak, A, Reiter-Owona, I. Recent trends in research on congenital toxoplasmosis. *Int. J. Parasitol.* 2001, 31, 115–144.

[88] Jenum, PA, Kapperud, G, Stray-Pedersen, B, Melby, KK, Eskild, A, Eng, J. Prevalence of *Toxoplasma gondii* specific immunoglobulin G antibodies among pregnant women in Norway. *Epidemiol. Infect.* 1998, 120, 87–92.

[89] Hershey, W, McGregor, JA. Low prevalence of *Toxoplasma* infection in a Rocky Mountain prenatal population. *Obstet. Gynecol.* 1987, 70, 900–902.

[90] Rai, SK, Shibata, H, Sumi, K, Kubota, K, Hirai, K, Matsuoka, A, *et al.* Seroepidemiological study of toxoplasmosis in two different geographical areas in Nepal. *Southeast Asian J. Trop. Med. Public Health* 1994, 25, 479–484.

[91] Montoya, JG, Liesenfeld, O. Toxoplasmosis, *Lancet* 2004, 363, 1965–1976.

[92] Nowakowska, D, Stray-Pedersen, B, Spiewak, E, Sobala, W, Malafiej, E, Wilczynski, J. Prevalence and estimated incidence of *Toxoplasma* infection among pregnant women in Poland: a decreasing trend in the younger population, *Clin. Microbiol. Infect.* 2006, 12, 913–917.

[93] Smith, KL, Wilson, M, Hightower, AW, Kelley, PW, Struewing, JP, Juranek, DD, McAuley, GB. Prevalence of *Toxoplasma gondii* antibodies in US military recruits in 1989: comparison with data published in 1965. *Clin. Infect. Dis.* 1996, 23, 1182–1183.

[94] Forsgren, M, Gille, E, Ljungstrom, I, Nokes, DJ. *Toxoplasma gondii* antibodies in pregnant women in Stockholm in 1969, 1979, 1987. *Lancet* 1991, 337, 1413-1414.

[95] Signorell, LM, Seitz, D, Merkel, S, Berger, R, Rudin, C. Cord blood screening for congenital toxoplasmosis in northwestern Switzerland, 1982–1999. *Pediatr. Infect. Dis. J.* 2006, 25, 123–128.

[96] Wolf, A, Cowen, D. (1939) Human toxoplasmosis: occurrence in infants as an encephalomielitis. Verification by transmission to animals. pp. 282-284, In Kean BH, Mott KE, Russel AJ (eds). Tropical Medicine and Parasitology: Classical Investigations. Chapter 13. Ithaca, Cornell University Press.

[97] Dunn, D, Wallon, M, Peyron, F, Petersen, E, Peckham, C, Gilbert, R. Mother-to-child transmission of toxoplasmosis: risk estimates for clinical counseling. *Lancet* 1999, 353, 1829-1833.

[98] National Committee for Clinical Laboratory Standard. *Clinical use and interpretation of serologic tests for Toxoplasma gondii*; Approved guideline M36-A. Wayne, PA: NCCLS, 2004.

[99] Sensini, A. *Toxoplasma gondii* infection in pregnancy: opportunities and pitfalls of serologic diagnosis. *Clin. Microbiol. Infect*. 2006, 12, 504-512.

[100] Fortier, B, Aissi, E, Ajana, F, Dieusart, P, Denis, P, Martin de Vassalle, E, Lecomte-Houcke, M, Vinatier, D. Spontaneous abortion and reinfection by *Toxoplasma gondii* (letter to the editor). *Lancet* 1991, 338, 444.

[101] Hennequin, C, Dureau, P, N'Guyen, L, Thulliez, P, Gagelin, B, Dufier, JL. Congenital toxoplasmosis acquired from an immune woman. *Pediatr. Infect. Dis. J.* 1997, 16, 75-77.
[102] Gavinet, MF, Robert, F, Firtion, G, Delouvrier, E, Hennequin, C, Maurin, JR, Tourte-Schaefer, C, Dupouy-Camet, J. Congenital toxoplasmosis due to maternal reinfection during pregnancy. *J. Clin. Microbiol.* 1997, 35, 1276-1277.
[103] Silveira, C, Ferriera, R, Muccioli, C, Nussenblatt, R, Belfort, R Jr. Toxoplasmosis transmitted to a newborn from the mother infected 20 years earlier. *Am. J. Ophtalmol.* 2003, 136, 370-371.
[104] Lebas, F, Ducrocq, S, Mucignat, V, Paris, L, Mégier, P, Baudon, JJ, Gold, F. Congenital toxoplasmosis: infection during pregnancy in an immune and immunocompetent woman. *Arch. Pediatr.* 2004, 11, 926-928.
[105] Kodjikian, L, Hoigne, I, Adam, O, Jacquier, P, Aebi-Ochsner, C, Aebi, C, Garweg, JG. Vertical transmission of toxoplasmosis from a chronically infected immunocompetent woman. *Pediatr. Infec. Dis. J.* 2004, 23, 272-274.
[106] European Collaborative Study and Research Network on Congenital Toxoplasmosis. Low incidence of congenital toxoplasmosis in children born to women infected with human immunodeficiency virus. *Eur. J. Ostet. Gynecol. Reprod. Biol.* 1996, 68, 93-96.
[107] Minkoff, H, Remington, JS, Holman, S, Ramirez, G, Goodwin, S, Landesman, S. Vertical transmission of toxoplasma by human immunodeficiency virus-infected women. *Am, J, Obstet, Gynecol.* 1997, 176, 555-559.
[108] Liesenfeld, O, Press, C, Montoya, JG, Gill, R, Isaac-Renton, JL, Hedman, K, Remington, JS. False-positive results in immunoglobulin M (IgM) toxoplasma antibody tests and importance of confirmatory testing: the Platelia Toxo IgM test. *J. Clin. Microbiol.* 1997, 35, 174-178.
[109] Liesenfeld, O, Montoya, JG, Kinney, S, Press, C, Remington, JS. Effect of testing for IgG avidity in the diagnosis of *T. gondii* infection in pregnant women: experience in a U.S. reference laboratory. *J. Infect. Dis.* 2001, 183, 1248-1253.
[110] Desmonts, G, Baufine-Ducrocq, H, Couzinequ, P, Peloux, Y. Anticorps toxoplasmic naturels. *Nouv. Presse Med.* 1974, 3, 1547-1549.
[111] Franco, EL, Sulzer, AJ, Highy, RW, Peralta, JM. Immunoglobulin G and immunoglobulin M polar staining of *Toxoplasma gondii* in the indirect immunofluorescence test. *J. Clin. Microbiol.* 1980, 12, 780-784.
[112] Potasman, I, Araujo, FG, Remington, JS. *Toxoplasma* antigens recognized by naturally occurring human antibodies. *J. Clin. Microbiol.* 1986, 24, 1050-1054.
[113] Konishi, E. A pregnant woman with a high level of naturally occurring immunoglobulin M antibodies to *Toxoplasma gondii*. *Am. J. Obstet. Gynecol.* 1987, 157, 832-833.
[114] Gussetti, N, D'Elia, R, Mottola, A, Rigoli, E. Natural immunoglobulin M antibodies against *Toxoplasma gondii* during pregnancy. *Am. J. Obstet. Gynecol.* 1990, 162, 1359-1360.
[115] Press, C, Montoya, JG, Remington, JS. Use of a single serum sample for diagnosis of acute toxoplasmosis in pregnant women and other adults. *J. Clin. Microbiol.* 2005, 43, 3481-3483.

[116] Lefevre-Pettazzoni, M, Le Cam, S, Wallon, M, Peyron, F. Delayed maturation of immnunoglobulin G avidity: implication for the diagnosis of toxoplasmosis in pregnant women. *Eur. J. Clin. Microbiol. Infect. Dis*. 2006, 25, 687-693.

[117] Jenum, PA, Stray-Pedersen, B. Development of specific immunoglobulins G, M, and A following primary *Toxoplasma gondii* infection in pregnant women. *J. Clin. Microbiol.* 1998, 36, 2907-2913.

[118] Montoya, JG. Laboratory diagnosis of *Toxoplasma gondii* infection and toxoplasmosis. *J. Infect. Dis.* 2002, 185 (Suppl.1), S73-82.

[119] Decoster, A, Lecolier, B. Bicentric evaluation of Access Toxo Immunoglobulin M (IgM) and IgG assays and IMx Toxo IgM and IgG assays and comparison with Platelia Toxo IgM and IgG assays. *J. Clin. Microbiol.* 1996, 34, 1606-1609.

[120] Liesenfeld, O, Press, C, Flanders, R, Ramirez, R, Remington, JS. Study od Abbott Toxo IMx system for detection of immunoglobulin M Toxoplasma antibodies: value of confirmatory testing for diagnosis of acute toxoplasmosis. *J. Clin. Microbiol.* 1996, 34, 2526-2530.

[121] Wilson, M, Remington, JS, Clavet, C, Varney, G, Press, C, Ware, D, and The FDA Toxoplasmosis Ad Hoc Working Group. Evaluation of six commercial kits for detection of human immunoglobulin M antibodies to *Toxoplasma gondii. J. Clin. Microbiol.* 1997, 35, 3112-3115.

[122] Hofgärtner, W, Swanzy, SR, Bacina, RM, Condon, J, Gupta, M, Matlock, PE, Bergeron, DL, Plorde, JJ, Fritsche, TR. Detection of immunoglobulin G (IgG) and IgM antibodies to *Toxoplasma gondii*: evaluation of four commercial immunoassay systems. *J. Clin. Microbiol.* 1997, 35, 3313-3315.

[123] Aubert, D, Maine, GT, Villena, I, Hunt, JC, Howard, L, Sheu, M, Brojanac, S, Chovan, LE, Nowlan, SF, Pinon, JM. Recombinant antigens to detect *Toxoplasma gondii*-specific immunoglobulin G and immunoglobulin M in human sera by enzyme immunoassay. *J. Clin. Microbiol.* 2000, 38, 1144-1150.

[124] Lecordier, L, Fourmaux, M-P, Mercier, C, Dehecq, E, Masy, E, Cesbron-Delauw, M-F. Enzyme-linked immunosorbent assays using the recombinant dense granule antigens GRA6 and GRA1 of *Toxoplasma gondii* for detection of immunoglobulin G antibodies. *Clin. Diagn. Lab. Immunol.* 2000, 7, 607-611.

[125] Li, S, Galvan, G, Araujo, FG, Suzuki, Y, Remington, JS, Parmley, S. Serodiagnosis of recently acquired *Toxoplasma gondii* infection using an enzyme-linked immunosorbent assay with a combination of recombinant antigens. *Clin. Diagn. Lab. Immunol.* 2000, 7, 781-787.

[126] Suzuki, Y, Ramirez, R, Press, C, Li, S, Parmley, S, Thulliez, P, Remington, JS. Detection of immunoglobulin M antibodies to P35 antigen of *Toxoplasma gondii* for serodiagnosis of recently acquired infection in pregnant women. *J. Clin. Microbiol.* 2000, 38, 3967-3970.

[127] Giraldo, M, Portela, RWD, Snege, M, Leser, PG, Camargo, ME, Mineo, JR, Gazzinelli, RT. Immunoglobulin M (IgM)-glycoinositolphospholipid enzyme-linked immunosorbent assay: an immunoenzymatic assay for discrimination between patients with acute toxoplasmosis and those with persistent parasite-specific IgM antibodies. *J. Clin. Microbiol.* 2002, 40, 1400-1405.

[128] Pietkiewicz, H, Hiszczynska-Sawicka, E, Kur, J, Petersen, E, Nielsen, HV, Stankiewicz, M, Andrzejewska, I, Myjak, P. Usefulness of *Toxoplasma gondii*-specific recombinant antigens in serodiagnosis of human toxoplasmosis. *J. Clin. Microbiol.* 2004, 42, 1779-1781.

[129] Kaul, R, Chen, P, Binder, SR. Detection of immunoglobulin M antibodies specific for *Toxoplasma gondii* with increased selectivity for recently acquired infections. *J. Clin. Microbiol.* 2004, 42, 5705-5709.

[130] Beghetto, E, Spadoni, A, Bruno, L, Buffolano, W, Gargano, N. Chimeric antigens of *Toxoplasma gondii*: toward standardization of toxoplasmosis serodiagnosis using recombinant products. *J. Clin. Microbiol.* 2006, 44, 2133-2140.

[131] Golkar, M, Azadmanesh, K, Khalili, G, Khoshkholgh-Sima, B, Babaie, J, Mercier, C, Brenier-Pinchart, MP, Fricker-Hidalgo, H, Pelloux, H, Cesbron-Delauw, MF. Serodiagnosis of recently acquired *Toxoplasma gondii* infection in pregnant women using enzyme-linked immunosorbent assays with a recombinant dense granule GRA6 protein. *Diagn. Microbiol. Infect. Dis*. 2008, 61, 31-39.

[132] Carvalho, FR, Silva, DAO, Cunha-Junior, JP, Souza, MA, Oliveira, TC, Béla, SR, Faria, GG, Lopes, CS, Mineo, JR. Reverse enzyme-linked immunosorbent assay using monoclonal antibodies against SAG1-related sequence, SAG2A, and p97 antigens from *Toxoplasma gondii* to detect specific immunoglobulin G (IgG), IgM, and IgA antibodies in human sera. *Clin. Vaccine Immunol.* 2008, 15, 1265-1271.

[133] Bessieres, MH, Roques, C, Berrei, A, Barre, V, Cazaux, M, Sequela, JP. IgA antibody response during acquired and congenital toxoplasmosis. *J. Clin. Pathol.* 1992, 45, 605-8.

[134] Patel, B, Young, Y, Duffy, K, Tanner, RP, Johnson, J, Holliman, RE. Immunoglobulin-A detection and the investigation of clinical toxoplasmosis. *J. Med. Microbiol.* 1993, 38, 286-292.

[135] Francis, JM, Joynson, DH. Duration of specific immunoglobulin A antibody following acute toxoplasmosis as determined by enzyme immunoassay and immunosorbent agglutination assay. *Eur. J. Clin. Microbiol. Infect. Dis.* 1993, 12, 556-559.

[136] Takahashi, EE, Rossi, CL. Use of three immunological techniques for the detection of *Toxoplasma* spIgA antibodies in acute toxoplasmosis. *J. Clin. Pathol.* 1994, 47, 1101-1104.

[137] Montoya, JG, Remington, JS. Studies on the serodiagnosis of toxoplasmic lymphadenitis. *Clin. Infect. Dis.* 1995, 20, 781-789.

[138] Candolfi, E, Pastor, R, Huber, R, Filisetti, D, Villard, O. IgG avidity assay firms up the diagnosis of acute toxoplasmosis on the first serum sample in immunocompetent pregnant women. *Diagn. Microbiol. Infect. Dis*. 2007, 58, 83-88.

[139] Pinon, JM, Toubas, D, Marx, C, Mougeot, G, Bonnin, A, Bonhomme, A, Villaume, M, Foudrinier, F, Lepan, H. Detection of specific immunoglobulin E in patients with toxoplasmosis. *J. Clin. Microbiol.* 1990, 28, 1739-1743.

[140] Wong, SY, Hadju, MP, Ramirez, R, Thulliez, P, McLeod, R, Remington, JS. Role of specific immunoglobulin E in diagnosis of acute *Toxoplasma* infection and toxoplasmosis. *J. Clin. Microbiol.* 1993, 31, 2952-2959.

[141] Ashburn, D, Joss, AW, Pennington, TH, Ho-Yen, DO. Specificity and usefulness of an IgE immunosorbent agglutination assay for toxoplasmosis. *J. Clin. Pathol.* 1995, 48, 689.

[142] Gross, U, Keksel, O, Dardé, ML. Value of detecting immunoglobulin E antibodies for the serological diagnosis of *Toxoplasma gondii* infection. *Clin. Diagn. Lab. Immunol.* 1997, 4, 247-251.

[143] Foudrinier, F, Villena, I, Jaussaud, R, Aubert, D, Chemla, C, Martinot, F, Pinon, JM. Clinical value of specific immunoglobulin E detection by enzyme-linked immunosorbent assay in cases of acquired and congenital toxoplasmosis. *J. Clin. Microbiol.* 2003, 41, 1681-1686.

[144] Hedman, K, Lappalainen, M, Seppala, I, Makela, O. Recent primary Toxoplasma infection indicated by a low avidity of specific IgG. *J. Infect. Dis.* 1989, 159, 736-739.

[145] Lappalainen, M, Hedman, K. Serodiagnosis of toxoplasmosis: the impact of measurement of IgG avidity. *Ann. Ist. Super. Sanità* 2004, 40, 81-88.

[146] Lappalainen, M, Koskela, P, Koskiniemi, M, Ammala, P, Hiilesmaa V, Teramo, K, Raivio, KO, Remington, JS, Hedman, K. Toxoplasmosis acquired during pregnancy: improved serodiagnosis based on avidity of IgG. *J. Infect. Dis.* 1993, 167, 691-697.

[147] Cozon, GJ, Ferrandiz, J, Nebhi, H, Wallon, M, Peyron, F. Estimation of the avidity of immunoglobulin G for routine diagnosis of chronic *Toxoplasma gondii* infection in pregnant women. *Eur. J. Clin. Microbiol. Infect. Dis.* 1998, 17, 32-36.

[148] Beghetto, E, Buffolano, W, Spadoni, A, Del Pezzo, M, Di Cristina, M, Minenkova, O, Petersen, E, Felici, F, Gargano, N. Use of an immunoglobulin G avidity assay based on recombinant antigens for diagnosis of primary *Toxoplasma gondii* infection during pregnancy. *J. Clin. Microbiol.* 2003, 41, 5414-5418.

[149] Montoya, JG, Liesenfeld, O, Kinney, S, Press, C, Remington, JS. VIDAS test for avidity of *Toxoplasma*-specific immunoglobulin G for confirmatory testing of pregnant women. *J. Clin. Microbiol.* 2002, 40, 2504-2508.

[150] Petersen, E, Borobio, MV, Guy, E, Liesenfeld, O, Meroni, V, Naessens, A, Spranzi, E, Thulliez, P. European multicenter study of the Liaison automated diagnostic system for determination of *Toxoplasma gondii*-specific immunoglobulin G (IgG) and IgM and the IgG avidity index. *J. Clin. Microbiol.* 2005, 43, 1570-1574.

[151] Roberts, A, Hedman, K, Luyasu, V, Zufferey, J. *et al.* Multicenter evaluation of strategies for serodiagnosis of primary infection with *Toxoplasma gondii*. *Eur. J. Clin. Microbiol. Infect. Dis*. 2001, 20, 467-474.

[152] Sensini, A, Pascoli, S, Marchetti, D, Castronari, R, Marangi, M, Sbaraglia, G, Cimmino, C, Favero, A, Castelletto, M, Mottola, A. IgG avidity in the serodiagnosis of acute *Toxoplasma gondii* infection: a multicenter study. *Clin. Microbiol. Infect.* 1996, 2, 25-29.

[153] Jenum, PA, Stray-Pedersen, B, Gundersen, AG. Improved diagnosis of primary *Toxoplasma gondii* infection in early pregnancy by determination of antitoxoplasma immunoglobulin G avidity. *J. Clin. Microbiol*. 1997, 35, 1972-1977.

[154] Flori, P, Tardy, L, Patural, H, Bellete, B, Varlet, MN, Hafid, J, Raberin, H, Sung, RT. Reliability of immunoglobulin G antitoxoplasma avidity test and effects of treatment on

avidity indexes of infants and pregnant women. *Clin. Diagn. Lab. Immunol.* 2004, 11, 669-674.

[155] Lefevre-Pettazzoni, M, Bissery, A, Wallon, M, Cozon, G, Peyron, F, Rabilloud, M. Impact of spiramycin treatment and gestational age on maturation of *Toxoplasma gondii* immunoglobulin G avidity in pregnant women. *Clin. Vaccine Immunol.* 2007, 14, 239-243.

[156] Derouin, F, Thulliez, P, Candolfi, E, Daffos, F, Forestier, F. Early prenatal diagnosis of congenital toxoplasmosis using amniotic fluid samples and tissue culture. *Eur. J. Clin. Microbiol. Infect. Dis.* 1988, 7, 423-425.

[157] Thulliez, P, Daffos, F, Forestier, F. Diagnosis of *Toxoplasma* infection in the pregnant woman and the unborn child: current problems. *Scand. J. Infect. Dis.* Suppl 1992, 84, 18-22.

[158] Foulon, W, Pinon, JM, Stray-Pedersen, B, Pollak, A, Lappalainen, M, Decoster, A, Villena, I, Jenum, PA, Hayde, M, Naessens, A. Prenatal diagnosis of congenital infection: a multicenter evaluation of different diagnostic parameters. *Am. J. Obstet. Gynecol.* 1999, 181, 843-847.

[159] Burg, JL, Grover, CM, Pouletty, P, Boothroyd, JC. Direct and sensitive detection of a pathogenic protozoan, *Toxoplasma gondii*, by polymerase chain reaction. *J. Clin. Microbiol.* 1989, 27, 1787-1792.

[160] Homan, WL, Vercammen, M, De Braekeleer, J, Verschuern, H. Identification of a 200- to 300-fold repetitive 529 bp DNA fragment in *Toxoplasma gondii*, and its use for diagnostic and quantitative PCR. *Int. J. Parasitol.* 2000, 30, 69-75.

[161] Rorman, E, Zamir, CS, Rilkis, I, Ben-David, H. Congenital toxoplasmosis-prenatal aspects of *Toxoplasma gondii* infection. *Reprod. Toxicol.* 2006, 21, 458-472.

[162] Montoya, JG, Remington, JS. Management of *Toxoplasma gondii* infection during pregnancy. *Clin. Infect. Dis.* 2008, 47, 554-566.

[163] Hohlfeld, P, Daffos, F, Costa J-M, Thulliez, P, Forestier, F, Vidaud, M. Prenatal diagnosis of congenital toxoplasmosis with polymerase-chain-reaction test on amniotic fluid. *N. Engl. J. Med.* 1994, 331, 695-699.

[164] Romand, S, Wallon, M, Franck, J, Thulliez, P, Peyron, F, Dumon, H. Prenatal diagnosis using polymerase chain reaction on amniotic fluid for congenital toxoplasmosis. *Ostet. Gynecol.* 2001, 97, 296-300.

[165] Thalib, L, Gras, L, Romand, S, Prusa, A, Bessieres, MH, Petersen, E, Gilbert, RE. for the European Multicentre Study on Congenital Toxoplasmosis (EMSCOT). Prediction of congenital toxoplasmosis by polymerase chain reaction analysis of amniotic fluid. BJOG 2005, 112, 567-574.

[166] Romand, S, Chosson, Franck, J, M. Wallon, M, Kieffer, F, Kaiser, K, Dumon, H, Peyron, F, Thulliez, P, Picot, S. Usefulness of quantitative polymerase chain reaction in amniotic fluid as early prognostic marker of fetal infection with *Toxoplasma gondii*. *Am. J. Ostet. Gynecol.* 2004, 190, 797-802.

[167] Gay-Andrieu, F, Marty, P, Pialat, J, Sournies, G, Drier de Laforte, T, Peyron, F. Fetal toxoplasmosis and negative amniocentesis: necessity of an ultrasound follow-up. *Prenat. Diagn.* 2003, 23, 558-560.

[168] Villena, I, Aubert, D, Leroux, B *et al.* Pyrimethamine-sulfadoxine treatment of congenital toxoplasmosis: follow-up of 78 cases between 1980 and 1997. Reims Toxoplasmosis Group. *Scand. Infect. Dis.* 1998, 30, 295-300.

[169] Jaisson-Hot, I, Wallon, M, al Kurdi, M, Thulliez, P, Kahi, S, Cozon, G, Peyron, F. Congenital toxoplasmosis. Transitory negative serology. *Presse Med.* 2001, 30, 1001-1004.

[170] Wallon, M, Cozon, G, Ecochard, R, Lewin, P, Peyron, F. Serological rebound in congenital toxoplasmosis: long-term follow-up of 133 children. *Eur. J. Pediatr.* 2001, 160, 534-540.

[171] Decoster, A, Darcy, F, Caron, A *et al.* Anti-P30 IgA antibodies as prenatal markers of congenital toxoplasma infection. *Clin. Exp. Immunol.* 1992, 87, 310-315.

[172] Foudrinier, F, Marx-Chemla, C, Aubert, D, Bonhomme, A, Pinon, JM. Value of specific immunoglobulin A detection by two immunocapture assays in the diagnosis of toxoplasmosis. *Eur. J. Clin. Microbiol. Infect. Dis.* 1995, 14, 585-590.

[173] Petithory, JC, Reiter-Owona, I, Berthelot, F, Milgram, M, De Loye, J, Petersen, E. Performance of European laboratories testing serum samples for *Toxoplasma gondii. Eur. J. Clin. Microbiol. Infect. Dis.* 1996, 15, 45-49.

[174] Ashburn, D, Joss, AW, Pennington, TH, Ho-Yen, DO. Do IgA, IgE, and IgG avidity have any value in the diagnosis of toxoplasma infection in pregnancy? *J. Clin. Pathol.* 1998, 51, 312-315.

[175] Gilbert, RE, Thalib, L, Tan, HK, Paul, M, Wallon, M, Petersen, E. European Multicentre Study on Congenital Toxoplasmosis. Screening for congenital toxoplasmosis: accuracy of immunoglobulin M and immunoglobulin A tests after birth. *J. Med. Screen*. 2007, 14, 8-13.

[176] Remington, JS, Araujo, FG, Desmonts, G. Recognition of different *Toxoplasma* antigens by IgM and IgG antibodies in mothers and their congenitally infected newborns. *J. Infect. Dis.* 1985, 152, 1020-1024.

[177] Sharma, SD, Mullenax, J, Araujo, FG, Erlich, HA, Remington, JS. Western blot analysis of the antigens of *Toxoplasma gondii* recognized by human IgM and IgG antibodies. *J. Immunol.* 1983, 131, 977-983.

[178] Partanen, P, Turunen, HJ, Paasivuo, RTA, Leinikki, PO. Immunoblot analysis of *Toxoplasma gondii* antigens by human immunoglobulins G, M, and A at different stages of infection. *J. Clin. Microbiol.* 1984, 20, 133-135.

[179] Wong, SY, Remington, JS. Biology of *Toxoplasma gondii*. *AIDS* 1993, 7, 299-316.

[180] Weiss, LM, Udem, SA, Tanowitz, H, Wittner, M. Western blot analysis of the antibody response of patients with AIDS and toxoplasma encephalitis: antigenic diversity among *Toxoplasma* strains. *J. Infect. Dis.* 1988, 157, 7-13.

[181] Chumpitazi, BFF, Boussaid, A, Pelloux, H, Racinet, C, Bost, M, Goullier-Fleuret, A. Diagnosis of congenital toxoplasmosis by immunoblotting and relationship with other methods. *J. Clin. Microbiol.* 1995, 33, 1479-1485.

[182] Gross, U, Lüder, CGK, Hendgen, V, Heeg, C, Sauer, I, Weidner, A, Krczal, D, Enders, G. Comparative immunoglobulin G antibody profile between mother and child (CGMC test) for early diagnosis of congenital toxoplasmosis. *J. Clin. Microbiol.* 2000, 38, 3619-3622.

[183] Pinon, JM, Dumon, H, Chemla, C *et al.* Strategy for diagnosis of congenital toxoplasmosis: evaluation of methods comparing mothers and newborns and standard methods for postnatal detection of immunoglobulin G, M, and A antibodies. *J. Clin. Microbiol.* 2001, 39, 2267-2271.

[184] Rilling, V, Dietz, K, Krezal, F, Enders, G. Evaluation of a commercial IgG/IgM western blot assay for early postnatal diagnosis of congenital toxoplasmosis. *Eur. J. Clin. Microbiol. Infect. Dis.* 2003, 22, 174-180.

[185] Nielsen, HV, Remmer Schmidt, DR, Petersen, E. Diagnosis of congenital toxoplasmosis by two-dimensional immunoblot differentiation of mother and child immunoglobulin G profiles. *J. Clin. Microbiol.* 2005, 43, 711-715.

[186] Buffolano, W, Beghetto, E, Del Pezzo, M, Spadoni, A, Di Cristina, M, Petersen, E, Gargano, N. Use of recombinant antigens for early postnatal diagnosis of congenital toxoplasmosis. *J. Clin. Microbiol.* 2005, 43, 5916-5924.

[187] Villena, I, Aubert, D, Brodard, V *et al.* Detection of specific immunoglobulin E during maternal, fetal, and congenital toxoplasmosis. *J. Clin. Microbiol.* 1999, 37, 3487-3490.

[188] Buffolano, W, Lappalainen, M, Hedman, L, Ciccimarra, F, Del Pezzo, M, Rescaldani, R, Gargano, N, Hedman, K. Delayed maturation of IgG avidity in congenital toxoplasmosis. *Eur. J. Clin. Microbiol. Infect. Dis.* 2004, 23, 825-830.

[189] Fricker-Hidalgo, H, Brenier-Pinchart, MP, Schaal, JP, Equy, V, Bost-Bru, C, Pelloux, H. Value of *Toxoplasma gondii* detection in one hundred thirty-three placentas for the diagnosis of congenital toxoplasmosis. *Pediatr. Infect. Dis. J.* 2007, 26, 845-846.

[190] Gilbert, R, Gras, L, European Multicentre Study on Congenital Toxoplasmosis. Effect of timing and type of treatment on the risk of mother to child transmission of *Toxoplasma gondii*. *BJOG* 2003, 110, 112-120.

[191] Gras, L, Wallon, M, Pollak, A, Cortina-Borja, M, Evengard, B, Hayde, M, Petersen, E, Gilbert, R. European Multicentre Study on Congenital Toxoplasmosis. Association between prenatal treatment and clinical manifestations of congenital toxoplasmosis in infancy: a cohort study in 13 European centres. *Acta Paediatr.* 2005, 94, 1721-1731.

[192] Thiébaut, R, Leproust, S, Chêne, G, Gilbert, R. Effectiveness of prenatal treatment for congenital toxoplasmosis: a meta-analysis of individual patients' data. *Lancet* 2007, 369, 115-122.

[193] Petersen, E. Prevention and treatment of congenital toxoplasmosis. *Expert Rev. Anti Infect. Ther.* 2007, 5, 285-293.

[194] Liesenfeld, O, Montoya, JG, Tathineni, NJ, Davis, M, Brown, BW Jr, Cobb, KL, Parsonnet, J, Remington, JS. Confirmatory serologic testing for acute toxoplasmosis and rate of induced abortions among women reported to have positive *Toxoplasma* immunoglobulin M antibody titers. *Am. J. Obstet. Gynecol.* 2001, 184, 140-145.

In: Infectious Pregnancy Complications
Editor: Richard N. Canfield
ISBN 978-1-60741-038-6

Chapter 11

Screening for *Toxoplasma gondii* Infection in Pregnancy in an Urban Area of Northern Italy: Management and Problems

Massimo De Paschale and Pierangelo Clerici
Microbiology Unit, Hospital of Legnano,
Milan, Italy

Abstract

Italian law requires serological screening for toxoplasmosis by the 13th week of pregnancy, with further screenings for seronegative women every 30-40 days until delivery (a total of 5-7). In order to make this protocol effective, full cooperation is required between physician and patient, and its implementation is particularly problematic in the case of women coming from countries with different languages, cultures and health conditions. Italy has recently seen an increase in immigration from countries outside the European Union, which means that a growing number of extra-Community women are involved in the screening programme. An audit of how such screening is carried out is of paramount importance in order to assess its effectiveness, identify its weaknesses, and plan focused interventions.

We considered the data regarding 3395 pregnant women referred for serological screening for anti-*Toxoplasma* IgG antibodies in the three years 2005-2007: 2465 Italians (72.6%) and 930 (27.4%) of foreign origin. Among the latter, 337 (36.2%) came from Eastern Europe, 213 (22.9%) from the Middle East and the Maghreb, 158 (17.0%) from Latin America, 94 (10.1%) from China and the Far East, 66 (7.1%) from the Indian subcontinent, and 62 (6.7%) from Equatorial and Southern Africa.

By the end of the first trimester, 85.0% of the Italians and 81.2% of the foreign women ($p<0.01$) had undergone their first screening. With reference to origin, the differences from Italians were statistically significant only in the case of the African (96.8%), Latin American (77.2%) and Chinese women (71.3%). The prevalence of anti-*Toxoplasma* IgG ranged from 3.2% in the women of Chinese origin to 54.4% in those of

Latin America: comparison with the Italian prevalence (19.4%) showed that all of the differences were statistically significant ($p<0.01$) except for that relating to the women of the Indian subcontinent (13.6%). Five or more screenings (as indicated by the Italian Ministry of Health) were undergone by 32.2% of the seronegative Italians and 30.4% of the seronegative foreign women, among whom the differences from the Italians were statistically significant only in the case of the Latin American (20.8%, $p<0.05$) and Chinese women (18.7%, $p<0.01$). In conclusion, our study shows that screening is active in recruiting both Italian and foreign women by the end of the first trimester of pregnancy, when it is easier to assess and manage a possible acute infection. However, it seems to be more difficult to implement the full screening programme as indicated by the Ministry of Health as only about one-third of the seronegative women underwent five or more screenings. Furthermore, the management of screening is particularly problematic in the case of Chinese and Latin American women, which should stimulate more health education campaigns.

Introduction

Toxoplasma gondii is an obligate intracellular parasite whose final host is the cat and whose intermediate hosts are various warm-blooded animals including humans. Humans can become infected by eating raw or poorly cooked foods contaminated with cysts [1, 2], or by means of contact with infected material, especially soil in which the oocysts expelled by cats' intestine are deposited [3].

Only 10% of the infections are symptomatic in immunocompetent subjects [4], and their clinical pictures are similar to those caused by cytomegalovirus (CMV) infection or mononucleosis. They are generally benign, but their course is more serious (and sometimes fatal) in immunodepressed subjects. Congenital infections are particularly important as their clinical manifestations range from non-specific forms comparable with CMV, rubella or *Herpes simplex* infection to more severe events such as corioretinitis, epilepsy, and psychomotor or mental retardation. Children with sub-forms at birth may also develop symptoms of full-blown toxoplasmosis in subsequent years.

The incidence and severity of the infection varies with the trimester of pregnancy in which it was contracted. The frequency of transmission increases proportionately with the trimester, and is estimated to be 10-15% in the first, 40% in the second, and 70% in the third with peaks of 90% in the ninth month [5-7], but the severity of co-natal infection decreases, with children born to mothers infected in the first or second trimester showing more severe forms of toxoplasmosis than those whose mothers infected in the third trimester. It has been estimated that congenital toxoplasmosis affects 1-10 infants in Europe every 10,000 births [8] and, given the importance of the problem, preventive campaigns aimed at screening pregnant or pre-pregnant women or infants have been proposed, as more general health education campaigns [9, 10].

The implementation of serological screening during pregnancy is related to the prevalence of infection: toxoplasmosis is widespread throughout the world, but its frequency varies from country to country, and has been attributed to climatic, hygienic, socio-economic and dietary factors [1, 5, 11-13], and it could reflect different exposure to the two main sources of contagion: cyst tissue in meat, or oocysts in soil contaminated by infected faeces.

Antibody prevalence in humans increases with age, with no gender differences. The seroprevalence of anti-*Toxoplasma* IgG among women has been reported to be 15% in the USA [14], 10-18% in Great Britain [15, 16], 19-29% in Spain [17, 18], 27% in Denmark [19], 10% in Norway [5], 14-26% in Sweden [20, 21], 55% in France [22], and 24% in Greece [23]. There has been a significant reduction in antibody prevalence over recent years [20, 23-25], which may be responsible for the variations found when comparing data from studies carried out at different times. In terms of incidence, the reported values in Europe range from 0.51 and 0.82 x 1000 pregnant women in Sweden [21] and Norway [26], to 2.9 and 3.04 x 1000 in Denmark [17] and Finland [28], and 5.4 and 8.1 x 1000 in The Netherlands [29] and France [22]. On the basis of these data, serological screening during pregnancy is not recommended in some countries such as Britain, Holland, Norway and the USA, where it is not justified in cost-benefit terms [29-32], but it is recommended (in different forms) in others, such as France, Belgium, Switzerland, Germany and Austria [33-35].

In Italy, IgG antibody prevalence rates range from 21% to 48% [25, 36-40], and have clearly decreased over recent years, whereas incidence rates are high: 9.1 x 1000 [41], with peaks of 35 x 1000 [42]. Current Italian health legislation (Official Gazette No. 245 of 20/10/98) includes serology for toxoplasmosis among the scheduled examinations during pregnancy and indicates that the first screening should be performed by the 13th week, after which seronegative women should be screened every 30-40 days until delivery (a total of 5-7 screenings).

However, it is not sure that the screening is implemented adequately: a knowledge, attitude and practice (KAP) study developed in Italy in the 1990s found that only 65% of the interviewed gynaecologists periodically re-screened women who were seronegative at their first screening during pregnancy [43], and there are published reports from both screening and non-screening countries indicating that 30-35% of initially seronegative women do not complete the follow-up during pregnancy [44, 45]. Finally, the recent increase in immigration to Italy [25] has meant that more immigrant women are involved in pregnancy screening programmes, but managing such screening can be difficult because of differences in culture and language.

The aim of this study was to assess serological screening in the three years 2005-2007 among pregnant Italian and foreign women on the basis of their geographical origin because their different cultural backgrounds may effect screening in different ways.

Materials and Methods

We retrospectively reviewed data relating to 3395 pregnant women with a mean age of 31.5 years (range 15-46) who started and concluded a pregnancy in the period 2005-2007, during which women underwent serological screening for anti-*Toxoplasma* IgG and IgM antibodies (ETI-TOXOK-G-PLUS, ETI-TOXOK-M reverse PLUS; Dia Sorin, Saluggia, Italy).

Of these 3395 women, 2465 (72.6%) were Italian (mean age 32.2 years, range 15-46) and 930 (27.4%) were of foreign origin (mean age 28.3 years, range 15-44), including 337

(36.2%) from Eastern Europe, 213 (22.9%) from the Middle East and the Maghreb, 158 (17.0%) from Latin America, 94 (10.1%) from China and the Far East, 66 (7.1%) from the Indian subcontinent, and 62 (6.7%) from Equatorial and Southern Africa. The data considered were the trimester of pregnancy in which they underwent their first screening, the number of screenings carried out during pregnancy, and the trimester distribution of the screenings. The data were statistically analysed using the χ^2 test and Fisher's exact test.

Results

A total of 3395 women (84.0%) underwent their first screening in the first trimester of pregnancy, 354 (10.4%) in the second trimester, and 190 (5.6%) in the third: the differences between the Italian and foreign women were statistically significant for the first and second trimester (Table 1).

Table 1. Trimester of pregnancy in which the first screening for anti-*Toxoplasma* antibodies was carried out in Italian and foreign women (period 2005-2007)

	Italian women		Foreign women			Total	
Trimester of pregnancy	No.	%	No.	%	P	No.	%
I trimester	2096	85.0	755	81.2	<0.01	2851	84.0
II trimester	240	9.7	114	12.3	<0.05	354	10.4
III trimester	129	5.2	61	6.6	NS	190	5.6
Total	2465		930			3395	

NS = not significant.

Table 2 shows the same data stratified by country of origin. By the end of first trimester, 96.8% of the African, 77.2% of the Latin American, and 71.3% of the Chinese women had undergone their first screening: all of these percentages are significantly different (p <0.01) from the percentage of Italian women (85.0%). The differences between the Italians and the other subgroups of foreign women were not statistically significant (Table 2).

Table 2. Trimester of pregnancy in which the first screening for anti-*Toxoplasma* antibodies was carried out, by geographical area of origin (period 2005-2007)

Origin	I trimester	p	II trimester	p	III trimester	p
Eastern Europe	276 (81.9%)	NS	37 (11.0%)	NS	24 (7.1%)	NS
Middle East	174 (81.7%)	NS	22 (10.3%)	NS	17 (8.0%)	NS
Latin America	122 (77.2%)	<0.01	25 (15.8%)	<0.05	11 (7.0%)	NS
China	67 (71.3%)	<0.01	24 (25.5%)	<0.01	3 (3.2%)	NS
Indian subcontinent	56 (84.8%)	NS	6 (9.1%)	NS	4 (6.1%)	NS
Africa	60 (96.8%)	<0.01	0 (0%)	< 0.01	2 (3.2%)	NS
Italy	2096 (85%)		240 (9.7%)		129 (5.2%)	

NS = not significant.

Eight hundred and four women (23.7%) were anti-*Toxoplasma* IgG and/or IgM positive at the time of the first screening: 479 Italians (17.7%) and 325 foreign women (34.9%) ($p<0.01$) (Table 3). The prevalence of anti-*Toxoplasma* varied from 3.2% among the Chinese women to 54.4% among the women of Latin America (Table 4); comparison with the prevalence among the Italian women (19.4%) showed that the differences were statistically significant ($p<0.01$) for all of the subgroups except the Indian subcontinent subgroup (13.6%).

Table 3. Prevalence of anti-*Toxoplasma* antibodies in pregnant Italian and foreign women (period 2005-2007)

	Italian women		Foreign women			Total	
Anti-*Toxoplasma*	No.	%	No.	%	P	No.	%
Negative	1986	80.6	605	65.0	<0.01	2591	76.3
Positive	479	17.7	325	34.9	<0.01	804	23.7
Total	2465		930			3395	

Table 4. Prevalence of anti-*Toxoplasma* antibodies by geographical area of origin (period 2005-2007)

Origin	Anti-*Toxoplasma* IgG antibodies		
	Positive	Negative	p
Eastern Europe	104 (30.9%)	233 (69.1%)	<0.01
Middle East	95 (44.6%)	118 (55.4%)	<0.01
Latin America	86 (54.4%)	72 (45.6%)	<0.01
China	3 (3.2%)	91 (96.8%)	<0.01
Indian subcontinent	9 (13.6%)	57 (86.4%)	NS
Africa	28 (45.2%)	34 (54.8%)	<0.01
Italy	479 (19.4%)	1986 (80.6%)	

NS = not significant.

Table 5. Number of screenings of pregnant Italian and foreign women who were anti-*Toxoplasma* negative at the first screening (period 2005-2007)

	Italian women		Foreign women			Total	
No.of screenings	No.	%	No.	%	p	No.	%
1	314	15.8	107	17.7	NS	421	16.2
2-4	1033	52.0	314	51.9	NS	1347	52.0
≥5	639	32.2	184	30.4	NS	823	31.8
Total	1986		605			2591	

NS = not significant.

Among the initially seronegative women, 823 (31.8%) underwent five or more screenings (as indicated by the Ministry of Health), with no significant difference between the Italian women and the foreign women considered as a whole (Table 5).

Table 6. Number of screenings of seronegative pregnant Italian and foreign women by geographical area of origin (period 2005-2007)

Origin	Number of screenings					
	1	p	2-4	p	≥5	p
Eastern Europe	43 (18.5%)	NS	108 (46.4%)	NS	82 (35.2%)	NS
Middle East	16 (13.6%)	NS	60 (50.8%)	NS	42 (35.6%)	NS
Latin America	14 (19.4%)	NS	43 (59.7%)	NS	15 (20.8%)	< 0.05
China	17 (18.7%)	NS	57 (62.6%)	< 0.05	17 (18.7%)	<0.01
Indian subcontinent	12 (21.0%)	NS	29 (50.9%)	NS	16 (28.1%)	NS
Africa	5 (14.7%)	NS	17 (50.0%)	NS	12 (35.3%)	NS
Italy	314 (15.8%)		1033 (52.0%)		639 (32.2%)	

NS = not significant.

Table 7. Comparison of screenings Italian and foreign women by trimester of pregnancy (period 2005-2007)

Origin	Trimesters of pregnancy						
	I+II+III	I	I+II	I+III	II	II+III	III	Total
Italy	1151 (58.0%)	204 (10.3%)	211 (10.6%)	81 (4.1%)	81 (4.1%)	142 (7.1%)	116 (5.8%)	1986
Abroad	300 (49.6%)	69 (11.4%)	77 (12.7%)	39 (6.4%)	26 (4.3%)	54 (8.9%)	40 (6.6%)	605
p	<0.01	NS	NS	<0.05	NS	NS	NS	
Total	1451 (56.0%)	273 (10.5%)	288 (11.1%)	120 (4.6%)	107 (4.1%)	196 (7.6%)	156 (6.0%)	2591

NS = not significant.

Table 8. Comparison of screenings of seronegative pregnant Italian and foreign women by trimester of pregnancy and geographical area of origin (period 2005-2007)

Origin	Trimesters of pregnancy						
	I+II+III	p	I	I+II	I+III	II	II+III	III
Eastern Europe	126 (54.1%)	NS	29 (12.4%)	28 (12.0%)	7 (3.0%)	3 (1.3%)	21 (9.0%)	19 (8.2%)
Middle East	60 (50.8%)	NS	11 (9.3%)	9 (7.6%)	15 (12.7%)	4 (3.4%)	12 (10.2%)	7 (5.9%)
Latin America	33 (45.8%)	<0.05	5 (6.9%)	11 (15.3%)	5 (6.9%)	7 (9.7%)	5 (6.9%)	6 (8.3%)
China	33 (36.3%)	<0.01	7 (7.7%)	18 (19.8%)	7 (7.7%)	11 (12.1%)	12 (13.2%)	3 (3.3%)

Indian subcontinent	30 (52.6%)	NS	13 (22.8%)	5 (8.8%)	1 (1.7%)	1 (1.7%)	4 (7.0%)	3 (5.3%)
	I+II+III	p	I	I+II	I+III	II	II+III	III
Africa	18 (52.9%)	NS	4 (11.8%)	6 (17.6%)	4 (11.8%)	0 (0%)	0 (0%)	2 (5.9%)
Italy	1151 (58.0%)		204 (10.3%)	211 (10.6%)	81 (4.1%)	81 (4.1%)	142 (7.1%)	116 (5.8%)

However, comparison by subgroup of origin showed that there was a statistically significant difference between the Italians and the women from Latin America ($p<0.05$) or China ($p<0.01$) (Table 6). In relation to the trimesters of pregnancy in which the screenings took place, 1451 seronegative women (56.0%) underwent at least one screening every three months: 1151 Italians (58.0%) and 300 foreign women (49.6%) ($p<0.01$) (Table 7). The differences in comparison with the Italians statistically significant only in the case of the Chinese (36.3%, $p<0.01$) and Latin American women (45.8%, $p<0.05$) (Table 8).

Conclusion

The severity of congenital *Toxoplasma gondii* infection has prompted some countries to launch antibody screening campaigns as a means of promptly identifying possible acute infections with a risk of transmitting *Toxoplasma* to the foetus. The current Italian legislation indicates a protocol for access to laboratory tests including a search for anti-*Toxoplasma* antibodies at the beginning of pregnancy (before the end of the 13th week) and, in the case of IgG negativity, repeat screenings every 30-40 days until childbirth (for a total of 5-7 screenings). Ensuring that this protocol is appropriately implemented requires the full cooperation of physicians and patients, and efficiently organised healthcare facilities capable of allowing timely access and prompt results, and so it is worth conducting an audit in order to assess the effectiveness of the screening, identify its weaknesses, and plan any necessary targeted interventions.

The vast majority of the women in our survey began monitoring during the first trimester of pregnancy as indicated by the Ministry of Health. However, although the vast majority of seronegative women underwent more than one screening during the course of their pregnancy, only about one-third underwent the recommended number of 5-7, and only slightly more than half underwent at least one screening every three months.

Comparison of the Italian women with those of foreign origin (about one-fifth of the total) showed that there was no difference in the timing of the first screening, but the percentage of women who underwent screening in every trimester was significantly lower. This may be due to various reasons, ranging from socio-economic, cultural and linguistic differences, to problems of integration related to their more or less recent time of immigration. Furthermore, our study only considered women who had access to the National Health Service, and did not include clandestine immigrants who do not undergo normal screening procedures.

Our findings show that women from Eastern Europe, the Middle East, the Indian subcontinent and Africa behaved like the Italians (and, in some cases, the Africans performed better), but the Chinese and Latin American women underwent screening later and less frequently. Although it would take a more sociological study to understand this behaviour, it does seem that these groups merit a particularly concentrated health education campaign. Moreover, as the proportion of pregnant women of foreign origin in Italy continues to grow, the problems involved in managing their screening should be increasingly taken into account at the level of national health policy.

References

[1] Remington, JS; McLeod, R; Desmonts, G. Toxoplasmosis. In: Remington JS, Klein JO, editors. *Infectious diseases of the fetus and newborn infant.* Philadelphia: Saunders WB; 1995; 140-267.

[2] Stray-Pedersen, B. Toxoplasmosis in pregnancy. In: *Infectious diseases. Challenges for the 1990's.* London: Bailliere's Clinical Obstetrics and Gynaecology; 1993; 1-107.

[3] Holliman, R. Commentary: Congenital toxoplasmosis-further thought for food. *BMJ*, 2000, 321, 147.

[4] McCabe, RE; Brooks, RG; Dorfman, RF; Remington, JS. Clinical spectrum in 107 cases of toxoplasmic lymphadenopathy. *Reviews of Infectious Diseases*, 1987, 9, 754-774.

[5] Dunn, D; Wallon, M; Peyron, F; Petersen, E; Peckham, C; Gilbert, R. Mother to child transmission of toxoplasmosis: risk estimates for clinical counselling. *Lancet*, 1999, 353, 1829-1833.

[6] Daffos, F; Forestier, F; Capella-Pavlovsky, M; Thulliez, P; Aufrant, C; Valenti, D; Cox, WL. Prenatal management of 746 pregnancies at risk for congenital toxoplasmosis. *The New England Journal of Medicine,* 1988, 318, 271-275.

[7] Desmonts, G; Couvreur, J. Congenital toxoplasmosis. Prospective study of the outcome of pregnancy in 542 women with toxoplasmosis acquired during pregnancy. *Annales de Pédiatrie*, 1984, 31, 805-809.

[8] Gilbert, RE. Epidemiology of infection in pregnant women. In: Petersen E, Amboise-Thomas P, editors. *Congenital toxoplasmosis: scientific background, clinical management and control.* Paris: Springer-Verlag; 2000.

[9] Pawlowski, ZS; Gromadecka-Sutkiewicz, M; Skommer, J; Paul, M; Rokossowski, H; Suchocka, E; Schantz, PM. Impact of health education on knowledge and prevention behaviour for congenital toxoplasmosis: the experience in Poznan, Poland. *Health Education Research*, 2001, 16, 493-502.

[10] Foulon, W; Naessens, A; Ho-Yen, D. Prevention of congenital toxoplasmosis. *Journal of Perinatal Medicine*, 2000, 28, 337-345.

[11] Jenum, PA; Kapperud, G; Stray-Pedersen, B; Melby, KK; Eskild, A; Eng, J. Prevalence of *Toxoplasma gondii* specific immunoglobulin G antibodies among pregnant women in Norway. *Epidemiology and Infection,* 1998, 120, 87-92.

[12] Dupouy Camet, J; Gavinet, MF; Paugam, A; Tourte Schaeffer, C. Transmission, incidence and prevalence of toxoplasmosis. *Médecine et Maladies Infectieuses,* 1993, 23, 139-147.

[13] Gilbert, RE; Tookey, PA; Cubitt, WD; Ades, AE; Masters, J; Peckham, CS. Prevalence of *Toxoplasma* IgG among pregnant women in west London according to country of birth and ethnic group. *BMJ,* 1993, 306, 185.

[14] Jones, JL; Kruszon-Moran, D; Wilson, M. *Toxoplasma gondii* infection in the Unites States, 1999-2000. *Emerging Infectious Diseases,* 2003, 9, 1371-1374.

[15] Ades, AE; Parker, S; Gilbert, R; Tookey, PA; Berry, T; Hjelm, M; Wilcox, AH; Cubitt, D; Peckham, CS. Maternal prevalence of *Toxoplasma* antibody based on anonymous neonatal serosurvey: a geographical analysis. *Epidemiology and Infection,* 1993, 110, 127-133.

[16] Allain, JP; Palmer, CR; Pearson, G. Epidemiological study of latent and recent infection by *Toxoplasma gondii* in pregnant women from a regional population in the UK. *The Journal of Infection,* 1998, 36, 189-196.

[17] Gutiérrez-Zufiaurre, N; Sánchez-Hernández, J; Muñoz, S; Marin, R; Delgado, N; Sáenz, MC; Muñoz-Bellido, JL; Garcia-Rodriguez, JA. Seroprevalence of antibodies against *Treponema pallidum*, *Toxoplasma gondii*, rubella virus, hepatitis B and C virus, and HIV in pregnant women. *Enfermedades Infecciosas y Microbiología Clínica,* 2004, 22, 512-516.

[18] Muñoz Batet, C; Guardià Llobet, C; Juncosa Morros, T; Viñas Domenech, L; Sierra Soler, M; Sanfeliu Sala, I; Bosch Mestres, J; Dopico Ponte, E; Lite Lite, J; Matas Andreu, L; Juste Sánchez, C; Barranco Romeu, M. Toxoplasmosis and pregnancy. Multicenter study of 16,632 pregnant women in Barcelona. *Medicina Clínica,* 2004, 123, 12-16.

[19] Lebech, M; Larsen, SO; Petersen, E. Prevalence, incidence and geographical distribution of *Toxoplasma gondii* antibodies in pregnant women in Denmark. *Scandinavian Journal of Infectious Diseases,* 1993, 25, 751-756.

[20] Petersson, K; Stray-Pedersen, B; Malm, G; Forsgren, M; Evengård, B. Seroprevalence of *Toxoplasma gondii* among pregnant women in Sweden. *Acta Obstetricia et Gynecologica Scandinavica,* 2000, 79, 824-829.

[21] Evengård, B; Petersson, K; Engman, ML; Winklund, S; Ivarsson, SA; Teär-Fahnehjelm, K; Forsgren, M; Gilbert, R; Malm, G: Low incidence of *Toxoplasma* infection during pregnancy and in newborns in Sweden. *Epidemiology and Infection,* 2001, 127, 121-127.

[22] Ancelle, T ; Goulet, V ; Tirad-Fleury, V; Baril, L ; du Mazaubrun, C ; Thulliez, P ; Wcislo, M ; Carme, B. La toxoplasmose chez la femme enceinte en France en 1995. Résultats d'une enquête nationale périnatale. *Bulletin Epidémiologique Hebdomadaire,* 1996, 51, 227-229.

[23] Diza, E; Frantzidou, F; Souliou, E; Arvanitidou, M; Gioula, G; Antoniadis, A. Seroprevalence of *Toxoplasma gondii* in northern Greece during the last 20 years. *Clinical Microbiology and Infection,* 2005, 11, 719-723.

[24] Horion, M; Thoumsin, H; Senterre, J; Lambotte, R. 20 years of screening for toxoplasmosis in pregnant women. The Liège experience in 20,000 pregnancies. *Revue Médicale de Liège,* 1990, 45, 492-497.

[25] De Paschale, M; Agrappi, C; Clerici, P; Mirri, P; Manco, MT; Cavallari, S; Viganò, EF. *Toxoplasma gondii* infection seroprevalence in Italian and foreign female

population living in the area of Legnano (MI). *Microbiologia Medica,* 2006, 21, 322-327.

[26] Jenum, PA; Stray-Pedersen, B; Melby, KK; Kapperud, G; Whitelaw, A; Eskild, A; Eng, J. Incidence of *Toxoplasma gondii* infection in 35,940 pregnant women in Norway and pregnancy outcome for infected women. *Journal of Clinical Microbiology,* 1998, 36, 2900-2906.

[27] Lebech, M; Andersen, O; Christensen, NC; Hertel, J; Nielsen, HE; Peitersen, B; Rechnitzer, C; Larsen, SO; Nørgaard-Pedersen, B; Petersen, E. Feasibility of neonatal screening for *Toxoplasma* infection in the absence of prenatal treatment. Danish Congenital Toxoplasmosis Study Group. *Lancet*, 1999, 353, 1834-1837.

[28] Lappalainen, M; Koskela, P; Hedman, K; Teramo, K; Ammälä, P; Hiilesmaa, V; Koskiniemi, M. Incidence of primary *Toxoplasma* infections during pregnancy in southern Finland: a prospective cohort study. *Scandinavian Journal of Infectious Diseases*, 1992, 24, 97-104.

[29] Conyn van Spoondonek, MAE Prevention of congenital toxoplasmosis in The Netherlands Bilthoven: National Institute of Public Health and Enviromental Protection. 1991 ISBN 90-90004179-6.

[30] Royal College of Obstetricians and Gynaecologists. Antenatal care. Routine care for the healthy pregnant woman. London: RCOG 2003.

[31] Eskild, A; Oxman, A; Magnus, P; Bjørndal, A; Bakketeig, LS. Screening for toxoplasmosis in pregnancy: what is the evidence of reducing a health problem? *Journal of Medical Screening,* 1996, 3, 188-194.

[32] Gilbert, RE; Peckham, CS. Congenital toxoplasmosis in the United Kingdom: to screen or not to screen? *Journal of Medical Screening,* 2002, 9, 135-141.

[33] Agence Nationale d'Accréditation et d'Evaluation en Santé. La surveillance biologique de la femme enceinte en bonne santé et sans antécédents pathologiques. Paris : ANAES 1996.

[34] Aspöck, H; Pollak, A. Prevention of prenatal toxoplasmosis by serological screening of pregnant women in Austria. *Scandinavian Journal of Infectious Diseases. Supplementum,* 1992, 84, 32-37.

[35] Hengst, P. Screening for toxoplasmosis in pregnant women: presentation of a screening programme in the former "East"-Germany and the present status in Germany. *Scandinavian Journal of Infectious Disease. Supplementum,* 1992, 84, 38-42.

[36] Condorelli, F; Scalia, G; Stivala, A; Costanzo, MC; Adragna, AD; Franceschino, C; Santagati, MG; Furieri, PM; Marino, A; Castro, A. Seroprevalence to some TORCH agents in a Sicilian female population of fertile age. *European Journal of Epidemiology,* 1993, 9, 341-343.

[37] Adorisio, E; De Cicco, AL; Calandri, A; Simili, M; Annichiarico, LS. Prevalence of *Toxoplasma gondii* infections in groups of individuals in Rome and its environment. *La Clinica Terapeutica*, 1996, 147, 317-320.

[38] Valcavi, PP; Natali, A; Soliani, L; Montali, S; Dettori, G; Cheezi, C. Prevalence of anti-*Toxoplasma gondii* antibodies in the population of the area of Parma (Italy). *European Journal of Epidemiology*, 1995, 11, 333-337.

[39] Moschen, ME; Stroffolini, T; Arista, S; Pistoia, D; Giammanco, A; Azara, A; De Mattia, D; Chiaramonte, M; Rigo, G; Scarpa, B. Prevalence of *Toxoplasma gondii* antibodies among children and teenagers in Italy. *Microbiologica*, 1991, 14, 229-234.

[40] Vezzo, R; Vigorè, L; Goglio, A; Raglio, A; Vecchia, L; Terenziani, P; Fortina, G; Di Natale, C; Rescaldani, R. Sieroprevalenza per anticorpi anti-*Toxoplasma gondii* in 14.186 soggetti. *Microbiologia Medica*, 2001, 16, 220.

[41] De Paschale, M; Agrappi, C; Clerici, P; Mirri, P; Manco, MT; Cavallari, S; Viganò, EF. Seroprevalence and incidence of *Toxoplasma gondii* infection in the Legnano area of Italy. *Clinical Microbiology and Infection*, 2008, 14, 186-189.

[42] Ricci, M; Pentimalli, H; Thaller, R; Ravà, L; Di Ciommo, V. Screening and prevention of congenital toxoplasmosis: an effectiveness study in a population with a high infection rate. *The journal of Maternal-Fetal and Neonatal Medicine*, 2003, 14, 398-403.

[43] Buffolano, W; Gilbert, RE; Holland, FJ; Fratta, D; Palombo, F; Ades, AE. Risk factors for recent *Toxoplasma* infection in pregnant women in Naples. *Epidemiology and Infection*, 1996, 116, 347-351.

[44] Charrier, L; Moiraghi Ruggenini, A; Renga, G; Ditommaso, S; Lievre, MA; Zotti, C. Cost analysis of *Toxoplasma* infection control in pregnancy. *Annali d'Igiene*, 2003, 15, 505-514.

[45] Eskild, A; Fallås Dahl, G; Melby, KK; Nesheim, BI. Testing for toxoplasmosis in pregnancy: a study of the routines in primary antenatal care. *Journal of Medical Screening*, 2003, 10, 172-175.

In: Infectious Pregnancy Complications
Editor: Richard N. Canfield

ISBN 978-1-60741-038-6

Chapter 12

Rickettsioses in Pregnancy

Maria Bitsori and Emmanouil Galanakis
Department of Paediatrics, Infectious Diseases Unit,
University of Crete Greece

Abstract

The term "rickettsioses" traditionally has included the diseases caused by 23 species of the genus *Rickettsia* up-to-date recognized to be pathogenic to humans as well as diseases caused by *Coxiella*, *Ehrlichia, Anaplasma* and *Orientia* species, which belong to different genera, families or even orders. Infections caused by rickettsiae and related pathogens are of major morbidity worldwide; additionally, new pathogens are continuously recognized and consideration has recently been given to their potentiality as biological weapons.

Pregnant women, especially those living in endemic areas, are of considerable risk for rickettsioses, but very little is known about the natural course of infections caused by rickettsiae and related pathogens during pregnancy. Transplacental passage has not been documented for any of the pathogens of the genus *Rickettsia,* the youngest serologically confirmed case having been a *R. ricketsii* infection a 6-month-old infant. By contrast, transplacental transmission is likely, for *Orientia* and *Anaplasma* species, thus treatment of the newborn should be considered in such cases. *C burnettii*, a major cause of infertility and abortions in animals has been associated with obstetric complications, abortions and stillbirths in humans as well and perinatal infection with this pathogen is considered possible.

The treatment of infections caused by rickettsiae and related pathogens in pregnancy raises serious safety issues. Tetracyclines, which are the treatment of choice for non-pregnant adults can be toxic for both, the mother and the fetus and the alternative choice of chloramphenicol has been associated with the rare but life-threatening complication of "gray baby syndrome" if given near term. Macrolides have been safely used in pregnancy for the treatment of other infections and seem to be an attractive option but their efficacy against the most serious of these infections, i.e., *R rickettsii*, is questioned. Moreover, macrolides alone are not sufficient for the management of *C burnettii* infection, which has the potential of chronicity and can complicate future pregnancies.

Rickettsioses in pregnancy are associated with complications both for the mother and fetus/infant. Treatment of these infections remains challenging and controversial and should be carefully considered on case-by-case basis until further investigation elucidates the natural course of the infections in pregnancy and the efficacy and safety issues. Prevention, principally by avoiding ticks and contact to infected animals, is of paramount significance.

Introduction

The term "rickettsiosis", has traditionally included the diseases caused by 23 species of the genus Rickettsia up-to-date recognised to be pathogenic for humans as well as diseases caused by Coxiella, Ehrlichia, Anaplasma and Orientia species, which cause similar clinical manifestations but have been ultimately proven to belong to diverse genera, families, orders or even classes [1-3]. The identification and classification of these organisms and the elucidation of their clinical features occurred during the 20th century and is still ongoing, however the diseases have existed since antiquity and have greatly affected the history and evolution of humanity. These diseases were called rickettsioses in honour of the American pathologist Howard Taylor Ricketts (1871–1910), who in 1908 identified R rickettsii as the responsible pathogen for Rocky Mountain spotted fever and lost his life investigating epidemic typhus in Mexico two years later.

Rickettsiae and related pathogens are all obligate intracellular gram-negative coccobacilli and their life-cycle involves small mammal vertebrate hosts and arthropod vectors, with the exception of C. burnetii, which is a zoonosis infecting humans through contaminated soil. Humans are only incidental hosts and do not contribute to the persistence of the organisms in nature, with the exception of R prowazekii. Because of the common properties of these organisms the diseases they cause, similarly sharing common clinical characteristics, are often discussed together as "rickettsioses" "rickettsial infections", or "infections caused by rickettsiae and associated organisms" [2]. Although we kept herein the traditional term "rickettsioses", we believe that time has come to think of and manage these infections as distinct clinical entities. To avoid the confusion often occurring by the designation of these diseases by both the pathogen and some other term of geographical or historical origin, we in general preferred the designation by the pathogen.

Rickettsiae and related pathogens are present worldwide, their epidemiology being determined by the ecology of vectors, i.e., ticks, mites, fleas and lice and new pathogenic species are continuously recognised. Recently, consideration has been given on their potentiality as biological threat [4], as they are easy to mass-produce, may be released in aerosol form or through infected arthropods, present with nonspecific manifestations leading to delayed diagnosis and treatment, are highly virulent, and as resistant strains may be developed [5, 6]. The CDC experts committee has listed R prowazekii and C burnetii in category B and R rickettsii in category C [5, 7]. However, it has been argued that all three species alongside with R typhi belong in the highest-priority category A, and deserve more attention [5]

The infections caused by rickettsiae and associated pathogens are generally considered more common among men and children, however women are also at considerable risk for infection in endemic areas as many of them maintain their occupation and activity in the pregnant state. The pregnant patient with a rickettsiosis presents a special problem in that the illness maybe easily misdiagnosed and attributed to more common pregnancy-related diseases [8]. Moreover, pregnancy imposes puzzling therapeutic questions since tetracyclines, which are the antibiotics of choice for most infections caused by rickettsiae and related pathogens, are not considered safe in pregnancy [8, 9]. The appropriate management of the neonate after birth, not only in terms of appropriate investigation and antibiotic treatment but also in terms of nursing and follow-up, remains an open question for most of these infections. The existing guidelines for the management of rickettsioses during pregnancy include only very general recommendations for the pregnant patient, leaving the management details to be resolved on case basis [1, 8, 10]. We present an overview of rickettsioses in pregnancy focusing on the management of mother and neonate, based on all available published information.

Incidence and Impact of Rickettsioses in Pregnancy

Although rickettsiae and related pathogens are of major morbidity worldwide they have only very rarely been reported during pregnancy and thus they are considered unusual among pregnant women [11, 12]. However, since these infections have a non-specific clinical presentation [10] they may well go unrecognised and since many of them are mild and self-limited [13, 14], they may also be underreported. Hence, their true incidence during pregnancy cannot be estimated. Information is derived from sporadic case reports encountered in medical literature for pregnant patients with *R. rickettsii* [8, 9, 15], *R. conorii* [16, 17], *R. typhi* [18, 19] and *A. phagocytophilum* [20-23] infection and scarce case series, concerning mainly *O. tsutsugamush* [11, 24-27] and *C. burnettii* infection [28, 29].

In addition, their impact on pregnancy is unclear for most of them. The pathogens of the genus *Rickettsia* seem not to be transmitted transplacentally. An indication pointing against vertical transmission in humans is that these infections are exceptional in infants, the youngest serologically confirmed case being a 6-month-old infant with *R rickettsii* infection whose older sibling was also affected in the same period [29]. In the reported cases there were no clinical or laboratory signs of infection in any of the delivered infants [8, 9, 15-19]. In one of the cases polymerase chain reaction for rickettsia species was performed on the placenta of a pregnant woman with *R. rickettsii* infection, which was negative for the organism [15]. Experimental studies with murine models did not demonstrate transplacental passage of *O tsutsugamushi* and *R typhi* [31, 32], although perinatal *O tsutsugamushi* infection has been suggested in two clinical cases [25, 26]. In these cases the neonates were born to mothers with *O. tsutsugamushi* infection who were not treated until delivery. They both developed febrile illnesses suggestive of scrub typhus infection and elevated *O. tsutsugamushi*-specific IgM antibodies were in both detected [26, 27]. Uncontrolled *O. tsutsugamushi* infection has also been associated with stillbirths or foetal loss [25].

By contrast, transplancental passage of *C burnetii* and possibly *Anaplasma* species may happen [23, 28]. Perinatal infection with *A. phagocytophylum* was reported in one case. The mother presented with signs of infection just one day before delivery and gave birth to a normal female infant, who presented with signs of infection on her ninth day of life [20]. Although *A. phagocytophylum* is known to be transmitted across the placenta in animals, the route of infant's infection in this case has not been confirmed. The placenta had been discarded and the infant had been breastfed before the mother's diagnosis was suspected [20]. In another occasion, infection early in pregnancy resulted in foetal loss [12].

C. burnetii infection deserves a special consideration, as it is a well-known cause of abortion and infertility in animals, and of placentitis, obstetric complications and risk in subsequent pregnancies in human cases [33]. Spontaneous abortions, foetal death, growth retardation and premature delivery have been reported despite treatment [28, 33]. Infection in the first and second trimester of pregnancy bears a high risk of chronicity, regardless of treatment [28, 33]. The impact of the disease on the foetus seems to be so devastating that it usually results either in foetal loss from placental insufficiency or in prematurity and low birth weight, thus neonatal acute *C. burnetii* infection has only rarely been reported [34]. Some cases of uninfected neonates born to mothers with confirmed acquisition of *C. burnettii* infection during pregnancy have also been reported [35, 36].

Clinical Presentation and Diagnosis: Pregnancy-Related Considerations

Probably the main difficulty in the diagnosis of rickettsioses is their non-specific clinical presentation. In most of these diseases fever and flu-like symptoms occasionally accompanied by a rash are the most common early symptoms, which the pregnant patient might easily attribute to the pregnancy itself [9]. In many cases a suggestive history, such as tick-bite, animal contact or occupational exposure is lacking [1, 10, 14]. Even when the history is suggestive, clinicians are not always familiar with the transmission route and the diverse, even protean manifestations of these infections, especially in non-endemic areas.

The diagnostic approach of rickettsioses in pregnancy can be a demanding and complicated task. Infectious diseases lead the list of differential diagnosis, which also includes several non-infectious pregnancy-associated conditions [8, 9]. Infections associated with arthropod bites or infected domestic animals and similar clinical manifestations, such as Lyme disease, leptospirosis and brucellosis and infections with special implications for vertical transmission, such as rubella, measles, toxoplasmosis, secondary syphilis, Epstein-Barr virus infection and enteroviral infection should be considered [8, 9]. Additionally, in the third trimester of pregnancy severe preeclampsia with liver involvement and thrombocytopenia (haemolysis, elevated liver enzymes, low platelet, HELLP syndrome), Gram-negative sepsis and streptococcal toxic shock syndrome (TSS) in the postpartum setting might have a clinical presentation resembling an infection caused by rickettsiae and related pathogens [8, 9].

Therapeutic decision is commonly made on clinical grounds, since laboratory confirmation is often unavailable, and even useless for clinical decisions, as specific IgM and IgG antibodies for all rickettsiae and associated organisms are only detected after the first or the second week of the disease, a follow-up sampling is required, and interpretation is often tricky and confounded by cross-reactivity [14, 37]. The possibility of false-positive serologic tests during pregnancy cannot be entirely excluded, since it is known that false-positive serologic tests often obscure the diagnosis of many diseases in pregnant patients [38-40]. A rapid latex-agglutination test, which had been used for early detection of *R.rickettsii* infection yielded high rates of false-positive results reaching 12% in the third trimester of pregnancy [41]. The false-positivity rates of this test were concluded on clinical grounds and in comparison with the highly sensitive and specific immunofluorescent assay (IFA), which is currently the method of choice for the laboratory confirmation of most rickettsioses [41]. False-positive results of IFA associated with pregnancy have not been reported. More accurate methods, such as culture and Western blotting, and rapid molecular assays have been developed but are not widely available.

Treatment of Rickettsioses in Pregnancy

Second-generation tetracyclines, doxycycline and minocycline, are the antibiotics of choice for the treatment of rickettsioses in nonpregnant adults. Rickettsiae and associated organisms are totally susceptible to tetracyclines in vitro with the exception of some *O. tsitsugamushi* strains [42-44]. Although the optimal duration of treatment has not been established, a short course of treatment, ranging from a few days to 2 weeks, is adequate to cure most of these infections. [1, 10, 37]. However, tetracyclines have long been known to bind irreversibly in calcifying tissues, resulting in growth inhibition of bones and permanent teeth discolouration [45, 46], thus there have been serious concerns about their safety during pregnancy and in early childhood [8, 47]. The American Academy of Pediatrics amended its recommendation against the use of tetracyclines in early childhood and advised for their exceptional use for life threatening rickettsial and related infections [10]. The rationale was that morbidity from rickettsioses outweighs the risk of dental staining from a short course of doxycycline [1].

Tetracyclines and pregnancy. Unfortunately, the same safety with short courses of doxycycline or other tetracyclines cannot be assumed for pregnant women. Tetracycline use in pregnancy may induce maternal hepatotoxicity and affect not only deciduous teeth but also foetal skeleton [8, 9]. Early studies in animals and observational studies with neonates receiving or exposed to tetracyclines *in utero* demonstrated bone growth inhibition, associated with large doses and reversible after discontinuation of tetracyclines [45, 46]. However, since no proven permanent tetracycline-associated skeletal malformation has ever been reported and calcification of permanent teeth does not begin until after birth, CDC recommendations call for the consideration of doxycycline for life-threatening rickettsioses, such as *R rickettsii* infection, in pregnancy [10]. Experience is limited though, the only clinical case reported being a patient with *O. tsutsugamushi* infection treated with minocycline with favourable outcome for the mother and without side-effects for the neonate [11].

Chloramphenicol, one of the oldest broad-spectrum antibiotics, with almost equal efficacy to tetracyclines against rickettsiae and associated pathogens, remains the recommended antibiotic for the treatment of most of these infections acquired during pregnancy [8, 17]. There have recently been some concerns of resistance, however, since *C burnettii* strains and the newly recognised *Ehrlichiae* and *Anaplasma* species exhibited tetracycline resistance *in vitro* [48-50]. Chloramphenicol is well-tolerated and of a very low risk of teratogenicity [9]. Mild bone marrow suppression is the commonest side effect and is usually dose-related and reversible, but serious safety concerns are raised by wide interindividual variations in metabolism and by the potentiality of aplastic anaemia, a rare but fatal idiosyncratic reaction occurring weeks after therapy [51]. The risk of "grey baby syndrome" of cardiovascular collapse after administration of chloramphenicol late in pregnancy is a theoretical possibility but it has never been confirmed [8]. Chloramphenicol has been successfully used for the treatment of a 28 weeks pregnant woman with *R. rickettsii* infection and a near term woman with *R conorii conorii* infection, who both recovered without side-effects for them or their infants [15, 17], but failed to control *O tsutsugamushi* infection in a pregnant woman, who delivered a premature baby on the second day of treatment. The neonate died within 6 hours because of respiratory distress, without signs of perinatal infection [24].

Macrolides, which are considered safe in pregnancy and have proven efficacy against intracellular organisms could be an ideal alternative, especially the newer ones, clarithromycin, josamycin and azithromycin [52, 53]. They have been widely used for toxoplasmosis and chlamydial infections in pregnancy, with excellent safety and tolerance profiles [54]. Erythromycin was successfully used for *R typhi* infection in two pregnant women in Australia and Cyprus [18, 19], but controlled only partially *A. phagocytophilum* infection in a 34 weeks pregnant woman [21]. In this case the neonate was born and remained healthy but mother's fever relapsed after delivery and was eventually cured with doxycycline for 2 weeks [21]. Josamycin has been recommended as the macrolide of choice for pregnancy [16, 22], but this agent is not widely available. Azithromycin in a single dose of 500 mg was successfully used in 11 pregnant women with *O tsutsugamushi* infection who delivered healthy neonates [11]. The efficacy of macrolides against the most serious rickettsial infections, i.e *R. rickettsii*, is questioned, despite susceptibility of the agent to newer macrolides in vitro [52, 55-57]. Additionally, although macrolides were efficient against acute *C. burnetti* infection [58], it is doubtful whether they are sufficient to control *C. burnettii* infection acquired in pregnancy and prevent chronicity [28, 59].

Rifampin. In vitro studies have demonstrated variable susceptibility of rickettsiae to rifampin [42] but both rifampin and its derivative rifabutin exhibited *in vitro* activity against *Ehrlichia* and *Anaplasma* species [60, 61]. At the clinical level, rifampin was used either as monotherapy or in combination with erythromycin for the treatment of pregnant women with *A. phagocytophilum* and *R conorii conorii* infection, respectively [16, 22]. Such regimens should be considered with caution, however, in ensuring that *R rickettsii* infection can be ruled out [10].

Fluoroquinolones have shown adequate efficacy against rickettsial and associated pathogens, including *C burnetii* and ehrlichiae, *in vitro* [42, 60-63], however they are officially contra-indicated in pregnancy as they act through inhibition of nucleic acid formation [17] and as up to date clinical experience has been disappointing. Ciprofloxacin has been used in the UK for the treatment of a pregnant woman with *C burnetii* infection and allergy to erythromycin, without side effects for the newborn, but also without control of her infection [36]. Three pregnant women treated with ciprofloxacin for *O tsutsugamushi* infection in India had unfavourable outcome with one abortion and two stillborns [26].

Co-trimoxazole. Rickettsiae are not susceptible *in vitro* to co-trimoxazole [42] and, more importantly, concerns have been raised that sulfonamides may increase the severity of *R rickettsii, R conorii conorii, R typhi* and *E. chaffeensis* infection. [64-67].

However, co-trimoxazole is very useful for the management of *C. burnettii* infection acquired in pregnancy. Co-trimoxazole until delivery followed by doxycycline and hydroxychloroquine thereafter has been suggested as the most successful therapeutic approach of pregnant patients with *C. burnettii* infection for favourable pregnancy outcome and prevention of chronicity [28, 29].The available information about rickettsioses management are summarised in Table 1.

Table 1. Rickettsioses during pregnancy: available information for the management of mother and neonate

Pathogen (Disease)	Management of mother	Management of neonate
R conorii (Mediterranean spotted fever)	Chloramphenicol 50-75 mg/kg/day qid po x 3 days after fever resolution [17] Erythromycin 500 mg tid or qid and rifampin 600 mg/day x 14 days [16] Josamycin 1 g tid x 5 days [16] Azithromycin x 1-5 days (dose not determined) [17]	Transplacental transmission not confirmed, no preventive treatment required [16, 17] Breastfeeding avoided only when mother is on doxycycline or chloramphenicol
R rickettsii (Rocky Mountain spotted fever)	Chloramphenicol 50-75 mg/kg/day qid po x 3 days after fever resolution [8] A short course of doxycycline could be considered in life-threatening situations [10]	Transplacental transmission not confirmed, no preventive treatment required [8] Breastfeeding avoided only when mother is on doxycycline or chloramphenicol
R typhi (Murine typhus)	Erythromycin 500 mg tid or qid x 7 days [18, 19]	Transplacental transmission not confirmed, no preventive treatment required [18, 19]
O tsutsugamushi (Scrub typhus)	Azithromycin 500 mg single dose [11] Chloramphenicol 50-75 mg/kg/day qid or minocycline 100 mg/day bid po x 1-7 days depending on infection severity [24, 25,68]	Transplacental transmission possible; doxycycline or chloramphenicol can be considered in symptomatic neonates [11, 27]

Table 1. (Continued)

Pathogen (Disease)	Management of mother	Management of neonate
C burnetii (Q fever)	Trimethoprim-sulfamethoxazole 160 mg/day TMP + 800 mg/day SMZ bid until delivery, and afterwards doxycycline 100 mg/day bid and hydroxychloroquine 600 mg/day (adjustment with blood levels) for a year [28, 29]	Transplacental transmission possible; preventive treatment of neonate until perinatal infection is excluded Doxycycline or combination of ciprofloxacin with a macrolide can be considered [36] Avoid breastfeeding in confirmed cases
A phagocytophilum (Human Granulocytic Anaplasmosis)	Rifampin 600 mg/day [22] x 5-7 days A short course of doxycycline can be considered if diagnosis uncertain or in life-threatening conditions [12]	Perinatal infection possible; doxycycline can be considered in symptomatic neonates [20]

Bid: in 2 daily doses; qid: in 4 daily doses; tid: in 3 daily doses; IV: intravenously; po: orally.

Management of Neonate

Antibiotics. Since rickettsiae seem not to be transmitted transplacentally, treatment of healthy infants born to mothers who acquired infections from pathogens of the genus *Rickettsia* during pregnancy is not recommended [8]. By contrast, transplancental passage of *C burnetii* and possibly *O. tsutsugamushi, Ehrlichia* and *Anaplasma* species may happen [20-28]. In such cases prophylactic treatment of the newborn is warranted until infection is excluded. The combination of ciprofloxacin and erythromycin for two weeks has been used in a case of suspected perinatal *C burnetii* infection [36]. In the single reported case of perinatal *A phagocytophilum* infection, intravenous doxycycline for 5 days was used successfully [20]. In two cases of symptomatic neonatal *O. tsutsugamushi* infection treatment with doxycycline and chloramphenicol in each case has been tried [26, 27]. Healthy neonates born to mothers with *O. tsutsugamushi* infection have not been treated [11].

Breastfeeding. Transmission of infection through breast milk has only been confirmed for *C. burnettii* [34, 59] but has also been suspected in cases of neonatal *A. phagocytophilum* infection [20, 21]. Thus, mothers who acquired these particular infections during pregnancy should better be advised to forego breastfeeding, even if their treatment regimen does not include doxycycline. In all other cases of rickettsioses, breastfeeding is only discouraged for women on treatment with a tetracycline.

A summary of available information about postnatal management of neonates is included in Table 1.

Prevention of Rickettsioses in Childhood and During Pregnancy

Prevention is strongly recommended and includes avoidance of ticks and arthropod bites, protective clothing, application of repellents and inspection for tick or mite attachment and proper removal [37, 68]. The immune status of pregnant women against *C. burnettii* should be checked among populations of high risk for occupational exposure, such as abattoir workers, wool and hides handling workers and farmers and probably excluded if non-immune [59].

Vaccines. No appropriate vaccines are available for rickettsial pathogens. The so-called Cox vaccine *for R prowazekii* appeared at the outset of Word War II but was halted in 1944 because of limited efficacy and side-effects [69]. Acellular and whole-cell Q fever vaccines are available in Australia, the USA and some European countries, but are only recommended for non-immune high-risk adults after pre-vaccination screening. There is no information about the safety of these vaccines in pregnancy [59].

Prophylactic antibiotics. The possibility of acquiring a rickettsial infection after a tick bite is small, given the low prevalence of infected ticks, and the low affinity of ticks for humans [37]. In addition, asymptomatic individuals with recent tick bites seem not to benefit from prophylaxis. A single dose of azithromycin, however, seems to protect adults with history of tick-bite against *R conorii conorii* [70, 71], as in a randomised clinical trial no patient in the azithromycin group developed infection, which was developed in 10% of patients without azithromycin. This measure seems simple and safe and might be considered for children and pregnant women. A case of an obstetrician who acquired *C burnetii* pneumonia from infected placenta suggests that protection of exposed personnel should be considered [72]. Safe disposal of contaminated material, use of high-efficiency particulate air-filter respirators, and probably prophylaxis with doxycycline are recommended for professionals involved in confirmed or highly suspected *C. burnettii* infection cases [36].

Conclusions. Infections caused by Rickettsiae and related pathogens are prevalent worldwide and new agents are continuously emerging. Morbidity is underestimated as clinical presentations are non-specific and laboratory diagnosis is retrospective. The management of these infections during pregnancy remains challenging and controversial and should be carefully considered on case-by-case basis, in a multidisciplinary approach involving laboratory, epidemiology and infectious diseases specialists. Until further investigation elucidates the natural course of these infections in pregnancy and the relevant efficacy and safety issues, prevention, principally by avoiding ticks and contact to infected animals and their products is of paramount importance.

References

[1] American Academy of Pediatrics. Rickettsial diseases. In: Pickering LK, Baker CJ, Overturf GD, Prober CG, editors. *2006 Red Book: report of the Committee on Infectious Disease*, 26th ed. Elk Grove Village, Illinois: American Academy of Pediatrics, Committee on Infectious Diseases; 2006; 567-572.

[2] Hechemy, K; Oteo JA; Raoult D; Silverman DJ; Blanco JR. A century of rickettsiology: emerging, reemerging rickettsioses, clinical, epidemiological and molecular diagnostic aspects and emerging veterinary rickettsioses. *Ann. NY. Acad. Sci.,* 2006 1078,1-14.

[3] Raoult, D; Fournier, PE; Eremeeva, M; Graves, S; Kelly, PJ; Oteo, JA; Sekeyova, Z; Tamura, A; Tarasevich, I; Ahang, L. Naming of rickettsiae and rickettsial diseases. *Ann. NY Acad. Sci.*, 2005 1063, 1-12.

[4] Kelly, DJ; Richards, AL; Temenak, J; Strickman, D; Dasch, GA. The past and present threat of rickettsial diseases to military medicine and international public health. *Clin. Infect. Dis*, 2002 34(S4), S145-169.

[5] Wu, JJ; Huang, DB; Pang, KR; Tyring, SK. Rickettsial infections around the world, Part 2: rickettsialpox, the typhus group and bioterrorism. *J. Cutan. Med. Surg.*, 2005 19, 105-115.

[6] Madariaga, M; Rezai, K; Trenholme, GM; Weinstein, RA. Q fever: a biological weapon in your backyard. *Lancet Infect Dis*, 2003 3, 709-721.

[7] Pappas, G; Akritidis, N; Tsianos, EV. Attack scenarios with rickettsial species. Implications for response and management. Ann NY Acad Sci, 2005 1063, 451-458.

[8] Stallings, SP. Rocky Mountain spotted fever and pregnancy: a case report and review of the literature. *Obstet Gynecol. Surv.*, 2001 56, 37-42.

[9] Herbert, WN; Seeds, JW; Koontz, WL; Cefalo, RC. Rocky Mountain spotted fever in pregnancy: differential diagnosis and treatment. *South Med. J.*, 1982 75, 1063-1066.

[10] Chapman, AS; Bakken, JS; Folk, SM; Paddock, CD; Bloch, KC; Krusell, A; Sexton, DJ; Buckingham, SC; Marshall, GS; Storch, GA; Dasch, GA; McQuiston, JH; Swerdlow, DL; Dumler, SJ; Nicholson, WL; Walker, DH; Eremeeva, ME; Ohl, CA. Tickborne Rickettsial Diseases Working Group; CDC. Diagnosis and management of tickborne rickettsial diseases: Rocky Mountain spotted fever, ehrlichioses, and anaplasmosis- United States: a practical guide for physicians and other health-care. MMWR Recomm Rep, 2006 55(RR-4), 1-27.

[11] Kim, YS; Lee, HJ; Chang, MY; Son, SK; Rhee, YE; Shim, SK. Scrub typhus during pregnancy and its treatment: a case series and review of the literature. *Am. J. Trop. Med. Hyg,* 2006 75, 955-959.

[12] Muffly, T; McCormick, TC; Cook, C; Wall, J. Human granulocytic ehrlichiosis complicating early pregnancy. *Infect Dis. Obstetr. Gynecol.*, 2008 2008, 359172.

[13] Edwards, MS; Feigin, RD. Rickettsial diseases. In: Feigin RD, Cherry JD, Fletcher J, editors. *Textbook of Pediatric Infectious Diseases*. 4th ed. WB Saunders Co; 1997; 2239-2258.

[14] Parola, P; Paddock, CD; Raoult, D. Tick-borne rickettsioses around the world: emerging diseases challenging old concepts. *Clin. Microbiol. Rev.*, 2005 18, 719-756.

[15] Markley, KC; Levine, AB; Chan, Y. Rocky Mountain spotted fever in pregnancy. *Obstetr. Gynecol.*, 1998 91, 860.

[16] Cohen, J; Lasri, Y; Landau Z. Mediterranean spotted fever in pregnancy. *Scand. J. Infect Dis.*, 1999 31, 202-203.

[17] Bentov, Y; Sheiner, E; Kenigsberg, S; Mazor, M. Mediterranean spotted fever during pregnancy: case presentation and literature review. *Eur. J. Obstetr. Gynecol. Rep. Biol.*, 2003 107, 214-216.

[18] Graves, SR; Banks, J; Dwyer, B; King, GK. A case of murine typhus in Queensland. *Med. J. Aust*, 1992 156, 50-651.

[19] Koliou, M; Christoforou, C; Soteriades, ES. Murine typhus in pregnancy: a case report from Cyprus. *Scand. J. Infect. Dis*, 2007 39, 625-628.

[20] Horowitz HW, Kilchevsky E, Haber S, Aguero-Rosenfeld M, Kranwinkel R, James EK, Wong, SJ; Chu, F; Liveris, D; Schwartz, I. Perinatal transmission of the agent of human granulocytic ehrlichiosis. *New Engl. J. Med.,* 1998 339, 375-378.

[21] Casau, NC; Hewins, ME; Zaleznik, DF. Treatment of human granulocytic ehrlichiosis during pregnancy and risk of perinatal transmission. *Scand. J. Infect Dis*, 2002 34, 853-855.

[22] Buitrago, MI; Ijdo, JW; Rinaudo, P; Simon, H; Copel, J; Gadbaw, J; Heimer, R; Fikrig, E; Bia, FJ. Human granulocytic ehrlichiosis during pregnancy treated successfully with rifampin. *Clin. Infect. Dis*, 1998 27, 213-215.

[23] Dhand, A; Nadelman, RB; Aguero-Rosenfeld, M; Haddad, FA; Stokes, DP; Horowitz, HW. Human granulocytic anaplasmosis during pregnancy: case series and literature review. *Clin. Infect. Dis*, 2007 45, 589-593.

[24] Phupong, V; Srettakraikul, K. Scrub typhus during pregnancy: a case report and review of the literature. Southeast Asian J Trop Med Public Health, 2004 35, 358-360.

[25] Mathai, E; Rollain, JM; Verghese, L; Mathai, M; Jasper, P; Verghese, G; Raoult D. Case reports: scrub typhus during pregnancy in India. Trans R Soc Trop Med Hyg, 2003 97, 570-572.

[26] Suntharasaj, T; Janjindamai, W; Krisanapan, S. Pregnancy with scrub typhus and vertical transmission: a case report. *J. Obstetr. Gynaecol.*, 1997 23, 75-78.

[27] Wang, CL; Yang, KD; Cheng, SN; Chu, ML. Neonatal scrub typhus: a case report. *Pediatrics*, 1992 89, 965-968.

[28] Raoult, D; Fenollar, F; Stein, A. Q fever during pregnancy: diagnosis, treatment, and follow-up. *Arch. Intern. Med.*, 2002 162, 701-704.

[29] Carcopino, X; Raoult, D; Bretelle, F; Boubli, L; Stein, A. Managing Q fever during pregnancy: the benefits of long-term cotrimoxazole therapy. *Clin. Infect Dis.*, 2007 45, 548-555.

[30] Jacobs, WM. Rocky Mountain spotted fever in an infant: Diagnosis in siblings. *Am. J. Dis. Child,* 1978 132, 928-929.

[31] Shirai, A; Chan, TC; Gan, E; Groves, MG. Lack of transplacental infection with scrub typhus organisms in labor mice. *Am. J. Trop Med. Hyg,* 1984 33, 285-287.

[32] Arango-Jaramillo, S; Wisseman, CL Jr; Azad, AF. Newborn rats in the murine typhus enzootic infection cycle: studies on transplacental infection and passively acquired maternal antirickettsial antibodies. *Am. J. Trop. Med. Hyg*, 1988 39, 391-397.

[33] Stein, A; Raoult, D. Q fever during pregnancy: a public health problem in southern France. *Clin. Infect. Dis.*, 1998 27, 592-596.

[34] Richardus, JH; Dumas, AM; Huisman, J; Schaap, GJ. Q fever in infancy: a review of 18 cases. *Pediatr. Infect. Dis.*, 1985 4, 369-373.

[35] Jover-Díaz, F; Robert-Gates, J; Andreu-Gimenez, L; Merino-Sanchez, J. Q fever during pregnancy: an emerging cause of prematurity and abortion. *Infect. Dis. Obstet. Gynecol.*, 2001 9, 47-49.

[36] Ludlam, H; Wreghitt, TG; Thornton, S; Thomson, BJ; Bishop, NJ; Coomber, S; Cunniffe, J. Q fever in pregnancy. *J. Infect.*, 1997 34, 75-78.

[37] Brouqui, P; Parola, P; Fournier, PE; Raoult, D. Spotted fever rickettsioses in Southern Europe. *FEMS Immunol. Med. Microbiol.*, 2007 49, 2-12.

[38] Scott, JS. Connective tissue disease antibodies and pregnancy. *Am. J. Reprod. Immunol.*, 1984 6, 19-24.

[39] Meurman, O; Terho, P; Salmi, A. Activation of rheumatoid factor during pregnancy. *Lancet,* 1978 2, 685-686.

[40] Nandwani, R; Evans, DT. Are you sure it's syphilis? A review of false positive serology. *Int. J. STD AIDS*, 1995 6, 241-248.

[41] Welch, KJ; Rumley, RL; Levine, JA. False-positive results in serologic tests for Rocky Mountain spotted fever during pregnancy. *South Med. J.*, 1991 84, 307-311.

[42] Rolain, JM; Maurin, M; Vestris, G; Raoult, D. In vitro susceptibilities of 27 rickettsiae to 13 antimicrobials. *Antimicrob Agents Chemother*, 1998 42, 1537-1541.

[43] Goodman, JL. Ehrlichiosis-Ticks, Dogs and Doxycycline. *New Engl. J. Med.*, 1999 341, 195-197.

[44] Strickman, D; Sheer, T; Salata, K; Hershley, J; Dasch, G; Kelly, D; Kushner, R. In vitro effectiveness of azithromycin against doxycycline-resistant and –susceptible strains of Rickettsia tsutsugamushi, etiologic agent of scrub typhus. *Antimicrob Agents Chemother,* 1995 39, 2406-2410.

[45] Demers, P; Fraser, D; Goldbloom, RB; Haworth, JC, LaRochelle, J; MacLean, R; Murray, TK. Effects of tetracyclines on skeletal growth and dentition. A report by the Nutrition Committee of the Canadian Paediatric Society. *Can. Med. Assoc. J.*, 1968 99, 849-854.

[46] Johnson, RH; Mitchell, DF. The effects of tetracyclines on teeth and bones. *J. Dent. Res.*, 1966 45, 86-93.

[47] Abramson, JS; Givner, LB. Should tetracycline be contraindicated for therapy of presumed Rocky Mountain spotted fever in children less than 9 years of age? *Pediatrics*, 1990 86, 123-124.

[48] Brennan, RE; Samuel, JE. Evaluation of Coxiella burnetii antibiotic susceptibilities by real-time PCR assay. *J. Clin. Microbiol.*, 2003 41, 1869-1874.

[49] Brouqui, P; Raoult, D. In vitro antibiotic susceptibility of the newly recognized agent of ehrlichiosis in humans, Ehrlichia chaffeensis. *Antimicrob Agents Chemother*, 1992 36, 2799-2803.

[50] Klein, MB; Nelson, CM; Goodman, JL. Antibiotic susceptibility of the newly cultivated agent of human granulocytic ehrlichiosis: promising activity of quinolones and rifamycins. *Antimicrob Agents Chemother*, 1997 41, 76-79.

[51] Balbi, HJ. Chloramphenicol: a review. *Pediatr. Rev.*, 2004 25, 284-288.

[52] Drancourt, M; Raoult, D. In vitro susceptibilities of Rickettsia rickettsii and Rickettsia conorii to roxithromycin and pristinamycin. *Antimicrob Agents Chem.other*, 1989 33, 2146-2148.

[53] Strickman, D; Sheer, T; Salata, K; Hershley, J; Dasch, G; Kelly, D; Kushner, R. In vitro effectiveness of azithromycin against doxycycline-resistant and –susceptible strains of Rickettsia tsutsugamushi, etiologic agent of scrub typhus. *Antimicrob Agents Chemother,* 1995 39, 2406-2410.

[54] Adair, CD; Gunter, M; Stovall, TG; McElroy, G; Veille, JC; Ernest, JM. Chlamydia in pregnancy: a randomized trial of azithromycin and erythromycin. *Obstet. Gynecol.*, 1998 91, 165-168.

[55] Maurin, M; Raoult, D. In vitro susceptibilities of spotted fever group rickettsiae and Coxiella burnetti to clarithromycin. *Antimicrob Agents Chemother*, 1993 37, 2633-2637.

[56] Raoult, D; Roussellier, P; Tamalet, J. In vitro evaluation of josamycin, spiramycin, and erythromycin against Rickettsia rickettsii and R. conorii. *Antimicrob Agents Chemother*, 1988 32, 255-256.

[57] Breitschwerdt, EB; Papich, MG; Hegarty, BC; Gilger, B; Hancock, SI; Davidson, MG. Efficacy of doxycycline, azithromycin, or trovafloxacin for treatment of experimental Rocky Mountain spotted fever in dogs. *Antimicrob Agents Chemother*, 1999 43, 813-821.

[58] Gikas, A; Kofteridis, DP; Manios, A; Pediaditis, J; Tselentis, Y. Newer macrolides as empiric treatment for acute Q fever infection. *Antimicrob Agents Chemother*, 2001 45, 3644-3646.

[59] Parker, NR; Barralet, JH; Bell, AM. Q fever. *Lancet,* 2006 367, 679-688.

[60] Brouqui, P; Raoult, D. In vitro antibiotic susceptibility of the newly recognized agent of ehrlichiosis in humans, Ehrlichia chaffeensis. *Antimicrob Agents Chemother*, 1992 36, 2799-2803.

[61] Klein, MB; Nelson, CM; Goodman, JL. Antibiotic susceptibility of the newly cultivated agent of human granulocytic ehrlichiosis: promising activity of quinolones and rifamycins. *Antimicrob Agents Chemother*, 1997 41, 76-79.

[62] Raoult, D; Drancourt, M; Antimicrobial therapy for rickettsial diseases. *Antimicrob Ag Chemother*, 1991 35, 2457-2462.

[63] Gikas, A; Spyridaki, I; Psaroulaki, A; Kofterithis, D; Tselentis, Y. In vitro susceptibility of Coxiella burnetii to trovafloxacin in comparison with susceptibilities to pefloxacin, ciprofloxacin, ofloxacin, doxycycline, and clarithromycin. *Antimicrob Agents Chemother,* 1998 42, 2747-2748.

[64] Steigman, AJ. Rocky Mountain spotted fever and the avoidance of sulfonamides. *J. Pediatr.*, 1977 91, 163-164.

[65] Ruiz Beltrán, R; Herrero Herrero, JI. Deleterious effect of trimethoprim-sulfamethoxazole in Mediterranean spotted fever. *Antimicrob Agents Chemother*, 1992 36, 1342-1343.

[66] Peters, TR; Edwards, KM; Standaert, SM. Severe ehrlichiosis in an adolescent taking trimethoprim-sulfamethoxazole. *Pediatr. Infect Dis J.*, 2000 19, 170-172.

[67] Brantley, RK. Trimethoprim-sulfamethoxazole and fulminant ehrlichiosis. *Pediatr. Infect.Dis J.*, 2001 20, 231.

[68] Watt, G; Parola, P. Scrub typhus and tropical rickettsioses. *Curr. Opin. Infect. Dis.*, 2003 16, 429-436.

[69] Quintal, D. Historical aspects of the rickettsioses. *Clin. Dermatol.*, 1996 14, 237-242.

[70] Dzelalija, B; Morović, M; Avsic-Zupanc, T. Azithromycin in the prevention of Mediterranean spotted fever. *Lijec Vjesn*, 1997 119, 270-272.

[71] Dzelalija, B; Petrovec, M; Avsic-Zupanc, T; Strugar, J; Milić, TA. Randomized trial of azithromycin in the prophylaxis of Mediterranean spotted fever. *Acta Med. Croatica*, 2002 56, 45-47.

[72] Raoult, D; Stein, A. Q fever during pregnancy- a risk for women, fetuses and obstetricians. *N. Engl. J. Med.*, 1994 330, 371.

In: Infectious Pregnancy Complications
Editor: Richard N. Canfield
ISBN 978-1-60741-038-6

Chapter 13

Infectious Diseases of the Urinary Tract during Pregnancy

Nándor Ács, Ferenc Bánhidy and Andrew E. Czeizel
Second Department of Obstetrics and Gynaecology, Semmelweis University, School of Medicine, Budapest, Hungary
Foundation for the Community Control of Hereditary Diseases, Budapest, Hungary

Abstract

The objective of our studies was to estimate the association between maternal glomerulonephritis / urinary tract infections (UTI) during pregnancy and structural birth defects, i.e. congenital abnormalities or adverse pregnancy outcome. The prevalence of these maternal diseases during the first trimester of pregnancy in cases with different congenital abnormalities was compared to that of matched controls without congenital abnormalities in the population-based Hungarian Case-Control Surveillance System of Congenital Abnormalities. Of 22,843 cases with congenital abnormalities, 309 (1.35%) had mothers with glomerulonephritis during pregnancy, compared to 479 (1.26%) of 38,151 controls (adjusted POR with 95% CI = 1.0, 0.9-1.2). Specified groups of congenital abnormalities were also assessed versus controls. Cases with isolated intestinal atresia/stenosis (adjusted POR with 95% CI: 6.8, 1.3-37.4) based on five cases were more likely to have mothers with prospectively and medically recorded glomerulonephritis. A total of 1542 (6.75%) mothers in the case group had UTI during the entire pregnancy compared with 2188 (5.74%) mothers in the control group (adjusted prevalence odds ratios [POR] with 95% CI: 1.15, 1.06-1.24). We did not find a higher prevalence of UTI during the second and/or third months of pregnancy in total case group (adjusted POR with 95% CI: 1.1, 0.9-1.2) and in any group of CAs including atrial septal defect type II. In conclusion a higher rate of congenital isolated intestinal atresia/stenosis may be associated with maternal glomerulonephritis. However, this finding is considered only as signal and further studies are needed to confirm or reject this possible association. Maternal urinary tract infections during pregnancy increase pre-eclampsia and polyhydramnios, and in addition the rate of preterm birth; however, the latter is preventable by appropriate drug treatments. No evidence was found for the teratogenic effect of maternal UTI and related drug treatments during early pregnancy.

Introduction

Infectious diseases of the urinary tract frequently complicate pregnancy. One the one hand there are striking alterations in renal structure, tubular function and volume homeostasis in pregnancy due to the hemodynamic and hormonal changes. On the other hand the growing uterus of pregnant women has a direct effect on the urinary tract. Finally the neighborhood of urethra and vagina can explain the common occurrence of urogenital infections.

Only the structural changes of the urinary tract will be summarized here [1]. Kidney length increases by 1 cm while kidney volume increases by 30% during pregnancy. These changes in the size and weight of kidneys are caused by an increase in renal vascular and interstitial volume. However, there is a more drastic change in the urinary collection system, because caliceal and ureteral dilation occurs at about 85% of pregnant women. This caliceal dilation is 3 times (15 mm vs. 5 mm) more pronounced on the right side due to dextrorotation of the gravid uterus and the location of the right ovarian vein that crosses the ureter. Thus the physiological hydronephrosis and hydroureter is explained by the compression of the ureters due to enlarging uterus and ovarian vein plexus. The ureteral tone also increases progressively as a result of mechanical obstruction though ureteral peristalsis is not changing in pregnant women.

The above described dilation of the urinary collecting system and urinary stasis are important factors in the increases of ascending urinary tract infections.

Our first aim of to analyze the association between urinary tract infections in pregnant women and other pregnancy complications and adverse pregnancy/birth outcomes, mainly *preterm birth* and structural birth defects, *congenital abnormalities*, the two major factors of infant mortality and handicaps. This review is based mainly on the data set of the Hungarian Case-Control Surveillance of Congenital Abnormalities (HCCSCA) completed with the more important results of others studies [2].

Hungarian Case-Control Surveillance of Congenital Abnormalities

The HCCSCA was established in 1980 and at present it is the largest population-based data set of cases with different CAs and their matched controls in the world.

Cases with congenital abnormality (CA) were identified from the Hungarian Congenital Abnormality Registry (HCAR) [3] for the HCCSCA. Notification of cases with CAs to the HCAR is mandatory for physicians, and most of them are reported by obstetricians (in Hungary practically all deliveries occur in inpatient obstetric clinics, and the birth attendants are obstetricians) and pediatricians (who work in the neonatal units of inpatient obstetric clinics, in addition in various inpatient and outpatient pediatric clinics). Autopsy during the study period was obligatory for all infant deaths, and usually also performed in stillborn fetuses. Pathologists sent a copy of the autopsy report to the HCAR if defects were found in stillborn fetuses or dead infants. Fetal defects diagnosed in antenatal diagnostic centers with or without termination of pregnancy have been included in the HCAR since 1984. Cases with isolated minor anomalies such as hydrocele, sacral dimp and epicanthal folds were recorded but not evaluated at the calculation of rate of different CAs in the HCAR. The recorded total (birth + fetal) prevalence of cases with CA diagnosed from the second trimester of pregnancy to the end of the first postnatal year was 35 per 1000 *informative offspring* (liveborn infants, stillborn fetuses and electively terminated malformed fetuses), and about 90% of major CAs were reported to the HCAR during the study period.

Thus both *birth weight* and *gestational age* at delivery were medically documented in the discharge summary of mothers after delivery. Gestational age was calculated from the first day of the last menstrual period.

The definition of *preterm birth* was less than 37 completed weeks (less than 259 days), while the definition of low birth weight newborns was less than 2,500 gram.

At the evaluation of cases with CA, the so-called isolated CAs (e.g. cleft lip) and multiple-syndromic CAs (e.g. cleft lip with cardiovascular CAs and hypospadias) are differentiated because their severity and etiology differ significantly. 25 groups of isolated CAs are classified according to well-defined diagnostic criteria. Multiple CAs are classified as CA-syndromes and CA-association while the group of unclassified multiple CAs includes unidentified (though previously delineated) and undelineated CA-syndromes and CA-association, in addition random combinations of CAs.

Different CAs have different critical periods [4]. Previously the critical period of CAs was considered during the first 3 months of gestation, i.e. in the first trimester. However, *gestational time* is calculated from the first day of the last menstrual period and it is worth differentiating three time windows: (i) First month of gestation because it is before the organogenesis. The first two weeks are before conception while the third and fourth weeks comprise the pre- and implantation period of zygotes and blastocysts including omnipotent stem cells. Thus CAs cannot be induced by environmental agents in the first month of gestation and it explains the "all-or-nothing effect" rule, i.e. total loss or normal further development. (ii) The most sensitive, the so-called critical period for CAs. (iii) The "postcritical period" of CAs, i.e. pregnancy after the organ-forming period.

These facts explain why the previous use of first trimester concept is misleading, thus outdated [5]. The critical period of most major CAs occurs in the second and third gestational months; we used therefore this time window as the critical period of CAs in our population-based case-control studies [6-8]. However, it is well-known that human teratogens can induce CAs after the third gestational month, i.e. after the first trimester (e.g. cleft palate, hypospadias, undescended testis). This methodological problem encourages us to introduce a new critical time approach based on the specified critical periods of different CAs separately, and our previous study showed that this is feasible [4], but we have to wait for the international consensus [9].

There were three selection criteria of cases with CAs from the HCAR for the HCCSCA: (i) Cases with three mild CAs: congenital dysplasia of the hip based on the Ortolani click, congenital inguinal hernia, large hemangiomas, and (ii) CA-syndromes of Mendelian or chromosomal origin (i.e. due to preconceptional causes) were excluded from the data set of the HCCSCA. (iii) In addition only cases with CAs reported to the HCAR in the first three months after birth or pregnancy termination were selected for the HCCSCA. This shorter time between the end of pregnancy and data collection increases the accuracy of information regarding pregnancy history without undue loss of power, since 77% of cases were reported to the HCAR within this time window.

Controls without CA were selected from the National Birth Registry for the HCCSCA. In general two or three controls were matched to each case on the basis of three criteria: (i) same sex, (ii) same birth week and (iii) same district of parents' residence.

In addition, a *malformed control group* including cases with Down syndrome caused by non-disjunction before conception was also selected from the HCAR to estimate better the recall bias.

Three sources of information were used to obtain exposure data from the mothers of cases, controls and malformed controls:

(i) *Prospective medically recorded data.* The mothers were asked to send us prenatal care logbook and all other medical records (mainly discharge summaries). Prenatal care was mandatory for pregnant women in Hungary (if somebody did not visit prenatal care clinic, she did not receive a maternity grant and leave), thus nearly 100% of pregnant women visited prenatal care clinics, an average 7 times in their pregnancies. The task of obstetricians in the prenatal care is to record all pregnancy complications, maternal diseases and related drug prescriptions in the prenatal care logbook.

(ii) *Retrospective maternal self-reported information.* A structured questionnaire, a list of maternal diseases and drugs as memory aid and informed consent were mailed to the mothers immediately the selection of case, controls and malformed controls. Mother were asked to read the enclosed list of maternal diseases and drugs in order to refresh their memory, after this to complete the structured questionnaire, and to send them back with signed informed consent in our prepaid envelop.

The period between the birth or pregnancy termination and return of information package including questionnaire, antenatal logbook, etc. in our prepaid envelope was 3.5 ± 1.2 and 5.2 ± 2.9 months in cases and controls, respectively.

(iii) *Supplementary information from non-respondent mothers.* Regional nurses were asked to visit all non-respondent case and malformed control mothers, in addition 200 control mothers and to help mother fill-in the same questionnaire, to evaluate available medical records and to obtain lifestyle data through a personal interview [10]. Unfortunately the Ethics Committee did not allow visiting all non-respondent control mothers because – according to their opinion – this visit might disturb these families.

Overall, the necessary information was available in 96.3% (84.4% from reply, 11.9% from visit) of cases and in 83.0% (82.6% from reply, 0.4% from visit) of controls. The antenatal logbooks were available in 88.4% of cases and in 91.8% of controls. Informed consent was signed and returned by 98% of case mothers. The name and address were not recorded in the rest of cases and controls of the HCCSCA.

Most chronic diseases were prospectively and medically recorded mainly in antenatal logbooks. The proportion of medically recorded acute diseases depended on the severity of diseases.

At the evaluation of pregnancy complications and birth outcomes, thus among others, preterm birth we used only controls in the data set of the HCCSCA. Cases with CA were excluded because CAs may have a more drastic effect for the incidence of pregnancy complications and birth outcomes (e.g. rate of preterm birth) than the maternal diseases studied.

The evaluation of possible association of maternal diseases with the higher risk for different CAs was based on the comparison of cases with CA and their matched controls without CA in the data set of the HCCSCA. The diagnosis of CAs is based on the report of medical doctors in the Hungarian Congenital Abnormality Registry, in addition the quality of CA-diagnosis is improved and specified better due to the results of recent medical examination in the HCCSCA. CAs are evaluated in the so-called *informative offspring*: live-born babies, stillborn fetuses and electively terminated pregnancies in the second and/or trimester after the prenatal diagnosis of fetal defect.

Among confounders the possible folic acid and/or multivitamin supplementation in the periconceptional period or in early pregnancy have some preventive effect of some CA, thus we have to consider this recently recognized effect as well [11-15].

We have to consider recall bias at the comparison of cases and controls. The birth of an infant with CA is a serious traumatic event for most mothers who therefore try to find a causal explanation such as diseases or drug uses during pregnancy for CA of their babies. This does not occur after the birth of a healthy newborn infant. Thus recall bias might inflate an increased risk for CAs. Our previous analysis showed that a case-control surveillance of this type may cause a spurious association between drugs and CAs with biased risk (odds ratio) up to a factor of 1.9 [16]. There are three possibilities to restrict or exclude recall bias. (i) The evaluation of exposures only during the critical period of CAs because we expect an underreporting of exposure in both the critical and non-critical periods of CAs in the control group. (ii) The use of prospectively and medically recorded data as a gold standard. (iii) Comparison between cases with CA and malformed control (cases affected with Dow syndrome caused by numerical chromosomal aberration in the preconceptional period) because the mother of malformed controls have similar recall.

The strengths of the HCCSCA is the large and population-based data set from an ethnically homogeneous European (Caucasian) population, most maternal diseases and related drug treatment are prospectively and medically recorded, potential confounders are known, finally there is a good validity of CA diagnoses due to the medically reported CAs to the HCAR, the critical evaluation of the reported CA-diagnoses in the HCAR and the postnatal medical examinations in the HCCSCA.

Here we evaluate the data set of the HCCSCA, 1980-1996 because after 1996 the collection of data has been changed (all mothers are visited at home by regional nurses) but the data have not been validated. Thus our previous publications were based on the data set of 17 years between 1980 and 1986.

Diseases of the Urinary System

At the evaluation of urinary system diseases we followed the International Classification of Diseases (ICD) published by WHO.

Table 1 shows the main category of urinary tract's diseases followed by number and percentage rate of urinary tract's diseases in the data set of the HCCSCA including the mothers of 22,843 cases and 38,151 controls (the data of 834 malformed controls are not shown here).

Non infectious diseases of the urinary tract are excluded from this analysis.

Table l. The name of urinary tract's diseases in the ICD, in addition number and rate (%) of these diseases in the case and control groups in the data set of the HCCSCA

Diseases of the urinary tract	Case group No.	%	Control group No.	%
Acute/chronic glomerulonephritis/nephritis	309	1.35	479	1.26
Nephrotic syndrome	0		0	
Nephropathy, not specified as acute or chronic	0		0	
Acute/chronic/unspecified renal failure	0		0	
Renal sclerosis, unspecified	0		0	
Disorders resulting from impaired function	0		0	
Small kidney of unknown causes	0		0	
Infections of kidney incl. acute pyelonephritis	143	0.63	243	0.64
Hydronephrosis	0		0	
Calculus of kidney and ureter	63	0.30	147	0.39
Other disorders of kidney and ureter (nephroptosis)	1	0.0	0	
Cystitis	149			
Other disorders of bladder	0		0	
Urethritis, not sexually transmitted	0		0	
Urethral stricture	0		0	
Others (vesicoureteric reflux)	0		2	0.01
Asymptomatic true bacteriuria	1,250	5.47	1,767	4.63

Urinary Tract Infections and Congenital Abnormalities

The urinary tract represents one of the most common sites of bacterial infections, particularly in women [17-19]. According to epidemiological studies, 10-15% of the adult female population are affected with urinary tract infection (UTI) at some time during their lives [19]. UTI is one of the most frequently seen complications in pregnant women because pregnancy is considered as a risk factor for UTI [20]. Several previously mentioned changes in the urinary tract predispose to infection during pregnancy mainly from the third month of gestation particularly in primiparae [1]. The above described changes allow bacteria, mainly Escherichia coli, in addition Enterobacter, Klebsiella, Pseudomonas and Proteus in the bladder to ascend to the upper tract. Bacteriuria occuring in about 5% of pregnant women, usually appears during the first trimester and predisposes to the development of acute pyelonephritis, associated with low birth weight and preterm birth [21], though previously published results on UTI and preterm birth/delivery require cautious interpretation due to the statistical methodological problems [22].

No association between UTI and CAs has not been found/published previously [23]. However, as an exception to a rule, Wilson et al. [24] reported in 1998 that UTI was an attributable risk factor (6.4%) in the origin of atrial septal defect.

We therefore decided to check the relative risk of CAs in the offspring of mothers affected with UTI and related drug treatments during pregnancy in the population-based large data set of the HCCSCA.

Methods

Maternal disorders including UTI were evaluated according to the *source of information,* the *severity, time and duration* of maternal diseases during pregnancy. Route (oral, parenteral, topical), dose, and duration of treatments were considered at the evaluation of *drug* administration.

Three diagnoses of UTI were accepted for evaluation:

(i) Urinary tract infection based on the so-called *significant or true bacteriuria* (i.e. more than 10^5 bacteria per ml) diagnosed by quantitative bacterial culture of fresh midstream urine collected after cleaning the urethral region [25-28]. There are two forms of true bacteriuria: (I) Symptomatic UTI and (II) asymptomatic or covert bacteriuria, i.e. without the symptoms of UTI. This laboratory investigation was performed in most pregnant women with any symptoms of genital infections mainly fluor, vaginosis, vulvovaginitis, etc. at the visits of antenatal care.

(ii) *Acute cystitis*, or lower UTI : The inflammation of the bladder produces typical symptoms such as dysuria, urgency, and frequency with or without suprapubic tenderness.

(iii) *Acute pyelonephritis*, or upper UTI. Formerly it was called pyelitis of pregnancy, however, the parenchyma of the kidney is also involved, so now the term pyelonephritis is used [25]. The typical symptoms include fever and flank tenderness/pain with or without accompanying symptoms of cystitis.

Pregnant women with UTI, including true bacteriuria were treated by antimicrobial drugs [25].

The above described three forms of UTI were evaluated in the study if UTI were diagnosed during the study pregnancy. If UTI occurred before the conception of the study pregnancy or the diagnosis was chronic cystitis or pyelonephritis, pregnant women were excluded from this analysis. Of course, pregnant women with other diseases of the urinary tract, such as glomerulonephritis, nephritis, calculus of kidney/ureter, vesicoureteric reflux, etc. were also excluded from the study.

Results

Of 22,843 cases with CA, 1,542 (6.75%). pregnant women were affected with UTI during pregnancy. During the study period, 2,146,574 total births were recorded in Hungary, so 38,151 controls without CAs represented 1.8% of the births and among them 2,188 (5.74%) had mothers with UTI (crude OR with 95% CI = 1.2, 1.1-1.3). The crude OR with 95% CI for the analysis of UTI only in the 2nd and/or 3rd months of pregnancy was 1.2 (1.0-1.4). These UTI rates were calculated on the basis of both medically recorded and maternal self-reported information.

The distribution of different manifestations of UTI is shown in Table 2. The group of mothers with true bacteriuria had a predominance.

Table 2. Prevalence and distribution of different manifestations/diagnoses of urinary tract infections during the study pregnancy

Different groups of urinary tract infections	Case group		Prevalence	Control group		Prevalence
	No.	%	%	No.	%	%
True bacteriuria with symptoms of genital infections	1,250	81.1	5.47	1,767	80.8	4.63
Acute cystitis	149	9.7	0.65	178	8.1	0.47
Acute pyelonephritis	143	9.3	0.63	243	11.1	0.64
Total	1,542	100.0	6.75	2,188	100.0	5.74

Of 1,542 case mothers, 1,277 (82.8%) and of 2,188 control mothers, 1,969 (90.0%) had medically recorded UTI in the prenatal care logbooks and/or discharge summaries. Of 3,023 non-respondent case mothers evaluated after the home visit, 181 (6.0%) had UTI during the study pregnancy and only 12 reported high fever (over 38.5 Celsius degree) due to UTI. Of these 12 pregnant women, 8 had acute pyelonephritis.

The occurrence of UTI according to gestational months depended on the type of UTI. Most true bacteriurias were diagnosed at the first prenatal visit. Most pregnant women with acute cystitis and pyelonephritis were recorded in the third-fourth and seventh gestational month, respectively. However, there was no significant difference in the onset of UTI by the gestational months between the case and control groups.

Basic characteristics of case and control mothers with UTI, in addition case and control mothers without UTI as referent are shown in Table 3. The mean maternal age and mean birth order was somewhat lower in pregnant women with UTI than in pregnant women without UTI due to the higher proportion of young and primiparae. The proportion of unmarried women and the distribution of employment status did not show obvious differences between pregnant women with or without UTI. On the other hand, the mean birth order was higher, the proportion of unmarried women was larger while the proportion of professional, managerial and skilled workers were smaller in case mothers with UTI compared to the control mothers with UTI.

Table 3. Characteristics of pregnant women with urinary tract infections (UTI) and without UTI

Variables	Case mothers				Control mothers				Comparison	
	Without UTI (N = 21,301)		With UTI (N = 1,542)		Without UTI (N = 35,963)		With UTI (N = 2,188)		Between case and control mothers with UTI	
Quantitative	No.	%	No.	%	No.	%	No.	%		
Maternal age (yr)										
24 or less	10,076	47.3	869	56.3	16,775	46.6	1,219	55.7		
25 – 29	6,726	31.6	428	27.8	12,250	34.1	635	29.0	$\chi^2_2 = 0.8$	p = 0.67
30 or more	4,499	21.1	245	15.9	6,938	19.3	334	15.3		
Mean ± S.D.	25.5±5.3		24.4±5.1		25.5±4.9		24.6±4.9		t = 1.0	p = 0.32
Birth order										
1	9,853	46.3	855	55.4	16,951	47.1	1,258	57.5	$\chi^2_1 = 1.5$	p = 0.21
2 or more	11,448	53.7	687	44.6	19,012	52.9	930	42.5		
Mean ± S.D.	1.9±1.1		1.7±1.1		1.7±0.9		1.6±0.9		t = 3.8	p = 0.0002
Categorical										
Unmarried	1,179	5.5	90	5.8	1,401	3.9	70	3.2	$\chi^2_1 = 15.3$	p < 0.0001
Employment status										
Professional	1,793	8.4	108	7.0	4,145	11.5	208	9.5		
Managerial	4,647	21.8	321	20.8	9,598	26.7	536	24.5		
Skilled worker	5,899	27.7	430	27.9	10,978	30.5	712	32.5		
Semiskilled worker	3,585	16.8	284	18.4	5,423	15.1	360	16.5	$\chi^2_6 = 56.2$	p < 0.0001
Unskilled worker	1,377	6.5	126	8.2	1,738	4.8	121	5.5		
Housewife	1,965	9.2	163	10.6	1,900	5.3	138	6.3		
Others	2,035	9.5	110	7.1	2,181	6.1	113	5.2		

Among case and control mothers with UTI, 469 (35.3%) and 537 (29.2%) had no other diseases during the study pregnancy, respectively. The prevalence of other acute and chronic maternal diseases was similar between case and control mothers with UTI with extremely high proportion (over 90%) of mild infectious diseases of genital organs (vulvoivaginitis, vaginosis, etc.). However, the prevalence of kidney stones (0.27% vs. 0.75%, OR with 95% CI: 2.8, 1.9-4.2) occurred more frequently in the combined case + control pregnant women with UTI than in pregnant women without UTI.

Among frequently used drugs, urinary tract antiseptics (nitrofurantoin, nalidixic acid), antimicrobial drugs (ampicillin,, cefalexin, sulfamethoxazole + trimethoprim) and drugs for genital infectious diseases (clotrimazole, metronidazole) showed a higher frequency in case and control mothers with UTI compared with pregnant women without UTI. However, the use of these three drugs did not show significant difference between case and control mothers with UTI in the second and/or third gestational months.

The use of folic acid supplementation was somewhat lower in case mothers (49.0%) than control mothers (53.6%) with UTI (OR with 95% CI: 0.8, 0.7-0.9). A similar pattern was found at the use of folic acid during the periconceptional period (i.e. first and second gestational month).

Cases with different CA-groups were compared with their matched controls according to the prevalence of UTI during the second and/or third months of pregnancy, i.e. in the critical period of most major CAs (Table 4). There was no CA group with a higher occurrence of UTI in pregnant women. This finding was confirmed at the evaluation of only medically recorded UTI cases as well (data not shown).

Table 4. Matched analysis to estimate the association between maternal urinary tract infections during the second and/or third months of pregnancy and congenital abnormalities

Study groups	Grand total	Second and/or third months of gestation			
	N	N	%	Crude OR(95%CI)	Adjusted OR(95%CI)*
Isolated CAs					
Neural-tube defects	1,202	24	2.0	1.2 (0.5 - 3.1)	1.1 (0.4 - 3.0)
Cleft lip± palate	1,374	31	2.3	1.7 (0.8 - 3.9)	1.7 (0.7 - 4.3)
Cleft palate only	582	10	1.7	0.9 (0.3 - 3.1)	0.5 (0.1 - 2.3)
Esophageal atresia/stenosis	217	2	0.9	0.6 (0.1 - 7.7)	0.5 (0.0 - 8.3)
Congenital pyloric stenosis	241	4	1.7	1.8 (0.2 - 19.8)	2.4 (0.1 - 39.5)
Intestinal atresia/stenosis	153	2	1.3	0.5 (0.0 - 6.7)	0.8 (0.0 - 14.4)
Rectal/anal atresia/stenosis	220	6	2.7	1.9 (0.3 - 12.9)	1.8 (0.2 - 16.9)
Renal a/dysgenesis	104	1	1.0	0.9 (0.0 - 42.3)	0.8 (0.0 - 58.7)
Obstructive urinary CAs	271	7	2.6	2.5 (0.3 - 18.1)	3.4 (0.4 - 33.6)
Hypospadias	3,038	48	1.6	1.2 (0.6 - 2.1)	1.2 (0.6 - 2.3)
Undescended testis	2,051	25	1.2	0.7 (0.3 - 1.6)	0.6 (0.3 - 1.5)
Exomphalos/gastroschisis	238	6	2.5	1.6 (0.3 - 9.7)	1.0 (0.1 - 8.4)
Microcephaly, primary	109	3	2.8	7.2 (0.2 - 270.9)	2.9 (0.1 - 142.9)
Congenital hydrocephaly	314	6	1.9	2.9 (0.3 - 27.7)	3.0 (0.2 - 39.1)
Eye CAs	99	1	1.0	0.3 (0.0 - 10.4)	0.2 (0.0 - 39.6)
Ear CAs	354	2	0.6	0.5 (0.0 - 5.9)	0.4 (0.0 - 5.9)
Cardiovascular CAs	4,479	61	1.4	1.1 (0.6 - 1.8)	0.9 (0.5 - 1.6)
CAs of genital organs	123	1	0.8	0.9 (0.0 - 42.3)	0.7 (0.0 - 52.5)
Clubfoot	2,424	39	1.6	1.1 (0.6 - 2.1)	0.9 (0.4 - 1.9)
Limb deficiencies	548	11	2.0	2.8 (0.6 - 12.8)	2.5 (0.5 - 13.8)
Poly/syndactyly	1,744	31	1.8	1.5 (0.7 - 3.3)	1.2 (0.5 - 2.9)
CAs of skeletal system	211	1	0.5	0.5 (0.0 - 18.7)	0.4 (0.0 - 15.5)
Diaphragmatic CAs	243	5	2.1	2.3 (0.3 - 18.5)	2.8 (0.2 - 38.5)
Other isolated CAs	1,155	15	1.3	1.2 (0.4 - 3.6)	1.1 (0.3 - 3.4)
Multiple CAs	1,349	21	1.6	1.2 (0.5 - 2.8)	1.2 (0.4 - 3.2)
Total cases	22,843	363	1.6	1.2 (1.0 - 1.4)	1.1 (0.9 - 1.2)
Total controls	38,151	514	1.4	-	

* Matched OR adjusted for maternal employment status and use of drugs for the treatment of UTI in the second and/or third months of pregnancy in conditional logistis regression model.

We compared the expected number of different subgroups of cardiovascular CAs based on the data set of the HCCSCA and observed number of cases with different cardiovascular CAs in the newborn infants born to mothers with UTI during the second and/or third month of gestation; however, we did not find any difference.

Finally, the different manifestations of UTI were evaluated separately with the possible association with CAs, however, there was no severity dependant effect of UTI.

Urinary Tract Infections in Pregnant Women and Pregnancy Complications, in Addition Pregnancy/Birth Outcomes

Previously an association between urinary tract infections (UTI) including significant bacteriuria and preterm birth/low birthweight was shown in several studies [21, 28, 19]. On the other hand kidney diseases in pregnant women are frequently associated with pregnancy complications [25].

The control data set (i.e. newborn infants without congenital abnormalities) of the Hungarian Case-Control Surveillance of Congenital Abnormalities (HCCSCA) [2] is appropriate to check the possible effect of UTI during pregnancy on pregnancy complications and birth outcomes particularly gestational age and birth weight, in addition preterm birth and low birthweight in the mirror of recent medical treatments of UTI.

Methods

Newborn infants without congenital abnormalities were selected from the National Birth Registry of the Central Statistical Office for the HCCSCA. These newborns were controls of cases with congenital abnormality who were identified from the Hungarian Congenital Abnormality Registry [3] for the HCCSCA. In general, two controls were matching individually to each case according to sex, week of birth and district of parents' residence of cases. If selected newborn controls were twins, only one of them was randomly included to the data set of the HCCSCA.

Immediately after the selection of newborns a letter was sent to the mothers explaining the purpose of the HCCSCA, the benefit of this public health activity for them and in general for the prevention of birth defects. Mothers were asked to send us their prenatal care logbook and every other medical record regarding their diseases and pregnancy complications during the study pregnancy for three weeks. In addition together with the above letter, a structured questionnaire with a list of medicines (drugs and pregnancy supplements) and diseases was also mailed to the mothers. The questionnaire requested information on, among other things, maternal personal (e.g. employment status) and medical (e.g. history of previous pregnancies) data, pregnancy complications, maternal diseases and medicine intakes during the study pregnancy according to gestational month. In order to standardize the answers, mothers were asked to read the enclosed lists of medicinal products and diseases (e.g. UTI) as a memory aid before they replied.

Thus exposure and other data regarding mothers were obtained prospectively through prenatal care logbooks and other medical records, and retrospectively by the questionnaire completed by mothers as previously described. If pregnant women showed the symptoms of genital infections (fluor, vaginosis, vaginitis without the symptoms of UTI such as dysuria, urgency and frequency with or without suprapubic tenderness, a quantitative bacterial culture was performed in the so-called fresh midstream urine collected after the cleaning of urethral region to estimate the types and number of bacteria and to diagnose the so-called true bacteriuria (more than 10^5 bacteria per one ml) or other types of UTI. If pregnant women complained on the symptoms of UTI, or diagnosed at the examination in the prenatal care clinics, UTI were differentiated into three groups: acute cystitis, cystopyelitis and pyelonephritis. All pregnant women who had UTI before the study pregnancy but they had no symptoms of UTI during the study pregnancy were excluded.

Pregnancy complications were recorded in the prenatal care logbook. Both *birth weight* and *gestational age* were medically recorded in the discharge summary of mothers connected with their delivery. Gestational age was calculated from the first day of the last menstrual period. The definition of preterm birth was less than 37 completed weeks (less than 259 days), while of low birth weight (less than 2500 g).

The interval between the end of pregnancy and return of the "information package" including prenatal logbook, questionnaire, etc. was 5.2 $\pm$ 2.9 months. In addition, 200 non-respondent mothers were visited and questioned at home [10] as part of a validation study. The main objective of the validation study was to check the exposure (drugs, diseases, etc.) data of non-respondent mothers in a home visit. There was no difference in the distribution and occurrence of frequently used drugs and diseases (e.g. UTI) between respondent and non-respondent mothers. Finally, the necessary information was obtained on 83.0% of mothers (82.6% from reply, 0.4% from visit). Prenatal care logbook was available in 93.8% of these mothers.

Results

The number of births was 2,146,574 during the study period. Thus 38,151 births in our study group represented 1.8% of Hungarian births during the study period. Of the 38,151 newborn infants, 2,188 (5.7%) had mothers with UTI during the study pregnancy and these pregnant women were differentiated into four groups: (i) true bacteriuria (N: 1,767) with symptoms of genital infections but without the symptoms of UTI. The main purpose of "true bacteriuria" examination was the identification and quantification of bacteria, mainly E.coli, Enterobacter, Klebsiella, Pseudomonas and Proteus agents in the urine in order to give appropriate treatment. (ii) Acute cystitis (N: 178), the diagnosis was based on the symptoms of inflammation of bladder such as dysuria, urgency and frequency with or without suprapubic tenderness. (iii-iv) Acute cystopyelitis (N: 171) and acute pyelonephritis (N: 72) based on the typical symptoms such as flank tenderness with or without symptoms of cystitis and fever. Several pregnant women showed a progression in the above groups of UTI, the most severe diagnosis was accepted at the evaluation.

Of 2,188 mothers, 1,969 (90.0%) had prospectively and medically recorded UTI in prenatal care logbooks and about 95% of these UTI were reported by mothers as well. Finally we evaluated medically recorded and maternal reported UTI together.

The basic characteristics of mothers with and without UTI (as referent) were shown previously in Table 3. Mother with UTI was younger with lower mean birth order due to the higher proportion of young (24 years or less) and primiparae. There was no obvious difference in the proportion of unmarried mothers between the two study groups. Maternal employment status showed some differences between mothers with or without UTI, because UTI were less frequent among professionals and managerials, while more frequent in other groups (except "others"). In Hungary most housewives belong to the lower socioeconomic class.

In general true bacteriuria was diagnosed after the first visit in the prenatal care, while acute cystopyelitis and acute pyelonephritis were diagnosed most frequently in the fourth and seventh gestational month, respectively. Of 2,188 pregnant women with UTI, 537 (29.2%) had no other diseases during the study pregnancy. The occurrences of other acute infectious maternal diseases are shown in Table 5.

Table 5. Other acute and chronic diseases in pregnant women with or without urinary tract infections (UTI)

Maternal diseases	Pregnant women				Comparison	
	without UTI (N = 35,963)		with UTI (N = 2,188)			
	No.	%	No.	%	OR	95% CI
Acute						
Influenza - common cold	6,651	18.5	410	18.7	1.0	0.9 - 1.1
Respiratory system	3,250	9.0	205	9.4	1.0	0.9 - 1.2
Digestive system	868	2.4	71	3.2	1.4	1.1 - 1.7
Urinary tract	113	0.3	20	0.9	2.9	1.8 - 4.7
Genital organs*	2,680	7.5	211	9.6	1.3	1.1 - 1.5
Others	488	1.4	24	1.1	0.8	0.5 - 1.2
Chronic						
Diabetes mellitus	44	0.1	8	0.4	2.4	1.3 - 4.4
Epilepsy	74	0.2	3	0.1	0.7	0.2 - 2.1
Others	5,603	15.6	334	15.3	1.0	0.9 - 1.1

* Without fluor, vaginosis and vulvovaginitis because these patients were included into the group of significant bacteriuria.

Threw acute diseases showed some difference between mothers with or without UTI. A higher occurrence of urinary tract particularly kidney stones, acute infections of digestive system and genital organs (without fluor, vaginosis and vulvovaginitis) was found in mothers with UTI. Among chronic maternal diseases insulin dependent diabetes mellitus was more frequent in mothers with UTI.

One of the main objectives of the study was the evaluation of pregnancy complications in pregnant women with UTI (Table 6). Three pregnancy complications: polyhydramnios, pre-eclampsia and anemia were more frequent in mothers with UTI than in mothers without UTI.

The most frequently used drugs were also evaluated. Obviously among antimicrobial drugs (ampicillin, cefalexin, cotrimoxazole), the so-called urinary tract antiseptics such as nitrofurantoin and nalidixic acid had a much more frequent use in mothers with UTI than in pregnant women without UTI. Pregnancy supplements including folic acid and multivitamins did not show an obvious difference between mothers with or without UTI.

Table 6. Prevalence of pregnancy complications in pregnant women with or without UTI

Pregnancy complications	Pregnant women				Comparison	
	without UTI (N = 35,963)		with UTI (N = 2,188)			
	No.	%	No.	%	OR	95% CI
Threatened abortion	6,124	17.0	388	17.7	1.1	0.9 - 1.2
Placental disorders*	559	1.6	33	1.5	1.0	0.7 - 1.4
Preeclampsia, eclampsia**	2,988	8.3	233	10.7	1.3	1.1 - 1.5
Nausea, vomiting (severe)	3,642	10.1	227	10.4	1.0	0.9 - 1.2
Threatened preterm delivery***	5,161	14.4	299	13.7	0.9	0.8 - 1.1
Polyhydramios	170	0.5	21	1.0	2.0	1.3 - 3.2
Olygohydramios	13	0.0	1	0.1	1.3	0.2 - 9.7
Prolonged pregnancy	482	1.3	26	1.2	0.9	0.6 - 1.3
Gestational diabetes	255	0.7	15	0.7	1.0	0.6 - 1.6
Anemia	5,946	16.5	410	18.7	1.2	1.0 - 1.3

* including placenta previa, premature separation of placenta, antepartum hemorrhage.
** including pregnancy hypertension, oedema and albuminuria.
*** including cervical incompetence.

Table 7. Main birth outcomes of 2,188 newborn infants born to mothers with urinary tract infections (UTI) and 35,963 newborn infants born to mothers without UTI

Quantitative	UTI group Mean S.D		No UTI group Mean S.D.		Adjusted t p	
Gestational age* (wk), boy	39.4	2.1	39.4	2.0	1.2	0.23
Girl	39.1	2.2	39.3	2.1	1.8	0.07
Total	39.3	2.2	39.4	2.0	2.1	0.04
Birth weight** (g), boy	3,304	514	3,325	514	1.7	0.08
Girl	3,154	497	3,189	494	1.6	0.11
Total	3,251	513	3,278	511	2.4	0.02
Categorical	No.	%	No.	%	Adjusted OR with 95% CI	
Preterm birth*, boy	136	9.6	1,933	8.3	1.2	0.9 – 1.4
Girl	92	11.8	1,335	10.6	1.1	0.9 – 1.4
Total	228	10.4	3,268	9.1	1.2	1.0 – 1.3
Low birthweight**, boy	82	5.8	1,156	4.9	1.1	0.9 – 1.4
Girl	64	8.2	865	6.9	1.1	0.9 – 1.5
Total	146	6.7	2,021	5.6	1.1	0.9 – 1.4

*adjusted for maternal employment status and use of pregnancy supplements during pregnancy.
**adjusted for maternal employment status, use of pregnancy supplements during pregnancy and gestational age.

Of 2,188 newborn infants born to mothers with UTI during pregnancy, 1,408 (64.35%) were boys, while the proportion of boys was 65.04% (23,391/35,963) among newborn infants of mothers without UTI during the study pregnancy. The higher proportion of boys among newborns is explained by one of the matching criteria: sex to cases with congenital abnormalities, because there is an obvious male excess among malformed cases due to the common defects of male genital organs, such as undescended testis and hypospadias.

Another main objective of the study was the analysis of birth outcomes (Table 7).

The figures of no UTI group correspond well to the Hungarian newborn population in the study period. The mean gestational age was somewhat shorter in newborn infants born to mothers with UTI compared to mothers without UTI as a reference group due to the subgroup of girls. The mean birth weight was slightly smaller in the babies of mothers with UTI. However, this statistical significant difference was caused by 0.1 week and 27 gram which are clinically not significant. The proportion of preterm births (10.4% vs. 9.1%) was larger in the group of mothers with UTI but the similar trend in the proportion of low birthweight (6.7% vs 5.6%) did not reach the level of significance.

We studied the possible correlation between severity of UTI including cystitis, cystopyelitis, pyelonephritis and mean gestational age and birth weight (Table 8).

Table 8. Major variables of birth outcomes according to the different group (severity) of UTI

Different group of UTI	No	%	Gestational age (wk)		Preterm birth		Birth weight (g)		Low birthweight	
			Mean	S.D.	No.	%	Mean	S.D.	No.	%
True bacteriuria with symptoms of genital infection	1,767	80.8	39.3	2.2	190	10.8	3250	509	115	6.5
Acute cystitis	178	8.1	39.4	2.0	14	7.9	3302	558	11	6.2
Acute cystopyelitis	171	7.8	39.2	2.0	16	9.4	3237	506	13	7.6
Acute pyelonephritis	72	3.3	39.1	2.1	9	12.5	3141	520	8	11.1
Total	2,188	100.0	39.3	2.2	228	10.4	3251	513	146	6.7

There was an obvious severity-effect association in the proportion of preterm birth and low birthweight. The exception is true bacteriuria which was connected with genital infections of pregnant women, with a high rate of preterm birth but a low rate of low birthweight. Thus preterm birth inducing effect of true bacteriuria associates with the infections of genital organs in our study.

Finally, we evaluated the preterm preventive effect of different drugs in mothers with UTI (Table 9).

Antimicrobial drugs such as ampicillin, cefalexin and cotrimoxazole seemed to be very effective in the prevention of preterm birth in mothers with UTI, while the so-called urinary tract antiseptics such as nitrofurantoin and nalidixic acid did not show any preventive effect. It is worth mentioning that pregnant women with UTI and appropriate antimicrobial treatment had a lower rate of preterm birth (7.4%) than the high preterm rate of the Hungarian pregnant population (9.1%) during the study period.

Table 9. Rate of preterm birth (%) in newborn infants born to mothers with different manifestation of urinary tract infecions and with or without antimicrobial drugs such as ampicillin, cefalexin and cotrimoxazole or urinary tract antiseptics such as nitrofurantoin and nalidixic acid treatment

Urinary tract infections	N.	Ampicillin, cefalexin, cotrimoxazole No Yes Preterm birth Preterm birth N. No. % N. No. %						Comparison POR** 95% CI		Nitrofurantoin-Nalidixic acid No Yes* Preterm birth Preterm birth N. No. % N. No. %						Comparison POR** 95% CI	
True bacteriuria	1,767	948	128	13.5	819	62	7.6	1.9	0.9 - 2.6	1,075	102	9.5	692	88	12.7	0.7	0.5 – 0.9
Cystitis	178	97	10	10.3	81	4	4.9	2.2	0.7 – 7.3	143	9	6.3	45	5	11.1	0.6	0.2 – 1.8
Cystopyelitis-pyelonephritis	243	154	17	11.0	98	8	8.2	1.4	0.6 – 3.4	144	16	11.1	108	9	8.3	1.4	0.6 – 4.3
Together	2,188	1,199	155	12.9	998	74	7.4	1.8	0.9 – 2.5	1,362	127	9.3	845	102	12.1	0.8	0.6 – 1.0

* without ampicillin, cefalexin and clotrimazole treatment.

** adjusted for maternal age, birth order, employment status, other maternal diseases and drug treatments.

Glomerulonephritis in Pregnant Women and CA in Their Offspring

Certain diseases of the urinary tract including kidney may cause a complication of pregnancy or a condition peculiar to it or may be only a concomitant disease [42, 43, 33, 25]. Thus the diseases of kidney belong to the common pathological conditions of pregnant women; and the objective of our project is to perform a systematic analysis regarding the possible association between all maternal kidney diseases and structural birth defects, i.e. congenital abnormalities (CAs).

Aim

The topic of glomerulonephritis [GN] and pregnancy was evaluated and discussed several times [e.g. 44], however, we did not find any publications regarding the possible association between GN and CAs [23], though all aspects of GN were discussed in the literature [45]. Acute poststreptococcal GN is a very rare complication of pregnancy, and if it occurs late in pregnancy, it can be mistaken for preeclampsia [25]. In general the term GN encompasses a range of immune-mediated disorders that cause inflammation within glomerules and other compartments of the kidney [46]. With chronic GN, one view warms of aggravation because of the hypercoagulable state accompanying pregnancy, with patients more prone to superimposed preeclampsia or hypertensive crises earlier in pregnancy. [25].

The data set of the Hungarian Case-Control Surveillance of Congenital Abnormalities (HCCSCA) [2] is appropriate for the study of possible association between GN and CAs.

Method

The protocol of the HCCSCA was presented previously.

Pregnant women were recorded and/or reported with different kidney diseases, however, we evaluated only mothers with GN and/or nephritis with the onset before the study pregnancy, in general for 3 or more months [46]. Pregnant women who had essential hypertension, infections of urinary tract, nephrolithiasis, lupus nephropathy, acute and chronic renal failure, renal sclerosis, renal osteodystrophy, nephronoptosis, cystic kidney diseases, gestational proteinuria and microscopic hematuria [47] and in general kidney diseases with the onset during the study pregnancy in the HCCSCA were excluded from this analysis.

Related *drug treatments and pregnancy supplements* were also evaluated. The latter may indicate the level of pregnancy care, and indirectly may show the socio-economic status and the motivation of mothers to prepare and/or to achieve a healthy baby. In addition it is necessary to consider folic acid and folic acid-containing multivitamins in the evaluation of preventable CAs [11-15]. Other *potential confounding factors* included maternal age, birth order, marital and employment status as indicators of socio-economic status, and influenza with high fever.

Results

The case group consisted of 22,843 malformed newborns or fetuses ("informative offspring"), of whom 309 (1.35%) had mothers with GN. The total number of births in Hungary was 2,146,574 during the study period between 1980 and 1996. Thus the 38,151 controls represented 1.8% of all Hungarian births, and among those controls, 479 (1.26%) were born to mothers with GN (crude OR with 95% CI: 1.1, 0.9-1.3).

Of 309 case and 479 control mothers, 243 (78.6%) and 373 (77.9%) had medically recorded GN in the prenatal logbooks (p = 0.80). Four case and six control mothers with GN were hospitalized during the study pregnancy. The onset of GN was after the first trimester of pregnancy in 5 case and 4 control mothers, they were excluded from this analysis. Thus, all pregnant women had GN with onset before the conception of the study pregnancy and lasted during the first trimester.

Table 10 summarizes the characteristics of mothers with GN and without GN, as reference.

Table 10. Characteristics of mothers with or without glomerulonephritis (GN) during pregnancy

Maternal variables	Case mothers without GN (N = 22,534)		Case mothers with GN (N = 309)		Control mothers without GN (N = 37,672)		Control mothers with GN (N = 479)		Comparison between case and control mothers with GN	
	No.	%	No.	%	No.	%	No.	%		
Quantitative										
Maternal age (yr)										
24 or less	10,752	47.7	193	62.5	17,710	47.0	284	59.3		
25 – 29	7,082	31.4	72	23.3	12,753	33.9	132	27.6	$\chi^2_2 = 1.8$	p = 0.41
30 or more	4,700	20.9	44	14.2	7,209	19.1	63	13.2		
Mean ± S.D.	25.5±5.3		23.8±5.0		25.5±4.9		24.2±4.6		t = 1.1	p = 0.26
Birth order										
1	10,526	46.7	182	58.9	17,909	47.5	300	62.6	$\chi^2_1 = 1.1$	p = 0.29
2 or more	12,008	53.3	127	41.1	19,763	52.5	179	37.4		
Mean ± S.D.	1.9±1.1		1.7±1.4		1.7±0.9		1.5±0.8		t = 2.8	p = 0.005
Categorical										
Unmarried	1,254	5.6	15	4.9	1,448	3.8	23	4.8	$\chi^2_1 = 0.001$	p = 0.97
Employment status										
Professional	1,877	8.3	24	7.8	4,313	11.5	40	8.4		
Managerial	4,897	21.7	71	23.0	10,010	26.6	124	25.9		
Skilled worker	6,260	27.8	69	22.3	11,530	30.6	160	33.4		
Semiskilled worker	3,805	16.9	64	20.7	5,698	15.1	85	17.8	$\chi^2_6 = 32.1$	p < 0.0001
Unskilled worker	1,486	6.6	17	5.5	1,832	4.9	27	5.6		
Housewife	2,076	9.2	52	16.8	2,010	5.3	28	5.9		
Others	2,133	9.5	12	3.9	2,279	6.1	15	3.1		

This comparison indicates a lower mean maternal age and birth order due to the higher proportion of younger primiparae in the GN groups. The distribution of employment status did not show obvious difference between pregnant women with or without GN. However, case and control mothers with GN showed some difference in mean birth order and the distribution of maternal employment status. Case mothers with GN had a lower socioeconomic status than control mothers with GN. It is worth mentioning the high proportion of housewives among case mothers particularly affected with GN. In general housewives belong to the lower social classes in Hungary.

The prevalence of pregnancy complications is shown in Table 11.

The prevalence of preeclampsia (9.9% vs. 7.3%; OR with 95% CI: 1.4, 1.1-1.8) and anemia (28.8% vs. 15.6%; OR with 95% CI: 2.2, 1.9-2.6) was higher in mothers with GN than in mothers without GN. However, case and control mothers with GN did not show significant difference with one exception. The latter was the lower occurrence of threatened preterm delivery in the case mothers with GN.

Of 309 case and 479 control mothers with GN, 96 (31.1%) and 128 (26.7%) had no other diseases during the study pregnancy, respectively. Among other acute maternal diseases, only the prevalence of infections in the urinary tract (93, 11.8% vs. 3,637, 6.0%, OR with 95% CI: 2.1, 1.7-2.6) and genital organs (75, 9.5% vs. 4,489, 7.5%, OR with 95% CI: 1.3, 1.0-1.7) was higher in pregnant women with GN than in pregnant women without GN. However, acute maternal diseases did not show difference between the case and control mothers with GN. The prevalence of chronic maternal diseases (such as diabetes mellitus, epilepsy) was similar in the study groups.

There was no difference in the distribution and frequency of drugs used by case and control mothers with GN.

Among pregnancy supplements the use of folic acid (47.6% vs. 51.6%) and multivitamins (3.9% vs. 4.6%) was less frequent in case mothers with GN than by pregnant women without GN but these differences were not significant.

The evaluation of cases with different CAs and their *all matched controls* is summarized in Table 12.

Table 11. Prevalence of pregnancy complications in mothers with or without GN

Pregnancy complications	Case mothers				Control mothers				Comparison	
	without (N = 22,534)		with GN (N = 309)		without (N = 37,672)		withGN (N = 479)		of case and control mothers with GN	
	No.	%	No.	%	No.	%	No.	%	POR	95% CI
Threatened abortion	3,463	15.4	38	12.3	6,438	17.1	74	15.5	0.8	0.5 – 1.2
Placental disorders*	28.3	1.3	1	0.3	583	1.6	9	1.9	0.2	0.0 – 1.3
Preeclampsia, eclampsia**	1,519	6.7	30	9.7	2,863	7.6	48	10.0	1.0	0.6 – 1.6
Nausea, vomiting (excessive)	1,721	7.6	25	8.1	3,827	10.2	42	8.8	0.9	0.5 – 1.5
Threatened preterm delivery***	2,605	11.6	29	9.4	5,387	14.3	73	15.2	0.6	0.4 – 0.9
Polyhydramnios	209	0.9	3	1.0	189	0.5	2	0.4	2.3	0.4 – 14.1
Olygohydramnios	32	0.1	1	0.3	14	0.0	0	0.0	-	-
Gestational diabetes	140	0.6	2	0.7	266	0.7	4	0.8	0.8	0.1 – 4.2
Anemia	3,159	14.0	81	26.2	6,210	16.5	146	30.5	0.8	0.6 – 1.1

* including placenta previa, premature separation of placenta, antepartum hemorrhage.

** including pregnancy hypertension, oedema and albuminuria.

*** including cervical incompetence.

Table 12. Results of conditional logistic regression analysis of cases and all matched controls to estimate the association between GN and different congenital abnormalities (CAs)

Study groups	Grand total	GN		
	N	No.	%	Adjusted OR(95%CI)*
Isolated CAs				
Neural-tube defects	1,202	17	1.4	0.6 (0.3 - 1.0)
Cleft lip± palate	1,374	14	1.0	0.9 (0.5 - 1.9)
Cleft palate only	582	10	1.7	2.2 (0.8 - 5.8)
Esophageal atresia/stenosis	217	3	1.4	3.3 (0.3 - 34.7)
Congenital pyloric stenosis	241	4	1.7	1.4 (0.4 - 5.6)
Intestinal atresia/stenosis	153	5	3.3	6.8 (1.3 - 37.4)
Rectal/anal atresia/stenosis	220	2	0.9	-
Renal a/dysgenesis	104	2	1.9	2.8 (0.2 - 36.2)
Obstructive urinary CAs	271	2	0.7	0.6 (0.1 - 4.0)
Hypospadias	3,038	32	1.1	0.7 (0.5 - 1.2)
Undescended testis	2,051	32	1.6	1.3 (0.8 - 2.1)
Exomphalos/gastroschisis	238	4	1.7	0.7 (0.2 - 2.4)
Microcephaly, primary	109	3	2.8	0.9 (0.2 - 4.4)
Congenital hydrocephaly	314	8	2.5	1.8 (0.6 - 5.5)
Ear CAs	354	7	2.0	0.7 (0.2 - 1.8)
Cardiovascular CAs	4,479	50	1.1	1.0 (0.6 - 1.4)
CAs of genital organs	123	3	2.4	0.9 (0.2 - 5.0)
Clubfoot	2,424	34	1.4	1.0 (0.6 - 1.6)
Limb deficiencies	548	11	2.0	1.7 (0.7 - 4.6)
Poly/syndactyly	1,744	22	1.3	0.8 (0.4 - 1.4)
Diaphragmatic CAs	243	6	2.5	6.5 (0.8 - 55.4)
Other isolated CAs	1,465	18	1.2	1.2 (0.6 – 2.2)
Multiple CAs	1,349	20	1.5	1.2 (0.7 - 2.3)
Total cases	22,843	309	1.4	1.0 (0.9 - 1.2)
Total controls	38,151	479	1.3	-

* Matched POR adjusted for maternal employment status and use of antimicrobial drugs any time during pregnancy in conditional logistic regression model.

Bold numbers show significant association.

A higher prevalence of GN in pregnant women associated with a higher risk for one CA-group: isolated intestinal atresia/stenosis. There was no positive family history in these 5 cases with isolated intestinal atresia/stenosis and GN was medically recorded in the prenatal logbook of these 5 case mothers.

The group of multiple CA included 20 cases but multimalformed offspring did not have intestinal atresia/stenosis.

Finally, we evaluated the birth outcomes of controls born to mothers with or without GN (Table 13). (Cases were excluded from this analysis because CAs may have a more drastic effect for birth weight and gestational age than GN itself).

There was a shorter mean gestational age and a higher rate of preterm birth of controls born to mothers with GN but these differences were not reflected in mean birth weight and proportion of low birthweight.

Table 13. Mean gestational age at delivery and birth weight, in addition rate of preterm births and low birthweight newborns without CA born to mothers with or without GN

Birth outcomes	Control infants without CA born to mothers with GN without GN (N=479) (N=37,672)				Comparison	
Quantitative variables	Mean	S.D.	Mean	S.D.	Adjusted t	p=
Gestational age, wk	39.1	2.2	39.4	2.0	**2.7**	**0.007***
Birth weight, g	3,252	477	3,276	512	0.6	0.53**
Categorical variables	No.	%	No.	%	Adjusted OR with 95% CI	
Preterm birth	71	14.8	3,425	9.1	**1.7**	**1.3 – 2.2***
Low birthweight	29	6.0	2,138	5.7	0.8	0.5 – 1.1**

* adjusted for maternal employment status and use of pregnancy supplements during pregnancy.
** adjusted for maternal employment status, use of pregnancy supplements and for gestational age.
Bold numbers show significant associations.

Interpretation of the Results of Our Study and Other Investigations

Urinary Tract Infections and Congenital Abnormalities

Some specific infections caused by rubella, varicella zoster, parvo-viruses, cytomegaloviruses, T. pallidum, Toxoplasma gondii, etc. during pregnancy have been associated with CAs. However, while the effects of the above mentioned microbial agents during pregnancy are well-known, the possible association of some common infections such as UTI with CAs was rarely studied. An improved understanding of the adverse effects of infections during pregnancy is important for the care and counseling of infected pregnant women, in addition for the prevention of CAs in the fetuses. Because of the relatively high occurrence of UTI during pregnancy, even a small elevated risk for CA and other adverse pregnancy outcomes have an important effect at the population level.

The analysis of maternal UTI was focused on specific CAs because teratogens can cause specific CAs without necessarily affecting the overall rate. We did not find an association between UTI and related drug treatments during the second and/or third months of pregnancy and any CA.

There are some weaknesses of our study:

(i) The diagnosis of maternal UTI was based on the reported clinical and/or laboratory data, in general without the microbiological proof of the infection. However, we were able to differentiate the primary infection of urinary tract in the study pregnancy and previous or chronic urinary tract's infection.

(ii) Case and control mothers did not have recorded CAs of urinary tract, but we were not able to exclude minor anatomical variation in their urinary tract [25, 29].

(iii) We had no data regarding fever in the total data set, however, among non-respondent mothers with UTI visited and questioned by regional nurses at home, only 6,0% had high temperature (over 38.5 Celsius) and two-third of these pregnant women had acute pyelonephritis.

Asymptomatic significant bacteriuria caused mainly by E.coli was found in 5.9% of the Hungarian female population of reproductive age [26], in 6.4% of pregnant women [27] and in 14.0% of pregnant women with preterm births [28]. The prevalence of asymptomatic significant bacteriuria with the symptoms of genital infections was 6.8 and 5.7% during pregnancy in case and control mothers in the study, respectively. These figures are within the range of asymptomatic significant bacteriuria (2-10%) in the international literature [25].

The occurrence of cystitis and pyelonephritis in pregnant women was found between about 1% and 2 % in other studies [25]. Our figures were somewhat lower (0.8% and 1.1% in the control group) because mainly only severe UTI were recorded in the prenatal care logbook.

UTI occurred mainly in the younger primiparae with lower socioeconomic status in the study. UTI were associated very frequently with the infections/diseases of the genital organs, however, it was the main indication of laboratory examinations of the urine in our data set. Among other maternal diseases, only kidney stones had an association with UTI, because kidney stones may predispose UTI during pregnancy as well.

We did not find any association between UTI and related drug treatments in the second and/or third month of gestation and any CA-group including atrial septal defect, thus we were not able to confirm the finding of Wilson et al. [24]. These authors evaluated the attributable fractions for 8 different cardiovascular CAs in the Baltimore-Washington Infant Study, 1981-1989. UTI had a small relative risk of 1.6 in the group of atrial septal defect, but the large percent exposed (20.3%) resulted in an extra attributable fraction of 6.4%. The expected number of atrial septal defect type II was 6.3 while the observed number was 3 (i.e. lower) in newborn infants born to mothers with UTI during the second and/or third gestational month (p=0.30) in our study.

Thus, our findings may indicate the lack of teratogenicity of microorganisms which cause UTI and related drug treatments in cardiovascular and other CAs. The detailed data of the study were published previously (30).

In conclusion, the higher occurrence of CAs was not found in the offspring of mothers with UTI and related drug treatments during the second and/or third months of pregnancy, thus the early treatment of UTI is strongly recommended.

Urinary Tract Infections in Pregnant Women and Pregnancy Complications, in Addition Pregnancy/Birth Outcomes

The purpose of our study was to evaluate the possible association between maternal UTI during pregnancy and pregnancy complications, in addition birth outcomes such as gestational age and/or birth weight, moreover the proportion of preterm birth and low birthweight and the efficacy of drug treatment.

Our study resulted in three important findings. First, maternal UTI showed an association with polyhydramnios and pre-eclampsia. The slightly higher rate of anemia was explained by the somewhat lower socioeconomic status of mothers with UTI. Second, there is an association between shorter gestational age of newborns and higher proportion of preterm births and the severity of UTI. Third, the higher rate of preterm birth in newborn infants born to mothers with UTI is preventable by antimicrobial drugs such as ampicillin, cefalexin and cotrimoxazole and their beneficial effect can explain the low rate of preterm birth in mothers with UTI.

It is a generally accepted opinion that renal diseases are associated with a higher risk for preeclampsia [31-33]. The possible association between polyhydramnios and UTI was also found [34]. True bacteriuria may be a marker for low socioeconomic status and sexually transmitted disorders which are associated with low birthweight and/or preterm birth. The main message of our study is that we confirmed the previous findings that UTI in pregnant women associate with a higher rate of preterm birth, but the association depends on the severity of maternal diseases and the efficacy of treatment. Up to 30% of mothers develop acute pyelonephritis if true bacteriuria is untreated, though antibiotic treatment is effective in reducing the risk of pyelonephritis in pregnancy and related preterm birth [35]. However, treated pyelonephritis associated with pregnancy does not appear to predispose to pretem birth or low birthweight [36] and this finding was confirmed in the milder form of UTI as well by our study.

Only a small number of women acquired UTI during the pregnancy [37]. UTI in unplanned pregnancies is not treated and it explains partly the higher rate of preterm birth in these pregnant women [38]. As our Hungarian experience showed, the preconceptional or early postconceptional screening is necessary particularly in women with symptoms of infections in genitourinary system followed by an effective treatment to prevent the higher risk for preterm birth [39, 40].

The detailed results of this study were published previously [41].

In conclusion, our study showed that maternal UTI increases the prevalence of preeclampsia and polyhydramnion, in addition the rate of preterm birth, however, available antimicrobial drugs provide an effective treatment for these adverse complications of pregnancies.

Glomerulonephritis in Pregnant Women and CA in Their Offspring

We examined the possible association between maternal GN during the study pregnancy and different CAs. A higher prevalence of GN was found only in one CA group and it included isolated intestinal atresia/stenosis.

The data set of the CCSCA has limitations.

(i) The diagnosis of GN was accepted on the basis of medical doctors' reports or maternal information in the HCCSCA. GN is a subject of confusion among health-care workers [45] because GN may have etiological, pathological, clinical descriptions and/or classification. We attempted to consider the latter approach, i.e.

nephritis syndrome, rapidly progressive GN, nephritic syndrome and chronic GN was included in the group of GN evaluated in the study, if it occurred during the first trimester of the study pregnancy. The persistent proteinuria was the principal marker of kidney damage in this group of kidney diseases. However, in general the precise diagnosis based on histological or other data was not available.

(ii) About 1.3% of pregnant women with GN were recorded in the HCCSCA. In general GN is underdiagnosed and undertreated [46], though the evidence of kidney damage based on proteinuria, low calculated glomerular filtration rate, or combination of these features may help to have an appropriate diagnosis of GN [45]. GN is more frequent in males and there is an increase in its prevalence parallel with advanced age [45, 46]. If we consider these facts, our 1.3% prevalence did not indicate an underascertainment.

(iii) Most women with GN were treated with several drugs, but their distribution and proportion was similar in case and control mothers with GN and they were considered at the calculation of adjusted OR with 95% CI.

(iv) Though the HCCSCA is the largest case-control data set of CAs in the world, the number of case mothers with GN is limited in the different CA groups.

(v) Finally, multiple comparisons between maternal diseases and various CA-groups may produce a chance association in every 20th analysis.

Our study showed that GN is more frequent in younger and primiparae women with a shorter gestational age and higher rate of preterm birth in newborn infants without CA born to mothers with GN. The somewhat higher occurrence of semiskilled workers and housewives among case mothers with GN may indicate their lower socioeconomic status. The well-known association of renal diseases with pre-eclampsia [31, 32, 48, 49] and genitourinary infectious diseases [19-21] was confirmed in the study. In addition we found a higher prevalence of anemia during the study pregnancy with GN. It is strange that the reported rate of threatened preterm delivery was lower while the rate of preterm birth was higher in pregnant women with GN. We did not find any data in the international literature which showed that GN can suppress the symptoms of threatened preterm delivery.

The association of GN and intestinal atresia/stenosis is noteworthy [51]. The question is whether this possible association is causal or explained by biases, confounders or by chance. The role of possible biases might be limited because all cases with isolated intestinal atresia/stenosis were born to mothers with prospectively and medically recorded GN during the first trimester of the study pregnancy. In addition the effect of confounders particularly related drug treatment was considered by the calculation of adjusted OR in our matched case-control approach. Previously a higher risk of infantile pyloric stenosis in infants exposed to nalidixic acid was observed [50], however, there was no mother with nalidixic acid treatment during the study pregnancy of 5 cases with intestinal atresia/stenosis. Nevertheless, the effect of other unknown confounders or residual confounders cannot be excluded.

Congenital intestinal atresia and stenosis is defined as total or partial obstruction of the intestine at any level (ileum is most common site followed by duodenum and jejunum, colon is least common) due to the lack or narrowing of continuity of the lumen in the fetus [51]. Of course, congenital hypertrophic pyloric stenosis, anal/rectal stenosis or atresia and diseases associated with intestinal atresia/stenosis (e.g., cases with Down syndrome ·may have duodenal atresia or cystic fibrosis may associate meconium ileus), in addition other CAs of the digestive system such as abnormal fixation, malrotation, duplication, diverticulum, etc. were excluded and evaluated separately. The etiology of isolated intestinal atresia and stenosis is probably similar but not well-known. In general isolated intestinal atresia/stenosis does not associate with other CAs beyond intestinal atresia/stenosis. Multiple intestinal atresia may have autosomal recessive inheritance [52]. In addition jejunal atresia (the so-called apple peel syndrome) due to obliteration of the superior mesenteric artery [53], duodenal atresia [54] and intestinal pseudoobstruction due to neuronal disease [55] with also autosomal recessive inheritance were not recognized in these cases. However, most isolated intestinal atresia/stenosis is thought to be due to fibrosis following intrauterine ischemia, i.e. vascular disruption. There are morphological and immunological evidence of coagulopathy in renal complications of pregnancy [26, 45]. Thus our hypothesis is that the pathomechanism of isolated intestinal atresia/stenosis in cases born to mothers with GN can be explained by the vascular lesion of the intestinal tract.

The absolute risk for isolated intestinal atresia/stenosis connected with GN is small. The expected number of cases with this CA is 16 per 100,000 births [3]. The estimated prevalence of GN during pregnancy is 1.3% and it may associate with 7 times higher risk for isolated intestinal atresia/stenosis. Thus, the estimated absolute excess number of isolated intestinal atresia/stenosis may be 1.5 cases among 100,000 newborn babies.

The detailed results of this study were published previously [57].

In conclusion, a higher occurrence of intestinal atresia/stenosis was found in the offspring of mothers with GN. However, these associations were based only on 5 cases, thus this finding is considered only as a *signal* and further studies are needed to confirm or reject this possible association.

Acknowledgement

This study was partly sponsored by a generous grant from Richter Gedeon Pharmaceuticals Ltd., Budapest, Hungary.

References

[1] Monga M. Maternal cardiovascular and renal adaptation to pregnancy. In: Creasy RK, Resnik MD (eds.): *Maternal-Fetal Medicine.* 5th ed. Saunders, Philadelphia, 2004.pp.111-120.

[2] Czeizel AE, Rockenbauer M, Siffel Cs, Varga E. Description and mission evaluation of the Hungarian Case-Control Surveillance of Congenital Abnormalities, 1980-1996. *Teratology* 2001; 63: 176-185.

[3] Czeizel AE. The first 25 years of the Hungarian Congenital Abnormality Registry. *Teratology* 1997; 55: 299-305.

[4] Czeizel AE, Puho HE, Ács N, Bánhidy F. Use of specified critical periods of congenital abnormalities instead of the first trimester concept. *Birth Def Res. Part A* 2008; 82: 139-146.

[5] Czeizel AE. The first trimester concept is outdated. *Cong Anom (Kyoto)* 2001; 41: 204.

[6] Ács N, Bánhidy F, Puho HE, Czeizel AE. Population-based case-control study of the common cold during pregnancy and congenital abnormalities. *Eur. J. Epidemiol.* 2006; 21: 65-75.

[7] Ács N, Bánhidy F, Puho HE, Czeizel AE. Acute respiratory infections during pregnancy and congenital abnormalities. A population-based case-control study. *Cong. Anom (Kyoto)* 2006; 46: 86-96.

[8] Ács N, Bánhidy F, Puho HE, Czeizel AE. Maternal influenza during pregnancy and rijk of congenital abnormalities in offspring. *Birth Defects Res. Part A* 2005; 73: 989-996.

[9] Czeizel AE. Specified critical period of different congenital abnormalities: A new approach fro human teratological studies. *Cong. Anom. (Kyoto)* 2008; 48: 103-109.

[10] Czeizel AE, Petik D, Vargha P. Validation studies of drug exposures in pregnant women. *Pharmacoepid Drug Safety*. 2003; 12: 409-416.

[11] Czeizel AE, Dudás I. Prevention of the first occurrence of neural-tube defects by periconceptional vitamin supplementation. *N. Engl. J. Med.* 1992; 327: 1832-1835.

[12] Czeizel AE. Prevention of congenital abnormalities by periconceptional multivitamin supplementation. *Brit. Med. J.* 1993; 306: 1645-1648.

[13] Czeizel AE. Reduction of urinary tract and cardiovascular defects by periconceptional multivitamin supplementation. *Am. J. Med. Genet.* 1996; 62: 179-183.

[14] Czeizel AE, Dobó M, Vargha P. Hungarian two-cohort controlled study of periconceptional multivitamin supplementation to prevent certain congenital abnormalities. *Birth Defects Res. Part A.* 2004; 70: 853-861.

[15] Botto LD, Olney RS, Erickson JD. Vitamin supplements and the risk for congenital anomalies other than neural tube defects. *Am. J. Med. Genet. Part C* 2004; 125C: 12-21.

[16] Rockenbauer M, Czeizel AE, Olsen J et al. Recall bias in a case-control study on the use of medicine during pregnancy. *Epidemiology* 2001; 12: 461-466.

[17] Roberts RB (ed). Infectious Diseases: Pathogenesis, Diagnosis and Therapy. Year Book Medical Publ. Chicago. 1986.

[18] Parker MT, Collier LH (eds). Topley Wilson Principles of Bacteriology, Virology and Immunity. Decker BC. 1990.

[19] Hart CC, Weisholtz SJ. Urinary tract infections. In: Roberts RB (ed). Infectious Diseases. Pathogenesis, Diagnosis and Therapy. Year Book Medical Publ. Chicago. 1986; pp: 73-96.

[20] Andriole VT. Urinary tract infection in pregnancy. *Urol. Clin. N. Am.* 1975; 2: 485-

[21] Kass EH. Bacteriuria and pyelonephritis of pregnancy. *Arch. Intern. Med.* 1960; 105: 42-46.

[22] O'Neill MS, Hertz-Picciotto I, Pastore LM, Wetherley BD. Have studies of urinary tract infection and pregerm delivery used the most appropriate methods? *Paediat Perinat Epidemiol* 2003; 17: 226-233.

[23] Shepard TH, Lemire RJ. Catalog of Teratogenic Agents. 11th ed. Johns Hopkins Univ Press Baltimore, 2004.
[24] Wilson PD, Loffredo CA, Correa-Villasenor A, Ferencz C. Attributable fraction for cardiac malformations. *Am. J. Epidemiol.* 1998; 148: 414-423.
[25] Davison JM, Lindheimer MD. Renal disorders. In: In:. In: Creasy RK, Resnik MD (eds.): *Maternal-Fetal Medicine.* 5th ed. Saunders, Philadelphia, 2004.pp.901-923.
[26] Czeizel AE, Berec M, Gerőfi J, et al. Study of asymptomatic significant bacteriuria in a population section of Budapest (Hungarian with English abstract). *Orvosi. Hetilap.* 1968; 109: 1985-1987.
[27] Czeizel AE, Hancsok M, Margitay Becht D, et al. Incidence of significant bacteriuria during pregnancy (Hungarian with English abstract). *Orvosi Hetilap* 1967; 108: 684-686.
[28] Czeizel AE, Hancsok M, Ormay L, Philipp G. The connection between significant bacteriuria during pregnancy and premature births (Hungarian with English abstract). *Orvosi Hetilap* 1967; 108: 101-102.
[29] Trembath DG, Rijhsinghani A. Possible maternal inheritance of a common obstructive urinary tract infections and two sons with posterior urethal valves. *J. Reprod. Med.* 2002; 47: 962-964.
[30] Bánhidy F. Ács N, Puho HE, Czeizel AE. Maternal urinary tract infection and related drug treatments during pregnancy and risk of congenital abnormalities in the offspring. *Br. J. Obstet. Gynaecol.* 2006. 113: 1465-1471.
[31] Kincaid-Smith P, Fairley KF. The differential diagnosis between preeclamptic toxemia and glomerulonephritis in patients with proteinuria during pregnancy. In: Lindheimer MD, Katz AI, Zuspan FP (eds). Hypertension in Pregnancy. Wiley. New York. 1976. pp. 157-171.
[32] Katz AI, Davison JM, Hayslett JP, Singson E, Lindheimer MD. Pregnancy in women with kidney diseases. *Kidney Int.* 1980; 18: 192-196.
[33] Heptinstall RH. Renal diseases in pregnancy. In: Heptinstall RH. Pathology of Kidney, 3rd ed. Little, Brown and Co. Boston. 1983. pp. 963-991
[34] Naeye RL. Causes of the excessive rates of perinatal mortality and prematurity in pregnancies complicated by maternal urinary tract infections. *N. Engl. J. Med.* 1979; 300: 819-823.
[35] Fan YD, Pastorek JG, Miller JM Jr, Mulvey J. Acute pyelonephritis in pregnancy. *Am. J. Perinatol.* 1987; 4: 324-326.
[36] Smaill F. 2001. Antibiotics for asymptomatic bacteriuria in pregnancy. *Cohrane Database Syst. Rev.* CD 000490.
[37] Norden CW, Kass EH. Bacteriuria of pregnancy – A critical appraisal. *Ann Rev Med* 1968; 19: 431-440.
[38] Yaris F. Kadioglu M, Kesim M, et al. Urinary tract infections in unplanned pregnancies and fetal outcome. *Eur. J. Contracep Reprod. Hlth* 2004; 9: 141-146.
[39] Czeizel AE. Ten years experience in periconceptional care. *Eur. J. Obstet. Gynecol. Reprod Biol* 1999; 84: 43-49.
[40] Czeizel AE, Dobó M, Dudás I, et al. The Hungarian Periconceptional Service as a model for community genetics. *Community Genetics* 1998; 1: 252-529.

[41] Bánhidy F, Ács N, Puhó E. Czeizel AE. Pregnancy complications and birth outcomes of pregnant women with urinary tract infections and related drug treatments. *Scand. J. Inf. Dis*. 2007; 37: 390-397.

[42] MacKey EV: Pregnancy and renal disease: A ten-year survey. *Aust. N. Z. J. Obstet. Gynecol.* 1963; 3: 21-26.

[43] Sims EAH: The kidney in pregnancy. In: Strauss MB, Welt LG (eds): Diseases of the Kidney (2nd ed). Little, Brown and Co. Boston, 1971, pp 1155. 1211.

[44] Fairley KF, Whitworth JA, Kincaid-Smith P: Glomerulonephritis and pregnancy. In: Kincaid-Smith P, Mathew TH, Becker ELC (eds): Glomerulonephritis: Morphology, Natural History, and Treatment. Wiley. New York, 1973. pp 997-1011.

[45] Chadban SJ, Atkins R: Glomerulonephritis. *Lancet,* 2005; 365: 1797-1806.

[46] Levey AS, Coresh J, Balk E, et al: National kidney foundation practice guidelines for chronic kidney disease: evaluation, classification and stratification. *Ann. Intern. Med.* 2000; 139: 137-147.

[47] Brown MA, Holt JL, Mangos GJ, et al: Microscopic hematuria in pregnancy: relevance to pregnancy outcomes. *J. Kidney Dis.* 2005; 45: 667-673.

[48] MacGillirray I: Some observations on the incidence of pre-eclampsia. *J. Obstet. Gynecol.* 1958; 65: 536-540.

[49] Altchek A, Albright NL, Sommers SC: The renal pathology of toxemia of pregnancy. *Obstet Gynecol* 1968; 31: 555-560.

[50] Czeizel AE, Rockenbauer M, Sorensen HT, Olsen J: Risk of infantile pyloric stenosis in infants exposed to nalidixic acid: a population-based case-control study. *Int. J. Gynec. Obstet*. 2001; 73: 221-228.

[51] Minor CL: Alimentary system. In: Rubin A (ed): Handbook of Congenital Malformations. W. B. Saunders Co. Philadelphia, 1969, pp. 1-14.

[52] Dallaire L, Perreault G: Hereditary multiple intestinal atresia. *Birth Defects Orig Art Ser X.* 1974; 10(4): 259-264.

[53] Mishalany HG, Najjar FB: Familial jejunal atresia: three cases in one family. *J. Pediat.* 1968; 73: 753-755.

[54] Fonkalsrud EW, de Lorimer AA, Hays DM: Congenital atresia and stenosis of the duodenum. *Pediatrics* 1969; 43: 79-83.

[55] Tanner MS, Smith B, Lloyd JK: Functional intestinal obstruction due to deficiency of argyrophil neurones in the myenteric plexus: familial syndrome presenting with short small bowel, malrotation, and pyloric hypertrophy. *Arch. Dis. Childh* 1976; 51: 837-841.

[56] Seymour AE, Petracco OM, Clarkson AR et al: Morphologic and immunological evidence of coagulopathy in renal complications of pregnancy. In: Lindheimer MD, Katz AI, Zuspan FP (eds): Hypertension in pregnancies. Wiley. New York, 1976. pp 139-145.

[57] Ács N, Bánhidy F, Puho HE, Czeizel AE. A possible association between maternal glomerulonephritis and congenital intestinal atresia/stenosis – a population-based case-control study. *Eur. J. Epidemiol.* 2007; 22: 557-564.

In: Infectious Pregnancy Complications
Editor: Richard N. Canfield
ISBN 978-1-60741-038-6

Chapter 14

Dengue Infection in Pregnancy: Pattern of Hematological Disturbance

Viroj Wiwanitkit
Wiwanitkit House, Bangkhae,
Bangkok Thailand 10160

Abstract

Dengue infection is a common arboviral infection that poses a significant threat to tropical countries. The serious forms of this infection are called dengue hemorrhagic fever and dengue shock syndrome. These serious forms of dengue infection can lead to a high rate of fatality. Pregnant women in the endemic area of dengue infection can be infected and can develop many signs and symptoms. In this chapter, the author will focus on dengue infection in pregnancy, especially on the pattern of hematological disturbance. The co-manifestation with other common hematological disorders in pregnancy will also be mentioned.

Introduction to Dengue Infection

Dengue infection is a common arboviral infection that poses a great threat to tropical countries. Since it is an arboviral infection, the disease is an important member of the arthropod-borne disease group. This viral infection is classified as a mosquito-borne viral infection. Mosquito bite is the main risk and cause of infection. *Aedes* species is the important corresponding vector. This infection is common in tropical countries, as previously mentioned. Southeast Asia is classified as a high endemic area for dengue infection. A wide spectrum of disease caused by four serotypes of this most prevalent arthropod-borne virus affects humans today, and its incidence has increased dramatically in the past half century [1]. Due in part to population growth and uncontrolled urbanization in tropical countries, breeding sites for the mosquitoes that transmit virus have proliferated, and successful vector control has still not been successful [1]. Dengue viruses have evolved rapidly, and genotypes associated with increased virulence have expanded from Southeast Asia into the Pacific, the Americas and other remote areas [1]. As previously mentioned, many thousands of cases of dengue and dengue hemorrhagic fever are reported in tropical regions of the Americas, Africas, Asia and Oceania every year [2]. In the absence of a safe and effective mass immunization, the best prevention and control of dengue outbreaks depend upon the surveillance of infected cases and the mosquito vector [3–5].

Dengue infection is a major cause of morbidity in tropical regions, bringing nearly 40% of the world population at risk and causing more than 20,000 deaths annually [6]. There is neither a vaccine for dengue disease nor antiviral drugs to treat the infection at present [6]. The classical simple form of dengue infection is called dengue fever. Dengue fever has the signs and symptoms of simple flu and patients can completely recover. The classical form of dengue infection has an incubation period of five to eight days followed by the onset of fever, violent headache, chill and rash developing after three to four days [7–9]. The fever usually lasts four to seven days, and most affected cases have a complete recovery without any complications [7–9]. However, there are other more serious forms of dengue infection. The serious forms of this infection are called dengue hemorrhagic fever and dengue shock syndrome. These serious forms of dengue infection can lead to a high rate of fatality.

Hematological Manifestation of Dengue

Dengue infection is an infection with dengue viruses producing a spectrum of clinical illness with several hematologic aberrations [10–12]. Thrombocytopenia and hemoconcentration are common in patients infected with dengue [10–12]. Generally, most of the dengue infections usually present with fever, constitutional symptoms and positive tourniquet test (the appearance of petichiae after the application tourniquet pressure for three to five minutes) [10–12]. Decrease platelet count and elevated hematocrit are the two hallmark hematologic disturbances of dengue infection [13]. Vasculopathy and thrombopathy due to immune mechanism are also reported to be responsible for those findings [14–15]. It is well known that the process of thrombocytopenia is a significant hemostasis disorder in dengue infection. The underlying pathogenesis of this condition is believed to be due to the immunological alteration. Immune mimicking is proposed as the key for development of hemorrhagic episode, and the difference in binding capacity of IgM and IgG are the clues for the self-resolving phenomenon of dengue in the recovery phase [16]. In clinical practice, platelet counts do not correlate well with clinical bleeding [17–18]. Recently, a summative report on the platelet count and its clinical correlation to duration of fever in infected Thai children was studied by Wiwanitkit [18]. In this series, most of the subjects visited the physician with a complaint of fever, and most patients went to see the physician between the third and the fifth day from the onset of fever [18]. There is no significant correlation between platelet count and duration of high fever; however, there is a positive trend of increased platelet count in the later days [18]. According to a recent study by Wiwanitkit and Munusvanich, the regression analysis revealed no significant statistical correlation between platelet count and the focused outcome [16]. This means that a platelet count in a routine complete blood count on admission cannot predict shock in the hospitalized dengue hemorrhagic patients [16]. There are only a few reports concerning the abnormal coagulation pathway among patients with dengue infections. Chua et al. reported that aPTT could be an index in predicting bleeding in DHF [19]. They noted that tendency to bleed was greater with prolongation of more than half a minute; platelet count can be a predictor of mortality, with death six times greater among those presenting with platelet counts higher than 50,000/microliter than those whose platelet count was less than 50,000/microliter [19]. Chua et al. also mentioned that PT could also predict bleeding in patients with DHF [19]. However, Chua et al. did not confirm that prolonged PT and aPTT were important hemastasis disorder indicators in dengue. There is no report on coagulation factor alteration in dengue.

Dengue in Pregnancy

The pregnant in the endemic area of dengue infection can become infected and can develop many signs and symptoms. In this section, the author will focus on dengue infection in pregnancy, especially for the pattern of hematological disturbance. Co-infection with other common hematological disorders in pregnancy will also be mentioned.

A. General Concern

Besides simple transmission by vector, there are other methods of simple transmission of dengue infection that can be seen in clinical practice. Some pregnant women can also be susceptible to dengue virus, and if they experience dengue fever virus infection, the vertical transmission of the virus their children is possible. There are some interesting prior reports on tropical intrapartum arboviral infection. Vertical transmission of dengue fever virus during pregnancy was first reported by Thaithumyanon et al. in 1994 [20]. The intrapartum infection can bring several complications, mainly disorders of coagulation. With regard to the clinical presentation of the affected pregnant subjects, a clinical presentation similar to the general population can be seen. It can be noted that the intrapartum and postnatal disorders of coagulation cascades can be corrected by standard replacement therapy. Of interest, intrapartum complications were dependant on postpartum complications. Besides, it seems that clinical complications did not relate to the method of delivery. Confirmation of intrapartum dengue infection is generally delayed due to the long turnaround time of the serological test. First, a bacterial infection was initially suspected in most cases. Nevertheless, the presumed diagnosis is generally due to combined presentation of fever and thrombocytopenia. Actually, in endemic areas of dengue virus infection, the diagnosis of dengue fever should be considered in neonates with signs of the bacterial infection [21–22]. When a high fever is suspected in a pregnant woman, laboratory investigation and prolonged observation of the newborn are advised [21–22]. Wiwanitkit recently presented a series of reports of pregnant with dengue infection [23]. This study was designed as a descriptive retrospective study with a literature review of the papers concerning DHF in pregnancy in Thailand using the database of published works cited in the Index Medicus and Science

Citation Index [23]. The key words for searching in this work were "pregnancy" and "dengue" [23] According to this work, seven reports on DHF in pregnancy were recruited for further study [23]. According to this study, there have been at least seven reports [23–29] in the literature of seven cases of DHF in pregnancy, of which no case was lethal [23]. All except one case (23 weeks pregnancy) had term pregnancy on presentation [23]. Considering the clinical manifestations, all had fever and some had other manifestations [23]. From physical examination, all had hepatosplenomegaly and petechiae. At the time of diagnosis, complete blood count demonstrated thrombocytopenia and hemoconcentration in all cases [23]. Due to possible long waiting times for results of laboratory tests, beginning standard replacement therapy in clinically suspected cases is recommended and useful for general practitioners. After the final diagnosis, mother and baby should be closely followed up for a year.

B. Pattern of Hematological Disturbance in Pregnant with Dengue Infection

About one-third of dengue infection cases are reported in adult patients; therefore, some pregnant women may also be susceptible to dengue infection [24]. Increased cases of dengue infection in pregnancy can be expected due to the increasing incidence during adulthood. Hematological disturbance in pregnant women with dengue infection can be modified due to the pregnancy. Pregnant women usually have some degree of anemia, which can alter the hemoconcentration detection in a routine hematocrit test in the medical laboratory. However, the recent series by Wiwanitkit reports no alteration in hematocrit and platelet count [23]. Hemoconcentration as well as thrombocytopenia were the two hallmark laboratory aberrations in the patients in this series [23]. Wiwanitkit noted that it should be suspected when a pregnant woman presents with symptoms and signs similar to a non-pregnant patient, and the triad of high fever, hemoconcentration and thrombocytopenia could be the clue for diagnosis in pregnancy [23]. Conclusively, Wiwanitkit found that dengue infection in pregnancy was similar to non-pregnant patients in the context of clinical presentation, treatment and outcome [23].

C. Treatment for Dengue Infection in Pregnancy

Treatment of dengue infection should be based on the severity of the infection. The concept of treatment is similar to other infections: eliminating the pathogen or control of the infection and supportive or symptomatic treatment. In dengue infection, the specific antiviral drug for dengue virus is not available at present. There are some recent reports on the possible antiviral drugs for dengue virus infection. Damonte et al. recently noted that drugs containing various alga sulfated polysaccharides posed high antiviral activity against dengue virus, and these polysaccharides should be further studied aiming at drug development [30]. With respect to supporting treatment, correction of vascular collapse in dengue should be a main consideration. In grade I or II of dengue fever, the blood pressure of patients has not yet seriously decreased; therefore, an extensive fluid replacement is not necessary. Oral fluid replacement is sufficient for these cases. Hospitalization in these cases is not necessary. To lower high fever, paracetamol table should be utilized in general. It should be noted that aspirin is contraindicated in these cases. A complication due to additional disturbance of platelet according to utilization of salicylate in dengue infection is extensively mentioned. Following up of patients with grade I or II of dengue fever should be put in 1 week according to course of viral illness. It should be noted that phase of the illness can go higher; therefore, advice to patients to observe their symptoms and to visit the physician again if the symptoms get worse is indicated. In severe cases of dengue infection (grade III or IV), fluid replacement should be considered with special care (hospitalization is required). Intravenous fluid replacement is indicated for all cases falling within these severe grades. The ideal fluid for administration should include cystalloids or colloids (inclusive albumen) [31]. Cystalloids are given as alimentary boluses as quickly as possible, and as much as two to three alimentary boluses are needed in cases of deep shock [31]. The colloidal liquids are indicated in patients with massive shrinkage of plasma and in whom a large volume of cystalloids has been administered [31]. In addition to a correction of electrolyte and metabolic disturbances, oxygen management is necessary in all patients with dengue shock [31]. As a guideline for the general practitioner, the author proposed the initiation of intravenous fluid replacement with 0.9% normal saline solution. The response of fluid replacement can be monitored from serial taking of blood pressure and manual hematocrit test. It should be noted that the fluid replacement should not exceed one day to avoid the redistribution of fluid and possible fluid intoxication in the convalescent phase. The intravenous administration of corticosteroids is not contraindicated and shown to be useful in some cases [32–33]. This principle for treatment of dengue infection can be applied to pregnancy. Conservative treatment by fluid replacement is the gold standard for treatment of pregnancy with dengue infection. According to a recent study by Wiwanitkit [23], conservative treatment should be conducted unless there are any complications, and appropriate fluid replacement can provide a positive maternal outcome. Considering the newborn, a positive outcome can be seen [23]. An important concern in fluid replacement therapy in pregnancy should also be mentioned. Because of the high possibility for water intoxication in pregnancy, careful monitoring of fluid replacement therapy is needed. Hofmeyr and Mohlala reported that hypovolaemic shock is a major cause of maternal mortality [34]. Hofmeyr and Mohlala noted that management of this conditioned required teamwork, co-ordination, speed and adequate facilities to be life-saving and the first priority was rapid fluid replacement [34]. Hofmeyr and Mohlala also reported that crystalloids were the fluids of choice over colloids, and particularly albumen, which was associated with increased mortality [34]. Recently, Martel et al. proposed that blood component transfusion was also indicated when overt deficiencies were documented by clinical assessment or hematological investigations, and those components should be warmed and infused through filtered lines with normal saline, free of additives and drugs [35].

D. Co-Manifestation with Other Common Hematological Disorders in Pregnancy

Co-manifestation with other common hematological disorders in pregnancy can be seen. A great concern is thalassemia. Beta-thalassemia trait is a common hemoglobin disorder in Southeast Asia [36]. This disease is one of the inherited hemoglobin disorders, with a high prevalence documented in Southeast Asia, the same area as dengue infection. Microcytic anemia is common in beta-thalassemia. Also, thrombocytosis, related to thromboembolism, is documented in the patients with beta-thalassemia [37–38]. The author hereby will present a short summary of the basic clinical information on hemostatic disorder in dengue, based on experience with two known cases of beta-thalassemia suffering from dengue fever. The effect of co-presentation of dengue infection and beta-thalassemia trait are discussed as well. Two patients were diagnosed with dengue infection during the endemic season, 2003. The diagnosis of dengue infection was made according to the WHO recommendation, while the patients had been diagnosed with beta-thalassemia trait due to previous hemoglobin electrophoresis study. The first case was a male patient who presented to the physician with the chief complaint of high fever for 10 days. He was a known case of beta-thalassemia trait. He reported that an over-the-counter antipyretic drug could not relieve his illness. This patient had a positive tourniquet test and thrombocytopenia. The second case was a female patient who presented to the physician with a chief complaint of dizziness and fatigue for two weeks. On routine physical examination she presented with high fever. She was a known case of beta-thalassemia trait. This patient had a positive tourniquet test and thrombocytopenia. These two cases still presented with high hematocrit and low platelet count. A difference in hematocrit and platelet count between thalassemic and non-thalassemic subjects in the author's setting can be demonstrated. It could be shown that the average hematocrit is lower and the average platelet count is higher in the thalassemic group. This can imply that investigation and interpretation of complete blood count in diagnosis and monitoring of dengue infection in thalassemic patients should be done carefully; error can be expected, especially in thalassemic cases with severe anemia in which hemoconcentration can be disguised. Nevertheless, the nature of hypochromic and microcytic red blood cell can be seen. This can confirm the real situation of co-manifestation of dengue and thalassemia. Although the two cases studies do not involve pregnancy, an implication can be made. The conservation of hemoconcentration and thrombocytopenia can still be seen and is a useful clinical hallmark for diagnosis. Thus, pregnancy with thalassemia, the focus on the mimicking effect of severe anemia to hide the hemoconcentration is a caution in coping with suspected dengue infection in pregnancy with thalassemia. The co-presentation of dengue infection and thalassemia can be detected in highly endemic areas such as Thailand. Due to the counter effect on the hematocrit and platelet of these two diseases, investigation and interpretation of complete blood count in the diagnosis and monitoring of dengue infection in thalassemic patients should be done carefully. In addition to thalassemia, another concern is other common blood infections. The focused diseases are malaria and filariasis. Co-infection between malaria and dengue infection can also be seen [39]. Pregnancy with both malaria and dengue infection can be expected and can be a serious complicated case [40].

E. Transmission of Dengue to Neonate

Transmission of dengue infection to the neonate is confirmed [23]. Neonatal dengue is considered a serious disorder in neonatal hematology. Tan et al. reported that a vertical transmission rate of 1.6% could be seen, and the pregnancy outcome of recently-infected women was not different [41]. Considering the nanostructure level in an explanation of vertical transmission, physiologically, the placental barrier, composed of the fetal endothelium and the syncytiotrophoblast and their fused basal laminae, plays important protective role, and the maternal blood bathes the syncytiotrophoblast only. It can be seen that the dengue virus has a smaller size compared with the placental filter (placental barrier pore size is equal to 10 nm [42]) and this allows vertical transmission. However, an important note is that viremia in the mother must be during the period near the time of labor to allow the virus to pass to infect the infant. It can be concluded that if a pregnant mother contracts the disease, is bitten by contaminated vector, and develops viremia in the week before term, this mother has a high risk for developing dengue infection in pregnancy and can pass the infection to her term infant in utero, which can result in vertical transmission and a case of neonatal dengue as a final outcome of this story of arbovirus transmission.

References

[1] Kyle JL, Harris E. Global Spread and Persistence of Dengue. Annu Rev Microbiol. 2008 Apr 22. [Epub ahead of print].

[2] Gubler DJ., Sc. D and Edward B.Hayes, MD. Dengue and dengue hemorrhagic fever. *Am. J. Trop. Med. Hyg.* 1992;25 (4):532-537.

[3] World Health Organization. Dengue haemorrhagic fever : Diagnosis, Treatment and Control. WHO, *Geniva*, 1986;1-15.

[4] Knudsen AB., Slooff R. Vector-borne disease problems in rapid urbanization: new approaches to vector control. *Bull World Health Organ*. 1992;70; 1-6.

[5] Gubler DJ., Clarke GG. Community-based integrated control of *Aedes aegypti*: a brief overview of current programs. *Am. J. Trop. Med. Hyg.* 1994;50(suppl);50-60.

[6] Qi RF, Zhang L, Chi CW. Biological characteristics of dengue virus and potential targets for drug design. Acta Biochim Biophys Sin (Shanghai). 2008 Feb;40(2):91-101.

[7] Guzman MG, Kouri G. Dengue: an update. *Lancet Infect. Dis*. 2002;2:33-42.

[8] da Fonseca BA, Fonseca SN. Dengue virus infections. *Curr. Opin. Pediatr*. 2002;14:67-71.

[9] Solomon T, Mallewa M. Dengue and other emerging flaviviruses. *J. Infect*. 2001;42:104-15.

[10] Thisyakorn U, Thisyakorn C. Diseases cuased by arboviruses-dengue hemorrhagic fever and Japanese B encephalitits. *Med. J. Aus*. 1994; 160: 22–6.

[11] Guzman MG, Kouri G. Dengue: an update. *Lancet Infect. Dis*. 2002;2:33-42.

[12] Srichaikul T, Nimmannitya S. Haematology in dengue and dengue haemorrhagic fever. *Baillieres Best Pract. Res. Clin. Haematol*. 2000 ;13:261-76.

[13] Vaughn DW, Green S, Kalayanarooj S, Innis BL, Nimmannitya S, Suntayakorn S, Endy TP, Raengsakulrach B, Rothman AL, Ennis FA, Nisalak A. Dengue viremia titer, antibody response pattern, and virus serotype correlate with disease severity. *J. Infect. Dis.* 2000;181:2-9.

[14] Bhamarapravati N. Hemostatic defects in dengue hemorrhagic fever. *Rev. Infect. Dis.* 1989;11 Suppl 4:S826-9.

[15] Wiwanitkit V. Weak binding affinity of immunoglobin G, an explanation for the immune mimicking theory in pathophysiologic findings in the recovery phase of dengue. Nanomedicine: *Nanotechnology, Biology, and Medicine* 2005; 1: 239-240.

[16] Wiwanitkit V, Manusvanich P. Can hematocrit and platelet determination on admission predict shock in hospitalized children with dengue hemorrhagic fever? A clinical observation from a small outbreak. *Clin. Appl. Thromb. Hemost.* 2004;10: 65-7.

[17] Schexneider KI, Reedy EA. Thrombocytopenia in dengue fever. *Curr. Hematol. Rep.* 2005;4:145-8.

[18] Wiwanitkit V. The importance of platelet counts in dengue infection: 35 cases and literature review. *Clin. Appl. Thromb. Hemost.* 2004;10:399-402.

[19] Chua MN, Molanida R, de Guzman M, Laberiza F. Prothrombin time and partial thromboplastin time as a predictor of bleeding in patients with dengue hemorrhagic fever. *Southeast Asian J. Trop. Med. Public Health.* 1993;24 Suppl 1:141-3.

[20] Thaithumyanon P, Thisyakorn U, Deerojnawong J, Innis BL. Dengue infection complicated by severe hemorrhage and vertical transmission in a parturient woman. *Clin. Infect. Dis.* 1994; 18: 248-9.

[21] Ahmed S. Vertical transmission of dengue: first case report from Bangladesh. *Southeast Asian J. Trop. Med. Public Health.* 2003; 34: 800-3.

[22] Chye JK, Lim CT, Ng KB, Lim JM, George R, Lam SK. Vertical transmission of dengue. *Clin. Infect. Dis.* 1997; 25: 1374-7.

[23] Wichmann O, Hongsiriwon S, Bowonwatanuwong C, Chotivanich K, Sukthana Y, Pukrittayakamee S. Risk factors and clinical features associated with severe dengue infection in adults and children during the 2001 epidemic in Chonburi, Thailand. *Trop. Med. Int. Health* 2004;9:1022-9.

[24] Witayathawornwong P. Parturient and perinatal dengue hemorrhagic fever. *Southeast Asian J. Trop. Med. Public Health.* 2003;34:797-9.

[25] Chotigeat U, Kalayanarooj S, Nisalak A. Vertical transmission of dengue infection in Thai infants: two case reports. *J. Med. Assoc. Thai.* 2003;86 Suppl 3:S628-32.

[26] Taechakraichana N, Limpaphayom K. Dengue hemorrhagic fever in pregnancy. *Chula Med. J.* 1989; 33: 213-218.

[27] Chawanpaiboon S, Titapant V, Puthavathana P, Chongkolwatana V. Antiplatelet transfusion in dengue haemorrhagic fever during pregnancy : a case report. *Siriraj Hosp. Gaz.* 1998; 50: 964-966.

[28] Sila'on J, Petdachai W. Dengue hemorrhagic fever during pregnancy. *Reg 6-7 Med. J.* 2004; 23: 15-21.

[29] Kungteerawat S. Dengue hemorrhagic fever in the pregnant. *Med. J. Srisaket. Surin. Buriram. Hosp.* 2002; 17: 93-100.

[30] Damonte EB, Matulewicz MC, Cerezo AS. Sulfated seaweed polysaccharides as antiviral agents. *Curr. Med. Chem*. 2004; 11: 2399-419.

[31] Soni A, Chugh K, Sachdev A, Gupta D. Management of dengue fever in ICU. *Indian. J. Pediatr.* 2001; 68: 1051-5.

[32] Sumarmo, Talogo W, Asrin A, Isnuhandojo B, Sahudi A. Failure of hydrocortisone to affect outcome in dengue shock syndrome. *Pediatrics*. 1982; 69: 45-9.

[33] Tassniyom S, Vasanawathana S, Chirawatkul A, Rojanasuphot S. Failure of high-dose methylprednisolone in established dengue shock syndrome: a placebo-controlled, double-blind study. *Pediatrics*. 1993; 92: 111-5.

[34] Hofmeyr GJ, Mohlala BK. Hypovolaemic shock. *Best Pract. Res. Clin. Obstet. Gynaecol*. 2001 Aug;15(4):645-62.

[35] Martel MJ, MacKinnon KJ, Arsenault MY, Bartellas E, Klein MC, Lane CA, Sprague AE, Wilson AK; Clinical Practice Obstetrics Committee and Executive and Council, Society of Obstetricians and Gynaecologists of Canada. Hemorrhagic shock. *J. Obstet. Gynaecol. Can.* 2002 Jun;24(6):504-20.

[36] Fucharoen S, Wanichagoon P. Thalassemia in SouthEast Asia: problems and strategy for prevention and control. *Southeast Asian J. Trop. Med. Public Health* 1992;23:647-55.

[37] Sonakul D, Fucharoen S. Pulmonary thromboembolism in thalassemic patients. *Southeast Asian J. Trop. Med. Public Health* 1992;23 Suppl 2:25-8.

[38] Sumiyoshi A, Thakerngpol K, Sonakul D. Pulmonary microthromboemboli in thalassemic cases. *Southeast Asian J Trop Med Public Health*. 1992;23 Suppl 2:29 -31.

[39] Carles G, Talarmin A, Peneau C, Bertsch M. Preparing your patients to travel abroad safely. Part 3: Reducing the risk of malaria and dengue fever. *Can. Fam. Physician*. 2000 May;46:1126-31.

[40] McGovern LM, Boyce TG, Fischer PR. Congenital infections associated with international travel during pregnancy. *J. Travel Med*. 2007 Mar-Apr;14(2):117-28.

[41] Tan PC, Rajasingam G, Devi S, Omar SZ. Dengue infection in pregnancy: prevalence, vertical transmission, and pregnancy outcome. *Obstet. Gynecol*. 2008 May; 111(5): 1111-7.

[42] Challier JC. The placental barrier: structure, resistance, asymmetry. *Reprod. Nutr. Dev*. 1989;29:703-16.

In: Infectious Pregnancy Complications
Editor: Richard N. Canfield
ISBN: 978-1-60471-038-6

Chapter 15

Infectious Diseases of the Respiratory System during Pregnancy

Andrew E. Czeizel[a]***, Nándor Ács***[b] ***and Ferenc Bánhidy***[b]
[a] Foundation for the Community Control of Hereditary Diseases, Budapest,Hungary
[b] Second Department of Obstetrics and Gynecology, Semmelweis University, School of Medicine, Budapest, Hungary

Abstract

Infectious diseases of respiratory system frequently complicate pregnancy. This review evaluates the possible association between maternal infectious diseases of the respiratory system during pregnancy and preterm birth or structural birth defects, i.e., congenital abnormalities (CAs), in addition to their pregnancy complications based on the data set of the Hungarian Case-Control Surveillance of Congenital Abnormalities.

At the evaluation of a *common cold*, it is necessary to differentiate the usual common cold (with short duration and without fever) and the common cold with secondary complications (i.e., with longer duration and frequently high fever). Pregnant women with a common cold mainly with secondary complications did not have a higher incidence of pregnancy complications. The gestational age at delivery was 0.1 week shorter with a somewhat higher rate of preterm birth, but these differences had no real clinical importance. However, an association of common cold (mainly with secondary complications) in the second and/or third gestational month of pregnancy with a higher rate of newborns with congenital cataract, cleft lip ± palate and possibly some other specific congenital abnormalities was found, and this association was preventable with antifever drug treatments.

Acute infectious diseases of the respiratory system cover a wide spectrum of diseases, from sinusitis to pneumonia. These diseases during pregnancy have no obvious effect of pregnancy complications. Infectious respiratory diseases in the severe lower catetory were associated with a higher risk for preterm birth, but their mild upper category seems to reduce indirectly the rate of preterm birth. Acute infectious diseases of the respiratory system during the second and third gestational months of pregnancy were not associated with a higher risk for the total group or any specific group/entity of congenital abnormalities. However, frequently high-fever–related tonsillitis in pregnant women was associated with a higher risk for congenital cataract, neural-tube defects, cleft lip ± palate and unclassified multiple congenital abnormalities. We may suppose that the association between these fever-sensitive defect groups and tonsillitis may be caused by high fever, because the parallel antifever treatment was able to prevent this risk.

Finally, *influenza* during pregnancy was evaluated. The short duration of influenza in pregnant women did not increase the risk for pregnancy complications. Our study showed that the appropriately treated pregnant women affected with influenza in the first and second trimester of pregnancy have no higher risk for preterm birth. However, the high- fever–related influenza in the second and/or third gestational month of pregnancy may associate with a higher risk of some hyperthermia-sensitive CAs such as neural-tube defects, congenital cataract, cleft lip ± palate, cleft palate only, cardiovascular CAs, and unclassified multiple CAs. The main finding of our study is that this higher risk for these major CAs can be prevented by the parallel use of antifever drugs.

Introduction

Infectious diseases of the respiratory system frequently complicate pregnancy. Here we focus on the two main adverse pregnancy outcomes of pregnant women affected with infectious diseases of respiratory system: *preterm birth* and structural birth defects, and *congenital abnormalities*; in addition, we evaluate their pregnancy complications.

In Hungary, practically all deliveries took place in inpatient obstetric clinics, and birth attendants were obstetricians during the study period. Thus, both *birth weight* and *gestational age* at delivery were medically documented in the discharge summary of mothers after delivery. Gestational age was calculated from the first day of the last menstrual period. The definition of *preterm birth* was less than 37 completed weeks (less than 259 days), while the definition of low birth weight newborns was less than 2,500 grams.

Three groups of preterm births are worth differentiation: (i) spontaneous (about 50%), (ii) preterm premature membrane rupture (30%), and (iii) medically-induced preterm birth due to maternal and genital complications (20%) [1].

Birth defects—or, according to the World Health Organization's (WHO) term, *congenital anomalies*—are structural, functional and/or biochemical-molecular defects present at birth, whether detected at that time or not. Among the different categories of birth defects, congenital abnormalities (CAs)—i.e., structural-morphological defects—represent the largest one. CAs have two main medical characteristics: (i) defect conditions with a limited chance for complete recovery, and (ii) the earliest (fetal-birth) onset. Thus, there is only one optimal medical solution, and this is prevention.

The causes of CAs can be classified into three groups:

1. *Genetic,* which includes chromosomal aberrations (e.g., Down syndrome) and Mendelian single-gene defects (e.g., achondroplasia).
2. *Environmental,* which includes infectious agents (e.g., rubella virus), maternal diseases (e.g., diabetes mellitus), teratogenic drugs, alcohol, smoking and environmental pollutants.

3. *Complex* (multifactorial) origin caused by gene-environmental interaction when the so-called polygenic liability (predisposition) is triggered by environmental "risk" factors.

The purpose of this review is to evalute the possible association between *maternal infectious diseases of the respiratory system* in pregnant women and preterm birth or CAs on their offspring, in addition the pregnancy complications of mothers during the pregnancy study based on the data set of the Hungarian Case-Control Surveillance of Congenital Abnormalities (HCCSCA).

Hungarian Case-Control Surveillance of Congenital Abnormalities

The HCCSCA was established in 1980, and at present it is the largest population-based data set in the world of cases with different CAs and their matched controls [2]. *Cases* with CA were identified from the Hungarian Congenital Abnormality Registry [3], while *controls* without CA from the National Birth Registry. In general, two or three controls were matched to each case on the basis of three criteria: (i) same sex, (ii) same birth week and (iii) same district of parents' residence. In addition, a *malformed control group,* including cases with Down syndrome caused by non-disjunction before conception, was also selected from the Hungarian Congenital Abnormality Registry to better estimate the recall bias.

Three sources of information were used to obtain exposure data in the mothers of cases, controls and malformed controls:

i. *Prospective medically recorded data*. The mothers were asked to send us a prenatal care logbook and all other medical records (mainly discharge summaries). Prenatal care was mandatory for pregnant women in Hungary (if somebody did not visit prenatal care clinic, she did not receive a maternity grant and leave), thus nearly 100% of pregnant women visited prenatal care clinics, an average 7 times in their pregnancies. The task of obstetricians in the prenatal care is to record all pregnancy complications, maternal diseases and related drug prescriptions in the prenatal care logbook.
ii. *Retrospective maternal self-reported information*. A structured questionnaire, a list of maternal diseases and drugs as a memory aid, and informed consent were mailed to the mothers immediately after the selection of cases, controls and malformed controls. Mothers were asked to read the enclosed list of maternal diseases and drugs in order to refresh their memory, after this to complete the structured questionnaire, and to send them back with signed informed consent in our prepaid envelope.
iii. *Supplementary information from non-respondent mothers*. Regional nurses were asked to visit all non-respondent cases and malformed control mothers, in addition to 200 control mothers, to help the mothers fill out the same questionnaire, to evaluate available medical records and to obtain lifestyle data through a personal interview. Unfortunately, the Ethics Committee did not allow visiting all non-respondent

control mothers because—according to their opinion—this visit might disturb these families.

Most chronic diseases were prospectively and medically recorded mainly in prenatal logbooks. The proportion of medically recorded acute diseases depended on the severity of diseases. As our validation study [4] showed mainly severe acute diseases were recorded medically in prenatal logbook.

At the evaluation of pregnancy complications and birth outcomes, thus among others, preterm birth we used only controls in the data set of the HCCSCA. Cases with CA were excluded because CAs may have a more drastic effect for the incidence of pregnancy complications and birth outcomes (e.g., rate of preterm birth) than the maternal diseases studied.

The evaluation of possible association of maternal diseases with the higher risk for different CAs was based on the comparison of cases with CA and their matched controls without CA in the data set of the HCCSCA. The diagnosis of CAs is based on the report of medical doctors in the Hungarian Congenital Abnormality Registry, in addition the quality of CA-diagnosis is improved and specified better due to the results of recent medical examination in the HCCSCA. CAs are evaluated in the so-called *informative offspring*: live-born babies, stillborn fetuses and electively terminated pregnancies in the second and/or trimester after the prenatal diagnosis of fetal defect.

At the evaluation of CAs we follow the following principles:

4. CA cannot be regarded as a single homogeneous birth outcome because teratogenic factors such as maternal diseases (e.g., diabetes mellitus) or chemical teratogens such as drugs (e.g., retinoid acid-isotretinoin, hydantoin-phenytoin, valproate, warfarin) do not uniformly increase the rates of all CAs but rather tends to increase the occurrence of one or a limited number of specific CAs, therefore we have to evaluate CA-entities or CA-groups separately. First, the so-called isolated CAs (e.g., cleft lip) and multiple-syndromic CAs (e.g., cleft lip with cardiovascular CAs and hypospadias) are differentiated because their severity and etiology differ significantly. Second, 25 groups of isolated CAs are classified according to well-defined diagnostic criteria. Third, multiple CAs are classified as CA-syndromes and CA-associations while the group of unclassified multiple CAs includes unidentified (though previously delineated) and undelineated CA-syndromes and CA-associations, in addition random combinations of CAs.
5. Different CAs have different critical periods [5]. Previously the critical period of CAs was considered during the first 3 months of gestation, i.e., in the first trimester. However, *gestational time* is calculated from the first day of the last menstrual period and it is worth differentiating three time windows: (i) First month of gestation because it is before the organogenesis. The first two weeks are before conception while the third and fourth weeks comprise the pre- and implantation period of zygotes and blastocysts including omnipotent stem cells. Thus CAs cannot be induced by environmental agents in the first month of gestation and it explains the "all-or-nothing effect" rule, i.e., total loss or normal further

development. (ii) The most sensitive, the so-called critical period for CAs. (iii) The "postcritical period" of CAs, i.e., pregnancy after the organ-forming period.

6. These facts explain why the previous use of first trimester concept is misleading, thus outdated [6]. The critical period of most major CAs occurs in the second and third gestational months; we used therefore this time window as the critical period of CAs in our population-based case-control studies [7-9]. However, it is well-known that human teratogens can induce CAs after the third gestational month, i.e., after the first trimester (e.g., hypospadias, undescended testis). This methodological problem encourages us to introduce a new critical time approach based on the specified critical periods of different CAs separately and our study showed that this is feasible [5], but we have to wait for the international consensus [10].
7. In general maternal diseases cannot be regarded homogeneous pathological conditions, e.g., pneumonia may have different etiology, thus we have to do our best to work homogeneous disease entities as much as possible.
8. At the evaluation of maternal diseases we have to consider related drug treatments, but we have to avoid the usual methodological errors in previous studies when drugs were combined as antibiotics, penicillins, tetracyclines, sulfonamides, etc because different drugs have different chemical structures, indications and routes of administration.
9. The validity of diagnosis of CAs and maternal diseases, in addition drug treatment can be improved with multiple sources of data, in addition extra validation studies.
10. Confounders such as maternal age, parity, socioeconomic status of pregnant women, etc. may modify the association studied, thus we have to calculate adjusted risk figures.
11. Among confounders the possible folic acid and/or multivitamin supplementation in the periconceptional period or in early pregnancy have some preventive effect of some CA, thus we have to consider this recently recognized effect as well [11-15].
12. We have to consider recall bias at the comparison of cases and controls. The birth of an infant with CA is a serious traumatic event for most mothers who therefore try to find a causal explanation such as diseases or drug uses during pregnancy for CA of their babies. This does not occur after the birth of a healthy newborn infant. Thus recall bias might inflate an increased risk for CAs. Our previous analysis showed that a case-control surveillance of this type may cause spurious association between drugs and CAs with biased risk (odds ratio) up to a factor of 1.9 [16]. There are three possibilities to restrict or exclude recall bias: (i) the evaluation of exposures only during the critical period of CAs because we expect an underreporting of exposure in both the critical and non-critical periods of CAs in the control group, (ii) the use of prospectively and medically recorded data as a gold standard, and (iii) comparison between cases with CA and malformed control (cases affected with Dow syndrome caused by numerical chromosomal aberration in the preconceptional period) because the mothers of malformed controls have similar recall.
13. Multiple comparisons may produce a non-causal association because a significant difference is expected in every 20th estimation as a result of chance.

14. The first thought after the recognition of an association should be the exclusion of all possible biases and chance.

Here we evaluate the data set of the HCCSCA, 1980–1996 because after 1996 the collection of data has been changed (all mothers are visited at home by regional nurses) but the data have not been validated. Thus our previous publications were based on the data set of 17 years between 1980 and 1986.

Table 1 shows the number and percentage rate of more frequent maternal infectious diseases of respiratory system (which occurred in 10 or more mothers in either group) in the group of cases (including 22,843 informative offspring) and controls (containing 38,151 newborn infants).

Table l. The number and rate (%) of more frequent maternal infectious diseases of respiratory system during pregnancy in the case and control groups of the HCCSCA

Infectious diseases of respiratory system	Case group		Control group	
	No.	%	No.	%
Acute respiratory infections				
Common cold (nasopharyngitis)	3,827	16.8	5,475	14.4
Acute sinusitis	141	0.6	250	0.7
Acute pharyngitis	641	2.8	1,048	2.8
Acute tonsillitis	674	3.0	1,165	3.1
Acute laryngitis-tracheitis	404	1.8	804	2.1
Acute bronchitis-bronchiolitis	339	1.5	398	1.0
Pneumonia	116	0.5	182	0.5
Others (pleurisy)	8	0.0	12	0.0
Influenza	1,328	5.8	1,838	4.8
Chronic infectious diseases				
Chronic bronchitis	13	0.1	16	0.1

Non-infectious diseases of respiratory system such as allergic rhinitis (hay fever), asthma bronchiale, emphysema, pneumothorax, epistaxis (from nose), in addition tuberculosis are excluded from this analysis. Influenza is the disease of the whole human body, but the predominance of symptoms is connected with the respiratory system, thus we evaluate this viral disease here.

Respiratory System and Function during Pregnancy

The proper function of respiratory system in collaboration with cardiovascular system is extremely important to achieve adequate oxygenation of the fetus therefore there are significant changes in the maternal cardiorespiratory system during pregnancy.

First the anatomic changes of the respiratory system in pregnant women are summarized [17]. The level of the diaphragm rises by 4 cm and the transverse diameter of the chest increases by 2 cm, in addition the so-called subcostal angle increases from 68 to 103 degrees. These changes together the enlarging uterus result in a decrease in residual volume because lungs are somewhat compressed. However, the decrease of residual lung volume does not associate with decreased ventilation because the excursion of the diaphragm in respiration increases by 1.5 cm.

Though there is no increase in respiratory rate, maternal minute ventilation is increased due to an increase of tidal volume (about 500 to 700 ml in each breath). This hyperventilation results in a compensatory alkalosis and an increase in arterial oxygenation tension in the third trimester of pregnancy. The residual volume is reduced by 20% during pregnancy, but the vital capacity (i.e., the maximum volume of gas that can be expired after a maximum inspiration) does not change during pregnancy [17]

Second, the oxygen delivery and consumption in pregnancy are also changed partly due to the physiological anemia of pregnancy because it results in a reduction in the hemoglobin concentration and arterial oxygen content. Oxygen consumption increases steadily during pregnancy.

Third, at the evaluation of infectious diseases of respiratory diseases we have to consider the immunology of pregnancy. In general, immune function is similar in pregnant and non-pregnant women. However, both T-cell and NK-cell function shows a decrease in pregnant women. Nevertheless there is no clear trend toward either the suppression or enhancement of systematic immune function during gestation [18].

Common Cold

The common cold is a conventional term for mild upper respiratory illnesses caused by different microorganisms mainly from the virus family of picornoviridae (rhinoviruses, echoviruses, coxsackie viruses) influenza, parainfluenza, metapneumovirus, adeno- and respiratory syncytial viruses [19]. The common cold is manifested such as acute coryza or nasopharingitis with the symptoms of nasal stuffiness and discharge, sneezing, sore throat, and cough, in general without fever [20]. However, common cold is frequently followed by secondary complications including fever.

The common cold is the most frequently reported maternal disorders during pregnancy in Hungary (Table 1). The data set of the HCCSCA included 3,827 cases with CA, 5,475 controls without CA and 144 malformed controls affected with Down syndrome (the total group includes 834 malformed controls). The seasonal monthly distribution of common cold showed a higher occurrence between October and February with a peak in December. The usual duration of common cold was one week without secondary complications. However, about two-third of our pregnant women affected with common cold had a longer duration due to secondary complications including sinusitis, otitis media, laryngitis, tracheitis, bronchitis, etc and in general these mothers had fever (and antifever therapy).

At the analysis of our data in the HCCSCA [7, 21, 22] showed that about 50% of common cold was medically recorded in the prenatal care logbook. Major part of these pregnant women had secondary complications on the basis of longer duration of diseases and high fever (over 38.5 degree Celsius) in 57% of pregnant women. Thus, data shown here may reflect mainly pregnant women with more severe common cold with secondary complications.

Common cold was diagnosed in all gestational months with the somewhat higher prevalence in third-fifth gestational months.

Table 2 shows the incidence of pregnancy complications in pregnant women with or without common cold as a reference group. The proportion of anemia was larger, while the rate of threatened preterm delivery was smaller in mothers with common cold than in the reference group. The higher rate of anemia was in agreement with the lower intake of iron in pregnant women with common cold.

Table 2. Incidence of pregnancy complications in pregnant women with or without common cold during pregnancy

Pregnancy complications	Pregnant women with common cold %	Pregnant women without common cold %	Comparison OR (95% CI)
Nausea and vomiting, severe	9.1	10.3	0.9 (0.8 – 1.0)
Threatened abortion	16.2	17.2	0.9 (0.9 – 1.0)
Pre-eclampsia	8.4	8.5	1.0 (0.9 – 1.1)
Threatened preterm delivery	10.4	15.0	0.7 (0.6 – 0.7)
Placental disorders	1.2	1.6	0.7 (0.6 – 1.0)
Poly/oligohydramnios	0.6	0.5	1.1 (0.7 – 1.5)
Gestational diabetes	0.5	0.7	0.7 (0.5 – 1.0)
Anemia	18.9	16.3	1.2 (1.1 – 1.3)

Table 3 summarizes the birth/pregnancy outcomes of pregnant women with or without common cold. There was no difference in the sex ratio and in the rate of twins between the two study groups. Mean gestation age was 0.1 week shorter and this finding was agreement with the somewhat higher rate of preterm birth in the babies of pregnant women with common cold compared to the reference group. However, the mean birth weight was larger by 34 gram and the rate of low birth weigh newborns was lower in babies of mothers with common cold during pregnancy.

Table 3. Data of birth outcomes of newborn infants born to mothers with or without common cold

Birth outcomes	Newborn infants born to mothers with common cold	Newborn infants born to mothers without common cold	Comparison
Quantitative	Mean (S.D.)	Mean (S.D.)	t-test
Gestational age at delivery	39.3 (2.0)	39.4 (2.1)	p=0.01
Birth weight	3,305 (487)	3,271 (51)	p=0.01
Categorical	%	%	OR (95% CI)
Preterm birth	9.6	9.1	1.2 (1.1 – 1.5)
Low birth weight	4.2	5.9	0.8 (0.7 – 0.9)

On one hand, the somewhat shorter gestational age at delivery and higher rate of preterm birth were in agreement with the symptoms of pregnant women with the fever-related common cold with secondary complications though a lower rate of threatened preterm delivery was recorded among these females. On the other hand there was a somewhat larger birth weight and lower rate of low birth weight in newborn infants born to mothers with common cold, in general with secondary complications. These surprising findings need confirmation or rejection in further studies. At present our hypothesis is that the anxiety caused by the severe but relatively short (2 weeks) common cold resulted in an improved lifestyle (a higher rate of smoking cessation and vitamin use) in the further part, mainly during the third trimester of pregnancy, when there is the most intensive fetal growth.

Antifever drugs (acetylsalicylic acid, paracetamol and dipyrone) and antimicrobial drugs (such as ampicillin, penamecillin, clotrimazole) were used more frequently by pregnant women with common cold. However, there was no significant difference in the use of these drugs between case and control mothers with common cold.

Among pregnancy supplement, the use of folic acid was somewhat lower in case mothers than control mothers with common cold (48.6% vs. 52.1%, OR with 95% CI: 0.9, 0.8-1.0). The intake of vitamin C was much more frequent in mother with common cold than in mothers without common cold.

Our main aim was to study the possible association of maternal common cold with a higher risk for CAs.

First, the possible association of maternal common cold (mainly with secondary complications) in the second and/or third gestational month with 25 isolated CA groups and 1 unclassified multiple CA group was evaluated in the cases-all matched control analysis and a higher risk for 8 CA-groups were found (Table 4). However, this risk disappeared in the group of neural-tube defects at the evaluation of only medically recorded common cold. At the comparison of all cases with malformed controls (i.e., Down syndrome) with similar recall (bias), only congenital cataract and cleft lip ± palate showed a higher risk.

Table 4. Estimation of the association of maternal common cold (in general with secondary complications) in the second and/or third gestational month of pregnancy with 7 CA groups/entities in all cases-matched control analysis with or without antifever drug treatments, in cases and their matched controls with only medically recorded common cold, finally in all cases-malformed control analysis

CA groups / entities	Cases—all matched controls OR (95% CI)	Antifever drugs* with OR (95% CI)	Antifever drugs* without OR (95% CI)	Medically recorded OR (95% CI)	Comparison with malformed controls OR (95% CI)
Isolated					
Neural-tube defects	1.7 (1.3 –2.4)	1.0 (0.6 – 1.7)	2.4 (1.9 – 3.0)	1.5 (0.9 – 2.4)	1.3 (0.9 – 1.9)
Congenital hydrocephaly	6.3 (2.7 – 14.8)	2.1 (0.7 – 6.8)	2.6 (1.7 – 4.0)	3.6 (1.3 – 9.7)	1.5 (0.9 – 2.5)
Congenital cataract**	4.0 (1.7 – 9.2)	0.6 (0.1 – 4.0)	11.1 (5.3 – 23.3)	3.6 (1.6 – 8.2)	4.0 (2.6 – 6.2)
Cleft lip ± palate	3.2 (2.3 – 4.3)	1.4 (0.9 – 2.2)	2.9 (2.4 – 3.6)	2.3 (1.5 – 3.6)	1.7 (1.2 – 2.5)
Cleft palate only	2.0 (1.3 – 3.3)	1.2 (0.6 – 2.4)	1.7 (1.2 – 2.5)	2.3 (1.2 – 4.1)	1.1 (0.7 – 1.8)
Cardiovascular CAs	1.5 (1.3 – 1.8)	1.0 (0.7 – 1.3)	1.5 (1.3 – 1.8)	1.5 (1.2 – 2.0)	1.0 (0.7 – 1.3)
Limb deficiencies	1.7 (1.1 – 2.7)	1.2 (0.6 – 2.3)	1.8 (1.2 – 2.6)	2.2 (1.1 – 4.1)	1.2 (0.8 – 1.9)
Unclassified multiple CAs	2.1 (1.6 – 2.9)	1.3 (0.8 – 2.0)	2.0 (1.6 – 2.6)	2.0 (1.4 – 2.9)	1.3 (0.9 – 1.9)
Grand total	1.5 (1.4 – 1.6)	-	-	1.4 (1.3 – 1.6)	1.0 (0.8 – 1.2)

*unmatched analysis

**common cold and influenza were combined

These analyses clearly demonstrated the importance of methodology in the human studies of teratogenic and maternal effects, e.g., the exclusion of recall bias by the comparison of case and malformed controls. However, our study showed an association of maternal common cold with congenital cataract and cleft lip + palate if maternal disease occurred in the critical period of this CA. The explanation for this association may be the high fever, because this association was prevented by the parallel antifever drug treatment (Table 4). We cannot exclude the possible association between maternal common cold with secondary complications and the previously mentioned other CAs but these possible associations were also prevented with antifever drug treatments.

At the evaluation of the association of maternal severe complicated common cold with congenital cataract and cleft lip + palate, in addition possible others CAs we have to differentiate the possible teratogenic effect of microbial agents of common cold, secondary complications with fever, medications and malnourishment. We did not find any report regarding the teratogenic effect of microbial agents having a role in the origin of common cold [23]. Antifever drugs used for the treatment of common cold did not show teratogenic effect [24, 25]. Severe malnourishment may cause folate deficiency thus indirectly predisposition for some CAs [26], but most common colds are not so severe and long that can induce real malnourishment. Thus we may suppose that fever may be the causal factor similar to influenza in the origin of "hyperthermia sensitive" CAs. The importance of high fever will be discussed in the Discussion part of this paper.

Previously Kruppa et al. [27] found a possible association between anencephaly (the most severe form of neural-tube defects) and maternal common cold, while Zhang and Cai [28] reported an association between common cold and neural-tube defects, hydrocephalus and cleft lip + palate.

In conclusion, at the evaluation of common cold, it is necessary to differentiate the usual common cold (with short duration and without fever) and common cold with secondary complications (i.e., with longer duration and frequently high fever). Pregnant women with common cold mainly with secondary complications had not a higher incidence of pregnancy complications. The gestational age at delivery was 0.1 week shorter with a somewhat higher rate of preterm birth, but these differences had no real clinical importance. However, an association of common cold with secondary complications in the second and/or third gestational month of pregnancy with a higher rate of newborns with congenital cataract, cleft lip + palate and possible some other specific congenital abnormalities was found and these associations were preventable with antifever drug treatments

Acute Infectious Diseases of the Respiratory System

Acute infectious diseases of respiratory system (AIDRS) represent a wide spectrum, and according to International Classification of Diseases, WHO, we differentiate sinusitis, pharyngitis, tonsillitis, laryngitis-tracheitis, bronchitis-bronchiolitis and pneumonia. As it appeared at the analysis of our data, it is worth separating upper/mild category of AIDRS including sinusitis, pharyngitis, tonsillitis, laryngitis-tracheitis and lower/severe category of AIDRS comprising of bronchitis-bronchiolitis, pneumonia.

AIDRS, particularly uncontrolled or poor controlled, may cause both maternal and fetal morbity and mortality [29], nevertheless the possible associations of AIDRS with birth outcomes and CAs, in addition pregnancy complications have not been frequently studied [30].

The data set of the HCCSCA included 2,118 cases, 3,455 controls and 92 malformed controls born to mothers with AIDRS during the study pregnancy [8, 22, 31] The duration of AIDRS was 1.2 $\pm$ 0.4 week in our pregnant women, though the duration of AIDRS and the proportion of medically recorded diseases depended on the severity of AIDRS (e.g., the latter was nearly 100% in the group of pneumonia). Hospitalization occurred only in pregnant women with pneumonia. AIDRS were recorded more frequently in the 3rd gestational month followed by 4th and 5th month. The monthly distribution of AIDRS showed some seasonality, the maximum was found in January followed by February, while the minimum occurred in July followed by August.

First the incidence of pregnancy complications in pregnant women with or without AIDRS as reference group was compared (Table 5).

The occurrence of pre-eclampsia was lower in pregnant women with AIDRS than in pregnant women without AIDRS. On the other hand, the rarely occurring poly/oligohydramnios was somewhat higher among pregnant women with AIDRS.

In the second step we evaluated the incidence of pregnancy complications in different groups of AIDRS.

Nausea and vomiting in pregnancy was evaluated in the whole groups (based on both medically recorded and maternal reported information) and in the subgroups based only on medically recorded nausea and vomiting in the prenatal logbook. The latter group represented the severe form with medical treatment. The groups of upper AIDRS category showed a somewhat higher value (52.4%) than the groups of lower AIDRS category (48.4%), and this trend occurred in the prevalence of severe nausea and vomiting as well (10.7% vs. 6.2%). These findings are worth mentioning because nausea and vomiting in pregnancy seems to have a protective affect of fetal death [32] and CAs [33].

The occurrence of both threatened abortion and pre-eclampsia reflected a U-shaped severity curve; they showed the highest prevalence in the groups of pneumonia and sinusitis. Threatened preterm delivery and gestational diabetes occurred most frequently in the group of sinusitis. The occurrence of placental disorders and poly/oligohydramnios was found most frequently in the group of pharyngitis. However, these differences can be explained mainly by the chance.

Table 6 summarizes the birth/pregnancy outcomes of pregnant women with or without AIDRS.

There was no difference in the sex ratio and in the rate of twins between the study groups. Mean gestation age was 0.3 week longer of pregnant women with AIDRS and this finding was agreement with the lower rate of preterm birth in their babies compared to the reference group. However, the mean birth weight was also by 57 gram larger and the rate of low birth weigh newborns was somewhat but not significantly lower in newborn infants born to mothers with AIDRS during pregnancy. However, the larger mean birth weight can be explained by the longer mean gestational age at delivery.

The detailed analysis of these variables in the different groups of AIDRS showed a different and interesting pattern. There was a significantly shorter mean gestational age at delivery and higher rate of preterm birth in lower AIDRS category while upper AIDRS category associated with a longer mean gestational age at delivery and lower rate of preterm birth compared to the reference group, i.e., pregnant women without AIDRS. We did not find significant differences in the mean birth weight and the rate of low birth weight newborns between upper and lower AIDRS categories at the calculation of adjusted risk figures, i.e., considered confounders (among them gestational age).

We repeated these calculations based on only medically recorded AIDRS, and similar associations were found among drugs, antimicrobial (ampicillin, penamecillin) and antifever (acetylsalicylic acid, paracetamol, aminophenazone) drugs had a more frequent use in mothers with AIDRS, but there was no significant difference in their use between case and control mothers affected with AIDRS. The use of pregnancy supplements such as folic acid and multivitamins was similar in pregnant women with or without AIDRS, only vitamin C was used more frequently by pregnant women affected with AIDRS.

Table 5. Incidence of pregnancy complications in pregnant women with different groups of acute infectious diseases of respiratory system and the reference group (pregnant women without these diseases)

Pregnancy complications	Sinusitis (N=250)	Pharyngitis (N=1,048)	Tonsillitis (N=1,165)	Laryngitis-tracheitis (N=804)	Bronchitis-broncholitis (N=308)	Pneumonia (N=182)	Total (N=3,455)* No.	%	Reference (N=34,696)		Comparison OR (95% CI)
Nausea/vomiting	53.2	50.9	53.6	52.5	48.0	49.5	1,994	51.3	18,175	52.4	1.0 (0.9 – 1.1)
medically recorded	8.8	11.2	10.3	11.6	5.0	8.8	329	9.9	3,540	10.2	0.9 (0.8 – 1.0)
Threatened abortion	20.4	17.5	14.7	18.3	13.1	23.1	573	16.6	5,939	17.1	1.0 (0.9 – 1.1)
Pre-eclampsia	9.6	7.5	5.9	7.5	8.0	9.3	254	7.4	2,904	8.4	0.8 (0.7 – 0.9)
Threatened preterm delivery	20.0	12.6	14.5	14.9	5.8	10.4	455	13.2	4,992	14.4	0.9 (0.8 – 1.0)
Placental disorders	2.0	2.4	1.6	2.0	0.3	1.6	58	1.7	535	1.5	1.1 (0.8 – 1.4)
Poly/oligohydramnios	0.0	1.2	0.9	0.7	0.3	0.1	2.6	0.8	179	0.5	1.2 (0.8 – 1.2)
Gestational diabetes	1.2	0.9	0.9	0.5	0.3	0.0	22	0.6	248	0.7	0.9 (0.6 – 1.4)
Anemia	14.4	19.1	14.2	19.5	11.3	18.7	55.3	16.0	5,803	16.7	0.5 (0.8 – 1.0

Table 6. Birth outcomes of pregnant women with different manifestations of AIDRS and without AIDRS as reference

Different AIDRS	Gestational age at delivery (wk)		Preterm births		Birth weight weight (g)		Low birth newborns	
	Mean	S.D.	No.	%	Mean	S.D	No.	%
Sinusitis	39.6	1.7	14	5.6	3,348	489	13	5.2
Pharyngitis	39.6	1.7	61	5.8	3,364	476	36	3.4
Tonsillitis	39.7	1.9	63	5.4	3,340	500	56	4.8
Laryngitis – tracheitis	39.8	1.7	32	4.0	3,349	512	39	4.9
Bronchitis – bronchiolitis	39.1	2.3	49	12.3	3,271	534	26	6.5
Pneumonia	38.9	2.2	28	15.4	3,217	525	16	8.8
Total	39.6	1.9	233	6.7	3,328	503	172	5.0
Mild/upper	39.7	1.8	161	5.5	3,343	496	134	4.6
Severe/lower	39.1	2.3	75	13.0	3,255	528	40	6.9
Total	39.6	1.9	233	6.7	3,328	503	172	5.0
Comparison	<0.0001		0.7 (0.6 – 0.8)		<0.0001		0.9 (0.8 – 1.0)	
Reference (without AIDRS)	39.3	2.1	3,263	9.4	3,271	512	1,195	5.8

The association between severe lower category of AIDRS and higher rate of preterm birth is plausible due to the pathological condition of mothers related to fever, drug treatments, etc. However, the association between mild upper category of AIDRS and lower rate of preterm birth would need further explanation. On the one hand we may hypothesize that pregnant women with mild AIDRS later may be more health consciousness. On the other hand most pregnant women were treated by antimicrobial drugs, and some of them (e.g., ampicillin) may have a beneficial effect for the parallel existing sexually transmitted infections/diseases [34] which can induce preterm birth.

The prevalence of AIDRS in the second and/or third gestational months of pregnant women who later delivered cases with 26 CA-groups and their matched controls did not show significant difference in the total groups of CAs or any CA-entities or groups (Table 7).

However, at the analysis of different groups of AIDRS separately, tonsillitis in the second and/or third gestational months of pregnancy did not show an association with the total group of CAs, but 4 CA-groups/entities showed an association with this fever-related maternal diseases. Our validation study showed that 47.7% of pregnant women with tonsillitis had high fever. (The proportion of pregnant women with high fever was lower than 20% in other groups of AIDRS.) The highest OR was found in the group of cases affected with congenital cataract, followed by cases with unclassified multiple CA. The other two CA-groups represented the "hyperthermia sensitive" neural-tube defects and cleft lip + palate. Again we checked these data in the subgroups with and without antifever drug treatments, and the previously found associations disappeared in the subgroups of pregnant women with antifever drug treatment while these risks increased in the subgroups without this treatment.

Table 7. Estimation of association of maternal acute infectious diseases of respiratory system and tonsillitis in the second and/or third gestational month of pregnancy with or without antifever treatment

CA groups / entities	Cases—all matched controls OR (95% CI)	Tonsillitis OR (95% CI)	Antifever with treatment OR (95% CI)	Antifever without treatment OR (95% CI)
Isolated CAs				
Neural-tube defects	0.8 (0.6 – 1.2)	1.9 (1.4 – 2.7)	1.2 (0.6 – 2.3)	2.0 (1.4 – 2.8)
Congenital cataract	3.0 (0.8 – 12.0)	4.4 (1.3 – 14.0)	0.6 (0.1 – 4.0)	8.6 (4.0 – 15.1)
Cleft lip ± palate	1.2 (0.9 – 1.7)	1.6 (1.1 – 2.4)	0.6 (0.3 – 1.2)	1.8 (1.3 – 2.4)
Unclassified multiple CAs	1.0 (0.8 – 1.4)	2.2 (1.3 – 3.9)	1.9 (0.8 – 7.5)	2.5 (1.9 – 3.7)
Total	0.9 (0.8 – 1.0)	1.2 (0.6 – 1.4)	–	–

Previously mainly pneumonias in pregnant women were reported in the international literature. Pneumonia is rare during pregnancy, occurring in 1 per 118 to 2,288 [17], our figure 1 in 210 is nearer to the upper limit of this range. In most cases pathogens were not identified, however, other studies showed that pneumococcus and Haemophilus influenza are the most common identifiable causes of pneumonia in pregnant women [35, 36]. In the lack of comprehensive serologic testing, the true incidence of viral pneumonia, Legionella and mycoplasma pneumonia is difficult to estimate. In our material aspiration and varicella pneumonia, in addition HIV patients with pneumonia caused by Pneumocystis carinii or other agents did not occur.

Preterm delivery was found as a common complication (up to 43%) in pregnant women with pneumonia after the introduction of antibiotic therapy as well [35–37] with lower mean birth weight (2,770 + 224 vs. 3,173 + 99 g) in one study [35]. Our recent experiences were better in Hungarian pregnant women affected with pneumonia.

In conclusion, in general AIDRS during pregnancy have no obvious effect for pregnancy complications. However, severe lower category of AIDRS associated with a higher risk for preterm birth, but the mild upper category of AIDRS seems to reduce indirectly the rate of preterm birth. The latter finding needs further studies whether this association is causal or can be explained by unevaluated confounders. Finally AIDRS during the second and third gestational months of pregnancy did not associated with a higher risk for the total group of CAs or any group of specific CA-groups/entities. However, the frequently high-fever–related tonsillitis associated with a higher risk for congenital cataract, neural-tube defects, cleft lip + palate and multiple CAs. We may suppose that the association between these fever sensitive CA-groups and tonsillitis may be caused by high fever, because the parallel antifever treatment was able to prevent this risk.

Influenza

Influenza is an acute infectious disease caused by influenza A, B and C viruses which occurs as an epidemic, in general winter [38, 39]. Most epidemic infections are due to influenza A, and influenza epidemics were recorded in Hungary between December and April. The latency period is about 2 (1–5) days, the usual duration of influenza is 5 days in general with high fever, coryza, headache, malaise and cough. However, if symptoms persist longer than 5 days, in general secondary bacterial infections of the respiratory system occur [40].

Pregnant women may have a higher risk for influenza pneumonia, partly in new pandemics [41, 42]. For example mortality rate of pregnant women with influenza pneumonia was about 50% in 1918-1919 [43, 44].

The data set of the HCCSCA included 1,328 cases with CA and.1,838 controls without CA, in addition 36,313 pregnant women without influenza were considered as reference group [9, 22, 45]. All pregnant women were affected with influenza during the epidemic periods, and 72% of them were recorded in the prenatal care logbook. The onset of influenza according to gestational months did not show any obvious difference with the exception of low prevalence in the 9th month. In our study 91.5 % of pregnant women had fever over 38.5 Celsius degree according to our validation study.

First we evaluated pregnancy complications (Table 8). These pregnancy complications did not show a higher incidence in pregnant women affected with influenza.

Table 8. Incidence of pregnancy complications in pregnant women with or without influenza during pregnancy

Pregnancy complications	Pregnant women with influenza %	Pregnant women without influenza %	Comparison OR (with 95% CI)
Nausea and vomiting severe	9.4	10.2	0.9 (0.8 – 1.1)
Threatened abortion	19.0	17.0	1.1 (0.9 – 1.3)
Pre-eclampsia (hypertension, edema, proteinuria)	10.6	12.2	0.9 (0.7 – 1.1)
Threatened preterm delivery (incl. cervical incompetence)	15.2	15.8	1.0 (0.9 – 1.1)
Placental disorders (placenta previa, premature separation of placenta, antepartum hemorrhage)	1.7	1.5	1.1 (0.8 – 1.6)
Poly/oligohydramnios	0.7	0.5	1.3 (0.7 – 1.6)
Gestational diabetes	0.9	0.7	1.3 (0.7 – 2.4)
Anemia	17.0	16.6	1.0 (0.9 – 1.2)

Table 9. Data of birth outcomes of newborn infants born to pregnant women with influenza or without influenza

Birth outcomes	Newborn infants born to pregnant women with influenza	without influenza	Comparison
Quantitative	Mean (S.D.)	Mean (S.D.)	Adjusted t
Gestational age at delivery	39.5 (1.9)	39.4 (2.1)	p=0.12
Birth weight	3,311 (492)	3,274 (512)	p=0.08
Categorical	%	%	Adjusted OR (95% CI)
Preterm birth	8.0	9.2	0.9 (0.8 – 1.1)
Low birth weight	4.7	5.7	0.9 (0.7 – 1.1)

The birth outcomes of newborn infants without CA born to mothers with influenza or without influenza as reference group during the study pregnancy were analyzed in the second step, and the results of this evaluation showed unexpected results (Table 9).

There was no difference in the sex ratio and in the rate of twins between the two study groups. Mean gestational age at delivery was 0.1 week longer, and in agreement with this finding, the rate of preterm birth was somewhat lower in newborn infants born to mother with influenza during pregnancy compared with the reference group, i.e., pregnant women without influenza. Mean birth weight was 37 g larger in live-born babies of pregnant women with influenza during pregnancy and this difference was reflected in the lower rate of low birth weight newborns as well. However, these differences were explained partly by the somewhat longer gestational age, partly maternal variables. The proportion of professionals was somewhat higher among pregnant women with influenza (14.2% vs. 11.3%), in addition pregnant women with influenza used more frequently vitamins (e.g., C. 9.1% vs. 4.2%, and multivitamins 7.6% vs. 6.5%). On the other hand, it is necessary to mention that influenza occurred rarely in the third trimester of pregnancy, thus our data are not appropriate to study the possible association of maternal influenza during the third trimester with higher risk for preterm birth.

Thus, the short duration of usual maternal influenza during the first and second trimesters of pregnancy does not induce a higher prevalence of unsuccessful birth/pregnancy outcomes. In fact we found a somewhat but significantly lower rate of preterm birth.

The major objective of our study was the evaluation of prevalence of maternal influenza in the second and/or third months of pregnancy, i.e., in the critical period of most major CAs (Table 10).

Of 26 CA-entities, five showed an association with maternal influenza. The higher risk for congenital cataract, cleft lip + cleft palate, neural-tube defects and cardiovascular CAs was significant, while cleft palate was near to the level of significance (and unmatched analysis resulted in a significant association).

Table 10. Estimation of the association (risk) of maternal influenza during the second and/or third gestational months of pregnancy with 5 CA groups in the cases-matched control analysis

Isolated CA-groups / entities	Case all matched controls OR (95% CI)	Antifever drugs with OR (95% CI)	Antifever drugs without OR (95% CI)
Neural-tube defect	1.9 (1.1 – 3.3)	0.7 (0.3 – 1.6)	2.7 (1.8 – 4.0)
Cong. cataract*	4.0 (1.7 – 9.2)***	0.6 (0.1 – 4.0)	11.1 (5.3 – 23.3)
Cleft lip ± palate	3.2 (2.0 – 5.3)	1.4 (0.8 – 2.5)	3.3 (2.4 – 4.7)
Cleft palate only	2.2 (0.9 – 5.1)*	1.3 (0.6 – 2.9)	2.5 (1.4 – 4.5)
Cardiovascular CA	1.7 (1.3 – 2.3)	1.4 (0.9 – 2.1)	1.7 (1.3 – 2.2)
Total	1.4 (1.3 – 1.6)	–	–

*Unmatched analyses showed OR (95% CI): 2.5 (1.6 – 4.0)
**Influenza and common cold were combined
***During entire pregnancy OR (95% CI): 7.4 (3.9 – 14.0)

In the next step we attempted to differentiate cases with the above five „candidate" CAs according to maternal influenza in the second and/or third months of gestation with or without antifever treatment. We did not find this association if maternal influenza was treated by antifever drugs (Table 9).

Our studies showed the importance of specificity of teratogens as one of the important rule of human teratology. At the evaluation of the possible association between maternal influenza and 26 different CAs, five showed a higher risk. Another important rule in human teratology is the time factor, i.e., critical period of different CAs. The previously mentioned association of maternal influenza with cleft lip + cleft palate, neural-tube defects, cardiovascular CAs and cleft palate was found if this maternal disease occurred in the critical period of these CAs. However, an obvious association was found between the maternal influenza and congenital cataract not only during the critical period of lens but during the entire pregnancy. Thus, congenital cataract is not only a defect of embryogenesis but it may be connected with the developmental disturbance of lens in the second and third trimesters of pregnancy.

At the evaluation of possible association between maternal influenza and neural-tube defects, cleft lip + cleft palate, cleft palate only, cardiovascular CAs, and congenital cataract, it is necessary to consider and differentiate the possible effect of pathogens (i.e., influenza viruses), symptoms of the disease, particularly high fever, medications and the secondary complications such as malnourishment. In the study by Shien et al. [46] influenza viruses did not cross the placenta until late in gestation period, i.e., after the critical period of CAs. In addition, influenza viruses caused fetal death in pregnant animals but not specific CAs. Thus, we may suppose that influenza viruses are not teratogenic. The different drugs used for the treatment for maternal influenza were evaluated in detail but these medications did not indicate any teratogenic effect [25]. In fact they showed an "anti-teratogenic" effect in our studies. The hazards of secondary complications of maternal influenza are difficult to exclude, but they exist in fetuses of all pregnant women and only 5 CAs showed association with maternal influenza. The common factor may be the high fever in the origin of these 5 CA-groups, and this hypothesis is confirmed by the protective effect of antifever drugs.

Hyperthermia-induced CAs were detected first in animal investigations [47, 48], however, later the evidences for human teratogenicity of high fever have been continuing to accumulate. Here only those CAs are mentioned which were found in our study associated with high fever-related influenza.

The association between high fever and isolated neural-tube defects was shown [48–60]. The spectrum of high fever-related CAs was expanded for cleft palate [61], cleft lip + palate [62] and cardiovascular CAs [63, 64]. However, to our best knowledge, the association of high fever with congenital cataract [22] and multiple CAs [65] were found by us, in addition we delineated the typical pattern of component CAs in high fever-related MCA-syndrome [66].

Previously Botto et al. [67] showed that the association of maternal fever with some CAs can be reduced by folic acid containing multivitamins. Our previous studies confirmed that the periconceptional high dose folic acid or folic acid containing multivitamin supplementation can also contribute to the prevention of neural-tube defects, oral clefts and cardiovascular CA due to influenza related hyperthermia [9, 68].

In conclusion, the short duration of influenza in pregnant women did not increase the risk for pregnancy complications. Our study showed that the appropriately treated pregnant women affected with influenza in the first and second trimester of pregnancy have no higher risk for preterm birth. However, the high fever-related influenza in the second and/or third gestational month of pregnancy may associate with a higher risk of some hyperthermia-sensitive CAs such as neural-tube defects, congenital cataract, cleft lip + palate, cleft palate only, cardiovascular CAs, and multiple CAs. The main finding of our study is that this higher risk for major CA can be prevented by the parallel use of antifever drugs.

Discussion

The evaluation of acute infectious diseases of the respiratory system in pregnant women was differentiated in three approaches.

The first approach included pregnancy complications, and our data did not detect any characteristic or clinically important association between maternal common cold, AIDRS, influenza and different pregnancy complications.

The second approach was connected with birth outcomes of newborn infants without CA born to mothers with common cold, AIDRS, and influenza during the pregnancy study. Our results were controversial, therefore unexpected. Pregnant women with a common cold (mainly with secondary complications), mild upper category of AIDRS and influenza were associated with a lower risk for preterm birth. Only the severe lower category of AIDRS was associated with a higher risk of preterm birth.

The third and main approach was the estimation of the possible association of acute infectious diseases of respiratory system in pregnant women (exactly in the second and/or third gestational months, i.e., the critical period of most major CAs) with CAs. Our studies showed some association of certain similar CAs with these maternal diseases, namely common cold with secondary complications, tonsillitis and influenza. We suppose that this CA pattern may be associated with the common denominator of these maternal diseases, i.e., high fever.

High temperature may result in arrest of mitotic activity and immediate death of cells in mitosis with threshold elevations (1.5–2.5 Celsius degrees) and a delayed death of cells, probably in S phase with higher elevation (3.5 or more Celsius degrees). Apoptosis is also affected by hyperthermia; in addition, high fever may cause micro-vascular disturbances leading to leakage, edema and hemorrhage. These pathological processes may be more obvious in embryos with extreme intensive development, particularly in certain critical locations, such as neural tube, eyes, face and cardiovascular system.

Of course, the teratogenic effect of maternal fever depends on the severity, duration and timing [68]. Over 40 degrees Celsius, there is no doubt regarding the teratogenic effect of fever; however, it is worth calculating a 38.5 degrees Celsius threshold. One or more days seem to be the critical duration of high fever. The timing of high fever determines the risk of specific CAs. If the neuronal cell population cannot recover from the antimitotic insult and heat stress response of high fever, mainly the development of the brain is affected. For example, if it occurs during the time of neural tube closure (i.e., between 21st and 28th postconceptional days, i.e., third postconceptional week), there is a higher risk for neural-tube defects [68].

"The prevention is better than cure"—we can translate this slogan for the prevention of CA due to high-fever–related acute infectious diseases of the respiratory system in pregnant women. Thus, it is worth recommending vaccination against influenza for women who are planning their pregnancy during the expected epidemic period. In addition, it is necessary to start the antifever therapy as soon as possible in pregnant women with fever-related acute infectious diseases of the respiratory system. This treatment may include both old-fashioned but not inefficient physical treatment (compress or Priessnitz method) and antifever drugs immediately after the diagnosis of fever-related respiratory diseases, particularly influenza in pregnancy, to prevent teratogenic hyperthermia. Finally, the periconceptional high dose folic acid or folic acid containing multivitamin supplementation can also contribute to the prevention of neural-tube defects, oral clefts and cardiovascular CA due to fever-related hyperthermia [9, 68].

General Conclusions

Maternal diseases are common during pregnancy, and some of them (e.g., diabetes mellitus and phenylketonuria) are well-known teratogenics. However, we have to widen the spectrum of these diseases with high-fever–related maternal diseases such as influenza, tonsillitis, and common cold with secondary complications.

In the past, the possible teratogenic effects of drugs have been studied frequently, but the potential hazards of underlying diseases were rarely evaluated. Our preliminary calculation is that the attributable risk of fever-related maternal diseases in the origin of CAs is obviously larger (about 5%) [68], while the attributable risk of all human teratogenic drugs used during pregnancy is 2% [25].

Thus, an important task is to systematically study the teratogenic and/or fetotoxic effects of all maternal diseases during pregnancy.

The teratogenic potential of high-fever–related maternal diseases is preventable with the reduction or avoidance of the teratogenic effect of hyperthermia using antifever therapy.

References

[1] Goldenberg RL, Culhane JF, Iams JD, Romero R. Epidemiology of preterm birth. *Lancet* 2008; 371: 75-84.

[2] Czeizel AE, Rockenbauer M, Siffel Cs, Varga E. Description and mission evaluation of the Hungarian Case-Control Surveillance of Congenital Abnormalities, 1980-1996. *Teratology* 2001; 63: 176-185.

[3] Czeizel AE. The first 25 years of the Hungarian Congenital Abnormality Registry. *Teratology* 1997; 55: 299-305.

[4] Czeizel AE, Petik D, Vargha P. Validation studies of drug exposures in pregnant women. *Pharmacoepid Drug Safety*. 2003; 12: 409-416.

[5] Czeizel AE, Puho HE, Ács N, Bánhidy F. Use of specified critical periods of congenital abnormalities instead of the first trimester concept. *Birth Def Res Part A* 2008; 82: 139-146.

[6] Czeizel AE. The first trimester concept is outdated. *Cong Anom (Kyoto)* 2001; 41: 204.

[7] Ács N, Bánhidy F, Puho HE, Czeizel AE. Population-based case-control study of the common cold during pregnancy and congenital abnormalities. *Eur J Epidemiol* 2006; 21: 65-75.

[8] Ács N, Bánhidy F, Puho HE, Czeizel AE. Acute respiratory infections during pregnancy and congenital abnormalities. A population-based case-control study. *Cong Anom (Kyoto)* 2006; 46: 86-96.

[9] Ács N, Bánhidy F, Puho HE, Czeizel AE. Maternal influenza during pregnancy and rijk of congenital abnormalities in offspring. *Birth Defects Res Part A* 2005; 73: 989-996.

[10] Czeizel AE. Specified critical period of different congenital abnormalities: A new approach fro human teratological studies. *Cong Anom (Kyoto)* 2008; 48: 103-109.

[11] Czeizel AE, Dudás I. Prevention of the first occurrence of neural-tube defects by periconceptional vitamin supplementation. *N Engl J Med* 1992; 327: 1832-1835.

[12] Czeizel AE. Prevention of congenital abnormalities by periconceptional multivitamin supplementation. *Br Med J* 1993; 306: 1645-1648.

[13] Czeizel AE. Reduction of urinary tract and cardiovascular defects by periconceptional multivitamin supplementation. *Am J Med Genet* 1996, 62: 179-183.

[14] Czeizel AE, Dobó M, Vargha P. Hungarian two-cohort controlled study of periconceptional multivitamin supplementation to prevent certain congenital abnormalities. *Birth Defects Res Part A.* 2004; 70: 853-861.

[15] Botto LD, Olney RS, Erickson JD. Vitamin supplements and the risk for congenital anomalies other than neural-tube defects. *Am J Med Genet Part C* 2004; 125C: 12-21.

[16] Rockenbauer M, Czeizel AE, Olsen J et al. Recall bias in a case-control study on the use of medicine during pregnancy. *Epidemiology* 2001; 12: 461-466.

[17] Whitty JE, Dombrowski MP. Respiratory disease in pregnancy. In: Creasy RK, Resnik MD (eds.): *Maternal-Fetal Medicine.* 5th ed. Saunders, Philadelphia, 2004.pp. 953-974.

[18] Silver RM, Peltier MR, Branch DW: The immunology of pregnancy. In: Creasy RK, Resnlk MD (eds.): *Maternal-Fetal Medicine.* 5th ed. Saunders, Philadelphia, 2004.pp.89-109.

[19] Makele MJ, Puhakka T, Ruskanen O et al. Viruses and bacteria in the etiology of common cold. *J Clin Microbiol* 1998; 36: 539-542.

[20] Heikkinen T, Jarvinen A. The common cold. *Lancet* 2003; 361: 51-59.

[21] Bánhidy F, Ács N, Puho HE, Czeizel AE. Pregnancy complications and delivery outcomes of pregnant women with common cold. *Cent Eur J Publ Health* 2006; 14: 12-16.

[22] Vogt G, Puhó E, Czeizel AE. Population-based case-control study of isolated congenital cataract. 2005. *Birth Defects Res Part A* 2005; 73: 997-1005.

[23] Roulston A, Marcellus RC, Branton PE. Viruses and apoptosis. *Ann Rec Microbiol* 1999; 53: 577-628.

[24] Heinonen OP, Slope D, Shapiro S. Birth Defects and drugs in Pregnancy. Publishing Sciences Group, Littleton, MA., 1977

[25] Bánhidy F, Lowry RB, Czeizel AE. Risk and benefit of drug use during pregnancy. *Int J Med Sci* 2005; 2: 100-106.

[26] Huang RF, Ho YH, Lin HL et al. Folate deficiency induces a cell-cycle-specific apoptosis in Hep62 cells. *J Nutr* 1999; 129: 25-31.

[27] Kruppa K, Holmberg PC, Kousma E et al. Anencephaly and maternal common cold. *Teratology* 1991; 44: 51-55.

[28] Zhang J, Cai WW. Association of the common cold in the first trimester of pregnancy with birth defects. *Pediatrics* 1993; 92: 559-563.

[29] Remington JS, Klein JO (eds.) Infectious Diseases in the fetus and newborn Infant. 4th ed., W. B. Saunders, Philadelphia.

[30] Hartert TV, Nenzil KM, Mitchel EE et al. Maternal morbidity and perinatal outcomes among pregnant women with respiratory hospitalization during influenza season. *Am J Obstet Gynecol* 2003; 189: 1705-1712.

[31] Bánhidy F, Ács N, Puho HE, Czeizel AE. Maternal acure respiratory infectious diseases during pregnancy and birth outcomes. *Eur J Epidemiol* 2008; 23: 29-35.

[32] Weigel MM, Weigel R. Nausea and vomiting o early pregnancy and pregnancy outcome. An epidemiological study. *Br J Obstet Gynaecol* 1989; 96: 1304-1311.

[33] Czeizel AE, Puho E, Ács N, Bánhidy F. Inverse association between severe nausea and vomiting in pregnancy and some congenital abnormalities. *Am J Med Genet* 2006; 140A: 453-462.

[34] Kazy Z. Puho HE, Czeizel AE. The possible preterm birth preventive effect of ampicillin during pregnancy. *Arch Gynecol* 2006; 274: 215-221.

[35] Madinger NE, Greenspoon JS, Gray-Ellrodt A. Pneumonia during pregnancy: Has modern technology improved maternal and fetal outcome? *Am J Obstet Gynecol* 1989; 161: 657-

[36] Berkovitz K, LaSala A. Risk factors associated with the increasing prevalence of pneumonia during pregnancy. *Am J Obstet Gynecol* 1990; 163: 981

[37] Benedetti TJ, Valle R, Ledger W. Antepartum pneumonia in pregnancy. *Am J Obstet Gynecol* 1982; 144: 412

[38] Roberts RB. Infectious Diseases: Pathogenesis, Diagnosis and Therapy. Years Book *Medical Publ, Chicago*, 1986.

[39] Parker MT, Collier LH. Topley Wilson Principle of Bacteriology, *Virology and Immunity.* Decker BC, Hamilton, Ontario, 1990.

[40] Berkow R, Fletchert AJ. The Merck Manual of Diagnosis and Therapy. 16th ed. *Merck and Co Inc*, Rahury, NY, 1992.

[41] Kort BA, Cefalo RC, Baker VV. Fatal influenza A pneumonia in pregnancy. *Am J Perinatol* 1986; 3: 179

[42] Mullooly JP, Barker WH, Nolan TF Jr. Risk of acute respiratory disease among pregnant women during influenza A epidemics. *Publ Health Rep* 1986; 101: 205-

[43] Harris JW. Influenza occurring in pregnant women. *Am J Med Ass* 1919; 72: 978-

[44] Freeman DW, Barno A. Death from Asian influenza associated with pregnancy. *Am J Obstet Gynecol* 1959; 78: 1172-

[45] Ács N, Bánhidy F, Puho E, Czeizel AE. Pregnancy complications and delivery outcomes of pregnant women with influenza. *J Mat-Fetal Neonat Med* 2006; 19: 135-140.

[46] Shien JH, Shiota K. Folic acid supplementation of pregnant mice suppresses heat-induced neural-tube defects in offspring. *J Nutr* 1999; 129: 2070-2073.

[47] Edwards MJ. Hyperthermia as a teratogen: A review of experimental studies and their clinical significance. *Terat Carcinog Mutag* 1986; 6: 563-582.

[48] Edwards MJ, Shiota K, Walsh DA, Smith MS. Hyperthermia and birth defects. *Reprod Toxicol* 1995; 411-425.

[49] Chance PF, Smith DW. Hyperthermia and meningomyelocele and anencephaly. *Lancet* 1978; 1: 769-770

[50] Halperin LR, Wilroy RS Jr. Maternal hyperthermia and neural-tube defects. *Lancet* 1978; 212-213.

[51] Miller P, Smith DW, Shepard TH. Hyperthermia as one possible etiology of anencephaly. *Lancet* 1978; 1: 519-521.

[52] Clarren SK, Smith DW, Harvey MAS, et al. Hyperthermia: A prospective evaluation of a possible teratogenic agent in man. *J Pediatr* 1979; 95: 81-83.

[53] Layde PM, Edmonds LD, Erickson JD. Maternal fever and neural-tube defects. *Teratology* 1980; 21: 105-108.

[54] Fisher NL, Smith DW. Occipital encephalocele and early gestational hyperthermia. *Pediatrics* 1981; 68: 480-483.

[55] Shiota K. Neural-tube defects and maternal hyperthermia in early pregnancy. Epidemiology in a human embryo population. *Am J Med Genet* 1982; 12: 281-288.

[56] Hunter AGW. Neural tube defects in eastern Ontario and western Quebec: Demography and family data. *Am J Med Genet* 1984; 19: 45-63.

[57] Milunsky A, Ulcickas M, Rothman KJ et al. Maternal heat exposure and neural-tube defects. *J Am Med Ass* 1992; 268: 882-885.

[58] Lynberg MC, Khoury MJ, Lu X, Cocian T. Maternal flu, fever and the risk of neural-tube defects: a population-based case-control study. *Am J Epidemiol* 1994; 140: 244-255.

[59] Shaw GM, Todoroff K, Velie EM, Lammer EJ. Maternal illness, including fever, and medication use as risk factors of neural-tube defects. *Teratology* 1998; 57: 1-7.

[60] Medveczky E, Puhó E, Czeizel AE. The evaluation of maternal illnesses in the origin of neural-tube defects. *Arch Obstet Gynec* 2004, 207: 244-251.

[61] Smith DW, Clarren SK, Harrey MA. Hyperthermia as a possible teratogenic agent. *J Pediatr* 1978; 92: 878-883.

[62] Métneki J, Puhó E, Czeizel AE. Maternal diseases and isolated orofacial clefts in Hungary. *Birth Defects Res Part A* 2005; 73: 617-623.

[63] Tikkanen J, Heinonen OP. Maternal hyperthermia during pregnancy and cardiovascular malformations in the offspring. *Eur J Epidemiol* 1991; 7: 628-635.

[64] Botto LD, Lynberg MC, Erickson JD. Congenital heart defects, maternal febrile illness, and multivamin use: a population-based study. *Epidemiology* 2001; 12: 485-490.

[65] Czeizel AE, Puho HE, Ács N, Bánhidy F. High fever-related maternal diseases as possible cause of multiple congenital abnormalities: A population-based case-control study. *Birth Defects Res Part A* 2007; 79: 544-551.

[66] Czeizel AE, Puho HE, Ács N, Bánhidy F. The delineation of a multiple congenital abnormality syndrome in the offspring of pregnant women with high fever related disorders – a population-based study. *Cong Anom (Kyoto)* 2008; 48:.

[67] Botto LD, Erickson JD, Mulinare J et al. Maternal fever, multivitamin use and selected birth defects: evidence or interaction. *Epidemiology* 2002; 13: 620-621.

[68] Czeizel AE, Ács N, Bánhidy F et al. Primary prevention of congenital abnormalities due to high fever related maternal diseases by antifever therapy and folic acid supplementation. *Current Woman's Health* 2007; 3: 1-12.

In: Infectious Pregnancy Complications
Editor: Richard N. Canfield
ISBN 978-1-60741-038-6

Chapter 16

Maternal Outcomes in Pregnancy with Smallpox: Epidemiologic Investigations of Case Fatality, Miscarriage and Premature Birth Based on Previous Outbreaks

Hiroshi Nishiura*
Theoretical Epidemiology, University of Utrecht
Yalelaan 7, 3584 CL, Utrecht, The Netherlands

Abstract

Objective: To assess the maternal outcomes and the characteristic features of pregnancy with smallpox.

Design: Retrospective collection and review of literature on previous smallpox outbreaks.

Setting: Case fatalities in 16 outbreaks and miscarriage and premature birth in 15 outbreaks in Europe, Australia and the United States during the 19th and 20th centuries.

Population: Pregnant smallpox cases at various gestational periods and with various vaccination histories.

Methods: Overall crude estimates of the outcomes were obtained based on the collected publications. Stratifications were then performed by gestational period, clinical classification of smallpox, and vaccination status.

Main outcome measures: Case fatality, and miscarriage and premature birth.

Results: Overall case fatality and the proportion of miscarriage and premature birth were estimated as 34.3% (95% confidence interval (CI); 31.4, 37.1) and 39.9% (36.5, 43.2), respectively. Although the estimate of case fatality was highest during the third trimester (40.5% (26.8, 54.2)), miscarriage and premature birth did not show a clear localised pattern according to gestational stage. Vaccination prior to pregnancy

* TEL: +31 30 253 1233 FAX: +31 30 252 1887, E-mail: h.nishiura@uu.nl

effectively reduced the risk of death in three outbreaks ($p < 0.01$, $p = 0.02$ and $p < 0.01$, respectively). Miscarriage and premature birth were frequently observed even among those with mild classifications of smallpox.

Conclusions: Despite the extremely high estimates of both outcomes, fatality can be lowered by vaccination prior to pregnancy. Nevertheless, it might be difficult to prevent cases from miscarriage and premature birth using vaccination only. The historical records appeared useful for clarifying the examined outcomes and in characterising the common patterns.

Introduction

Pregnant individuals are recognised as being at special risk of smallpox vaccine complications [1]. This topic has been discussed in detail based on published evidence, and consequently, vaccination of pregnant women is not recommended prior to the actual re-emergence of smallpox [2-4]. Although the epidemiologic parameters of smallpox have been extensively analysed and reviewed [5-6], maternal and perinatal outcomes have rarely been documented [7-9], despite the universal agreement that smallpox in pregnancy is much more severe than in non-pregnant individuals and adult males [5]. The understanding of this issue is supported by a limited number of epidemiologic studies during the mid-20th century that identified high case fatality [7-9] as well as an extremely severe course of pregnancy [7].

Being the first disease against which a vaccine became available and with the achievement of global eradication [5,10], and because outbreaks after the mid-20th century were accompanied by only a small number of pregnant cases except in limited areas in Africa and Central Asia, we lack a sufficient amount of statistical evidence on smallpox in pregnancy. The widely discussed possibility of a bioterrorist attack using variola virus makes re-evaluation and clarification of the epidemiology of smallpox essential. In line with this, historical records are a potentially valuable resource [11]. In this chapter, epidemiologic analysis of smallpox in pregnancy is performed based on outbreaks in Europe, Australia and the United States in the 19th and 20th centuries. Two maternal outcomes [12], (1) case fatality and (2) miscarriage and premature birth, were investigated and then stratified by gestational period, severity of smallpox, and vaccination prior to pregnancy to characterise key aspects of smallpox in pregnancy.

Methods

Search Strategy

Since the majority of documented large-scale outbreaks of smallpox were written before the mid-20th century, this chapter could not follow formal methods of systematic review, i.e., using MEDLINE or other databases. Consequently, this chapter firstly tracked selected references in major specialised books [5,13-15] and articles on smallpox or viral diseases after the mid-20th century [7,16-18]. These references [19-22] were subsequently reviewed and their references were further tracked, regardless of language, in search of potentially useful articles. This task was repeated as many times as necessary until no further references were identified (Figure 1). Consequently, references dating back to the 19th century were reviewed.

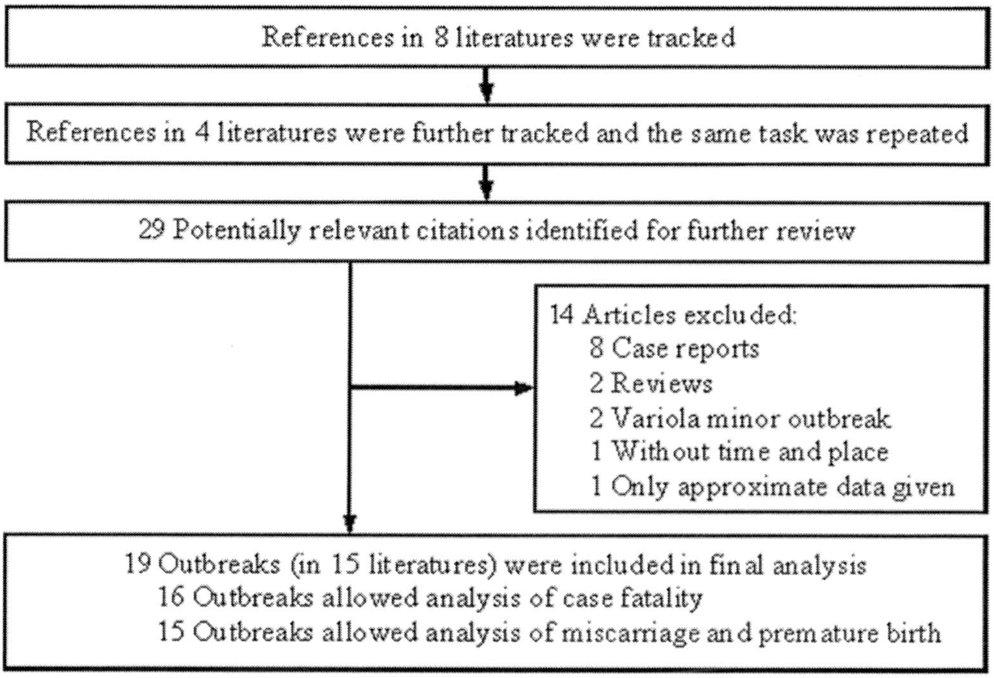

Figure 1. Flow diagram of study selection process.

Study Selection Criteria

First, all publications reporting either of the defined maternal outcomes of smallpox, i.e., case fatality and miscarriage and premature birth, were selected. Second, the obtained publications were limited by the following inclusion criteria: the publication (1) documents more than 8 smallpox cases during pregnancy (cxclusion of case reports), (2) clarifies the time as well as place of the outbreak, (3) reports an outbreak of variola major (not variola minor) and (4) explicitly defines and describes either of the outcomes as one of the major topics of discussion. All selected publications were retrospective studies based on epidemiologic observations of outbreaks.

Statistical Analysis

Since crude case fatalities and frequencies of miscarriage and premature birth could be biased by several serious underlying factors, i.e., vaccination and progress in obstetrics and medicine on a whole, the heterogeneity of which cannot be methodologically adjusted, interpretation of the obtained findings after combination of the data following statistical adjustment was deemed inappropriate in this study. Thus, the data analysis did not follow usual methods of meta-analysis for estimation of combined case fatality and the proportion of miscarriage and premature birth. Rather, the outcomes, except overall crude estimates, were investigated by each publication where possible. Both outcomes were then stratified by (1) gestational period at onset of smallpox (3 months precision), (2) clinical classification of smallpox and (3) vaccination history. The frequency of miscarriage and premature birth was also stratified by clinical stage of smallpox (dates after onset of fever), and comparisons of the outcome were made according to prior history of miscarriage and delivery. Case fatality was also compared between non-pregnant and pregnant individuals using univariate analysis. The χ^2 and Fisher's exact tests were used to evaluate univariate associations. Confidence intervals (CI) for a proportion, p, were obtained using the standard error, $\sqrt{\frac{p(1-p)}{N}}$, where N is the sample size. Statistical data were analysed using the statistical software JMP IN ver. 5.1 (SAS Institute Inc., Cary, NC).

Results

Identification of Previous Studies

A total of 19 outbreaks were identified from historical records [7,22-35], and of these, 16 and 15 enabled estimation of the case fatality and the proportion of miscarriage and premature birth, respectively (Figure 1). The original reports were written in Dutch, English, French, German and Italian. Half originated from a review article published in 1932 [20]. Thirteen literatures were firstly excluded: 8 were clinical case reports [36-43], one did not clarify time and place of the outbreak and showed the exactly same number of cases and deaths in another literature included for analysis [44], 2 were variola minor outbreaks [16,19], and the remaining 2 were review papers that did not provide the outcomes [45,46] (Figure 1). Further, a relatively recent study by Dixon in Tripolitania was also excluded because only approximate case fatalities (40% and 11% for pregnant and non-pregnant cases, respectively) were given [9]. Consequently, 368 deaths from a total of 1074 pregnant cases (Figure 2a) and 331 miscarriages or premature births from a total of 830 pregnant cases (Figure 2b) were identified. Accordingly, the mean number of smallpox deaths among a mean of 63.2 (standard deviation (SD) = 74.0; median = 36.5) pregnant cases was 21.6 (SD= 26.0; median = 13.5), while the mean number of miscarriages and premature births among a mean of 55.3 (SD = 61.4; median = 28.0) pregnant cases was 22.1 (SD = 19.1; median = 14.0). The raw data used for obtaining crude estimates are shown in Figure 2. Since individual case records were provided for the outbreaks in Philadelphia [25], Paris [33] and New South Wales [34], these data are also provided anonymously as supplementary material in the original publication (www.cdc.gov/ncidod/EID/vol12no07/05-1531.htm). Four individuals in the New South Wales report [34] were excluded from the following analyses because they contracted smallpox after delivery.

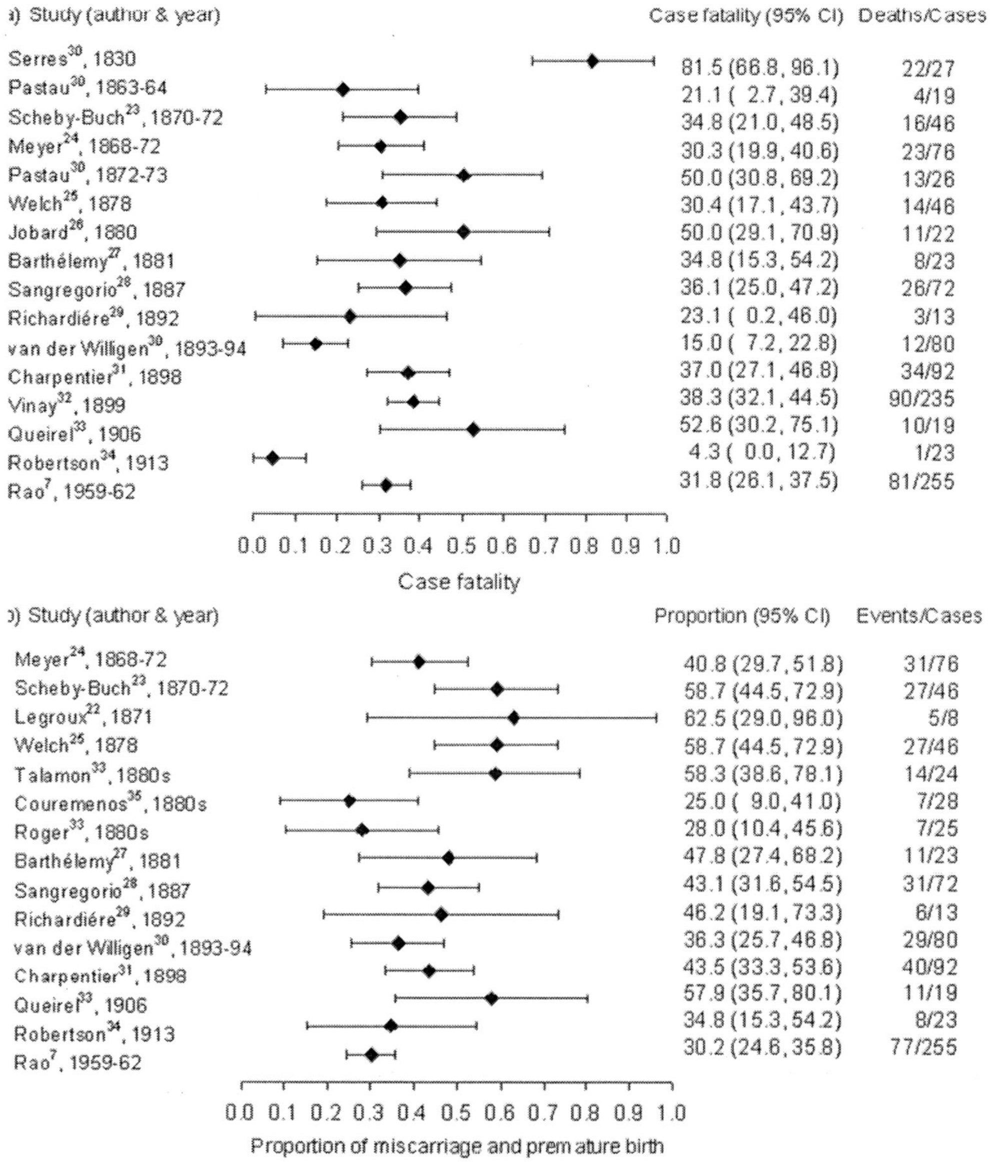

a) Case fatality and b) the proportion of miscarriage and premature birth are shown. Miscarriage and premature birth prior to maternal death are included.

Figure 2. Maternal outcomes in pregnancies complicated by smallpox, from data from the 19th and early 20th century outbreaks.

Case Fatality

Figure 2a shows the distribution of case fatalities for each outbreak estimated with corresponding 95% CI. Without adjustment for background characteristics, case fatalities varied widely among outbreaks: the earliest outbreak in 1830 (before compulsory vaccination practice) yielded the highest estimate (81.5%), while the outbreak in New South Wales in

1913 the lowest (4.3%). The overall crude case fatality was estimated to be 34.3% (95% CI; 31.4, 37.1). Case fatalities stratified by gestational age at onset of smallpox are given in Table 1a. Only four studies enabled stratification, and of these, only one, Rao's work [7] provided case fatalities by monthly intervals. Consequently, the results shown in the table are stratified by 3-month intervals of gestation following the remaining three studies. Despite the difficulty in direct comparisons due to the small sample sizes for each outbreak, case fatality showed the highest estimate during the third trimester except Queirel's study that was accompanied by scarcity of cases [33]. Table 2a shows case fatality stratified by the clinical classification of smallpox. Although Rao additionally took into account the speed of rash spread in his original clinical classifications, this was ignored and only the extent of rash on the patients' body was used for comparisons of severity (for details of Rao's classifications, see his original literature and review [7,14]). Whereas all hemorrhagic cases resulted in death, cases without a rash (variola sine eruptione, VSE) were not fatal.

Table 3a compares case fatality among pregnant and non-pregnant smallpox cases. Whereas case fatality was not significantly higher among pregnant cases than non-pregnant cases in Rotterdam ($p = 0.33$), where many VSE cases were observed (Table 2a), the risks of a fatal outcome among pregnant cases in Berlin and Madras were 2.5 and 4.2 times higher than that among non-pregnant cases ($p < 0.01$ for each).

Table 1. (a) Case fatality, and (b) miscarriage and premature birth among pregnant women with smallpox, by gestational period, from data from 19th and early 20th century outbreaks

a)	0-3 months		4-6 months		7-9 months	
Reference	D/C†	CF (95% CI) ‡	D/C	CF (95% CI)	D/C	CF (95% CI)
Meyer [24] 1868-72	3/33	9.0 (0.0, 18.9)	11/33	33.3 (17.2, 49.4)	8/10	80.0 (55.2, 100.0)
Welch [25], 1878	4/12	33.3 (6.7, 60.0)	4/22	18.2 (2.1, 34.3)	6/12	50.0 (21.7, 78.3)
Queirel [33], 1906	2/4	50.0 (1.0, 99.0)	7/10	14.5 (41.6, 98.4)	1/5	17.9 (0.0, 55.1)
Rao [7], 1959-62	7/21	33.3 (13.2, 53.5)	16/65	24.6 (14.1, 35.1)	34/94	36.2 (26.5, 45.9)
Total	16/70	22.9 (2.3, 43.4)	38/130	29.2 (14.8, 43.7)	49/121	40.5 (26.8, 54.2)
b)	0-3 months		4-6 months		7-9 months	
Reference	L/C ¶	PL (95% CI) $	L/C	PL (95% CI)	L/C	PL (95% CI)
Meyer [24], 1868-72	7/33	21.2 (7.3, 35.1)	16/33	48.5 (31.5, 65.4)	8/10	80.0 (55.3, 100.0)
Welch[25], 1878	8/12	66.7 (40.1, 93.2)	9/22	40.9 (20.5, 61.3)	10/12	83.3 (62.4, 100.0)
Queirel [33], 1906	3/4	75.0 (32.8, 100.0)	8/10	80.0 (55.3, 100.0)	0/5	0 (NC¶)
Robertson [34], 1913	1/2	50.0 (0.0, 100.0)	6/9	66.7 (36.0, 97.3)	1/12	8.3 (0.0, 23.9)
Rao [7], 1959-62	10/21	47.6 (26.4, 68.9)	16/65	24.6 (14.2, 35.0)	41/94	43.6 (33.6, 53.6)
Total	29/72	40.3 (29.0, 51.5)	55/139	39.6 (31.5, 47.7)	60/133	45.1 (36.7, 53.5)

†D/C, Smallpox deaths/cases; ‡CF, Case fatality with corresponding 95% confidence interval; ¶L/C, Miscarriage or premature birth / cases; $PL, Proportion of miscarriage and premature birth with corresponding 95% confidence interval; ¶NC, Not calculable.

Table 2. (a) Case fatality, and (b) miscarriage and premature birth among pregnant women with smallpox by clinical types of Variola major, from data from 19th and early 20th century outbreaks

a)	Hemorrhagic		Confluent		Discrete		VSE	
Reference	D/C†	CF (95% CI) ‡	D/C	CF (95% CI)	D/C	CF (95% CI)	D/C	CF (95% CI)
Meyer [24], 1868-72	13/13	100.0 (NC¶)	9/26	34.6 (16.3, 52.9)			0/37	0.0 (NC)
Sangregorio [28], 1887	3/3	100.0 (NC)	20/22	90.9 (78.9, 100.0)	3/40	7.5 (0.0, 15.7)	0/7	0.0 (NC)
van der Willigen [30], 1893-94	6/6	100.0 (NC)	4/4	100.0 (NC)	2/10	20.0 (0.0, 44.8)	0/60	0.0 (NC)
Charpentier [31], 1898	13/13	100.0 (NC)	17/34	50.0 (33.2, 66.80	4/45	8.9 (0.6, 17.2)		
Queirel [33], 1906	8/8	100.0 (NC)	2/3	66.7 (13.3, 100.0)	0/8	0.0 (NC)		
Rao [7], 1959-62	14/14	100.0 (NC)	12/32	37.5 (20.7, 54.3)	0/48	0.0 (NC)		

b)	Hemorrhagic		Confluent		Discrete		VSE	
Reference	L/C¶	PL (95% CI) $	L/C	PL (95% CI)	L/C	PL (95% CI)	L/C	PL (95% CI)
Meyer [24], 1868-72	13/13	100.0 (NC)	14/26	53.8 (34.7, 73.0)			4/37	10.8 (0.8, 20.8)
Sangregorio [28], 1887	3/3	100.0 (NC)	17/22	77.3 (59.8, 94.8)	10/40	25.0 (11.6, 38.4)	1/7	14.3 (0.0, 40.2)
Charpentier [31], 1898	13/13	100.0 (NC)	18/34	52.9 (36.2, 69.7)	9/45	20.0 (8.3, 31.7)		
Queirel [33], 1906	8/8	100.0 (NC)	3/3	100.0 (NC)	0/8	0.0 (NC)		

Hemorrhagic (widespread hemorrhages in the skin and mucous membranes); Confluent (confluent rash on the face and arms); Discrete (areas of normal skin visible between pustules, even on the face); and VSE (Variola sine eruptione: fever without rash caused by variola virus. Also known as varioloid) [14].

†D/C, Smallpox deaths/cases; ‡CF, Case fatality with corresponding 95% confidence interval; ¶L/C, Miscarriage or premature birth /cases;

$PL, Proportion of miscarriage or premature birth with corresponding 95% confidence interval; ¶NC, Not calculable.

Table 3. Comparison of the frequency of death in pregnant and non-pregnant cases, by vaccination history, from data from 19th and early 20th century outbreaks

a)	Non-pregnant		Pregnant			
Reference	Cases	Deaths	Cases	Deaths	p-value†	OR (95% CI) ‡
Meyer [24], 1868-72	1116	163	76	23	< 0.01	2.5 (1.5, 4.3)
van der Willigen[30], 1893-94	352	39	80	12	0.33	1.4 (0.7, 2.8)
Rao [7], 1959-62	348	29	94	26	< 0.01	4.2 (2.3, 7.6)
b)	Non-pregnant		Pregnant			
Reference	Cases	Hemorrhagic	Cases	Hemorrhagic	p-value†	OR (95% CI) ¶
van der Willigen[30], 1893-94	352	11	80	6	0.07	2.5 (0.9, 7.0)
Rao[7], 1959-62	348	13	94	14	< 0.01	4.5 (2.0, 10.0)
c)	Unvaccinated		Vaccinated			
Reference	Cases	Deaths	Cases	Deaths	p-value†	OR (95% CI) $
Welch[25], 1878	7	7	39	7	< 0.01	NC¶
van der Willigen[30], 1893-94	2	2	78	10	0.02	NC
Rao[7], 1959-62	12	9	82	17	< 0.01	11.5 (2.8, 47.1)

a) Fatality and b) severity stratified by pregnant and non-pregnant cases, and c) fatality among pregnant cases stratified by vaccination. †Two-sided; ‡Odds ratio of smallpox deaths and ¶odds ratio of hemorrhagic smallpox among pregnant women with corresponding 95% confidence intervals; $Odds ratio of smallpox deaths among unvaccinated cases; ¶NC, Not calculable.

Table 3b confirms that the difference in case fatality partly reflects the proportion of hemorrhagic cases. Comparisons between vaccinated and unvaccinated pregnant cases were also performed to assess whether vaccinated cases are protected, albeit even partially, from a fatal outcome (Table 3c). The risk of smallpox death was significantly higher among unvaccinated cases in these three outbreaks ($p < 0.01$, $p = 0.02$ and $p < 0.01$, respectively).

Miscarriage and Premature Birth

Crude proportions of miscarriage and premature birth are given in Figure 2b with corresponding 95% CI. No publication, except Rao's [7], explicitly distinguished between miscarriage and premature birth; in other words, in most studies they are described together. The overall crude proportion of miscarriage and premature birth was estimated to be 39.9% (95% CI; 36.5, 43.2). Five outbreaks allowed stratification by gestational period at onset of smallpox (Table 1b). The overall proportion of premature birth was highest during the last 3 months of pregnancy, but the frequency of miscarriage and premature birth did not show a clear localised pattern according to gestational period. The proportion of miscarriage and premature birth is stratified by severity of smallpox in Table 2b. All hemorrhagic cases given here resulted in either miscarriage or premature birth prior to the mother's death. It should be noted that even mild cases, those classified as discrete type and VSE, tended to result in miscarriage or premature birth.

Only the outbreak in Philadelphia in 1878 [25] allowed comparison between vaccinated and unvaccinated pregnant cases. Twenty-two (56.4%) and five (71.4%) cases experienced miscarriage or premature birth among 39 vaccinated and 7 unvaccinated cases, respectively, suggesting that in Philadelphia vaccination did not provide significant protection against either outcome (p = 0.68, odds ratio (OR) of miscarriage or premature birth while vaccinated = 0.5, 95% CI; 0.1, 3.0). Table 4 shows the frequency of miscarriage or premature birth by clinical stage of smallpox among a total of 27 cases in Philadelphia in 1878 [25]; all experienced miscarriage or premature birth at the given date of the illness. Fourteen cases (51.9%) experienced miscarriage or premature birth within 5 days after appearance of a rash, while the frequency among the remainder showed a long-tailed distribution.

Table 4. Frequency of miscarriage or premature birth with smallpox by clinical stage of symptoms in Philadelphia, 1878 (n = 27)†

Stage of illness	N
Prodromal period	1
Eruption day 1	4
Day 2	2
Day 3	3
Day 4	2
Day 5	2
Days 6-10	1
Days 11-20	1
Days 21-30	3
Day 31 onwards	3
No precise description	5
Total	27

†Frequencies were obtained from the records of ref.25.

Comparison of the outcomes by previous experience of miscarriage could only be performed for the outbreak in New South Wales in 1913 [35]. Two out of 3 (66.7%) cases with no experience and 6 out of 20 (30%) cases with previous experience of miscarriage resulted in miscarriage or premature birth, but this difference was not significant (p = 0.27, OR of miscarriage or premature birth among those with a previous experience of miscarriage = 4.7, 95% CI; 0.4, 61.8). Comparison by previous experience of normal delivery (primipara or multipara) could only be performed based on the outbreak in Rotterdam from 1893-94 [30]. Of 21 primipara and 53 multipara cases, 10 (47.6%) and 18 (34.0%) resulted in miscarriage or premature birth, respectively, suggesting that the frequency of the outcomes was not significantly influenced by previous delivery (p = 0.30, OR of miscarriage or premature birth among primipara cases = 1.8, 95% CI; 0.6, 4.9).

Conclusion

This chapter investigated the maternal outcomes of pregnancy with smallpox based on historical records. Estimates of the overall crude case fatality and proportion of miscarriage and premature birth were extremely high. Whereas case fatality was highest during the third trimester, the frequency of miscarriage and premature birth did not show a clear localised pattern according to gestation stage. With regard to the clinical classifications, hemorrhagic type showed a hopeless prognosis in all investigated outbreaks. Although fatal outcomes were very rare among mild types, miscarriage and premature birth were frequently observed. The outbreaks in Berlin and Madras confirmed that case fatality is higher among pregnant cases than non-pregnant cases, and the overall case fatality based on 16 outbreaks was rather high compared to that of the total population [47]. In contrast, no significant difference in case fatality between pregnant and non-pregnant cases was observed in the Rotterdam outbreak, mainly because of the high proportion of cases classified as VSE. Even after infection, vaccination prior to pregnancy appeared to reduce the risk of death effectively in three outbreaks. It is worth noting that the outbreak in 1830, before the introduction of compulsory vaccination programme, yielded the highest estimate of case fatality [30]. Analyses of miscarriage and premature birth in relation to vaccination status and previous experiences of miscarriage and delivery could only be conducted with one respective outbreak each. Although it is difficult to draw conclusions with a limited number of cases and single method, univariate analyses showed that miscarriage and premature birth were not significantly associated with these factors. No association between vaccination and miscarriage and premature birth was supported since the outcomes were observed even among mild cases. In Philadelphia, more than half the miscarriages and premature births were observed within the first 5 days after appearance of a rash.

Since the smallpox vaccination was effective in general and previous efforts achieved global eradication [1], outbreak sizes have been limited since the mid-20th century, and thus, only historical analyses allow epidemiologic clarification of maternal outcomes. This study improved our understanding of smallpox in pregnancy, in addition to the findings of Rao [7], highlighting the following: (1) case fatality was highest during the last 3 months of gestation, but the patterns of occurrence of miscarriage and premature birth were not clearly localised by gestational stage; (2) even mild cases were at high risk of miscarriage and premature birth; and (3) miscarriage and premature birth were not significantly associated with vaccination history and previous experiences of miscarriage and delivery. Consequently, it might be difficult to prevent cases from miscarriage and premature birth using vaccination only.

A few specific limitations of this study must be addressed. The first one is related to the underdiagnosis of pregnancy especially in the early gestational ages [48]. The definition of pregnancy-related deaths is still difficult to grasp the reality even in present days [49]. Whereas this could have led to overestimation of miscarriage, case fatality may hardly be influenced by this factor when the sample size is sufficiently large. Second, it is possible that waning vaccine-induced immunity also played a role. In addition to all-or-nothing effect (protection against disease) which may last for a few decades after vaccination [13,50,51], long-lasting residual protection (partial protection against smallpox death), which is thought to be sustained for some 50 years [51-53], could also be affected by pregnancy. The ignorance of time since successful vaccination could also partly explain why no significant difference in fatality between pregnant and non-pregnant cases was found in the Rotterdam outbreak. Third, regarding the validity of the statistical data, it should be noted that some of the earliest epidemiologic studies were performed prior to maturation of both the epidemiologic and statistical methods used in current epidemiological observations [54,55].

For example, technical problems arise when epidemiologic interpretation is needed: (1) adjustment of confounding variables was extremely difficult, and I refrained from performing further stratification for adjustment or multivariate analysis using the limited number of cases, and (2) the cases classified as VSE shown here did not follow virological confirmation, and diagnosis of this type was made mainly based on the trace of probable contacts. Nevertheless, other types of variola major can be confidently diagnosed compared to other infectious diseases, and thus, historical records still remain a useful tool as long as the literature appropriately documents the necessary data. This study was motivated by the relatively high reliability of diagnosis and determination of both fatality as well as miscarriage and premature birth, obvious events compared to fetal vaccinia, which is extremely difficult to diagnose, and neonatal outcomes, which could be rather biased by progress in neonatology and medicine on a whole. Although it was difficult to follow formal methods of meta-analysis and show combined estimates of the determined maternal outcomes with adjustment, this study successfully confirmed that smallpox is more severe with pregnancy, characterising several important features of the maternal outcomes.

Although it is well known that pregnant individuals are at higher risk of fatal and severe outcomes in several viral infections due to immune suppression [56,57], the actual biological mechanisms in smallpox have yet to be clarified, and the only fact known with certainty is that prior vaccination offers less protection to pregnant individuals than others [58]. However, it should be emphasised that vaccination might offer at least partial protection among pregnant cases; this study confirmed that the conditional probability of smallpox fatality (given infection) was lower among vaccinated pregnant cases. This finding implies that case fatality in the event of a bioterrorist attack could be lowered with vaccination prior to pregnancy and prior to the attack. This issue should be discussed further in the future, especially with regard to preparedness planning. In conclusion, given the notorious and extremely severe outcomes of smallpox in pregnancy in addition to the requirements of detailed stratification, I believe this chapter partly satisfies the needs to summarise the common patterns of maternal outcomes in pregnancy with smallpox.

Acknowledgements

I would like to thank Hiroshi Sameshima for his comments from the Obstetric point of view. Further thanks are due to Klaus Dietz, Birgit Kaiser, Martin Eichner and Chris Leary for their discussion and support in data collection. This chapter is a full description of an original study, published in Emerging Infectious Diseases [59].

References

[1] Henderson DA, Inglesby TV, Bartlett JG, Ascher MS, Eitzen E, Jahrling PB, et al. Smallpox as a biological weapon: medical and public health management. Working Group on Civilian Biodefense. *JAMA* 1999;281:2127-2137.

[2] Suarez VR, Hankins GD. Smallpox and pregnancy: from eradicated disease to bioterrorist threat. *Obstet. Gynecol.* 2002;100:87-93.

[3] Amstey MS, Gall SA. Smallpox vaccine and pregnancy. *Obstet. Gynecol.* 2002;100.1356.

[4] Levine MM, Edsall G, Bruce-Chwatt LJ. Live-virus vaccines in pregnancy. Risks and recommendations. *Lancet* 1974;2:34-8.

[5] Fenner F, Henderson DA, Arita I, Ladnyi ID. Smallpox and its eradication. Geneva: World Health Organization, 1988. Available at http://whqlibdoc.who.int/smallpox/.

[6] Eichner M, Dietz K. Transmission potential of smallpox: estimates based on detailed data from an outbreak. *Am. J. Epidemiol.* 2003;158:110-117.

[7] Rao AR, Prahlad I, Swaminathan M, Lakshmi A. Pregnancy and smallpox. *J. Indian Med. Assoc.* 1963;40:353-363.

[8] Rao AR. Haemorrhagic smallpox: A study of 240 cases. *J. Indian Med. Assoc.* 1964;43:224-229.

[9] Dixon CW. Smallpox in Tripolitania, 1946: an epidemiological and clinical study of 500 cases, including trials of penicillin treatment. *J. Hyg.* 1948;46:351-377.

[10] Breman JG, Arita I. The confirmation and maintenance of smallpox eradication. *N. Engl. J. Med.* 1980;303:1263-1273.

[11] Ferguson NM, Keeling MJ, Edmunds WJ, Gani R, Grenfell BT, Anderson RM, et al. Planning for smallpox outbreaks. *Nature* 2003;425:681-685.

[12] Horstmann DM. Viral infections in pregnancy. *Yale J. Biol. Med.* 1969;42:99-112.

[13] Dixon CW. Smallpox. London: Churchill, 1962.

[14] Rao AR. Smallpox. Bombay: Kothari Book Dept, 1972.

[15] Hanshaw JB, Dudgeon JA. Viral diseases of the fetus and newborn. Philadelphia: Saunders, 1978.

[16] Megale P, Angulo JJ, Pederneiras CA. Variola minor in Braganca Paulista county, 1956. Observations on the clinical course of variola minor and on pregnancy in women with the disease. *Bull Soc. Pathol. Exot. Filiales* 1979;72:11-20.

[17] Marsden JP. Variola minor; a personal analysis of 13,686 cases. *Bull Hyg.* 1948;23:735-746.

[18] Saxen L, Cantell K, Hakama M. Relation between smallpox vaccination and outcome of pregnancy. *Am. J. Public Health Nations Health* 1968;58:1910-1921.

[19] Marsden JP, Greenfield CRM. Inherited smallpox. *Arch. Dis. Child* 1934;9:309-314.

[20] Lynch FW. Dermatologic conditions of the fetus with particular reference to variola and vaccinia. *Arch. Derm. Syphilol.* 1932;26:997-1019.

[21] Bancroft IR. Clinical observations on variola. *Journal of medical research* 1904;11:322-344.

[22] Voigt L. Über den Einfluss der Pockenkrankheit auf Menstruation, Schwangerschaft, Geburt und Fötus. Sammlung klinischer Vortraege / *Gynaekologie* 1894-1897; 112:249-272 (in German).

[23] Scheby-Buch. Bericht über das Material des Hamburger Pockenhauses vom August 1871 bis Februar 1872. *Arch. Derm. Syphi* 1872-1873; 4:506-532 (in German).

[24] Meyer L. Über Pocken beim weiblichen Geschlecht. Beiträge zur Geburtshülfe und Gynäkologie / hrsg. von d. Gesellschaft für Geburtshülfe in Berlin (Berlin: Crede) 1873; 2: 186-198 (in German).

[25] Welch WM. Smallpox in the pregnant woman and in the foetus. *Philadelphia medical times*. 1877-1878;8:390-398.

[26] Jobard. Influence de la variole sur la grossesse. Paris: Université de Paris (Thése), 1880 (in French).

[27] Barthélemy. Recherches sur l'influence de lavariole sur la grossesse. Paris: Université de Paris (Thése), 1880 (in French).

[28] Sangregorio G. Vaiuolo e gravidanza. Cenni statistici (1). I Morgagni (Guardia Ostetrica di Milano) 1887;29:793-796 (in Italian).

[29] Richardière. La variole pendant la grossesse. *Arch. de tocol et de gynecol* 1893;20:611-615 (in French).

[30] van der Willigen AM. Pokken in de Zwangerschap, 80 gevallen van variolae gravidarum. *Nederlands tijdschrift voor geneeskunde* 1895;11:485-499 (in Dutch).

[31] Charpentier JB. Variole et vaccine dans la grossesse. Paris: Université de Paris (Thése), 1900 (in French).

[32] Viany C. Vaccine et variole au cours de la grossesse. *Lyon méd* 1900;93:397-401 (in French).

[33] Queirel. Variole et grossesse. *Annales de gynecologie et d''obstetrique* 1907;4:137-147 (in French).

[34] Robertson DG. Small-pox epidemic in New South Wales, 1913. Melbourne: issued under the authority of the Minister for Trade and Customs, 1914.

[35] Couréménos M. Influence de la variole sur la grossesse et le produit de la conception. Paris: Université de Paris (Thése), 1901 (in French).

[36] Lop PA. Variole et vaccine dans la grossesse. Paris: Université de Paris (Thése), 1893 (in French).

[37] Jenner E. Two cases of Small-pox infection communicated to the Foetus in Utero under particular circumstances, with additional remarks. *Medico-Chirurgical Transactions* 1809; 1:269-275.

[38] Davidson W. Small-pox in utero. *Lancet* 1837-1838; 2: 628.

[39] Marsden JP, Chir B. Metastatic calcification. Notes on twins born shortly after an attack of smallpox in the mother. *Brit. J. Child Dis*. 1930; 27:193-200.

[40] Rigden G. Influence of maternal small-pox on the fetus. *Brit Med J* 1877; 1: 229-230.

[41] Robinson H. Occurrence of confluent small-pox at the seventh month of pregnancy. *Brit. Med. J.* 1877;1:163.

[42] Cowie JM, Forbes D. Intrauterine influence of the fetus in small-pox. *Brit. Med. J.* 1904; 1: 1485.

[43] Paranjothy D, Samuel I. Pregnancy associated with haemorrhagic smallpox. *J. Obstet. Gynaecol. Br. Emp.* 1960;67:309-313.

[44] Pfeiffer L. Behandlung und Prophylaxe der Blattern. Handbuch der speciellen Therapie. Jena: Fischer, 1894 (in German).

[45] von Jarrier. De la menstruation dans la variole. Paris: Université de Paris (Thése), 1880 (in French).

[46] von Obermeier. Beiträge zur Kenntnis der Pocken. *Virchow's Archiv* 1872;IV: S345 (in German).

[47] Shafa E. Case fatality ratios in smallpox. WHO/SE/72.35. Geneva: World Health Organization, 1972.

[48] Ryan MA, Seward JF, Smallpox Vaccine in Pregnancy Registry Team. Pregnancy, birth, and infant health outcomes from the National Smallpox Vaccine in Pregnancy Registry, 2003-2006. *Clin. Infect. Dis.* 2008; 46: S221-S226.

[49] Deneux-Tharaux C, Berg C, Bouvier-Colle MH, Gissler M, Harper M, Nannini A, et al. Underreporting of pregnancy-related mortality in the United States and Europe. *Obstet. Gynecol.* 2005;106:684-692.

[50] Arita I. Duration of immunity after smallpox vaccination: a study on vaccination policy against smallpox bioterrorism in Japan. *Jpn J. Infect. Dis*. 2002;55: 112-116.

[51] Nishiura H, Schwehm M, Eichner M. Still protected against smallpox? Estimation of the duration of vaccine-induced immunity against smallpox. *Epidemiology*. 2006; 17: 576-581.

[52] Eichner M. Analysis of historical data suggests long-lasting protective effects of smallpox vaccination. *Am. J. Epidemiol*. 2003;158:717-723.

[53] Nishiura H, Eichner M. Estimation of the duration of vaccine-induced residual protection against severe and fatal smallpox based on secondary vaccination failure. *Infection*. 2006; 34: 241-246.

[54] Nishiura H, Brockmann SO, Eichner M. Extracting key information from historical data to quantify the transmission dynamics of smallpox. *Theor. Biol. Med. Model.* 2008; 5: 20.

[55] Susser E, Bresnahan M. Origins of epidemiology. *Ann N Y Acad Sci*. 2001;954:6-18.

[56] Waterson AP. Virus infections (other than rubella) during pregnancy. *Br. Med. J.* 1979;2:564-566.

[57] Grossman JH III. Viral infections in obstetrics and gynecology. *Obstet. Gynecol. Annu.* 1980;9:55-76.

[58] Hassett DE. Smallpox infections during pregnancy, lessons on pathogenesis from nonpregnant animal models of infection. *J. Reprod. Immunol*. 2003;60:13-24.

[59] Nishiura H. Smallpox during pregnancy and maternal outcomes. *Emerg. Infect. Dis*. 2006;12:1119-1121.

In: Infectious Pregnancy Complications
Editor: Richard N. Canfield
ISBN 978-1-60741-038-6

Chapter 17

Chicken Pox Infection in Pregnancy

Viroj Wiwanitkit
Wiwanitkit House, Bangkhae,
Bangkok Thailand 10160

Abstract

Chicken pox infection is a common viral infection. Fever with skin abnormality is the common presentation. Pregnant women in areas with poor hygienic conditions can become infected and can develop many signs and symptoms. In this chapter, the author will focus on chicken pox infection in pregnancy. Important reports are reviewed and presented.

Introduction to Chicken Pox Infection

Chicken pox infection is a common viral infection that presents a serious threat in tropical countries. Since it is a viral infection, the disease is an important member of the group of highly contagious diseases. This viral infection is classified as an infection with skin manifestation. Contact with infected patients is the main risk and cause of infection. This infection is common in tropical countries, as previously mentioned. However, it can be seen around the world [1]. A wide spectrum of diseases caused by this virus affects humans today and its incidence has persisted in many countries for decades [1]. Due in part to population growth and uncontrolled urbanization in tropical countries, contact with infected cases becomes easier, and successful control of this viral infection has still not been successful. In the presence of a safe and effective mass immunization, the best prevention and control of chicken pox depends upon the vaccination program. Chicken pox infection is a major cause of infantile fever with skin manifestation in tropical regions. The classic discrete skin lesion looking like clear vesicle in a moist heat wound brings the name "Sook Sai" in Southeast Asia, which means "moist burnt clear vesicle".

Clinical Manifestation of Chicken Pox

Chicken pox is a viral infection with chicken pox virus producing a spectrum of clinical illnesses with a prominent skin manifestation [2–3].

The chicken pox virus is the same as varicella-zoster virus (VZV), which is a herpesvirus [4]. This virus is responsible for two distinct clinical disorders: primary varicella (chickenpox) and zoster (shingles) [4]. Primary varicella is a common pediatric disease that presents as pruritic macules, papules, vesicles, pustules, and crusts, usually on the back, chest, face, and abdomen [4]. In generally immunocompetent healthy infected children, chickenpox is usually a mild disease with little morbidity and rare mortality; however, primary varicella is associated with more morbidity in adults [4]. The chicken pox virus is a member of enveloped alpha herpesviruses and can cause highly contagious airborne infections. Even careful hygienic measures in the hospital can hardly prevent the spread of infections, and such infections may be severe and lethal for newborns [5]. Both the primary disease and the secondary reactivation—shingles—can bring complications, both in the form of serious effects on organs by the virus itself, and through secondary bacterial infections owing to temporary immune deficiency [6]. For natural history, the virus has a respiratory port of entry [7]. After two successive viremias, it reaches the skin, where it causes typical lesions, and it then penetrates the peripheral nervous system and it remains latent in dorsal root ganglia [7]. Structurally, the virion has a nucleocapsid surrounding a core that contains the linear, double-stranded DNA genome; a protein tegument separates the capsid from the lipid envelope, which incorporates the major viral glycoproteins [8]. It is noted for relatively frequent complications which include secondary bacterial skin infections, pneumonitis, complications affecting the central nervous system, and hepatitis [6]. Herpes zoster, caused by viral reactivation, is a localized, painful vesicular rash involving one or adjacent dermatomes [8]. The incidence of herpes zoster usually increases with age or immunosuppression [8]. In the era of acquired immunodeficiency virus (AIDS), the reoccurrence of herpes zoster is classified as a clue for further workup of AIDS.

Chicken Pox in Pregnancy

Pregnant women in nonendemic regions of chicken pox infection can become infected and can develop signs and symptoms of primary infection of this virus; most pregnant women in endemic areas usually acquire a primary infection, since they are still in the childhood period. In this chapter, the author will focus on chicken pox infection in pregnancy, especially for the pattern of hematological disturbance.

A. General Concern

Besides simple transmission by respiratory contact, there are other ways of simple transmission for chicken pox infection that can be seen in clinical practice. Some pregnant women can also be susceptible to chicken pox virus and if they acquire the infection, vertical transmission of the virus to their child can be possible. Intrapartum infection is an interesting obstetric infection. There are some prior reports on this kind of intrapartum viral infection. With regard to the clinical presentation of the affected pregnant subjects, a clinical presentation similar to that of the general population can be seen. Of interest, intrapartum complications were also dependant on postpartum complications. Moreover, it seems that clinical complications did not relate to the method of delivery. Confirmation of intrapartum chicken pox infection is generally delayed due to the long turnaround time of the serological test. However, a correct diagnosis of chicken pox infection can be performed initially in most cases due the classical skin appearance in this disease. Nevertheless, the presumed diagnosis is generally made with a history of contact, high fever and typical skin rash. Truly, in nonendemic areas of chicken pox virus infection, the diagnosis of chicken pox should be rare in pregnancy because most pregnant women should be past the age of primary infection. When a high fever is suspected in a pregnant woman, laboratory investigation and prolonged observation of newborn are advised.

Transmission of chicken pox infection to neonates has been confirmed. Neonatal chicken pox is considered a serious disorder. Considering the nanostructure level for an explanation of vertical transmission, physiologically, the placental barrier, composed of fetal endothelium and the syncytiotrophoblast and their fused basal laminae, plays important protective role, and maternal blood bathes the syncytiotrophoblast only. In the case of dengue virus infection, the virus is smaller in size than the placental filter (placental barrier pore size is equal to 10 nm [9]) and this allows vertical transmission. However, an important note is that viremia in the mother must be present close to the time of labor, which can allow the virus to infect the infant. It can be concluded that if a pregnant mother contracts the disease, is bitten by a contaminated vector, and develops viremia in the week before term, this mother has a high risk for developing dengue infection in pregnancy and can pass the infection to her term infant in utero, which can bring a vertical transmission and a case of neonatal dengue.

B. Clinical Pattern of Pregnant Women with Chicken Pox Infection

In nonendemic regions, some pregnant women may also be susceptible to chicken pox. Increased cases of chicken pox infection in pregnancy can be expected due to the increasing incidence during adulthood. Good sanitatary conditions that prevent childhood infection can be the clue to this new finding. For pregnant women with chicken pox, clinical symptoms are high fever and generalized vesicle eruptions [10]. During the first trimester, primary chicken pox infection may result in stillbirth or a baby born with congenital varicella syndrome, while infection in the peripartum period can result in neonatal chicken pox, which carries a very high mortality rate despite appropriate antiviral therapy [11]. Chicken pox in pregnant women can progress to pneumonitis and other severe sequelae that may also compromise the viability of the fetus in utero [11]. For infected pregnant women with severe pneumonitis, treatment in an intensive care unit with ventilatory support is suggested. An exposure to chicken pox most commonly occurs in the community or from children in the household, but occasionally, exposure may occur in the hospital environment during the antenatal visit to the physician at the hospital [11]. Daley et al. proposed that detection for serostatus prior to pregnancy is useful because an effective vaccine is available and can be administered to non-pregnant seronegative women of child-bearing age [11]. It has also been shown that infection during the second or third trimester of pregnancy may have serious consequences for infants [12]. Gidia et al. said that it was necessary to clarify previous disease in the history of every woman before their planned pregnancy, and it was also necessary to recommend the administration of a varicella vaccine before conception in cases of negative or unsure history [13]. Manten et al. recommended that if a pregnant woman without a prior history of infection was exposed to a patient with chicken pox, passive immunisation with varicella-zoster immunoglobulin should be administered, and this protocol helps reduce the risk of maternal complications and prevent fetal varicella syndrome [14]. For confirmation of fetal infection, prenatal diagnosis can be confirmed by serology and fetal damage by ultrasonography [15]. In fetal death in utero, autopsy of the fetus usually shows multiorgan manifestation with disseminated foci of necrosis and microcalcifications, encephalitis and unilateral segmental skin scarring with an underlying hypoplastic fixed lower limb, and the placenta usually shows a multifocal chronic villitis with multinucleated giant cells [15].

C. Treatment for Chicken Pox Infection in Pregnancy

Chicken pox infection in pregnant women can result in severe maternal illness, and it is five times more likely to be fatal than in non-pregnant women [16]. Although most women who have chicken pox in pregnancy give birth to healthy children, in other cases the baby is affected by in-utero infection or severe infection of the newborn [16]. Treatment of chicken pox infection should be based on the severity of the infection. The concept of treatment is similar to other infections: eliminating the pathogen or control of the infection and supportive or symptomatic treatment. In chicken pox infection, a specific antiviral drug for chicken pox virus is available at present. There are some recent reports on possible antiviral drugs for chicken pox virus infection. Intravenous acyclovir is recommended for severe maternal pneumonia and severely affected neonates; however, no controlled study has yet evaluated the effectiveness of acyclovir or valacyclovir for postexposure prophylaxis to pregnant women or neonates [17]. A more useful protocol is the administration of immunoglobulin, as previously mentioned. Tan and Koren recommended that varicella-zoster immune globulin (VZIG) should be administered as soon as possible, preferably within 96 hours from exposure, to prevent maternal infection or subsequent complications [17].

D. Neonatal Chicken Pox

Generally, the risk for fetal disease is low (1%) [13]. Usually, the neonatal blood IgM against varicella-zoster virus is negative. However, newborns of infected pregnant women should be given varicella-zoster immunoglobulin within 24 hours and isolated in a neonatal care unit. Despite this protocol if the baby still develops skin lesions post delivery, intravenous acyclovir should be administered for seven days [10].

It can be observed that neonatal varicella is more severe if a maternal rash appears five days prior to or two days after delivery [17].

E. Chicken Pox Vaccination and Pregnancy

It is recommended that pre-pregnancy chicken pox vaccination should be administered in cases without a history of primary infection. There are many reports on the usefulness of pre-pregnancy vaccine. For example, Plans et al. showed that a varicella-zoster vaccination programme aimed at women of childbearing age could be necessary in Catalonia to prevent all varicella-zoster infections during pregnancy [18]. Talukder et al. reported that women arriving in the United Kingdom in adulthood should be screened routinely during pregnancy, and vaccination should be offered postpartum if they were susceptible [19]. Watson et al. noted that a self-reported history of varicella seemed to be a strong predictor of VZV IgG antibodies in pregnant women; however, negative or uncertain histories were poorly predictive of negative serostatus [20]. In pregnant women, the vaccine may be used for postexposure prophylaxis, and is most effective if given within three days after exposure, but can be used up to five days from exposure [21]. For a postpartum scenario, there is no evidence of varicella vaccine virus excretion in breast milk; therefore, it can be suggested that postpartum vaccination of varicella-susceptible women need not be delayed because of breastfeeding [22].

References

[1] Suga S, Asano Y. Varicella. *Nippon Rinsho*. 2001 Nov;59 Suppl 7:68-72.

[2] Brigden D. Skin infections. *Br. Med. Bull.* 1985 Oct;41(4):357-60.

[3] Raimer SS. Controversies in pediatric dermatology. *Adv Dermatol.* 1994;9:193-203

[4] Tyring SK. Natural history of varicella zoster virus. *Semin. Dermatol.* 1992 Sep;11(3):211-7.

[5] Eggers HJ. Nosocomial virus infections. *Zentralbl. Bakteriol. Mikrobiol. Hyg.* [B]. 1986 Dec;183(2-3):114-9.

[6] Chelsom J, Langeland N. Varicella zoster complications. *Tidsskr Nor Laegeforen*. 1994 Sep 10;114(21):2486-8.

[7] Rentier B, Piette J, Baudoux L, Debrus S, Defechereux P, Merville MP, Sadzot-Delvaux C, Schoonbroodt S. Lessons to be learned from varicella-zoster virus. *Vet Microbiol.* 1996 Nov;53(1-2):55-66.

[8] Grose C. Varicella Pathogenesis: from Hox to Mutated gE glycoproteins. *Herpes*. 2006 Nov;13(3):59.

[9] Challier JC. The placental barrier: structure, resistance, asymmetry. *Reprod. Nutr. Dev.* 1989;29:703-16.

[10] Pattanasuttinont S. Maternal chickenpox in peripartum period: a case report and review. *J. Med. Assoc. Thai*. 2008 Jan;91(1):110-6.

[11] Daley AJ, Thorpe S, Garland SM. Varicella and the pregnant woman: prevention and management. *Aust. N. Z. J. Obstet. Gynaecol.* 2008 Feb;48(1):26-33.

[12] Narkeviciute I. Consequences of varicella in pregnancy: a report of four cases. *Acta Paediatr.* 2007 Jul;96(7):1099-100.

[13] Gidai J, Bács E, Czeizel E. Fetal varicella syndrome. *Orv. Hetil.* 2007 Jul 22;148(29):1373-9

[14] Manten GT, Derks JB, van Loon AM, Gerards LJ, Bruinse HW. Chickenpox in pregnancy with serious consequences for both mother and child. *Ned. Tijdschr. Geneeskd.* 2003 Oct 11;147(41):2029-32.

[15] Petignat P, Vial Y, Laurini R, Hohlfeld P. Fetal varicella-herpes zoster syndrome in early pregnancy: ultrasonographic and morphological correlation. *Prenat. Diagn.* 2001 Feb;21(2):121-4.

[16] Chickenpox, pregnancy and the newborn. *Drug Ther. Bull.* 2005 Sep;43(9):69-72.

[17] Tan MP, Koren G. Chickenpox in pregnancy: revisited. *Reprod. Toxicol.* 2006 May;21(4):410-20.

[18] Plans P, Costa J, Espuñes J, Plasència A, Salleras L. Prevalence of varicella-zoster antibodies in pregnant women in Catalonia (Spain). Rationale for varicella vaccination of women of childbearing age. *BJOG.* 2007 Sep;114(9):1122-7.

[19] Talukder YS, Kafatos G, Pinot de Moira A, Aquilina J, Parker SP, Crowcroft NS, Brown DW, Breuer J. The seroepidemiology of varicella zoster virus among pregnant Bangladeshi and white British women in the London Borough of Tower Hamlets, UK. *Epidemiol. Infect.* 2007 Nov;135(8):1344-53.

[20] Watson B, Civen R, Reynolds M, Heath K, Perella D, Carbajal T, Mascola L, Jumaan A, Zimmerman L, James A, Quashi C, Schmid S. Validity of self-reported varicella disease history in pregnant women attending prenatal clinics. *Public Health Rep.* 2007 Jul-Aug;122(4):499-506.

[21] Litt J, Burgess M. Varicella and varicella vaccination. An update. *Aust. Fam. Physician.* 2003 Aug;32(8):583-7.

[22] Bohlke K, Galil K, Jackson LA, Schmid DS, Starkovich P, Loparev VN, Seward JF. Postpartum varicella vaccination: is the vaccine virus excreted in breast milk? *Obstet. Gynecol.* 2003 Nov;102(5 Pt 1):970-7.

Index

A

AAA, 143
AAT, 6, 204
ABC, 219
abdomen, 37, 43, 47, 50, 76, 154, 422
abnormalities, xiv, xv, 13, 15, 27, 30, 31, 33, 57, 80, 133, 237, 345, 346, 354, 355, 359, 361, 364, 370, 371, 383, 384, 393, 403, 404, 406
abortion, viii, xi, 8, 12, 13, 17, 20, 21, 24, 25, 30, 33, 37, 45, 46, 53, 87, 88, 89, 92, 102, 108, 109, 111, 112, 117, 118, 119, 120, 128, 137, 140, 142, 147, 148, 192, 199, 200, 201, 203, 236, 244, 245, 310, 334, 337, 342, 358, 363, 390, 394, 395, 398
accidental, 172, 296
accounting, 24, 243
accuracy, ix, 77, 140, 142, 153, 155, 297, 316, 348
acetate, 125, 252
acetic acid, 250, 252
achievement, 283, 408
achondroplasia, 384
acid, 6, 11, 13, 15, 20, 29, 36, 37, 42, 74, 114, 121, 136, 173, 179, 180, 204, 224, 250, 252, 336, 349, 353, 357, 359, 360, 361, 363, 368, 372, 386, 387, 391, 394, 401, 402, 405, 406
acidic, 21
acidification, 175
acidity, 21, 179
acidosis, 155, 158, 207, 208, 232
acquired immunity, 236, 237, 241, 266
acquired immunodeficiency syndrome, 308
ACR, 80
activation, ix, 7, 8, 9, 22, 58, 111, 112, 116, 117, 123, 124, 125, 126, 129, 132, 214, 270, 279
acute, xii, xiii, 3, 14, 15, 18, 25, 28, 32, 33, 39, 43, 44, 46, 56, 67, 75, 76, 89, 116, 118, 132, 133, 135, 151, 152, 153, 157, 158, 171, 203, 204, 223, 224, 278, 289, 291, 294, 295, 296, 297, 298, 301, 305, 307, 311, 312, 313, 314, 317, 320, 325, 334, 336, 343, 349, 350, 351, 352, 353, 356, 357, 361, 363, 366, 367, 386, 389, 395, 397, 398, 401, 402, 405
acute infection, xii, xiii, 25, 28, 203, 204, 224, 289, 291, 295, 296, 297, 298, 320, 325, 357
acute respiratory distress syndrome, 33
adaptation, 99, 135, 369
adaptive functioning, 169
additives, 377
adenine, 117
adenopathy, 38, 39
adhesion, 35, 125, 126, 127, 173, 237
adjustment, 338, 410, 411, 417
administration, 15, 22, 41, 49, 50, 117, 171, 180, 187, 188, 265, 336, 351, 377, 387, 424
adolescence, 300
adolescents, 25, 27, 39, 44, 60
adult, 9, 15, 16, 28, 34, 38, 58, 68, 244, 270, 278, 306, 350, 376, 408
adult population, 16
adulthood, 376, 423, 425
adults, xiv, 10, 14, 16, 23, 24, 25, 27, 28, 29, 38, 39, 40, 44, 45, 67, 70, 73, 78, 146, 149, 243, 278, 279, 287, 295, 301, 311, 331, 335, 339, 380, 422
adverse event, 181, 264
Aedes, 373, 379
aerobe, 36
aerobic, 47, 56, 172, 173, 190, 192
aerobic bacteria, 47
aerosol, 29, 332
afebrile, 33, 42, 49

Africa, xi, xiii, 15, 16, 18, 34, 35, 37, 39, 70, 71, 72, 78, 113, 199, 200, 203, 209, 211, 216, 218, 220, 221, 222, 223, 225, 227, 231, 232, 236, 237, 238, 239, 240, 241, 242, 243, 244, 245, 248, 252, 263, 264, 267, 268, 270, 271, 272, 273, 274, 276, 277, 278, 279, 280, 282, 283, 284, 286, 292, 319, 322, 323, 324, 325, 408
African continent, 274
Ag, 223, 343
agent, xii, 3, 4, 5, 21, 26, 48, 55, 179, 181, 289, 336, 341, 342, 343, 405, 406
agents, ix, 3, 7, 43, 56, 117, 139, 193, 283, 328, 339, 347, 356, 365, 381, 384, 386, 392, 397
agglutination, 21, 252, 297, 313, 314, 335
agglutination test, 21, 335
aggregation, 9, 115
aid, 14, 43, 52, 56, 348, 355, 385
AIDS, 4, 19, 62, 72, 195, 219, 221, 222, 223, 224, 225, 226, 227, 228, 230, 231, 232, 243, 275, 276, 277, 278, 279, 281, 286, 287, 288, 297, 299, 308, 316, 342, 422
air, 36, 40, 96, 159, 160, 161, 163, 164, 339
airway epithelial cells, 114
albumin, 37
albuminuria, 358, 363
alcohol, 140, 170, 384
alcohol consumption, 140
alkaline, 252
alkalosis, 389
allergens, 9
allergic reaction, 52
allergic rhinitis, 388
allergy, 336
allograft, 170, 214
alopecia, 5
alpha, ix, 130, 139, 141, 219, 422
ALT, 14
alternative, xiv, 24, 33, 36, 178, 204, 214, 217, 219, 331, 336
alternatives, 208
alveoli, 117, 163
Amazon, 307
amebiasis, 8
American Academy of Pediatrics, 15, 60, 73, 335, 339
amino, 14, 121
amniocentesis, 11, 25, 26, 41, 42, 94, 188, 299, 300, 315
amnion, viii, 22, 41, 89, 111, 112, 119, 121, 122, 124, 125, 131
amniotic, xiii, 7, 11, 18, 22, 25, 37, 41, 42, 46, 47, 63, 68, 74, 75, 84, 86, 91, 94, 102, 107, 118, 120, 123, 124, 129, 131, 132, 171, 172, 181, 188, 192, 290, 295, 299, 300, 315
amniotic fluid, xiii, 7, 11, 18, 22, 25, 37, 41, 42, 46, 63, 68, 75, 118, 120, 123, 124, 131, 132, 171, 181, 188, 192, 290, 295, 299, 300, 315
anaemia, vi, xi, xii, 67, 71, 200, 203, 206, 207, 208, 218, 220, 231, 235, 236, 237, 239, 240, 241, 242, 244, 245, 246, 248, 250, 251, 262, 263, 264, 265, 269, 270, 271, 275, 276, 277, 278, 279, 280, 281, 282, 283, 284, 285, 286, 288, 336
anaerobes, 22, 47
anaerobic, 21, 22, 42, 47, 56
anaerobic bacteria, 22, 47
anaesthesia, 9, 165
anal atresia, 354, 364
analgesia, 44, 48
analgesics, 26, 28
analysis of variance, 143
anatomy, 152
ANC, xii, 200, 235, 256, 259, 260, 264, 265, 272, 274
anemia, 4, 5, 25, 26, 32, 34, 35, 36, 37, 40, 46, 71, 231, 300, 357, 358, 363, 367, 368, 376, 378, 389, 390, 395, 398
anencephaly, 393, 405
animal models, 16, 420
animal studies, 53, 155
animals, xiv, 2, 5, 9, 28, 53, 54, 57, 171, 282, 290, 292, 304, 307, 310, 320, 331, 332, 334, 335, 339, 400
anorexia, 14, 35, 39, 47
antagonist, 120
antibiotic, 22, 40, 42, 47, 48, 49, 50, 64, 75, 94, 171, 179, 180, 298, 333, 335, 342, 343, 367, 397
antibiotic resistance, 94
antibiotics, 32, 37, 40, 42, 44, 45, 49, 56, 76, 94, 118, 177, 180, 195, 333, 335, 339, 387
antibodies, 281, 296, 297, 301, 303
antibody, 6, 10, 11, 14, 15, 21, 23, 27, 29, 30, 56, 65, 67, 68, 69, 119, 127, 141, 145, 147, 148, 149, 203, 204, 246, 267, 297, 298, 301, 302, 307, 311, 313, 316, 317, 321, 325, 327, 380
anticoagulant, 50
anticoagulation, 50
antigen, 6, 10, 11, 15, 18, 24, 39, 40, 65, 116, 117, 128, 204, 223, 275, 281, 297, 298, 299, 302, 312
anti-HIV, 223
anti-inflammatory drugs, 74, 128

antimalarial agents, 283
antimalarial drugs, 35, 273, 274, 283
antimalarials, 273
antimicrobial therapy, 33, 45
antioxidant, 121
antipyretic, 378
antiretroviral, 19, 209, 210, 211, 212, 213, 215, 226, 227, 230, 272
antiretrovirals, xi, 19, 200, 218, 220, 221
antiviral, 27, 122, 123, 374, 376, 381, 423, 424
antiviral agents, 381
antiviral drugs, 374, 376, 424
antiviral therapy, 423
anus, 20
anxiety, 52, 391
aorta, 163
apicomplexa, 290
aplastic anemia, 25
apoptosis, viii, 8, 9, 24, 31, 65, 111, 112, 113, 114, 116, 121, 122, 123, 124, 125, 126, 128, 129, 130, 131, 132, 133, 134, 136, 137, 138, 404
apoptotic, 112, 116, 117, 120, 122, 123, 124, 125, 126, 128, 129, 132, 133, 134, 136
apoptotic cells, 117, 120, 123, 124, 128, 136
appendectomy, 43, 44, 76, 77, 153, 155, 156, 157, 158
appendicitis, x, 8, 43, 76, 77, 151, 152, 153, 154, 155, 156, 157, 158
appendix, 43, 76, 152, 153, 154, 155, 156, 157
appetite, 32
application, 18, 94, 274, 339, 374
Argentina, 221
armed conflict, 274
Armenia, 309
arrest, 402
ART, 205, 206, 207, 214, 218, 219, 274
arteries, 135
arteriosclerosis, 30
artery, 26, 56, 369
arthralgia, 5, 35
arthritis, 5, 8, 27, 30, 40, 56
arthropods, 332
ascites, 2, 21, 26, 29
aseptic, 3
aseptic meningitis, 3
asexual, 34
ash, 116
Asia, 15, 16, 18, 34, 39, 71, 113, 374, 378, 381, 408, 421
Asian, 112, 116, 118, 130, 131, 135, 137, 310, 341, 380, 381, 405
aspartate, 120
aspergillosis, 8
aspiration, 37, 397
aspirin, 377
assessment, x, 6, 50, 77, 91, 167, 177, 182, 183, 188, 190, 268, 269, 271, 282, 284, 377
asthma, 118, 163, 388
astrocytes, 119
asymmetry, 381, 425
asymptomatic, ix, xiii, 2, 3, 5, 13, 14, 16, 17, 21, 22, 23, 24, 28, 32, 33, 34, 37, 39, 42, 49, 62, 63, 70, 140, 142, 147, 171, 172, 177, 180, 194, 219, 236, 239, 275, 286, 289, 292, 294, 295, 298, 300, 304, 306, 339, 351, 366, 371
ATC, 143
atresia, xiv, 345, 354, 364, 367, 368, 369, 372
atrial septal defect, xv, 345, 351, 366
atrophy, 4, 23, 27
attachment, 114, 339
attacks, 246
attitudes, 203, 222
attributable fraction, 366
auditing, 220
Australia, xvi, 336, 339, 407, 408
Austria, 93, 296, 321, 328
authority, 419
autism, 9, 23
autocrine, 133
autoimmune, 30, 41
autoimmune disease, 41
autopsy, 27, 347, 424
autosomal recessive, 369
availability, 36, 203, 214, 248, 273
avian influenza, 112, 113, 116, 119, 129, 131, 135, 136, 137
Avian influenza, 113, 129, 136, 138
avoidance, xi, 199, 205, 214, 220, 339, 343, 403
awareness, 118, 203, 248, 304
Azerbaijan, 113

B

B cell, 123, 134
B cells, 123
B19 infection, 24, 25, 26, 65, 66, 67
babies, xii, 15, 17, 20, 21, 37, 228, 236, 241, 242, 252, 253, 255, 259, 260, 261, 262, 264, 265, 266, 267, 268, 269, 270, 271, 281, 349, 359, 369, 386, 387, 390, 394, 399

bacilli, 36, 37
back pain, 45
bacteremia, 39
bacteria, 22, 31, 39, 41, 45, 47, 73, 118, 146, 149, 171, 176, 350, 351, 356, 404
bacterial, vii, 2, 3, 11, 13, 22, 23, 27, 31, 32, 44, 45, 48, 50, 51, 59, 63, 64, 75, 78, 93, 104, 121, 146, 172, 173, 174, 176, 177, 178, 179, 180, 181, 188, 190, 192, 193, 194, 195, 196, 350, 351, 356, 375, 398, 422
bacterial infection, 23, 27, 31, 32, 350, 375, 398, 422
bacterium, 20, 40
Bangladesh, 113, 380
barium, 153
barium enema, 153
barrier, viii, 41, 83, 84, 90, 104, 170, 177, 187, 270, 379, 381, 423, 425
barriers, viii, 15, 111, 112, 128
basal lamina, 239, 379, 423
basement membrane, 35, 238, 269
baths, 48
battery, 96
B-cell, 16, 131, 298
B-cell lymphoma, 16
BCG, 51
Bcl-2, 131
behavior, xii, 222, 289
behavioral problems, 169
Belgium, 321
beliefs, 76, 158
benchmark, ix, 140, 141
beneficial effect, 88, 367, 396
benefits, xi, 28, 51, 52, 54, 89, 106, 155, 200, 203, 207, 208, 214, 220, 273, 304, 341
benign, xii, 28, 289, 320
Best Practice, 58, 64
beverages, xii, 289
bias, 348, 349, 370, 385, 387, 391, 392, 403
binding, 35, 113, 114, 117, 237, 374, 380
biological consequences, 116
biological weapons, xiv, 331
biomarkers, xiii, 289
biopsies, 56, 137
biopsy, 37, 40, 56, 73, 116, 146, 240
bioterrorism, 340, 420
birds, 114
birth rate, 184, 185, 187
birth weight, vii, xi, xii, 1, 2, 5, 12, 21, 22, 30, 32, 33, 37, 44, 64, 71, 76, 84, 101, 168, 169, 170, 183, 184, 185, 187, 191, 199, 200, 203, 218, 226, 235, 236, 237, 241, 242, 243, 244, 245, 246, 250, 255, 259, 260, 264, 265, 266, 267, 268, 273, 275, 277, 279, 280, 281, 282, 287, 334, 347, 351, 355, 356, 359, 364, 365, 366, 384, 390, 391, 394, 396, 397, 399
births, viii, x, xii, 46, 83, 84, 85, 86, 87, 88, 90, 92, 93, 101, 103, 105, 118, 167, 168, 169, 170, 171, 175, 184, 186, 187, 189, 190, 203, 269, 289, 293, 320, 352, 356, 359, 362, 365, 366, 367, 369, 371, 384, 396, 410, 416
birthweight, 17, 20, 34, 35, 232, 245, 248, 250, 255, 259, 260, 261, 264, 265, 267, 269, 276, 277, 280, 281, 282, 283, 285, 355, 358, 359, 364, 365, 366, 367
bladder, 8, 27, 31, 39, 44, 350, 351, 356
bleeding, 23, 30, 39, 40, 94, 95, 96, 117, 182, 374, 380
blindness, 5, 13, 18, 142, 219
blood, xii, 6, 7, 10, 11, 14, 15, 16, 18, 21, 23, 24, 25, 26, 32, 33, 34, 35, 40, 41, 46, 56, 57, 60, 75, 94, 115, 119, 126, 129, 134, 136, 141, 154, 155, 156, 158, 160, 163, 206, 219, 235, 237, 238, 239, 241, 242, 246, 247, 248, 250, 251, 252, 255, 256, 258, 260, 266, 267, 268, 269, 270, 271, 273, 275, 278, 279, 280, 281, 283, 284, 285, 286, 287, 294, 295, 296, 299, 303, 306, 310, 338, 375, 376, 378, 379, 423, 424
blood collection, 284
blood flow, 7, 21, 32
blood group, xii, 24, 235, 246, 248, 250, 251, 252, 255, 258, 260, 266, 267, 278, 279, 280, 281, 283, 285, 286
blood monocytes, 126
blood pressure, 155, 160, 163, 376
blood sampling, 25, 26, 41, 75
blood smear, 11, 35, 238, 239, 250, 251, 267, 296
blood stream, 294
blood transfusion, 6, 16, 219
blood urea, 56
blood urea nitrogen, 56
blood vessels, 34
bloodstream, 15, 31, 124, 290
blot, 6, 19, 68, 147, 302, 316, 317
body fluid, 46
body mass index, 242
body temperature, 7, 154
body weight, 54, 277
bomb, 80
bone growth, 57, 335
bone marrow, 39, 40, 56, 65, 73, 117, 123, 336

bone marrow biopsy, 40, 56
borate, 252
borderline, 298
Boston, 230, 371, 372
Botswana, 212, 221, 222, 229
bowel, 2, 27, 32, 36, 47, 152, 372
bowel obstruction, 152
boys, 358
bradycardia, 39
brain, 4, 9, 17, 23, 36, 40, 45, 46, 54, 55, 57, 58, 115, 116, 117, 119, 123, 132, 170, 291, 299, 402
brain abscess, 40, 46
brain damage, 45, 57, 170
brain injury, 9
Brazil, 221, 229, 275, 284, 292, 306, 308, 310
Brazilian, 306
breaches, 20
breakdown, 48, 57
breast feeding, xi, 39, 199
breast milk, 7, 16, 24, 39, 216, 217, 338, 425, 426
breastfeeding, xi, 4, 15, 18, 23, 39, 48, 51, 62, 199, 200, 204, 205, 206, 214, 215, 216, 217, 218, 220, 225, 227, 229, 230, 293, 338, 425
breathing, 160
breeding, 373
Britain, 321
bronchial tree, 161
bronchiolitis, 388, 393, 396
bronchitis, 388, 390, 393
bronchoscopy, 116
bronchus, 116, 163
brucellosis, 8, 334
bubbles, 161
buffer, 142, 252
Burkina Faso, 71, 222, 227, 231, 240, 264, 268, 282, 308
burning, 182

C

C. trachomatis, 13
caecum, 152
caesarean section, xi, 19, 62, 153, 199, 204, 205, 214, 220, 252
calcification, 4, 5, 335, 419
calcium, 56
calculus, 351
CAM, 252
Cambodia, 113
Cameroon, 240, 264, 267, 274, 277, 286
campaigns, xiv, 320, 325
Canada, 381
canals, 90
cancer, 54
candida, 93
Candida, 41, 172, 173, 174, 176
candidates, 128
candidiasis, 308
Cape Town, 222
capillary, 33
capsule, 49
CAR, 141, 346
carbohydrates, 114
carbon, 158
carboxylic, 121
carcinogenesis, 53
carcinoma, 3, 15, 16
cardiac muscle, 291
cardiac output, 25, 44
cardiac tamponade, 163
cardiomyopathy, 208
cardiopulmonary, 133
cardiovascular system, 389, 402
carrier, 3, 39
caspase, 120, 122, 132
caspases, 120
catalase, 121
cataract, xv, xvi, 383, 384, 391, 392, 393, 396, 397, 399, 400, 401, 404
cataracts, 27, 30
category a, 394
catheter, 164
catheterization, 49
cats, xii, 5, 28, 289, 290, 291, 293, 294, 305, 307, 309
Caucasian, 349
causal relationship, 171
cavitation, 54
cavities, 57
CCC, 143
CD8+, 115
CDC, 6, 7, 13, 15, 19, 21, 36, 50, 73, 77, 80, 149, 192, 332, 335, 340
cDNA, 132
CDR, 63, 135
cefazolin, 33
cell, 9, 16, 18, 25, 31, 35, 38, 42, 44, 45, 53, 56, 65, 112, 113, 114, 115, 117, 119, 120, 122, 123, 124, 125, 126, 128, 129, 130, 131, 133, 134, 136, 146, 156, 214, 247, 250, 251, 252, 266, 271, 274, 275,

276, 277, 279, 281, 282, 283, 284, 286, 287, 288, 290, 298, 299, 304, 339, 378, 389, 402, 404
cell adhesion, 125
cell culture, 299
cell cycle, 9, 31
cell death, 9, 53, 65, 112, 117, 120, 122, 123, 129, 130, 133, 134, 290
cell division, 31
cell invasion, 304
cell line, 125, 131, 136
cell lines, 125, 136
cell surface, 113, 124, 126
cellulitis, 27, 33, 46, 48, 79
cellulose, 252
Census, 283
Centers for Disease Control, 6, 7, 19, 20, 35, 51, 58, 60, 63, 67, 71, 80, 281
Central America, 294
Central Asia, 408
central nervous system, vii, 1, 2, 23, 26, 142, 247, 422
cephalosporin, 45
cerebral palsy, 9, 22, 23, 42, 64, 76, 169, 170, 180
cerebrospinal fluid, 18, 46, 115, 116, 130, 303
cervicitis, 13
cervix, viii, 7, 20, 47, 83, 85, 86, 87, 88, 89, 90, 91, 93, 94, 96, 99, 100, 101, 102, 105, 107, 108, 118, 120, 132, 160, 170, 172, 177, 183, 188
cesarean section, 42, 47, 49, 50, 78, 101, 102, 118, 119
CGT, 143
chancre, 5
Checkpoints, 133
chemical structures, 387
chemicals, 73
chemoattractant, 124
chemotactic cytokines, 269
chemotherapy, 27, 38, 73, 137
chest radiograph, 37, 38
chest radiography, 37, 38
chicken, xvi, 52, 67, 421, 422, 423, 424, 425
chicken pox, xvi, 52, 421, 422, 423, 424, 425
chickens, 123, 131
child development, 272
child mortality, 227
childbearing, 17, 51, 149, 239, 294, 425, 426
childbirth, xii, 46, 75, 235, 248, 252, 253, 254, 255, 256, 257, 258, 259, 260, 262, 271, 279, 325
childcare, 6
childhood, 17, 24, 27, 53, 54, 71, 73, 145, 148, 282, 300, 335, 422, 423
children, 6, 9, 16, 17, 18, 19, 23, 24, 27, 29, 39, 44, 53, 57, 60, 66, 67, 68, 73, 80, 81, 134, 148, 158, 174, 185, 191, 200, 223, 225, 226, 227, 228, 229, 232, 242, 243, 247, 265, 267, 270, 272, 274, 281, 282, 283, 295, 297, 302, 303, 311, 316, 320, 329, 332, 339, 342, 374, 375, 380, 422, 423, 424
Chile, 307
China, xiii, 113, 135, 319, 322, 323, 324, 325
Chinese women, xiii, 319, 322, 323
Chlamydia trachomatis, 7, 13, 32, 59, 62, 78, 79, 171, 172
chloride, 126
chloroquine, 36, 71, 283
cholangitis, 8, 40
cholecystectomy, 44, 77
cholecystitis, 8, 44, 77, 152
cholelithiasis, 77
cholestasis, 14, 117
chorioamnionitis, 9, 22, 41, 45, 63, 74, 75, 76, 120, 123, 124, 130, 131, 132, 171
choriomeningitis, 4
chorion, viii, 22, 31, 41, 111, 112, 119, 120, 121, 122, 124, 125, 126, 127, 128, 130, 132, 133, 136, 137, 138
chorioretinitis, 5, 17, 23, 27, 29, 294, 300
chromatography, 75
chronic active hepatitis, 16
chronic disease, 60, 218, 349, 357, 386
chronic diseases, 349, 357, 386
chronic granulomatous disease, 128, 129
chronic illness, 52, 250
chronic renal failure, 40, 361
cilia, 116
ciprofloxacin, 337, 338, 343
circulation, 7, 9, 18, 31, 94, 95, 241, 294
cirrhosis, 3, 15, 16, 60
civil service, 254
civil society, 220
classes, 332, 363
classical, 34, 87, 152, 153, 296, 374, 423
classification, xvi, 277, 332, 367, 372, 407, 410, 412
classroom, 25
cleaning, 351, 356
cleavage, 115, 120, 122
cleft lip, xv, xvi, 4, 347, 383, 384, 386, 391, 392, 393, 396, 397, 399, 400, 401
cleft palate, xvi, 347, 384, 399, 400, 401
clients, xi, 168

clinical assessment, 377
clinical diagnosis, 30, 41
clinical disorders, 422
clinical presentation, x, 37, 89, 151, 171, 333, 334, 339, 375, 376, 423
clinical symptoms, 244, 299, 423
clinical trial, 19, 62, 74, 89, 181, 185, 194, 225, 228, 339
clinical trials, 181
clinically significant, 155
clinician, 46, 56
clinics, 104, 106, 219, 244, 272, 287, 346, 348, 356, 384, 385, 426
clonality, 305
closure, 49, 86, 160, 181, 291, 402
clotting factors, 15
clusters, 17, 20
CMV, ix, x, 6, 11, 23, 24, 139, 140, 142, 143, 144, 145, 146, 148, 320
CNS, vii, 1, 2, 4, 290
Co, 37, 39, 81, 96, 135, 218, 245, 273, 306, 337, 340, 341, 371, 372, 375, 378, 405
coagulation, 17, 23, 141, 375
coagulation factor, 375
coagulopathy, 15, 369, 372
Cochrane, 13, 59, 62, 64, 70, 72, 74, 75, 77, 279
codes, 113
coding, 113
co-existence, 36, 116
cognition, 44
cognitive development, 241
cognitive impairment, 45
cohort, 57, 58, 62, 64, 86, 88, 175, 200, 203, 209, 214, 222, 225, 226, 277, 280, 287, 300, 317, 328, 370, 403
colds, 393
collaboration, 62, 181, 225, 272, 389
collagen, 131
colloids, 377
Colombia, 292, 306, 309
colon, 368
colonisation, 64, 193
colonization, 22, 75, 146, 172
colony-stimulating factor, 125
colostrum, 10
coma, 17, 129
combination therapy, 205, 214
commensals, 32
common symptoms, 24, 153, 156
communication, 304
communities, 272
community, 34, 44, 104, 119, 195, 221, 222, 272, 275, 309, 310, 371, 423
co-morbidities, 200
comorbidity, 35
complete blood count, 56, 375, 376, 378
complexity, 43
compliance, 250
complications, ix, x, xiv, xv, xvi, 19, 21, 22, 27, 30, 32, 33, 34, 37, 40, 43, 45, 47, 50, 51, 60, 62, 69, 71, 73, 75, 76, 89, 111, 112, 118, 122, 123, 128, 139, 141, 146, 147, 151, 152, 155, 156, 157, 159, 160, 164, 169, 172, 180, 244, 273, 331, 332, 334, 346, 348, 349, 350, 355, 356, 357, 358, 363, 366, 367, 369, 372, 374, 375, 377, 383, 384, 385, 386, 389, 390, 391, 392, 393, 394, 395, 397, 398, 400, 401, 402, 404, 405, 408, 422, 423, 424, 425
components, 113, 377
computed tomography, 17, 53, 56
concentration, xii, 30, 39, 75, 89, 115, 124, 173, 235, 250, 251, 257, 259, 260, 262, 265, 271, 389
conception, vii, 1, 2, 6, 29, 30, 46, 53, 64, 102, 299, 347, 348, 351, 362, 385, 386, 419, 424
concrete, 84
confidence, xvi, 407, 412, 413, 414
confidence interval, xvi, 407, 412, 413, 414
confidence intervals, 410, 414
confidentiality, 249
conflict, 274
conformity, 270
confounders, 349, 368, 387, 394, 397
confounding variables, 417
confusion, 332, 367
congenital cataract, xv, xvi, 383, 384, 391, 392, 393, 396, 397, 399, 400, 401, 404
congenital dysplasia, 347
Congress, 196
conization, 86
conjunctivitis, 5, 29
connective tissue, 50, 86
Connective tissue, 8, 342
consciousness, 45, 396
consensus, 22, 299, 347, 387
consent, 7, 142, 224, 250, 348, 349, 385
conservation, 378
constipation, 39
constraints, 273
consumption, xii, 140, 289, 294, 389
contaminated food, 39
contamination, 28, 47, 299, 309

continuity, 368
contractions, 15, 18, 22, 86, 118, 160, 170, 177
contracts, 379, 423
contrast agent, 56
control, ix, x, xv, 19, 58, 60, 67, 71, 72, 102, 104, 105, 122, 125, 140, 142, 143, 144, 145, 146, 158, 161, 186, 209, 212, 214, 217, 221, 230, 231, 238, 244, 245, 248, 249, 263, 267, 272, 273, 274, 278, 279, 282, 287, 288, 291, 295, 296, 307, 309, 326, 329, 336, 345, 347, 348, 349, 350, 352, 353, 355, 362, 363, 365, 366, 368, 370, 372, 374, 376, 379, 381, 385, 387, 388, 391, 392, 394, 400, 403, 404, 406, 421, 424
control group, ix, xv, 102, 104, 105, 140, 143, 144, 186, 217, 345, 348, 349, 350, 352, 366, 385, 387, 388
controlled studies, 104
controlled trials, 88, 104, 230, 264, 267
conversion, 298
cooking, 309
Copenhagen, 151
corneal ulcer, 13
coronary arteries, 135
correlation, 9, 75, 265, 268, 292, 293, 299, 305, 359, 374, 426
corticosteroids, 297, 377
cost-effective, 203, 204, 248, 273
costs, 106, 217, 218, 273, 274
cough, 29, 37, 163, 219, 389, 398
counsel, 7
counseling, 16, 25, 80, 207, 222, 224, 225, 265, 272, 310, 365
countermeasures, 177
country of origin, 322
couples, 206
cracking, 48
cranberry, 33, 70
cranial nerve, 5
craniofacial, 26
CRC, 285, 304
C-reactive protein, 32
creatinine, 56
crepitation, 160, 163
Crete, 331
critical period, 347, 349, 354, 370, 386, 387, 392, 399, 400, 401, 403
critical state, 91
CRM, 418
cross-sectional, 222
CRP, 180
CRS, 29, 30, 31, 145
crust, 26
cryotherapy, 20
cryptococcosis, 8
CSF, 18, 125, 295
CT, 17, 48, 50, 53, 55, 56, 80, 81, 155, 163, 307, 380
CT scan, 48, 155
C-terminal, 285
cues, 58
culture, viii, ix, 6, 11, 13, 18, 21, 32, 38, 42, 46, 49, 56, 94, 111, 122, 125, 127, 135, 140, 141, 147, 188, 299, 302, 315, 321, 335, 351, 356
curettage, 160
curing, 309
cyanosis, 163
cycles, 143
cyclooxygenase, 121, 138
cyclooxygenase-2, 138
Cyprus, 336, 341
cyst, 28, 291, 305, 320
cysteine, 121
cystic fibrosis, 369
cystitis, 11, 31, 32, 351, 352, 356, 359, 366
cysts, 28, 290, 291, 292, 293, 299, 304, 320
cytochrome, 131
cytokine, 22, 136, 137, 146, 214, 218
cytokine response, 218
cytokines, viii, 8, 9, 106, 111, 112, 120, 124, 125, 127, 128, 131, 136, 171, 192, 214, 269, 279
cytomegalovirus, ix, x, 6, 64, 65, 139, 140, 142, 144, 145, 146, 148, 149, 320
cytoplasm, 115, 125
cytotoxicity, 137

D

danger, 141
data analysis, 410
data collection, 348, 417
data set, xv, 346, 347, 349, 350, 351, 354, 355, 361, 366, 367, 368, 383, 385, 386, 388, 389, 393, 398
database, 375
dating, 409
de novo, 301
deafness, 30, 31, 39, 57, 69, 142
death, vii, ix, xi, xii, xvi, 2, 3, 4, 5, 8, 9, 20, 21, 24, 25, 26, 27, 31, 33, 34, 35, 41, 44, 45, 46, 52, 53, 57, 65, 72, 81, 112, 113, 117, 120, 122, 123, 129, 130, 133, 134, 138, 139, 199, 201, 203, 212, 214, 239, 243, 244, 245, 281, 289, 290, 334, 375, 394, 400, 402, 408, 411, 412, 414, 416, 424

death rate, 27, 113
deaths, vii, 1, 2, 5, 27, 34, 36, 37, 39, 44, 45, 46, 67, 112, 163, 203, 212, 219, 229, 236, 240, 243, 346, 374, 410, 412, 413, 414, 416
debridement, 49
deciduous, 335
decisions, 334
decompression, 164
defects, vii, xiv, xv, xvi, 1, 2, 3, 4, 8, 23, 26, 30, 33, 52, 54, 58, 141, 142, 169, 345, 346, 347, 354, 355, 359, 361, 364, 370, 380, 383, 384, 391, 392, 393, 396, 397, 399, 400, 401, 402, 403, 404, 405, 406
defense, 129
deficiency, 8, 18, 30, 57, 241, 271, 275, 277, 278, 282, 283, 372, 392, 404, 422
deficit, 169
definition, 46, 86, 125, 238, 251, 267, 302, 347, 356, 384, 416
deformities, 4
degradation, 22, 112, 123, 125, 129
degrading, 171
dehiscence, 79
dehydration, 14
dehydrogenase, 57, 122, 131, 132, 138
dementia, 5
demography, 253
denaturing gradient gel electrophoresis, 280
dendritic cell, 146
Dendritic cells, 128
dengue, xv, 373, 374, 375, 376, 378, 379, 380, 381, 423
dengue fever, 374, 375, 376, 378, 380, 381
dengue hemorrhagic fever, xv, 373, 374, 379, 380
Denmark, 151, 321, 327
density, 35, 236, 239, 242, 244, 251, 270
deoxyribonucleic acid, 15
Department of Health and Human Services, 62, 80
deposition, 242
deposits, 238
depression, 25, 155
dermatology, 96, 425
desensitization, 21
destruction, 247, 271, 290
detachment, 122, 138
detection, ix, x, xiii, 10, 11, 16, 18, 37, 75, 85, 140, 143, 144, 145, 147, 148, 167, 175, 182, 189, 200, 204, 223, 224, 227, 243, 280, 285, 290, 295, 296, 297, 298, 299, 301, 302, 303, 312, 313, 314, 315, 316, 317, 335, 376, 423
detection techniques, 11
developed countries, 145, 205, 227, 270
developing countries, xi, 20, 34, 39, 46, 47, 59, 142, 169, 199, 204, 214, 219, 237, 269, 270, 274, 280, 294
developmental delay, 169
deviation, 410
dexamethasone, 45
dextrocardia, 27
diabetes, 30, 120, 357, 358, 363, 384, 386, 390, 394, 395, 398, 402
diabetes mellitus, 357, 363, 384, 386, 402
diagnostic criteria, 86, 179, 347, 386
diagnostic ultrasound, 54
diaphragm, 115, 389
diarrhea, 39, 117, 129
diarrhoea, 216
dichotomy, 237
dietary, 6, 41, 265, 320
differential diagnosis, 334, 340, 371
differentiation, viii, 111, 112, 125, 126, 128, 133, 136, 137, 302, 317, 384
diffusion, 291
dilation, 346
diphtheria, 50, 51
disability, 45, 191, 281
disclosure, 217
discomfort, 52, 160
discordance, 238, 267
discrimination, 312
disease progression, 19, 219
diseases, vii, xiv, xv, 1, 2, 37, 57, 58, 63, 65, 66, 67, 69, 70, 87, 148, 157, 158, 220, 221, 227, 229, 243, 244, 273, 274, 307, 326, 331, 332, 333, 334, 335, 339, 340, 345, 346, 348, 349, 350, 351, 353, 355, 356, 357, 360, 361, 363, 366, 367, 368, 369, 371, 378, 383, 384, 385, 386, 387, 388, 389, 390, 393, 395, 396, 397, 401, 402, 403, 404, 406, 408, 418, 421
disinfection, 94
disorder, 43, 86, 169, 374, 378, 379, 423
displacement, 153
disseminated intravascular coagulation, 17, 23
distilled water, 143
distress, 5, 21, 42, 71, 75, 169, 245, 336
distribution, 143, 237, 253, 274, 279, 292, 322, 327, 352, 356, 362, 363, 368, 389, 393, 411, 415
disulfide, 115
divergence, 306
diversity, 292, 305, 316

diverticulitis, 8
division, 31, 107, 291
dizygotic, 293
dizygotic twins, 293
dizziness, 378
DNA, ix, xiii, 13, 15, 17, 23, 24, 25, 26, 53, 79, 122, 130, 140, 142, 143, 144, 146, 147, 290, 299, 315, 422
DNA polymerase, 143
doctors, 52, 349, 386
dogs, 343
donor, 121
donors, 275, 293
doppler, 26
Doppler, 54
dosimetry, 56, 80
dosing, 303
DOT, 38
Down syndrome, 348, 369, 384, 385, 389, 391
down-regulation, 45
drainage, 48, 49
drinking, xii, 33, 289, 293, 309
drinking water, 293, 309
drug abuse, 200
drug design, 379
drug exposure, 370, 403
drug history, 206
drug interaction, 219, 273
drug resistance, 73, 270, 274
drug treatment, xv, 346, 349, 351, 360, 361, 365, 366, 368, 371, 372, 383, 387, 392, 393, 396
drug use, 6, 14, 16, 170, 349, 387, 404
drugs, xi, xvi, 19, 35, 38, 39, 40, 62, 72, 73, 74, 128, 170, 199, 208, 220, 227, 273, 274, 283, 297, 348, 349, 351, 353, 354, 355, 356, 357, 359, 360, 363, 364, 367, 368, 374, 376, 384, 385, 386, 387, 391, 392, 394, 396, 400, 401, 402, 404, 424
ductus arteriosus, 30, 181
duodenum, 368, 372
duplication, 369
duration, vii, xv, xvi, 1, 2, 8, 19, 28, 33, 34, 41, 44, 142, 175, 179, 204, 205, 216, 217, 226, 242, 245, 298, 335, 351, 374, 383, 384, 390, 393, 398, 399, 401, 402, 420
dyslexia, 54
dysplasia, 27, 347
dysuria, 17, 32, 351, 356

E

ears, 35, 239, 334
East Asia, 18, 71
Eastern Europe, xiii, 319, 322, 323, 324, 325
eating, 5, 294, 320
echocardiogram, 56
eclampsia, xv, 220, 239, 276, 345, 357, 358, 363, 367, 368, 372, 390, 394, 395, 398
ecology, 308, 332
economic status, 250, 293, 294, 361
ecosystem, x, 167, 177, 189
ectopic pregnancy, 165
edema, 26, 33, 48, 49, 119, 236, 398, 402
education, 59, 79, 80, 128, 287, 326
efavirenz, 219
effusion, 38
egg, 93, 94, 106, 188
Egypt, 60, 113, 139, 142
ehrlichiosis, 340, 341, 342, 343
election, 298
electrolyte, 15, 377
electrolytes, 56, 160
electromagnetic, 55
electromagnetic fields, 55
electron, 137
electrophoresis, 252, 280, 285, 302, 378
ELISA, xii, 67, 142, 235, 297
elongation, 115
e-mail, 1
embolism, 50, 55, 81
embolus, 50
embryo, 8, 9, 53, 405
embryogenesis, 2, 400
embryos, 402
emphysema, x, 159, 160, 161, 162, 163, 164, 165, 388
employment, 352, 354, 355, 357, 358, 360, 361, 362, 364, 365
employment status, 352, 354, 355, 357, 358, 360, 361, 362, 364, 365
empyema, 8, 44
encapsulation, 39
encephalitis, 18, 27, 28, 51, 296, 316, 424
encephalopathy, 15, 26, 30, 66, 116, 118, 130, 132
endocarditis, 46, 50, 56
endocrine, 140, 170
endocrinological, 22
endocytosis, 114
endometritis, 12, 13, 22, 42, 47, 50, 63, 75, 78, 142, 148
endonuclease, 115
endoplasmic reticulum, 115

endothelial cell, 31, 114, 115, 119, 123, 246
endothelial cells, 31, 114, 115, 119, 123, 246
endothelium, 237, 379, 423
endotoxins, 7
enemas, 153
energy, 53, 54
England, 282, 326
enlargement, 154
enterocolitis, 169
environment, 47, 48, 85, 120, 204, 266, 292, 328, 423
environmental conditions, 292
environmental factors, 141, 263
enzyme immunoassay, 6, 19, 147, 302, 312, 313
enzyme-linked immunosorbent assay, 223, 312, 313, 314
enzymes, 22, 115, 121, 171, 291, 334
epidemic, 37, 72, 112, 119, 130, 134, 149, 243, 245, 286, 288, 332, 380, 398, 402, 419
epidemics, 112, 119, 132, 398, 405
epidemiologic studies, 54, 408, 416
epidemiology, 59, 60, 61, 67, 106, 141, 192, 196, 231, 280, 308, 332, 339, 408, 420
epigenetic, 308
epilepsy, 23, 169, 320, 363
episiotomy, 48, 49, 79
epistaxis, 388
epithelial cell, 114, 115, 116, 117, 123, 178, 290, 291
epithelial cells, 114, 115, 116, 117, 123, 178, 290, 291
epithelium, viii, 20, 83, 89, 90, 91, 96, 98, 99, 101, 104, 116
epitopes, 267, 302
Epstein-Barr virus, 65, 334
erythema infectiosum, 4, 24, 65
erythematous, 27, 40, 48
erythrocyte, 26, 277
erythrocytes, 15, 34, 35, 237, 246, 247, 281, 286
erythroid, 24, 65
erythroid cells, 24
erythropoietin, 219, 277, 278
*Escherichia coli(*E. coli), 32, 41, 47, 48, 173, 356, 350, 366
esophagoscopy, 163
esophagus, 163
ESR, 37, 56
esterase, 32, 75
estimating, 29
Estonia, 308
estriol, 194
ethical issues, viii, 84, 104
ethics, 105, 142
Ethiopia, 230, 243
ethnicity, 37
ETI, 321
etiologic agent, 342, 343
etiology, ix, x, 9, 59, 112, 140, 159, 164, 169, 187, 241, 270, 347, 369, 386, 387, 404, 405
Europe, xiii, xvi, 15, 16, 18, 63, 113, 148, 224, 226, 292, 294, 304, 306, 319, 320, 321, 322, 323, 324, 325, 342, 407, 408, 420
European Union, xiii, 319
evening, 179
evolution, 63, 113, 134, 283, 332
ewe, 158
examinations, 26, 41, 47, 54, 87, 93, 321, 349, 366
excitotoxicity, 58
exclusion, 85, 242, 388, 392, 409
excretion, 30, 291, 425
exercise, 41, 163
expertise, 35, 43
exposure, 6, 7, 10, 18, 19, 22, 23, 24, 25, 26, 27, 28, 30, 33, 34, 41, 52, 53, 54, 55, 58, 68, 69, 80, 81, 86, 138, 141, 227, 228, 236, 246, 270, 293, 296, 304, 307, 320, 334, 339, 348, 349, 355, 356, 385, 387, 405, 423, 424, 425
exposure, 10, 25, 53, 138, 226
expulsion, 9
extraction, 142
eyelid, 160
eyes, 17, 18, 291, 402

F

faecal, 11
failure, 15, 21, 25, 38, 40, 44, 45, 57, 65, 74, 215, 238, 269, 273, 350, 420
falciparum malaria, 35, 36, 71, 236, 237, 240, 245, 246, 264, 266, 267, 268, 274, 278, 279, 281, 284, 288
falciparum malaria infection, 240
false positive, 10, 342
familial, 372
family, ix, 17, 29, 51, 58, 113, 139, 141, 206, 219, 220, 272, 290, 364, 372, 389, 405
family history, 364
family physician, 51
family planning, 206, 219, 220, 272
Far East, xiii, 319, 322
farmers, 309, 339

farming, 258
farms, 309
Fas, 134
fascia, 48, 49
fatalities, xvi, 407, 409, 410, 411
fatigue, 5, 14, 37, 52, 378
FDA, 232, 312
fear, 203
feces, 28, 291, 292
fee, 106
feeding, xi, xii, 39, 48, 62, 199, 200, 204, 207, 212, 214, 216, 225, 227, 229, 230, 289, 290, 307
females, 21, 145, 243, 252, 293, 391
ferritin, 278
fertility, 47, 93, 281
fertilization, vii, 291
fetal brain, 9, 54
fetal death, ix, 2, 4, 21, 25, 26, 41, 57, 139, 394, 400, 424
fetal demise, 26
fetal distress, 21, 245
fetal growth, 146, 282, 391
fetal nutrition, 242, 268
fetal tissue, 9, 58, 119
fetus, vii, ix, xii, xiv, 1, 2, 3, 4, 5, 7, 9, 10, 11, 12, 16, 17, 18, 19, 20, 21, 23, 24, 25, 29, 30, 31, 33, 37, 39, 41, 42, 43, 45, 50, 51, 53, 54, 55, 56, 57, 64, 65, 66, 69, 75, 81, 112, 118, 119, 139, 141, 142, 152, 238, 270, 271, 289, 292, 294, 295, 296, 297, 298, 299, 300, 301, 303, 304, 307, 326, 331, 332, 368, 389, 404, 418, 419, 423
fetuses, 25, 26, 27, 31, 57, 142, 180, 243, 244, 344, 347, 349, 362, 365, 386, 400
fever, vii, xv, xvi, 2, 3, 5, 7, 8, 9, 17, 23, 24, 26, 28, 29, 32, 34, 35, 37, 39, 40, 42, 44, 45, 46, 47, 48, 49, 50, 51, 52, 56, 58, 73, 74, 79, 88, 117, 181, 236, 244, 279, 295, 332, 334, 336, 337, 338, 339, 340, 341, 342, 343, 344, 351, 352, 356, 361, 366, 373, 374, 375, 376, 377, 378, 379, 380, 381, 383, 384, 388, 389, 390, 391, 392, 393, 396, 397, 398, 400, 401, 402, 403, 405, 406, 410, 413, 421, 423
fibrin, 238, 242, 269
fibroblast, 133, 136
fibronectin, 132, 187, 188
fibrosis, 369
fifth disease, 24, 65
filariasis, 378
film, 35, 56, 242, 254, 255, 256, 260, 268, 269, 270, 284
films, 251, 284
filtration, 32, 368
fingerprinting, 79
Finland, 321, 328
firms, 313
fistulas, 89
fixation, 369
flank, 50, 154, 351, 356
flare, 37
flaviviruses, 379
flora, 11, 22, 32, 42, 47, 64, 94, 104, 173, 175, 176, 192, 193, 194
flow, 7, 21, 32, 160
fluid, xiii, 8, 11, 15, 18, 22, 25, 37, 41, 42, 46, 63, 64, 68, 75, 94, 115, 116, 119, 120, 123, 124, 130, 131, 132, 134, 163, 171, 174, 178, 181, 188, 192, 222, 290, 295, 299, 300, 303, 315, 377
fluorescence, 135
fluorescence in situ hybridization, 135
fluoroquinolones, 33, 40
focusing, 333
folate, 33, 206, 219, 241, 264, 392, 404
folic acid, 29, 349, 353, 358, 361, 363, 387, 391, 394, 401, 402, 406
food, xii, 5, 28, 39, 45, 280, 289, 292, 293, 294, 326
Food and Drug Administration, 13, 232
food products, 45
foodborne illness, 45
forceps, 164
forebrain, 58
formal education, 255, 258
fragmentation, 122, 130
France, 209, 230, 292, 296, 321, 327, 341
free radical, 53
free radicals, 53
freedom, 252
freezing, 309
fresh frozen plasma, 15
FTA, 21
fulminant hepatitis, 14
funds, 104
fungi, 129
fusion, 114, 115

G

Gabon, 71, 238, 242, 268, 276
gall bladder, 39, 44
gametocytes, 34, 291
ganglia, 27, 422
gas, 42, 54, 75, 163, 389
gastroenteritis, xi, 200

gastrointestinal, 3, 5, 31, 46, 116
gastrointestinal tract, 116
gastroschisis, 354, 364
gel, 143, 180, 280, 302
gels, 299
gender, 321
gender differences, 321
gene, viii, 8, 111, 112, 113, 121, 125, 126, 131, 134, 136, 137, 143, 275, 299, 300, 302, 384, 385
gene expression, viii, 111, 112, 121, 125, 126, 136, 137
general practitioner, 376, 377
general practitioners, 376
generation, 40, 45, 48, 204, 223, 335
genes, 112, 131, 132, 293, 308
genetic diversity, 292
genetic factors, 19
genetic marker, 284
genetic mutations, 53
genetic traits, 279
genetics, xii, 140, 289, 371
Geneva, 63, 75, 78, 79, 276, 286, 288, 418, 420
genital herpes, 18, 61, 62, 141, 147, 148, 149
genital warts, 20
genitourinary tract, 59
genome, 16, 114, 422
genomic, 114
genotype, xii, 235, 247, 248, 250, 251, 252, 255, 258, 260, 266, 267, 281, 286, 292, 293, 305, 306
genotypes, 266, 278, 292, 306, 374
gentamicin, 33, 42, 46, 47
germ cells, 53
German measles, 4
Germany, viii, xi, 83, 84, 86, 89, 93, 102, 104, 105, 142, 167, 168, 178, 184, 187, 190, 321, 328
gestation, viii, ix, x, 2, 9, 15, 17, 18, 20, 21, 25, 27, 28, 30, 37, 53, 55, 76, 83, 84, 86, 88, 90, 92, 99, 102, 103, 118, 120, 134, 139, 140, 142, 151, 156, 160, 167, 168, 177, 184, 185, 203, 207, 215, 238, 240, 249, 273, 294, 297, 299, 300, 303, 304, 347, 350, 354, 366, 386, 389, 390, 394, 400, 412, 416
gestational age, xv, 21, 26, 29, 43, 71, 85, 107, 156, 171, 174, 179, 181, 184, 187, 191, 196, 232, 282, 300, 315, 347, 355, 356, 358, 359, 364, 365, 366, 367, 368, 383, 384, 391, 393, 394, 399, 412, 416
gestational diabetes, 394
Gibbs, 61, 74, 75, 78, 129, 172, 192, 193
girls, 142, 146, 359
gland, 34, 115
glass, 276
glaucoma, 30
glia, 58
glial, 116
glial cells, 116
gliosis, 9
globalization, 305
globulin, 10, 15, 28, 67, 424
glomerulonephritis, xiv, 345, 350, 351, 361, 362, 371, 372
glottis, 163
gloves, 178, 190
glucocorticoids, 121
glucose, 35, 42, 56, 57, 75, 232
glucose tolerance, 232
glutamate, 58
glutathione, 121
glutathione peroxidase, 121
glycogen, 35
glycolipids, 114
glycoprotein, 114, 141, 147
glycoproteins, 29, 112, 113, 114, 422, 425
glycosylation, 115
GM-CSF, 125
goals, 274
gold, 18, 35, 42, 104, 269, 272, 297, 349, 377, 387
gold standard, 18, 35, 42, 104, 269, 272, 297, 349, 377, 387
gonorrhea, 7, 13, 59, 62
governance, xi, 200
government, iv, 220, 249, 250, 272
GPx, 121
grades, 377
gram stain, 196
Gram-negative, 32, 42, 47, 334
Gram-positive, 36, 42, 47
grants, 128
granulocyte, 125
granulomas, 37
Great Britain, 321
Greece, 321, 327, 331
Grenada, 307
grouping, 252
groups, xiv, xvi, 14, 37, 38, 101, 103, 104, 105, 142, 143, 179, 190, 241, 246, 247, 263, 278, 279, 281, 283, 285, 286, 290, 298, 305, 326, 328, 345, 347, 350, 352, 354, 356, 357, 362, 363, 364, 368, 384, 386, 388, 390, 391, 392, 394, 395, 396, 397, 399, 400, 401
growth, vii, ix, 1, 2, 3, 4, 5, 8, 21, 23, 27, 30, 53, 57, 117, 139, 146, 173, 174, 181, 218, 236, 244, 246,

247, 265, 269, 275, 282, 285, 334, 335, 342, 373, 391, 421
growth hormone, 30
growth inhibition, 335
guessing, 152, 157
guidelines, 20, 55, 58, 63, 70, 79, 205, 249, 272, 273, 333, 372
Guinea, 264, 276
gums, 117
gut, 34, 39

H

H1, 113
H1N1, viii, 111, 112, 117, 118, 122, 123
H3N2, 112, 118, 132, 134
H5N1, 112, 113, 116, 117, 119, 129, 130, 131, 133, 135, 136, 137, 138
H7N7, 113
HA, 106, 112, 113, 114, 115, 119, 192, 307, 316
HA1, 115
haemoglobin, 218, 247, 250, 251, 257, 259, 262, 264, 266, 270, 271, 272, 274, 278, 280, 284, 285
haemoglobin concentration, 250, 251, 257, 259, 262, 271
half-life, 301
handedness, 54
handling, 339
hands, 6
harm, 51, 56, 214, 291
harmful effects, 39, 53, 54
hay fever, 388
hazards, 74, 400, 402
HBV, 15, 16, 206, 308
HBV infection, 15
headache, 5, 29, 32, 35, 39, 47, 52, 295, 374, 398
healing, 99
health, xi, xii, xiii, xiv, 6, 19, 20, 37, 47, 54, 57, 62, 73, 113, 132, 142, 168, 185, 186, 190, 192, 193, 199, 200, 203, 205, 206, 214, 220, 221, 223, 225, 226, 227, 230, 231, 232, 236, 239, 241, 243, 244, 248, 249, 250, 266, 272, 273, 274, 275, 277, 284, 287, 288, 289, 296, 304, 307, 319, 320, 321, 326, 328, 340, 341, 355, 367, 396, 417, 420
Health and Human Services, 62, 80
health care, xi, 20, 54, 142, 200, 203, 249, 272, 275
health care professionals, 203
health care workers, 54
health education, xiv, 304, 320, 326
health information, 220
health insurance, xi, 168, 185, 186, 190
health problems, xii, 225, 235, 241, 248
health services, 272, 274
healthcare, xi, 200, 325
hearing, 23, 24, 29, 30, 44, 45, 169
hearing loss, 23, 24, 29, 30, 44, 45
heart, 30, 41, 115, 119, 155, 290, 406
heart disease, 30
heart rate, 41, 155
heat, 9, 54, 112, 122, 126, 127, 402, 405, 421
heating, 54, 127
height, 37, 169, 249
hemagglutinin, 112, 131, 134
hematocrit, 251, 374, 376, 377, 378, 380
hematologic, 33, 374
hematological, xv, 308, 373, 375, 377, 378, 422
hematology, 37, 379
hematomas, 48
hematuria, 32, 361, 372
hemodynamic, 346
hemoglobin, 242, 247, 252, 266, 274, 282, 285, 286, 378, 389
hemoglobin (Hb), 247, 252, 281
hemoglobin electrophoresis, 378
hemoglobinopathies, 285
hemoglobinopathy, 24
hemoptysis, 37
hemorrhage, 40, 42, 169, 239, 271, 358, 363, 380, 398, 402
hemorrhages, 413
hemostasis, 95, 374
hemostatic, 378
Heparin, 79
hepatic failure, 15
hepatic injury, 16
hepatic necrosis, 3
hepatitis, 3, 4, 6, 7, 14, 15, 16, 25, 27, 28, 50, 59, 60, 296, 327, 422
Hepatitis A, 14, 16, 28, 51, 52, 60
Hepatitis B, 3, 6, 7, 15, 16, 50, 51, 52, 60, 327
Hepatitis C, 6, 16, 60
hepatocellular, 3, 16
hepatocellular carcinoma, 3, 16
hepatocytes, 115
hepatomegaly, 21, 300
hepatosplenomegaly, 3, 5, 21, 23, 28, 40, 142, 376
hepatotoxicity, 208, 213, 232, 335
hernia, 347
herpes, ix, x, 11, 12, 17, 18, 26, 28, 61, 62, 139, 140, 141, 142, 144, 145, 146, 147, 148, 149, 219, 231, 422, 426

herpes infections, 61
herpes labialis, 141
herpes simplex, ix, x, 12, 18, 61, 62, 139, 140, 141, 142, 144, 145, 146, 147, 148, 149, 219, 231
herpes virus, 26, 148
herpes zoster, 27, 28, 147, 422, 426
herpesviruses, 422
heterogeneity, 179, 298, 409
heterogeneous, 293
heterozygotes, 247
HHS, 80
high risk, viii, xi, 6, 7, 19, 20, 37, 51, 52, 83, 84, 88, 102, 103, 108, 141, 145, 167, 179, 220, 236, 267, 334, 339, 379, 416, 423
high temperature, 366
Highly active antiretroviral therapy (HAART), xi, 1219, 199, 200, 203, 205, 207, 209, 213, 214, 215, 218, 220, 230, 272
high-risk, 22, 88, 101, 103, 108, 179, 183, 339
high-risk populations, 179
high-speed, 96
hip, 48, 347
Hiroshima, 80
Hispanic, 149
histidine, 281
histological, 41, 117, 120, 171, 238, 269, 280, 368
histology, 269, 284
histopathology, 282
histoplasmosis, 8
HIV infection, xi, xii, 18, 19, 36, 37, 38, 62, 199, 200, 203, 204, 216, 221, 223, 224, 227, 231, 235, 239, 241, 243, 244, 245, 246, 248, 250, 251, 253, 254, 256, 257, 259, 262, 263, 265, 271, 272, 273, 274, 275, 276, 279, 280, 284
HIV test, 203, 204, 207, 220, 222, 223, 224, 274
HIV/AIDS, 219, 221, 243, 286
HIV-1, 4, 62, 64, 206, 210, 219, 221, 222, 223, 225, 226, 227, 228, 229, 230, 231, 232, 244, 277, 279, 281, 287
HIV-2, 4
HLA, 293, 308
Holland, 307, 309, 321, 329
homeostasis, 346
Hong Kong, 112, 118, 130
hookworm, 219, 251, 264
hormone, 30
hospital, 28, 32, 47, 79, 93, 101, 148, 161, 164, 174, 249, 250, 251, 285, 309, 422, 423
hospitalization, 27, 44, 118, 377, 404
hospitalizations, 130, 133
hospitalized, 15, 118, 362, 375, 380
hospitals, 47, 101, 224, 272
host, xii, 19, 20, 23, 113, 114, 115, 131, 181, 218, 237, 263, 289, 290, 292, 295, 304, 305, 320
hot spots, 39
House, 278, 373, 421
household, 25, 423
HPV, 6, 19, 66
HR, 217
HSV-1, 17, 141, 142, 143, 144, 147
human exposure, 54, 81
human milk, 60, 73
human papillomavirus, 6
human parvovirus B19, 65, 66, 67
human subjects, 288
humanity, 332
humans, xiv, 29, 33, 39, 45, 53, 54, 58, 112, 113, 114, 129, 131, 137, 138, 282, 290, 292, 293, 306, 320, 321, 331, 332, 333, 339, 342, 343, 373, 421
humidity, 291
Hungarian, xiv, xv, 345, 346, 349, 355, 356, 359, 361, 362, 366, 367, 369, 370, 371, 383, 385, 386, 397, 403
Hungary, 345, 346, 348, 352, 357, 362, 363, 369, 383, 384, 385, 389, 398, 406
hybridization, 13, 119, 135, 136
hydramnios, 21, 26
hydration, 7, 49
hydrocele, 347
hydrocephalus, 2, 5, 26, 29, 300, 393
hydrocephaly, 354, 364, 392
hydrocortisone, 381
hydrogen, 54, 173, 193
hydrogen peroxide, 173, 193
hydronephrosis, 346
hydrops, 2, 3, 4, 21, 25, 26, 65, 66, 67
hydroxide, 178
hydroxyl, 121
hygiene, 278, 293
hygienic, xvi, 24, 294, 320, 421, 422
hyperbilirubinemia, 5, 300
hypercoagulable, 50, 361
hyperesthesia, 151
hyperglycaemia, 208
hyperinsulinemia, 35
hyperplasia, 119
hypertension, 30, 32, 33, 358, 361, 363, 371, 372, 398
hypertensive, 361

hyperthermia, xvi, 8, 9, 54, 58, 384, 393, 396, 401, 402, 403, 405, 406
hyperthyroidism, 55
hypertrophy, 372
hyperventilation, 389
hypoglycemia, 35, 71, 236
hypoplasia, 27, 86
hypospadias, 347, 359, 386, 387
hypotension, 9, 43, 154
hypotensive, 118
hypothalamic, 7
hypothermia, 58
hypothesis, 22, 84, 128, 238, 281, 292, 369, 391, 401
hypotonia, 23
hypoventilation, 155
hypoxia, 9, 25, 58
hypoxic, 9, 266, 270

I

IAC, 277
ICD, 46, 350
ice, 48
ICU, 381
id, xvi, 88, 179, 191, 333, 352, 359, 362, 365, 384, 396, 397, 401, 410, 415
identification, xi, 48, 141, 148, 199, 204, 220, 304, 332, 356
identity, 134
idiopathic, 66
idiosyncratic, 336
IFA, 299, 335
IgE, xiii, 290, 298, 303, 314, 316
IgG, x, xiii, 6, 10, 11, 24, 27, 28, 29, 30, 31, 40, 67, 68, 140, 142, 143, 144, 146, 284, 290, 295, 296, 297, 298, 301, 302, 303, 308, 311, 312, 313, 314, 316, 317, 319, 321, 323, 325, 327, 334, 374, 425
IL-1, 9, 120, 125, 128, 129
IL-6, viii, 9, 111, 120, 125, 127, 128, 129, 188
IL-8, 85, 89, 188
ileum, 39, 368
ilium, 153
Illinois, 80, 309, 339
illumination, 143
images, 54
imaging, 45, 50, 52, 53, 54, 55, 56, 79, 80, 81, 154, 155
imaging modalities, 52
immigrants, 325
immigration, xiii, 319, 321, 325
immune activation, 8, 270, 279
immune function, 45, 389
immune globulin, 10, 15, 28, 67, 424
immune response, 9, 23, 29, 31, 45, 124, 125, 131, 146, 147, 226, 228, 238, 247, 274, 276, 278, 284, 285, 290, 291, 293, 295, 301
immune system, xii, 9, 27, 34, 58, 218, 289, 300
immunity, xii, 6, 9, 10, 14, 25, 27, 28, 31, 34, 45, 58, 69, 134, 145, 149, 216, 236, 237, 239, 241, 244, 247, 263, 266, 289, 298, 416, 420
immunization, 30, 51, 60, 65, 67, 80, 141, 145, 146, 374, 421
immunoassays, 302
immunocompromised, 26, 45, 46, 291, 295, 297
immunodeficiency, 6, 7, 12, 56, 58, 61, 62, 72, 223, 224, 225, 228, 231, 232, 243, 273, 275, 277, 283, 286, 308, 311, 422
immunodeficient, 37
immunofluorescence, 19, 297, 311
immunoglobulin, ix, 15, 16, 23, 24, 26, 27, 35, 40, 68, 125, 140, 146, 302, 308, 310, 311, 312, 313, 314, 315, 316, 317, 326, 424
immunoglobulin G, 27, 35, 40, 125, 146, 302, 308, 310, 312, 313, 314, 315, 316, 317, 326
immunoglobulins, ix, 140, 142, 296, 301, 312, 316
immunohistochemical, 116, 119, 280
immunological, 7, 104, 145, 226, 237, 238, 269, 313, 369, 372, 374
immunology, 109, 284, 389, 404
immunoreactivity, 124
immunosuppression, 37, 218, 272, 287, 308, 422
immunosuppressive, 297
immunosuppressive drugs, 297
implementation, x, xiii, 146, 167, 182, 185, 186, 200, 222, 264, 272, 273, 319, 320
in situ, 119, 130, 135
in situ hybridization, 119, 135
in utero, vii, ix, 1, 2, 10, 18, 21, 23, 25, 31, 53, 58, 66, 67, 135, 139, 142, 146, 204, 224, 226, 246, 302, 335, 379, 419, 423
in vitro, viii, 65, 111, 121, 133, 134, 138, 247, 284, 302, 335, 336, 337
in vivo, 117, 134, 135
incidence, vii, x, xv, 1, 2, 22, 24, 28, 36, 39, 42, 43, 44, 49, 50, 53, 63, 66, 132, 134, 151, 152, 159, 185, 194, 200, 204, 221, 222, 231, 232, 246, 269, 274, 282, 310, 311, 320, 321, 326, 327, 329, 333, 349, 372, 373, 376, 383, 386, 390, 393, 394, 397, 398, 421, 422, 423
inclusion, 23, 85, 148, 249, 250, 251, 271, 409
income, 20, 220, 251, 310

incubation, 23, 26, 28, 29, 45, 121, 125, 126, 127, 133, 374
incubation period, 23, 26, 29, 45, 374
India, 36, 72, 74, 145, 222, 223, 230, 231, 232, 337, 341
Indian, xiii, 69, 148, 222, 283, 285, 286, 319, 320, 322, 323, 324, 325, 381, 418
indication, viii, 51, 53, 55, 84, 333, 366
indicators, 361, 375
indices, 54, 158, 298
indomethacin, 121, 181
Indonesia, 113, 135
inducer, 129
inducible enzyme, 121
induction, 99, 112, 114, 116, 121, 122, 125, 126, 127, 128, 132, 135, 137, 138, 181
industrialized countries, 29
infancy, 287, 300, 303, 317, 341
infant mortality, 70, 221, 246, 273, 274, 276, 282, 287, 346
infant mortality rate, 221
infarction, 9
infectious, vii, xv, 1, 2, 7, 8, 9, 14, 15, 20, 24, 30, 39, 41, 48, 63, 64, 78, 79, 117, 141, 148, 151, 156, 173, 187, 216, 219, 227, 229, 273, 275, 290, 291, 334, 339, 350, 353, 357, 368, 383, 384, 385, 388, 389, 393, 395, 397, 398, 401, 402, 404, 417
infectious disease, vii, xv, 1, 2, 8, 148, 151, 173, 219, 227, 229, 273, 275, 339, 350, 353, 368, 383, 384, 385, 388, 389, 393, 395, 397, 398, 401, 402, 404, 417
infectious diseases, vii, xv, 1, 2, 8, 148, 151, 173, 227, 229, 339, 350, 353, 368, 383, 384, 385, 388, 389, 393, 395, 397, 401, 402, 404, 417
infectious mononucleosis, 64
inferiority, 213
infertility, xiv, 47, 219, 331, 334
inflammation, 7, 9, 21, 22, 31, 41, 43, 48, 58, 74, 79, 85, 89, 105, 116, 117, 124, 133, 134, 151, 170, 171, 180, 188, 274, 351, 356, 361
inflammatory, viii, 7, 9, 24, 29, 31, 47, 74, 111, 112, 120, 124, 125, 128, 132, 135, 136, 154, 170, 171, 181, 189, 192, 219, 237, 290, 291
inflammatory cells, 9, 237
inflammatory disease, 47, 219
inflammatory mediators, 237
inflammatory response, 7, 24, 31, 125, 170, 181, 192, 290, 291
influenza, viii, xvi, 9, 50, 59, 111, 112, 113, 114, 115, 116, 117, 118, 119, 122, 123, 124, 125, 126, 127, 128, 129, 130, 131, 132, 133, 134, 135, 136, 137, 138, 181, 361, 370, 384, 389, 392, 393, 397, 398, 399, 400, 401, 402, 403, 404, 405
influenza a, 130, 397, 398, 399, 400, 401, 405
informed consent, 142, 224, 250, 348, 385
infrastructure, 203, 220, 274
ingestion, xii, 10, 37, 39, 45, 289, 291, 292, 296
inguinal, 347
inguinal hernia, 347
inheritance, 369, 371
inherited, 378
inhibition, 114, 121, 123, 136, 138, 216, 335, 336
inhibitor, 121, 122, 126, 205, 208, 226, 232
inhibitors, 121, 137, 205, 208, 220
inhibitory, 124, 129, 131, 133
initiation, 123, 124, 226, 238, 268, 377
injection, 6, 10, 16, 52
injuries, 163
injury, 7, 9, 16, 33, 42, 58, 135, 155, 163, 164, 170
innate immunity, 58
innominate, 158
inoculation, 18, 115, 120, 122, 299, 302, 303
inoculum, 41, 48
iNOS, 121
insecticide, 35, 231, 248, 250, 255, 256, 263, 274
insemination, 206
insight, 113, 174
inspection, 20, 48, 339
inspiration, 389
insulin, 357
insulin dependent diabetes, 357
insults, 9
insurance, xi, 168, 185, 186, 190
insurance companies, xi, 168, 185, 190
integration, 273, 325
integrity, 49
intensive care unit, 423
interaction, 119, 200, 243, 245, 277, 385, 406
interactions, 135, 219, 273, 277, 288
interface, 113, 146, 237
interference, 31, 263
interferon (IFN), viii, 111, 112, 125, 127, 134, 214, 279
interferons, 138
interleukin, viii, 108, 111, 133, 134, 137
interleukin-1, 134
interleukin-6, 133, 137
interleukin-8, 108
interleukins, 42
International Classification of Diseases, 46, 350, 393

international standards, 220
interstitial, 119, 163, 346
interval, xvi, 42, 45, 156, 182, 202, 356, 407, 412, 413
intervention, 43, 137, 156, 177, 182, 216, 225, 248, 264, 273
interview, 348, 385
interviews, 142
intestinal obstruction, 372
intestinal perforation, 40
intestinal tract, 164, 369
intestine, 116, 123, 291, 320, 368
intoxication, 377
intracranial, 2, 5, 300
intramuscular, 59
intramuscularly, 12, 13, 21
intrauterine growth retardation, ix, 139, 181, 218, 236, 244, 246, 265, 269, 275, 285
intravascular, 17, 23
intravenous, 6, 14, 18, 24, 26, 28, 41, 42, 44, 207, 338, 377, 424
intravenous fluids, 41, 44
intravenously, 338
intrinsic, 271
introitus, 177, 178
invasive, 25, 26, 28, 94, 172
Investigations, vi, 276, 310, 365, 407
investment, 220
iodine, 55, 56, 179
ionizing radiation, 53, 54, 55, 81, 155
IPV, 51, 52
Iraq, 113
Ireland, 226
iritis, 5
iron, 218, 241, 264, 271, 272, 275, 277, 278, 279, 280, 282, 283, 390
iron deficiency, 241, 271, 275, 277, 278, 282, 283
irritation, 21
ischemia, 9, 58, 170, 369
Islam, 74
isolation, 148, 149, 154, 171, 299, 303
isoniazid, 38, 219
isotopes, 55, 56
Israel, 69
Italy, vi, xiii, 142, 289, 296, 319, 321, 322, 323, 324, 325, 326, 328, 329
IUGR, 244, 269
IVIg, 26
Ivory Coast, 228

J

JAMA, 62, 64, 65, 71, 72, 76, 80, 147, 157, 165, 225, 226, 229, 232, 233, 417
Jamaica, 221
Japan, 111, 128, 309, 420
Japanese, 51, 149, 379
Japanese encephalitis, 51
jaundice, 14, 21, 23, 142, 247
jejunum, 368
joints, 52
Jordan, 66, 69, 131, 306
Jun, 223, 381

K

KAP, 321
Kashmir, 148
Kenya, 218, 230, 242, 245, 263, 264, 266, 270, 271, 275, 284, 285, 286, 287
kidney, 8, 31, 115, 116, 123, 346, 350, 351, 353, 355, 357, 361, 366, 368, 371, 372
kidney stones, 353, 357, 366
kidneys, 32, 36, 163, 291, 346
kinase, 125, 137
Korean, 306

L

labeling, 122, 130
labor, vii, x, 1, 13, 14, 15, 18, 19, 22, 36, 41, 42, 43, 45, 46, 47, 60, 61, 74, 75, 86, 87, 89, 90, 93, 99, 100, 101, 106, 107, 108, 120, 124, 129, 131, 134, 147, 155, 156, 159, 160, 161, 163, 164, 165, 169, 170, 171, 172, 177, 180, 181, 188, 191, 192, 195, 222, 224, 269, 341, 379, 423
laboratory studies, 56
labor-intensive, 269
labour, xii, 2, 7, 18, 22, 36, 37, 59, 76, 131, 132, 165, 204, 205, 214, 215, 220, 235, 249, 253, 254, 255
lack of control, 205
lactate dehydrogenase, 122, 131, 132, 138
lactic acid, 173, 179, 207, 208, 232
lactobacillus, x, 70, 94, 167, 173, 174, 177, 178, 179, 180, 189
lamina, 239
lamivudine, xi, 19, 200, 214, 227, 228, 229, 272
language, 321, 408
laparoscopic, 43, 44, 77, 155, 157, 158
laparoscopic cholecystectomy, 44

laparoscopic surgery, 43, 155, 158
laparoscopy, 43, 77, 156, 157, 158, 163, 165
laparotomy, 43
large-scale, 408
laryngitis, 388, 390, 393
larynx, 116, 161
latency, 398
latex, 126, 335
Latin America, xiii, 15, 39, 319, 322, 323, 324, 325, 326
law, xiii, 319
LDH, 122
leadership, xi, 200
leakage, 15, 60, 122, 402
learning, 18, 23, 169, 247
learning disabilities, 18, 23
lectin, 119, 277
Legionella, 397
legislation, 321, 325
lens, 400
lesion, 11
lesions, 6, 17, 18, 20, 23, 27, 29, 37, 38, 89, 138, 163, 241, 284, 422, 424
lethargy, 23
leukaemia, 67
leukemia, 53, 56, 125, 133, 136, 137
leukemia cells, 133, 136
leukocyte, 9, 22, 32, 35, 42, 75, 146
leukocyte esterase, 32, 42
leukocytes, 7, 117, 120, 124, 135
leukocytosis, 23, 42
levator, 49
liberation, 115
lice, 332
life cycle, xii, 289, 290, 295, 303
life-cycle, 332
lifestyle, 348, 385, 391
life-threatening, xiv, 28, 49, 75, 208, 214, 331, 335, 337, 338
lifetime, 151
likelihood, 177, 266
limitation, 269, 271
limitations, 84, 171, 367, 416
linear, 53, 252, 422
linguistic, 325
linkage, 114
links, 70
lipid, 113, 115, 422
lipopolysaccharide, 121
lipoprotein, 29
liquid chromatography, 75
liquids, 377
Listeria monocytogenes, 41, 45
literacy, 266
liver, 8, 15, 16, 23, 34, 35, 37, 39, 56, 57, 115, 116, 117, 123, 206, 208, 291, 334
liver cells, 34
liver cirrhosis, 15
liver damage, 16
liver enzymes, 334
liver failure, 57
liver function tests, 23, 56
livestock, 290
local government, 249, 250
localised, xvi, 407, 414, 416
London, 69, 78, 106, 129, 195, 196, 199, 214, 223, 277, 278, 279, 284, 305, 326, 327, 328, 418, 426
long period, 298
longitudinal study, 148, 275
Los Angeles, 230
loss of appetite, 32
losses, 84, 140
low birthweight, 17, 20, 34, 35, 245, 264, 265, 267, 276, 283, 355, 359, 364, 365, 366, 367
low molecular weight, 302
low platelet count, 378
low risk, 25, 88, 179, 336
low-income, 310
low-level, 80
LPS, 121
lumbal, 164
lumbar, 56, 165
lumbar puncture, 56
lumen, 39, 116, 291, 368
lung, 8, 37, 116, 117, 119, 123, 135, 389
lungs, 36, 117, 119, 133, 161, 163, 291, 389
lupus, 8, 361
lymph, 5, 17, 24, 28, 29, 36, 39, 56, 115, 117, 295, 300, 326
lymph node, 29, 36, 39, 56, 115, 117
lymphadenitis, 313
lymphadenopathy, 5, 17, 24, 28, 295, 300, 326
lymphocyte, 134, 224
lymphocytes, 115, 117, 119, 131
lymphocytosis, 23, 296
lymphoid, 119, 123
lymphoid cells, 123
lymphomas, 16
lysis, 122

M

M.O., 67, 283
MI, 113, 114, 115
macromolecules, 112
macrophage, ix, 111, 112, 116, 117, 124, 125, 126, 127, 134
macrophage inflammatory protein, 124
macrophages, viii, 10, 111, 114, 116, 118, 121, 124, 125, 126, 128, 130, 133, 135, 136, 138, 146, 238, 269
macules, 422
magnetic, 50, 52, 55, 81
magnetic field, 55
magnetic resonance, 50, 52, 81
magnetic resonance imaging, 50, 52, 54, 81
magnets, 54
Maine, 312
maintenance, 136, 263, 271, 418
malaise, 14, 17, 23, 26, 28, 29, 32, 35, 37, 47, 295, 398
malaria, xi, xii, 5, 33, 34, 35, 36, 56, 70, 71, 72, 171, 173, 200, 203, 206, 218, 220, 230, 231, 235, 236, 237, 238, 239, 240, 241, 242, 243, 244, 245, 246, 247, 248, 250, 251, 253, 254, 255, 256, 257, 258, 259, 260, 261, 262, 263, 264, 265, 266, 267, 268, 269, 270, 271, 272, 273, 274, 275, 276, 277, 278, 279, 280, 281, 282, 283, 284, 285, 286, 287, 288, 378, 381
males, 252, 293, 368, 408
malignancy, 20, 50, 308
malnutrition, xi, 200, 214, 216, 220, 242
mammal, 332
management, xi, xiv, 12, 35, 36, 44, 48, 50, 53, 61, 63, 68, 69, 70, 72, 74, 75, 76, 77, 78, 79, 88, 107, 132, 147, 155, 157, 158, 200, 204, 219, 238, 276, 320, 326, 331, 333, 337, 338, 339, 340, 377, 417, 426
manufacturer, 204
Marfan syndrome, 87
marrow, 39, 40, 56, 65, 73, 117, 123, 134, 336
Marx, 313, 316
Maryland, 130, 131
MAS, 1, 405
masking, 219
mastitis, 8, 46, 48, 79, 204, 217
mastoiditis, 44
maternal age, 168, 239, 256, 263, 352, 360, 361, 362, 387
maternal care, 250, 251
maternal inheritance, 371
maternofetal, 303
matrix, 22, 113, 171
matrix metalloproteinase, 22
matrix protein, 113
maturation, 136, 298, 303, 312, 315, 317, 416
maxillary, 164
maxillary sinus, 164
MCA, 401
MCP, 124
MDI, 112, 124, 125, 126, 127, 137
MDR, 40
measles, 4, 31, 50, 149, 334
measurement, ix, x, 91, 140, 167, 174, 175, 176, 177, 178, 179, 182, 186, 187, 188, 190, 195, 196, 303, 314
measures, x, xi, xvi, 24, 28, 36, 85, 91, 94, 104, 105, 141, 167, 168, 170, 176, 177, 181, 187, 188, 190, 238, 264, 267, 282, 294, 304, 307, 407, 422
meat, 5, 6, 28, 292, 293, 294, 320
meconium, 9, 60, 369
media, 6, 13, 44, 216, 390
median, 143, 202, 215, 216, 217, 265, 410
mediastinum, 159, 161, 163, 164
mediators, 237
medication, 36, 38, 406
medications, 35, 39, 43, 392, 400
medicine, viii, x, 52, 55, 81, 83, 84, 104, 167, 168, 191, 278, 279, 340, 355, 370, 403, 409, 417
Mediterranean, 337, 340, 341, 343, 344
MEDLINE, 408
mefloquine, 36
membrane permeability, 33
membranes, viii, 13, 18, 19, 22, 41, 42, 46, 76, 88, 89, 92, 104, 108, 111, 112, 118, 120, 124, 128, 129, 130, 131, 132, 134, 135, 136, 160, 169, 170, 171, 172, 174, 180, 185, 187, 188, 193, 195, 204, 413
memory, 348, 355, 385
men, 81, 152, 157, 244, 332
meninges, 115
meningitis, 3, 5, 40, 42, 44, 45, 46, 56, 78
meningoencephalitis, 3, 4, 5
meningomyelocele, 405
menstruation, 180, 419
mental retardation, 23, 29, 30, 53, 80, 320
merozoites, 34
meta-analysis, 62, 63, 74, 107, 179, 194, 196, 200, 215, 217, 218, 221, 225, 228, 229, 245, 317, 410, 417

metabolic, 9, 377
metabolic disturbances, 377
metabolic rate, 9
metabolism, 7, 32, 279, 336
metalloproteinase, 129
metalloproteinases, 22
methylprednisolone, 381
metropolitan area, 118
Mexico, 309, 332
mice, 116, 118, 120, 123, 129, 133, 135, 138, 285, 292, 299, 305, 341, 405
microbes, 22, 89, 132, 133, 284, 306
microbial, x, 9, 41, 84, 86, 107, 124, 129, 167, 171, 172, 177, 181, 192, 365, 392
microbial agents, 365, 392
microcephaly, 2, 3, 4, 17, 23, 27, 53
microflora, 193
microglial, 9, 132
microorganisms, 41, 105, 172, 173, 174, 188, 366, 389
microscopy, xii, 11, 35, 56, 126, 235, 254, 267, 272
microvasculature, 237
microwave, 309
microwaves, 80
Middle East, xiii, 319, 322, 323, 324, 325
midwives, x, 167, 190
migration, 124, 129, 131, 133, 138
military, 310, 340
milk, 7, 16, 24, 39, 45, 48, 60, 73, 79, 216, 217, 225, 230, 338, 425, 426
mimicking, 132, 374, 378, 380
Ministry of Education, 128
minority, 14
MIP, 124
mirror, 355
miscarriage, vii, xvi, 1, 2, 22, 40, 52, 64, 85, 103, 107, 146, 193, 294, 407, 408, 409, 410, 411, 412, 413, 414, 415, 416
miscarriages, 85, 88, 89, 101, 105, 183, 410, 416
misleading, 347, 387
Missouri, 86
mites, 332
mitochondria, 113, 114
mitochondrial, 9, 129
mitogen, 125, 137
mitogen-activated protein kinase, 125, 137
mitosis, 402
mitotic, 9, 402
modalities, ix, 52, 140, 141
modality, 54
models, 16, 120, 171, 243, 333, 420
modulation, 226
molecular biology, 131
molecular mechanisms, 58
molecular pathology, 130
molecular weight, 302
molecules, viii, 111, 114, 126, 127, 137, 173, 291
monkeys, 208
monoclonal, 313
monoclonal antibodies, 313
monocyte, 112, 124, 125, 137
monocyte chemoattractant protein, 124
monocytes, viii, 111, 124, 126, 128, 136, 242
monolayers, 299
mononuclear cell, 115, 119, 136
mononuclear cells, 115, 119, 136
mononucleosis, 23, 64, 295, 320
monotherapy, 36, 201, 209, 214, 220, 336
morbidity, vii, x, xi, xiv, 1, 2, 13, 15, 18, 23, 25, 36, 37, 42, 44, 46, 49, 56, 70, 78, 79, 81, 130, 148, 151, 152, 156, 157, 168, 169, 172, 173, 199, 218, 220, 236, 241, 245, 247, 268, 269, 275, 280, 283, 285, 331, 333, 335, 374, 404, 422
morning, 179
morphological, 132, 369, 384, 426
morphology, 23, 54, 64
mortality, vii, x, xi, 1, 2, 4, 13, 15, 23, 27, 28, 31, 32, 33, 37, 42, 43, 44, 45, 46, 47, 49, 56, 57, 70, 72, 78, 88, 102, 130, 148, 151, 152, 155, 156, 168, 169, 199, 200, 202, 216, 219, 220, 225, 227, 229, 232, 236, 237, 239, 241, 243, 244, 245, 246, 247, 265, 269, 273, 274, 275, 276, 278, 282, 283, 284, 287, 346, 371, 375, 377, 393, 398, 420, 422, 423
mortality rate, 15, 23, 27, 28, 42, 45, 152, 221, 265, 398, 423
mosquito bites, 34, 36
mosquitoes, 373
motherhood, 272
motion, 54
motivation, 361
motor function, 169
mouse, 115, 116, 132, 135, 302, 303
mouse model, 115, 117
mouth, 3, 17, 18, 24, 298
movement, 43
Mozambique, 270
MRI, 52, 54, 55, 81, 155
mRNA, 113, 114, 115, 124, 125, 126, 127, 128, 136
mucosa, 40
mucous membranes, 413

mucus, 87, 104, 108, 109
multidisciplinary, 339
multigravidae, 230, 237, 239, 256, 259, 262, 263, 264, 285
multiplication, 34
multiplicity, 281
multivariate, 417
mumps, 31, 50
murine model, 333
murine models, 333
muscle, 27, 39, 48, 56, 115, 151, 290
muscle atrophy, 27
muscles, 291
muscular tissue, 291
mutations, 53, 112, 215, 228
myalgia, 5, 14, 17, 23, 35, 48, 116
Myanmar, 113
mycobacterium, 5, 36
myelination, 23
myeloid, 136
myocarditis, 3, 4, 25, 296
myometrium, 22, 50
myopathy, 208

N

N-acety, 121
NAD, 135
naloxone, 74
Namibia, 221
narcotic, 155
Nash, 307
National Health Service, 325
National Institute of Neurological Disorders and Stroke, 58
national policy, 274
National Research Council, 80
natural, xiv, 27, 53, 60, 239, 247, 297, 298, 306, 331, 332, 339, 422
nausea, 14, 39, 153, 156, 394, 404
Nebraska, 149
neck, 44, 52, 160, 161, 163, 164, 295
necrosis, viii, 3, 31, 111, 112, 117, 119, 123, 129, 130, 134, 137, 238, 424
necrotizing fasciitis, 48, 79, 158
needles, 164
negative consequences, 245
negativity, 325
neonatal, vii, ix, xi, xiii, 1, 2, 3, 4, 5, 9, 13, 17, 21, 24, 27, 34, 37, 40, 41, 42, 45, 56, 57, 58, 59, 61, 63, 69, 75, 88, 101, 137, 139, 141, 146, 147, 180, 200, 211, 212, 215, 216, 219, 226, 227, 228, 242, 243, 244, 245, 248, 250, 259, 260, 261, 265, 268, 270, 283, 287, 290, 295, 300, 301, 304, 327, 328, 334, 338, 346, 379, 417, 423, 424, 425
neonatal sepsis, 3, 42, 75, 180, 216
neonate, 3, 10, 12, 18, 19, 45, 141, 215, 296, 301, 333, 335, 336, 337, 338, 379
neonates, vii, xi, 1, 2, 12, 15, 17, 23, 148, 167, 168, 169, 215, 219, 255, 269, 272, 275, 283, 300, 301, 303, 333, 334, 335, 336, 337, 338, 375, 423, 424
Neoplasms, 8
Nepal, 310
nephritic syndrome, 368
nephritis, 27, 350, 351, 361, 368
nephrolithiasis, 361
nephropathy, 361
nerve, 49
nerves, 5
nervous system, vii, 1, 2, 23, 26, 142, 247, 422
nested PCR, 143, 299, 300
Netherlands, 321, 328, 407
neuraminidase, 112, 115, 131, 138
neuritis, 5
neurodegeneration, 58, 132
neurological condition, 9
neurological disorder, 116
neurons, 115, 116, 119, 123, 132
neuropathy, 208
neuroprotective, 9
neurotoxic, 9
neurotoxic effect, 9
neutropenia, 24, 208
neutrophil, 131, 188
neutrophils, 117, 119, 133, 154
New England, 282, 326
New Jersey, 73
New South Wales, 410, 411, 415, 419
New York, 59, 61, 70, 80, 106, 109, 130, 147, 192, 193, 194, 195, 196, 371, 372
New Zealand, 1
Newton, 74
nicotinamide, 117
Nielsen, 76, 157, 313, 317, 328
Niger, 278
Nigeria, vi, xii, 73, 113, 235, 248, 249, 255, 256, 259, 260, 261, 262, 272, 275, 277
NIH, 218
nitrate, 32
nitric oxide, 9, 58, 121, 135, 138
nitric oxide synthase, 121, 135, 138

nitrogen, 56
NK-cell, 389
nodes, 29, 36, 39, 161
non-infectious, 8, 334
non-pharmacological, 195
non-profit, 106
non-random, 216, 218
normal, viii, ix, x, 7, 8, 14, 21, 22, 23, 26, 30, 31, 32, 64, 76, 91, 94, 101, 111, 112, 124, 131, 140, 145, 151, 152, 153, 155, 156, 157, 160, 167, 173, 174, 175, 176, 180, 181, 183, 190, 243, 270, 282, 288, 325, 334, 347, 377, 386, 413, 415
normal conditions, 173
North America, 15, 16, 292
North Carolina, 224
Norway, 308, 309, 310, 321, 326, 328
nuclear, 9, 52, 55, 81, 113, 130
nuclei, 116
nucleic acid, 6, 11, 13, 204, 224, 336
nucleoside reverse transcriptase inhibitors, 205
nucleus, 115
nulliparous, 160
nurses, 348, 349, 366, 385, 388
nursing, 39, 79, 333
nutrient, 35, 269
nutrition, 37, 46, 206, 216, 220, 227, 242, 264, 268, 273, 286
nutritional deficiencies, 218

O

objective criteria, 56
obligate, 36, 290, 320, 332
observations, 124, 160, 176, 185, 240, 247, 265, 372, 409, 416, 418
obstetricians, 104, 250, 304, 344, 346, 348, 384, 385
obstruction, 33, 152, 346, 368, 372
occlusion, 89, 90, 91, 93, 94, 101, 102, 104, 105, 109, 192
occupational, 334, 339
Oceania, 374
odds ratio, xv, 345, 349, 387, 414, 415
oedema, 164, 358, 363
ofloxacin, 74, 343
oil, 5, 143
old-fashioned, 402
omentum, 43
online, 71, 78, 159, 194
optic neuritis, 5
optimism, 221
optimization, 145
oral, 13, 14, 35, 39, 46, 59, 68, 163, 215, 216, 222, 227, 351, 401, 402
oral cavity, 163
orchitis, 27
organ, 6, 16, 27, 30, 34, 37, 123, 127, 134, 135, 238, 267, 293, 347, 387
organelles, 304
organism, 20, 45, 114, 180, 181, 290, 292, 333
osteodystrophy, 361
osteomyelitis, 40
otitis media, 44, 216, 390
outpatient, 142, 346
over-the-counter, 378
oxidative, 116, 121, 134
oxidative damage, 116
oxidative stress, 121, 134
oxide, 9, 58, 121, 135, 138
oxygen, 9, 25, 35, 121, 133, 135, 160, 164, 173, 269, 377, 389
oxygenation, 389
oxytocin, 160, 164

P

P. falciparum, xii, 34, 35, 235, 236, 237, 238, 240, 242, 245, 246, 263, 266, 267, 268, 269, 270
p38, 125
pain, 14, 17, 32, 39, 43, 45, 46, 47, 48, 50, 52, 117, 151, 153, 154, 156, 163, 164, 351
Pakistan, 113
palpation, 91, 160
pancreas, 8, 115, 123
pancreatic, 35
pancreatitis, 44, 208
pandemic, 112, 113, 116, 118, 131, 133
Pap, 93
Papillomavirus, 19
Papua New Guinea, 264, 276
paracrine, 133
paramagnetic, 56
parameter, 252
parasitaemia, 236, 243, 245, 267, 269, 275, 278, 284, 287
parasite, xii, 28, 34, 35, 218, 237, 238, 239, 242, 245, 247, 250, 251, 255, 256, 258, 261, 263, 266, 270, 273, 287, 289, 290, 291, 292, 294, 295, 296, 297, 299, 302, 303, 305, 312, 320
parasitemia, 34, 35, 238, 239, 240, 242, 244, 246, 254, 268, 270, 273, 285, 287, 294

parasites, 34, 35, 56, 237, 238, 239, 240, 241, 247, 254, 255, 256, 260, 263, 269, 270, 273, 278, 279, 294, 300
parasitic diseases, 286
parasitic infection, 219, 308
parenchyma, 31, 351
parenchymal, 38
parenteral, 40, 41, 51, 60, 351
paresis, 160, 161
Paris, 74, 230, 287, 305, 311, 326, 328, 410, 419
partial thromboplastin time, 380
particles, 15, 117, 123, 126, 127, 133
passive, 10, 16, 216, 424
pathogenesis, ix, 7, 58, 78, 111, 112, 116, 117, 120, 122, 123, 124, 130, 131, 133, 137, 138, 237, 238, 247, 305, 374, 420
pathogenic, xiv, 41, 113, 117, 146, 149, 173, 315, 331, 332
pathogens, xiv, 45, 47, 124, 125, 146, 173, 331, 332, 333, 334, 335, 336, 338, 339, 397, 400
pathologic diagnosis, 43
pathologist, 332
pathologists, 347
pathology, 30, 70, 117, 130, 161, 163, 269, 280, 372
pathophysiological, 22, 26
pathophysiological mechanisms, 22
pathways, 57, 70, 128, 129, 170, 172
patient care, 81
PCR, 6, 11, 16, 35, 136, 142, 143, 144, 146, 148, 202, 207, 238, 280, 281, 292, 295, 299, 300, 303, 306, 315, 342
pediatric, 16, 18, 42, 346, 422, 425
pelvic, 8, 13, 32, 46, 47, 50, 53, 79, 154, 160, 182, 219
pelvic inflammatory disease, 47, 219
pelvic pain, 46, 47, 154
pelvis, 50, 154
penicillin, 12, 21, 42, 47, 63, 418
PEP, 218
peptide, 15, 115, 306
perforation, x, 13, 39, 40, 43, 44, 151, 153, 154, 155, 156, 157, 163, 164
perfusion, 55
pericardial, 2, 26, 163
pericardial sac, 163
pericarditis, 27
perinatal, vii, viii, x, xi, xii, xiv, 1, 2, 3, 4, 5, 14, 15, 16, 20, 21, 22, 26, 32, 33, 57, 62, 64, 66, 70, 71, 72, 83, 84, 85, 102, 105, 109, 130, 141, 149, 167, 168, 191, 200, 203, 221, 224, 225, 227, 228, 229, 232, 233, 235, 236, 241, 243, 265, 267, 269, 272, 275, 280, 282, 284, 286, 287, 331, 333, 336, 338, 341, 371, 380, 404, 408
perineum, 47
periodic, 34
periodontal, 171, 173, 177, 181
periodontal disease, 171, 173, 177, 181
periodontitis, 193
peripheral, xii, 11, 235, 240, 257, 259, 260, 262, 268
peripheral blood, 115, 126, 136, 237, 238, 239, 241, 242, 250, 255, 256, 268, 269, 270, 296, 303, 306
peripheral blood mononuclear cell, 115, 136
peripheral nervous system, 422
peristalsis, 346
peritoneal, 38, 135, 172
peritoneal cavity, 172
peritoneum, 43, 156
peritonitis, 47, 60, 153
peri-urban, 280
periventricular, 29, 58
periventricular leukomalacia, 58
permeability, 33, 122
permit, 105, 190
peroxide, 173, 193
peroxynitrite, 121, 134
person-to-person contact, ix, 139
petechiae, 23, 376
pH, x, 21, 113, 115, 167, 173, 174, 175, 176, 177, 178, 179, 181, 182, 183, 186, 187, 188, 190, 193, 195, 196, 252
pH values, 174, 175, 179, 183
phagocyte, 117, 129
phagocytic, 7
phagocytosis, 116, 124, 127, 130, 133, 135, 138, 290
phalanx, 178
pharmacological, 195
pharyngitis, 5, 116, 388, 393, 394
pharynx, 17
phenotype, xii, 247, 289
phenotypes, 224, 246, 266, 281
phenylketonuria, 402
phenytoin, 386
Philadelphia, 57, 59, 65, 66, 69, 76, 81, 307, 326, 369, 371, 372, 404, 410, 414, 415, 416, 418, 419
Philippines, 229
phlebitis, 46
phorbol, 136
phosphate, 36, 47, 57, 117
phosphatidylserine, 117, 138
photons, 53

phylogenetic, 292
phylum, 290
physical properties, 54
physicians, x, 7, 22, 50, 51, 85, 135, 167, 170, 176, 178, 190, 220, 325, 340, 346
physics, 80, 81
physiological, 9, 10, 32, 58, 120, 247, 346, 389
pig, 119, 135
pigments, 238
pilot study, 148
pitch, 53
placebo, 28, 61, 68, 180, 194, 209, 210, 211, 214, 215, 227, 230, 231, 381
placenta, viii, xii, 3, 18, 19, 21, 28, 30, 31, 35, 37, 39, 40, 45, 55, 111, 112, 118, 119, 130, 131, 142, 146, 149, 160, 172, 205, 227, 236, 237, 238, 239, 240, 241, 242, 243, 246, 250, 261, 268, 269, 276, 279, 281, 282, 284, 285, 287, 290, 292, 303, 333, 334, 339, 358, 363, 398, 400, 424
placenta previa, 358, 363, 398
placental, xii, 9, 15, 21, 35, 36, 71, 74, 89, 119, 120, 140, 142, 146, 210, 218, 235, 236, 237, 238, 239, 240, 241, 242, 243, 244, 245, 246, 248, 250, 251, 255, 260, 261, 265, 266, 267, 268, 269, 270, 273, 275, 276, 277, 280, 281, 282, 283, 284, 286, 294, 303, 334, 379, 381, 394, 423, 425
placental abruption, 89
placental barrier, 15, 270, 379, 381, 423, 425
planning, 39, 206, 219, 220, 272, 402, 417
plasma, 6, 14, 15, 18, 21, 56, 115, 124, 205, 217, 218, 377
plasma membrane, 115
plastic, 250
platelet, 334, 374, 376, 377, 378, 380
platelet count, 374, 376, 378, 380
platelets, 15
play, viii, 78, 111, 112, 120, 124, 146, 173, 175, 219, 269, 270, 271
pleura, 163
pleural, 2, 26, 38, 163
pleural cavity, 163
pleural effusion, 2, 26, 38
pleurisy, 388
plexus, 49, 115, 346, 372
PLUS, 206, 207, 210, 212, 213, 218, 230, 321
pneumococcus, 397
pneumonia, xv, 4, 27, 28, 40, 42, 67, 116, 118, 131, 171, 181, 216, 339, 383, 387, 393, 394, 397, 398, 404, 405, 424
pneumonitis, 13, 17, 296, 422, 423
pneumothorax, 163, 165, 388
point mutation, 112
Poland, 292, 306, 310, 326
polarity, 113, 136
policy makers, 266
polio, 51, 52
pollutants, 384
polygenic, 385
polyhydramnios, xv, 21, 345, 357, 367
polymer, 133
polymerase, ix, xiii, 6, 16, 18, 35, 68, 113, 114, 115, 116, 119, 121, 126, 140, 142, 143, 145, 146, 147, 148, 149, 238, 290, 315, 333
polymerase chain reaction, ix, xiii, 6, 16, 18, 35, 116, 119, 126, 140, 142, 145, 146, 147, 148, 149, 238, 290, 315, 333
polymorphism, 280, 292, 305
polymorphisms, 293
polymorphonuclear, 7
polymyositis, 296
polysaccharides, 376, 381
poor, xi, xii, xvi, 10, 14, 22, 34, 37, 46, 90, 93, 102, 103, 105, 169, 200, 203, 204, 218, 219, 237, 273, 277, 289, 301, 303, 393, 421
poor performance, 301
population, vii, x, xiv, 1, 2, 15, 16, 27, 29, 43, 53, 66, 68, 85, 86, 120, 141, 146, 149, 151, 152, 153, 155, 184, 214, 221, 224, 243, 248, 249, 264, 269, 287, 292, 305, 309, 310, 327, 328, 329, 345, 346, 347, 349, 350, 351, 359, 365, 366, 370, 371, 372, 373, 374, 375, 385, 387, 402, 403, 405, 406, 416, 421, 423
population growth, 373, 421
pore, 379, 423
port of entry, 422
positive correlation, 265
postmortem, 123
postoperative, 155, 156
postpartum, xi, 7, 12, 13, 17, 22, 27, 31, 42, 44, 46, 47, 48, 49, 50, 78, 79, 88, 146, 200, 202, 204, 205, 207, 209, 210, 211, 212, 213, 215, 216, 218, 219, 220, 221, 228, 232, 239, 334, 375, 423, 425, 426
postpartum period, xi, 17, 44, 49, 200, 219
potassium, 178
poverty, 203, 220, 274
power, 348
pragmatic, 272
preclinical, 41, 188, 208
prediction, 107, 132, 196

predisposing factors, 46, 266
pre-eclampsia, xv, 32, 120, 146, 220, 239, 276, 334, 345, 357, 361, 363, 368 367, 372, 394
pre-existing, 236, 239, 244
preference, 103, 294
pregnancy test, 6
premature contraction, 170
premature delivery, vii, viii, 1, 2, 5, 13, 32, 34, 43, 111, 112, 118, 214, 226, 237, 334
premature infant, 58, 191
premature labor, vii, 1, 13, 89, 90, 155, 169, 177
prematurity, viii, x, 3, 5, 12, 17, 19, 21, 33, 63, 64, 74, 83, 84, 85, 91, 102, 104, 105, 109, 167, 185, 192, 195, 236, 245, 265, 275, 285, 334, 342, 371
prenatal care, x, 85, 167, 175, 177, 182, 190, 274, 284, 348, 352, 355, 356, 357, 366, 385, 390, 398
preparedness, 417
pressure, 54, 153, 155, 160, 163, 164, 182, 290, 374, 377
preterm delivery, 21, 33, 59, 63, 64, 88, 107, 108, 120, 132, 156, 157, 172, 177, 181, 184, 193, 194, 196, 205, 226, 244, 269, 358, 363, 368, 390, 391, 394, 398
preterm infants, 76, 168
pre-term labor, 15, 36
Pretoria, 78
prevention, x, xi, xii, 60, 62, 63, 67, 70, 72, 73, 78, 85, 87, 88, 89, 91, 104, 105, 107, 108, 117, 120, 167, 170, 173, 175, 176, 185, 188, 189, 190, 192, 195, 199, 200, 203, 204, 218, 221, 222, 223, 225, 226, 227, 228, 231, 232, 264, 265, 266, 272, 273, 274, 277, 281, 282, 283, 284, 285, 286, 289, 304, 326, 329, 337, 339, 344, 355, 359, 365, 374, 381, 384, 401, 402, 406, 421, 426
prevention of infection, 170
preventive, viii, xi, 35, 83, 90, 93, 94, 102, 104, 170, 187, 199, 230, 231, 248, 264, 266, 267, 273, 320, 337, 338, 349, 359, 387, 404
primary care, 70
primates, 283
primigravidae, xii, 235, 239, 256, 259, 262, 263, 264, 278, 282, 285
probability, 56, 252, 417
probe, 13
probiotic, 178
prodrome, 17
production, 7, 9, 10, 22, 25, 26, 34, 45, 106, 115, 117, 121, 125, 126, 127, 128, 138, 269, 297, 301
production costs, 106
professions, 106
profit, 106
progenitor cells, 24
progesterone, 45, 86, 170, 180, 187, 196
prognosis, 265, 416
prognostic marker, 300, 315
program, x, 71, 85, 125, 143, 167, 176, 177, 182, 183, 184, 185, 186, 187, 189, 190, 192, 195, 273, 296, 302, 421
programming, 273
proinflammatory, 9
pro-inflammatory, viii, 8, 111, 112, 120, 125, 128, 136, 171, 237
prolapse, 91, 104
proliferation, 122, 123, 238
promyelocytic, 126
propagation, 292
property, 237
prophylactic, 18, 32, 36, 88, 102, 108, 156, 214, 338
prophylaxis, xi, 19, 33, 61, 200, 204, 206, 211, 212, 213, 214, 217, 219, 220, 221, 223, 224, 227, 228, 229, 230, 240, 279, 339, 344, 424, 425
prostaglandin, 7, 22, 181
prostaglandins, 64
prostanoids, 135
protease inhibitors, 205, 220
proteases, 115, 133
protection, 35, 36, 51, 145, 173, 216, 225, 229, 247, 266, 281, 288, 339, 415, 416, 417, 420
protective clothing, 339
protective role, 379, 423
protein, 9, 29, 32, 113, 114, 115, 116, 122, 124, 125, 127, 129, 137, 141, 238, 241, 281, 285, 313, 422
protein aggregation, 115
protein synthesis, 9
proteins, 9, 29, 34, 113, 115, 116, 119, 120, 121, 125, 137, 146, 147
proteinuria, 361, 368, 371, 398
proteolytic enzyme, 291
protocol, xiii, 214, 249, 299, 319, 325, 361, 424
protocols, 47
protons, 54
protozoa, 33
pruritus, 17
Pseudomonas, 350, 356
psychological problems, 84
public health, xii, 113, 192, 227, 235, 248, 272, 284, 288, 289, 340, 341, 355, 417
Public Health Service, 19, 62, 226
puerperium, vii, 1, 2, 33, 46, 49, 77, 78, 79, 101
pulmonary edema, 33, 236

pulmonary embolism, 50, 55
pulse, 160
Purkinje cells, 115
purpura, 30
pyelonephritis, 11, 31, 32, 33, 49, 70, 171, 350, 351, 352, 356, 357, 359, 360, 366, 367, 370, 371
pyloric stenosis, 354, 364, 368, 372
pyogenic, 27
pyuria, 31, 32

Q

Q fever, 338, 339, 340, 341, 342, 343, 344
quality control, 249, 295
Quebec, 405
questionnaire, 250, 348, 355, 356, 385
questionnaires, 186
quinidine, 36
quinine, 36, 285

R

Rabies, 51
race, xii, 284, 289
radiation, 52, 53, 54, 55, 80, 81, 155
radioactive isotopes, 56
radiofrequency, 55
radiography, 37, 38
radioisotope, 55
radiological, 153, 157, 160, 161
radius, 96
rain, 115, 249
rain forest, 249
rainfall, 249
random, 79, 347, 386
random amplified polymorphic DNA, 79
range, vii, 1, 2, 22, 29, 53, 143, 176, 183, 245, 246, 271, 273, 290, 302, 320, 321, 361, 366, 397
RANTES, 124
rapid plasma reagin, 6, 21
rash, 4, 5, 21, 24, 26, 28, 29, 39, 52, 69, 208, 300, 334, 374, 412, 413, 415, 416, 422, 423, 425
rat, 121, 134, 138
rats, 9, 58, 341
RAW, 127
reactive oxygen species (ROS), 121, 135
reactivity, 145, 302, 335
reading, 113, 178, 251, 302
reagent, 56, 121, 122
reagents, 121, 123, 133, 252, 298
real time, 299, 300
reality, 416
rebound tenderness, 151, 154
recall, 348, 349, 385, 387, 391, 392
receptors, 9, 35, 113, 119, 120, 128, 133, 237
recognition, xi, 7, 44, 199, 247, 248, 263, 273, 388
recombination, 292, 305
recovery, xii, 15, 40, 155, 289, 303, 374, 380, 384
recruiting, xiii, 320
rectum, 18, 154
recurrence, 18, 61, 85, 103, 107, 147, 184, 187, 196
red blood cell, 25, 57, 115, 125, 246, 247, 271, 286, 378
red blood cells, 25, 57, 115, 125, 246, 247, 286
redistribution, 377
redness, 52
regeneration, 96, 101, 102
registry, 346, 348, 349, 355, 369, 385, 386, 403, 420
regression, 74, 164, 354, 364, 374
regression analysis, 74, 364, 374
regular, x, 118, 154, 160, 167, 176, 177, 236, 296
regulation, 7, 45, 131, 133, 137, 146, 247, 293
rehabilitation, 161
rejection, 391
relapse, 38, 300
relationship, 78, 116, 171, 172, 193, 239, 240, 242, 243, 246, 247, 248, 266, 268, 270, 271, 277, 279, 282, 286, 316
relationships, 246
relevance, 248, 372
reliability, 81, 196, 314, 417
remodeling, 117, 131
renal, 31, 32, 33, 40, 45, 55, 206, 346, 350, 361, 367, 368, 369, 372
renal disease, 367, 368, 371, 372
renal dysfunction, 33
renal failure, 40, 45, 350, 361
renal osteodystrophy, 361
renal scan, 55
repair, 79
reparation, 284
replication, viii, 70, 111, 113, 116, 120, 136, 137, 146, 238, 269
reproductive age, 5, 36, 69, 243, 366
reservoir, ix, 29, 139, 146
resistance, 36, 42, 73, 94, 206, 207, 215, 220, 224, 228, 230, 247, 266, 270, 274, 275, 279, 281, 336, 381, 425
resolution, 66, 135, 337
resources, xi, 67, 142, 199
respiration, 58, 389

respiratory, xv, 5, 7, 24, 26, 29, 33, 42, 46, 58, 71, 75, 116, 117, 118, 119, 130, 132, 135, 163, 164, 169, 229, 336, 370, 383, 384, 385, 388, 389, 393, 395, 397, 398, 401, 402, 403, 404, 405, 422
respiratory distress syndrome, 33, 42, 169
respiratory rate, 389
respiratory syncytial virus, 389
restitution, 179
restriction fragment length polymorphis, 292
retardation, ix, 8, 18, 23, 27, 29, 30, 31, 53, 80, 139, 181, 218, 236, 244, 246, 265, 269, 275, 285, 320, 334
reticulum, 115
retinitis, 23
retroviral, 230
reverse transcriptase, 119, 205
Reye's syndrome, 27
Reynolds, 155, 158, 221, 231, 426
RFLP, 306
rheumatoid arthritis, 56
rheumatoid factor, 342
rhinitis, 116, 388
ribose, 121
ribosomal, 299
ribosome, 115
risk assessment, 188
risk factors, x, xii, 6, 16, 19, 49, 50, 66, 74, 103, 149, 158, 167, 200, 205, 219, 222, 238, 274, 279, 285, 286, 289, 293, 294, 304, 307, 309, 406
risks, vii, xi, 1, 2, 16, 33, 35, 36, 43, 50, 51, 52, 53, 60, 61, 65, 80, 93, 155, 157, 170, 200, 207, 208, 214, 236, 244, 245, 273, 276, 299, 396, 412
RNA, 3, 11, 14, 16, 18, 29, 113, 114, 115, 116, 136, 202, 204, 205, 206, 207, 217, 218, 225
rodent, 285
roentgen, 53
Rome, 328
ROS, 121, 128, 138
routines, 329
Royal Society, 274, 275, 278, 279, 280, 281, 282, 283, 285, 286, 288
RPR, 6, 21, 56
RTA, 316
RTI, 205
rubella, ix, x, 3, 6, 29, 30, 31, 50, 52, 69, 70, 139, 140, 141, 142, 143, 144, 145, 146, 148, 149, 206, 320, 327, 334, 365, 384, 420
rubella virus, ix, x, 30, 139, 140, 141, 145, 146, 327, 384
ruptured appendix, 155
ruptured membranes, 19, 41, 42
rural, 149, 216, 221, 222, 232, 243, 265, 273, 274, 278, 281, 282, 285, 286, 287, 307, 308
rural women, 274
Russia, 145, 149
Russian, 118, 221
Rutherford, 64
Rwanda, 263, 265, 266, 280, 281

S

S phase, 402
safety, xiv, 51, 52, 54, 55, 62, 81, 273, 283, 331, 332, 335, 336, 339
saline, 21, 49, 377
saliva, 23, 24
Salmonella, 39, 73, 74
salpingitis, 8
sample, viii, 29, 83, 85, 103, 142, 204, 238, 250, 251, 252, 261, 297, 302, 311, 313, 410, 412, 416
sampling, 25, 26, 41, 75, 251, 334
sanitation, 14
SAS, 410
savings, 185
scalp, 26
scarcity, 274, 412
scavenger, 126, 133
schistosomiasis, 219, 251
schizophrenia, 9, 58, 59
Schmid, 63, 426
school, 65
sclerosis, 350, 361
scores, 44, 160
sea level, 249
search, xiii, 37, 289, 299, 325, 408
searching, 376
seasonality, 393
seaweed, 381
secondary syphilis, 20, 334
secrete, 112, 128
secretion, 125, 127
sedatives, 164
sedimentation, 47
seed, 28
seeds, 31
seizures, 18, 23, 29, 39, 44, 45
selectivity, 313
self, xi, 103, 168, 177, 179, 181, 182, 183, 184, 185, 186, 187, 189, 190, 196, 231
self monitoring, 190
self-assessment, 182

self-care, x, 167, 177, 181, 186, 190
self-report, 348, 352, 385, 425, 426
Senegal, 267, 278
sensitivity, 13, 40, 56, 73, 144, 154, 155, 297, 299, 301, 302, 303
sensitization, 134
separation, 358, 363, 398
sepsis, 3, 42, 45, 46, 47, 49, 74, 75, 78, 79, 134, 180, 216, 244, 334
septicemia, 32, 40, 47
sequelae, vii, 1, 2, 12, 21, 23, 24, 29, 44, 45, 68, 71, 169, 192, 300, 304, 423
sequencing, 292
serologic test, 14, 18, 21, 28, 141, 145, 296, 310, 317, 335, 342, 397
serological marker, 145
serology, 6, 11, 12, 21, 30, 56, 149, 219, 316, 321, 342, 424
serum, ix, xiii, 10, 11, 15, 16, 30, 37, 116, 140, 149, 204, 278, 290, 292, 297, 298, 301, 302, 303, 311, 313, 316
serum albumin, 37
serum erythropoietin, 278
service provider, 220
services, xii, 203, 216, 220, 236, 249, 251, 270, 272, 273, 274
severity, xii, 4, 16, 27, 29, 203, 219, 236, 239, 242, 247, 266, 276, 284, 286, 289, 294, 300, 320, 325, 337, 347, 349, 351, 355, 359, 367, 376, 380, 386, 393, 394, 402, 408, 412, 414, 424
sewage, 39
sex, 6, 7, 250, 348, 355, 359, 385, 390, 394, 399
sex ratio, 390, 394, 399
sexual activity, 20
sexual contact, 6, 7, 17, 20, 23
sexual risk behavior, 222
sexuality, 305
sexually transmitted disease (STD), 20, 58, 63, 59, 195, 221, 223, 275, 342
sexually transmitted infections (STIs), xi, 6, 7, 12, 15, 17, 19, 61, 63, 200, 204, 206, 218, 219, 220, 231, 272, 396
Shanghai, 379
shape, 50
sharing, 332
sheep, 125
shingles, 422
shock, xv, 9, 33, 41, 47, 163, 334, 373, 374, 375, 377, 380, 381
short period, 240
short-term, 227
sialic acid, 113, 114, 119
sibling, 333
siblings, 341
sickle cell, 44, 247, 266, 275, 277, 279, 286, 288
side effects, 52, 94, 336
Sierra Leone, 267, 283
sign, 20, 21, 50, 95, 152, 154, 303
signal transduction, 127
signs, x, xv, xvi, 14, 20, 21, 23, 27, 29, 32, 41, 42, 43, 44, 45, 47, 84, 93, 101, 142, 153, 156, 158, 167, 177, 178, 180, 182, 295, 333, 334, 336, 373, 374, 375, 376, 421, 422
signs of dehydration, 14
sine, 412, 413
sinus, 164
sinuses, 163
sinusitis, xv, 44, 383, 388, 390, 393, 394
sites, 71, 116, 137, 239, 350, 373
skeletal muscle, 115
skeleton, 335
skills, 250
skin, xvi, 4, 17, 18, 20, 26, 27, 37, 38, 39, 48, 56, 160, 413, 421, 422, 423, 424
small intestine, 291
smallpox, xvi, 407, 408, 409, 410, 411, 412, 413, 414, 415, 416, 417, 418, 419, 420
smoking, 140, 170, 309, 384, 391
smoking cessation, 391
smoothing, 96
social class, 363
social costs, 217
social development, 278
socioeconomic, 46, 357, 363, 366, 367, 368, 387
socioeconomic status, 46, 363, 366, 367, 368, 387
sociological, 326
SOD, 126, 133
sodium, 121
software, 54, 410
soil, xii, 5, 6, 28, 289, 291, 293, 320, 332
sounds, 47
South Africa, 199, 200, 203, 209, 211, 215, 216, 219, 221, 222, 225, 227, 230, 232
South America, 292, 306
Southeast Asia, 310, 341, 373, 378, 380, 381, 421
Southern blot, 299
Spain, 142, 321, 426
spasticity, 18

species, ix, xii, xiv, 5, 10, 33, 34, 35, 41, 48, 113, 121, 135, 139, 148, 172, 235, 281, 331, 332, 333, 336, 338, 340, 373
specificity, 13, 40, 43, 56, 73, 114, 144, 154, 155, 223, 238, 297, 299, 300, 302, 400
spectrophotometer, 251
spectrum, xv, 44, 49, 58, 67, 76, 326, 335, 373, 374, 383, 393, 401, 402, 421, 422
speculation, 247
speech, 54, 81
speed, 53, 96, 377, 412
S-phase, 9
spinal cord, 115
spine, 164
spleen, 34, 39, 115, 116, 117, 247
splenic rupture, 40
splenomegaly, 300
spontaneous abortion, ix, xi, 12, 13, 17, 21, 25, 30, 31, 33, 45, 118, 135, 139, 140, 142, 147, 148, 177, 199, 200, 201, 203, 244
sporadic, 32, 333
sputum, 11, 37, 38, 56
sputum culture, 38
stages, ix, 5, 20, 27, 69, 120, 139, 163, 175, 176, 177, 188, 189, 190, 290, 291, 305, 316
stainless steel, 95
standard deviation, 410
standard error, 410
standardization, 67, 313
standards, 220
staphylococcal, 8
staphylococcus, 32, 47, 48
Staphylococcus aureus, 48
stasis, 48, 79, 346
statistical analysis, 252, 261, 264
statistics, 39, 78, 191
status asthmaticus, 163
steel, 95
stem cells, 347, 386
stenosis, xiv, 345, 354, 364, 367, 368, 369, 372
stent, 33
sterile, 46, 47, 96, 143, 171, 250
stiffness, 44, 52
stigma, 203, 222
stillbirth, vii, viii, xi, 1, 2, 3, 4, 5, 12, 13, 21, 25, 33, 45, 63, 111, 112, 118, 119, 138, 199, 200, 201, 203, 219, 226, 236, 243, 245, 282, 423
stock, 220
stomach, 291
stool culture, 39, 40
stool cultures, 39, 40
strabismus, 23
strain, xii, 23, 119, 122, 123, 137, 145, 174, 246, 289, 292, 297, 300, 302, 306
strains, 40, 112, 134, 174, 178, 292, 305, 306, 316, 332, 335, 336, 342, 343
strategies, x, xi, 56, 59, 62, 145, 151, 152, 170, 200, 203, 205, 220, 221, 232, 248, 250, 273, 277, 286, 314
stratification, 372, 412, 414, 417
strength, 55
streptococci, 11, 47, 48, 79
stress, 37, 122, 128, 134, 170, 402
stretching, 43
structural changes, 346
Student t test, 143
students, 285
subacute, 50
subcellular, 304
subcutaneous emphysema, x, 159, 160, 161, 162, 163, 164
subcutaneous tissue, 48, 163, 164
subgroups, 88, 103, 322, 323, 354, 394, 396
subjective, 161
sub-Saharan Africa, xi, 37, 70, 71, 72, 199, 200, 218, 220, 221, 222, 236, 237, 238, 239, 240, 241, 242, 243, 244, 245, 248, 252, 263, 264, 267, 268, 270, 271, 272, 273, 274, 276, 280, 283, 284, 286
Sub-Saharan Africa, 35, 279
success rate, viii, 83, 102, 104, 175, 177
Sudan, 247, 263, 266, 274, 277
suffering, 32, 156, 178, 378
sugar, 138
sulfonamide, 303
sulfonamides, 302, 337, 343, 387
sulphate, 35
summaries, 348, 352, 385
superiority, 215
supernatant, 125
superoxide, 117, 121, 125, 126, 127, 128, 133, 135
superoxide dismutase, 135
supplements, 219, 355, 358, 361, 363, 365, 370, 394, 403
supply, 203, 293
support services, 272
suppression, 206, 207, 215, 219, 231, 263, 336, 389, 417
suprapubic, 351, 356
surgeries, 152, 156

surgery, x, 43, 44, 47, 76, 77, 151, 152, 153, 155, 156, 157, 158, 159
surgical, xi, 43, 46, 48, 49, 77, 89, 152, 155, 156, 157, 158, 160, 163, 164, 199
surgical debridement, 49
surgical intervention, 43, 156
surveillance, 145, 148, 220, 221, 224, 265, 301, 328, 349, 374, 387
survival, viii, xi, 25, 66, 83, 103, 199, 202, 216, 217, 220, 229, 231, 264, 272, 281, 283, 294
survival rate, viii, 83, 103
surviving, viii, 12, 83, 101, 102, 105
survivors, 18, 23, 45, 80, 191
susceptibility, 5, 9, 10, 32, 38, 40, 41, 45, 57, 74, 169, 237, 245, 246, 247, 263, 266, 284, 336, 342, 343
suture, 104, 109
Sweden, 308, 321, 327
swelling, 48, 52, 160, 163
switching, 55
Switzerland, 68, 78, 93, 310, 321
symptom, 10, 41, 45, 156, 163
symptomatic treatment, 376, 424
symptoms, xv, xvi, 4, 5, 12, 14, 17, 20, 21, 23, 24, 28, 31, 32, 35, 37, 39, 42, 44, 45, 49, 65, 116, 117, 153, 156, 159, 160, 161, 163, 164, 177, 179, 180, 182, 189, 219, 244, 247, 251, 296, 299, 320, 334, 351, 352, 355, 356, 359, 366, 367, 368, 373, 374, 375, 376, 377, 388, 389, 391, 398, 400, 415, 421, 422, 423
syncytium, 237
syndrome, xiv, xv, 4, 5, 8, 23, 27, 29, 30, 42, 56, 57, 69, 74, 86, 87, 106, 132, 145, 148, 163, 169, 170, 171, 191, 192, 295, 308, 331, 334, 336, 348, 349, 350, 368, 369, 372, 373, 374, 381, 384, 385, 387, 389, 391, 401, 406, 423, 426
synergistic, 245
synthesis, 9, 22
syphilis, 6, 7, 8, 11, 12, 20, 21, 63, 206, 219, 231, 334, 342
systemic circulation, 9

T

T cell, 124, 146
T cells, 146
T lymphocytes, 115, 117
tachycardia, 37, 39, 41, 43, 154, 163
Taiwan, 307
Tanzania, 209, 212, 213, 222, 227, 229, 230, 231, 242, 264, 266, 268, 275, 281
targets, 220, 379
T-cell, 282, 389
teaching, 79
teenagers, 329
teeth, 57, 335, 342
temperature, 2, 7, 8, 9, 41, 46, 54, 56, 154, 160, 249, 291, 366, 402
temporal, 56
Tennessee, 118
tension, 389
teratogen, 2, 145, 405
teratogenesis, 28
teratogenic, xv, 23, 26, 39, 53, 206, 346, 384, 386, 392, 400, 402, 403, 405, 406
teratogens, 347, 365, 386, 387, 400
teratology, 400
testis, 347, 354, 359, 364, 387
tetanus, 8, 50, 52, 52, 206
tetracycline, 36, 335, 336, 338, 342
tetracyclines, 333, 335, 342, 387
Thai, 374, 380, 425
Thailand, 113, 129, 210, 211, 221, 223, 224, 228, 373, 375, 378, 380, 421
thalassemia, 378, 381
therapeutic interventions, 265
therapy, xi, 12, 13, 18, 19, 22, 26, 32, 33, 37, 45, 48, 50, 60, 61, 64, 73, 74, 79, 89, 93, 94, 108, 156, 175, 177, 179, 180, 181, 194, 195, 196, 199, 204, 205, 206, 214, 218, 219, 221, 226, 228, 230, 232, 233, 272, 274, 297, 301, 303, 336, 341, 342, 343, 375, 377, 390, 397, 402, 403, 406, 423
thermal index, 54
thermoregulation, 58
thin film, 35
third-generation cephalosporin, 40, 45, 48
thoracic, 27, 164
thorax, 163, 164
threat, xv, 113, 175, 332, 340, 373, 418, 421
threatened, 89, 363, 368, 390, 391, 394
threatened abortion, 89, 394
threatening, xiv, 28, 49, 75, 195, 196, 208, 214, 331, 335, 337, 338
threshold, 9, 54, 122, 402
threshold level, 122
throat, 24, 29, 39, 56, 160, 163, 295, 389
thrombocytopenia, 24, 32, 40, 142, 300, 334, 374, 375, 376, 378
thrombocytopenic purpura, 30
thrombocytosis, 378
thromboembolic, 81

thromboembolism, 378, 381
thrombophlebitis, 50, 79
thymocytes, 121, 134
thymus, 161
thyroid, 55
thyroiditis, 30
ticks, xiv, 332, 339
time consuming, 301
timing, 44, 217, 219, 225, 300, 317, 325, 402
tissue, 7, 8, 9, 31, 42, 48, 49, 50, 54, 58, 86, 87, 95, 96, 99, 100, 101, 112, 117, 119, 120, 124, 127, 163, 164, 210, 290, 291, 292, 293, 304, 305, 315, 320, 342
titration, 298
TMP, 338
TNF, viii, 9, 111, 112, 120, 125, 127, 128, 132, 134
TNF-α, 9
Tokyo, 111
tolerance, 122, 227, 232, 336
toll-like, 9
tonsillitis, xv, 384, 388, 393, 396, 397, 402
tourniquet, 374, 378
toxemia, 33, 37, 371, 372
toxic, xiv, 7, 9, 50, 117, 128, 331, 334
toxic effect, 9, 117
toxic shock syndrome, 334
toxicity, 19, 39, 49, 74, 80, 207
toxin, 121
toxoplasmosis, ix, xii, xiii, 6, 11, 29, 68, 69, 140, 289, 292, 293, 294, 298, 299, 300, 301, 302, 303, 304, 305, 306, 307, 308, 309, 310, 311, 312, 313, 314, 315, 316, 317, 319, 320, 321, 326, 327, 328, 329, 334, 336
TPA, 125
TPH, 21
trachea, 116, 161, 163
traction, 95
traits, 279, 283
trans, 34
transcriptase, 119, 126, 205
transcription, 9, 113, 116, 136
transcription factor, 9
transcription factors, 9
transcriptional, 114, 125, 131
transducer, 135
transduction, 127
transfer, 7, 10, 68, 73, 75, 138, 163, 216, 246
transfusion, 6, 16, 25, 26, 41, 67, 219, 279, 293, 377, 380
transfusions, 18
transgenic, 285
transition, 220
transition period, 220
transmembrane, 113
transparent, 250
transplant, 6, 16
transplantation, 293
transport, 25, 35, 269
trauma, 9, 15, 141, 165
travel, 35, 36, 39, 56, 381
treatment programs, 79
trial, 13, 19, 50, 59, 61, 62, 64, 68, 70, 74, 76, 81, 88, 103, 105, 108, 185, 190, 194, 195, 202, 205, 215, 217, 218, 223, 225, 227, 228, 229, 230, 231, 233, 240, 277, 339, 343, 344
triggers, 9, 135
trophoblast, 119, 120, 121, 127, 128, 133, 138, 146, 149
tropical areas, 28, 34
trypsin, 115
tuberculosis, xi, 5, 8, 36, 37, 38, 39, 56, 72, 73, 200, 206, 218, 220, 231, 232, 251, 272, 388
tubular, 346
tumor, viii, 111, 112, 129, 137
tumor necrosis factor, viii, 111, 112, 129, 137
Turkey, 113, 146, 149, 196, 307, 309
twins, 187, 253, 293, 308, 355, 390, 394, 399, 419
two-dimensional, 302, 317
typhoid, 39, 40, 73, 74
typhoid fever, 39, 40, 73, 74
typhus, 332, 333, 337, 340, 341, 342, 343

U

U.S. Agency for International Development, 281
U.S. Preventive Services Task Force, 19, 62
Uganda, 203, 209, 211, 221, 222, 227, 228, 230, 231, 276, 280, 287
Ukraine, 221
ulcer, 219
ulceration, 13, 39, 40
ultrasonographic examination, 299
ultrasonography, xiii, 21, 52, 54, 55, 76, 81, 92, 155, 290, 424
ultrasound, 2, 26, 27, 54, 56, 80, 81, 88, 89, 108, 156, 206, 300, 315
ultraviolet, 143
umbilical cord, 9, 119, 250, 266, 273, 281, 287
umbilical cord blood, 119, 250, 266, 273, 281, 287
UN, 221
uncertainty, 40

unclassified, xvi, 347, 384, 386, 391, 396
underreported, 333
United Kingdom (UK), 21, 30, 63, 141, 199, 214, 226, 252, 285, 307, 327, 328, 336, 425, 426
United States, xvi, 13, 17, 19, 35, 36, 39, 44, 45, 46, 52, 59, 60, 62, 67, 71, 72, 141, 145, 146, 168, 169, 205, 223, 224, 226, 292, 340, 407, 408, 420
univariate, 410, 416
unmarried women, 352
unplanned pregnancies, 367, 371
updating, 299
urbanization, 373, 379, 421
urea, 56, 298
urea nitrogen, 56
ureter, 346, 350, 351
ureters, 32, 346
urethra, 31, 177, 346
urethritis, 31, 32
urinalysis, 56
urinary, xiv, 31, 32, 40, 46, 49, 70, 85, 171, 173, 177, 182, 251, 345, 346, 350, 351, 352, 353, 354, 355, 357, 358, 359, 360, 361, 363, 364, 365, 370, 371, 372, 403
urinary tract, xiv, 31, 32, 40, 46, 49, 70, 85, 171, 173, 177, 182, 345, 346, 350, 351, 352, 353, 354, 355, 357, 358, 359, 360, 361, 363, 365, 370, 371, 372, 403
urinary tract infection, xiv, 31, 40, 46, 49, 70, 85, 171, 173, 177, 182, 345, 346, 350, 352, 353, 354, 355, 357, 358, 370, 371, 372
urine, 11, 13, 14, 18, 23, 24, 31, 32, 33, 40, 56, 115, 295, 303, 351, 356, 366
uterus, 7, 32, 37, 41, 43, 44, 46, 47, 53, 89, 146, 149, 154, 155, 156, 181, 346, 389
uveitis, 5

V

vaccination, ix, xvi, 6, 14, 29, 50, 51, 52, 59, 60, 77, 139, 141, 145, 148, 149, 339, 402, 407, 408, 409, 411, 414, 415, 416, 417, 418, 420, 421, 425, 426
vaccinations, 6
vaccine, 15, 16, 24, 31, 44, 45, 50, 51, 52, 73, 221, 339, 374, 408, 416, 418, 419, 420, 424, 425, 426
vacuole, 290
vagina, 20, 21, 41, 47, 172, 173, 178, 183, 346
vaginitis, 22, 172, 173, 178, 190, 192, 194, 356
Valdez, 308
Valencia, 277
validation, 356, 386, 387, 396, 398
validity, 349, 387, 416
values, 174, 175, 179, 183, 243, 252, 255, 271, 321
vancomycin, 45
variability, 297, 302
variables, 143, 250, 252, 359, 362, 365, 394, 399, 417
variance, 143
variation, 7, 56, 241, 278, 365
vascular disease, 170
vascular system, 8
vasculitis, 21, 26
vasomotor, 7
VDRL, 6, 21
vector, 34, 225, 373, 375, 379, 423
vegetables, 6
vegetation, 249
vein, 37, 79, 346
venereal wart, 19
ventilation, 55, 389
very low birth weight, 183, 265
vesicle, 114, 421, 423
vesico-ureteric reflux, 32
vessels, 7, 34, 44
Vietnam, 113, 135, 136
village, 276
villus, 146
violence, 203
violent, 374
viral diseases, 67, 408
viral envelope, 15
viral infection, x, xvi, 11, 50, 57, 129, 140, 146, 373, 417, 421, 422, 423
virological, ix, 116, 140, 144, 215, 417
virology, 147
virulence, ix, xii, 41, 111, 112, 118, 122, 128, 246, 289, 292, 293, 300, 305, 374
virus infection, viii, ix, 60, 61, 62, 65, 67, 111, 112, 115, 116, 119, 120, 122, 123, 124, 125, 126, 127, 128, 130, 132, 133, 134, 135, 136, 137, 138, 140, 147, 148, 223, 277, 283, 286, 334, 375, 376, 379, 423, 424, 425
virus replication, 70, 116, 120
viruses, ix, 4, 56, 112, 113, 115, 118, 119, 122, 131, 139, 141, 143, 145, 146, 147, 148, 365, 374, 389, 398, 400
visible, 161, 413
vision, 29, 39
visualization, 18
vitamin C, 391, 394
vitamin E, 121
vitamin supplementation, 370, 403

vitamins, 399
vomiting, 39, 44, 117, 153, 156, 163, 358, 363, 390, 394, 395, 398, 404
vRNA, 113, 114
vulnerability, 273
vulva, 20

W

waiting times, 376
Wales, 410, 411, 415, 419
warfarin, 386
warrants, 154
warts, 19, 20
water, xii, 7, 39, 121, 143, 289, 291, 292, 293, 309, 377
water-soluble, 121
weakness, 39, 87
weapons, xiv, 331
weight gain, 37
weight loss, 5, 37, 219
well-being, 45, 53
wells, 309
West Africa, 227, 276, 282, 287
West Indies, 307
western blot, 295, 302, 317
western countries, 24
Western Europe, 16, 63
white blood cell count, 156
white matter, 9, 23
windows, 347, 386
winter, 398
wool, 339
workers, 6, 37, 54, 113, 119, 174, 309, 339, 352, 367, 368
World Health Organization (WHO), xi, 20, 21, 35, 36, 46, 57, 63, 67, 71, 72, 73, 75, 78, 79, 113, 129, 136, 138, 149, 200, 203, 204, 206, 207, 214, 217, 218, 221, 222, 224, 227, 229, 230, 231, 232, 240, 243, 244, 251, 272, 273, 274, 276, 279, 284, 286, 288, 350, 378, 379, 384, 393, 418, 420
worm, 152
worms, 241
wound infection, 46, 49, 78

X

x-rays, 54, 55, 56

Y

yield, 18, 40, 266, 303
young adults, 39, 44
young men, 81
young women, 32, 152, 157, 236, 239

Z

Zimbabwe, 221, 247, 263, 265, 276
zoonosis, 332
zygote, 291, 305
zygotes, 347, 386